HEALTH

Contributing Authors

Joseph D. Brain, Sc.D.
William J. Curran, J.D., LL.M., S.M.Hyg.
Melvin W. First, Sc.D.
Paul Goldhaber, D.D.S.
Lewis B. Holmes, M.D.
Robert H. Holtrop, M.D.
John B. Little, M.D.
Robert B. McGandy, M.D., M.P.H.
Ralph E. Minear, Jr., M.D., M.P.H.
Richard R. Monson, M.D., Sc.D.
Duncan Neuhauser, Ph.D.
Elinor Neuhauser, M.D.
John M. Peters, M.D., M.P.H.
Elizabeth P. Rice, M.S.
Barbara Gutmann Rosenkrantz, Ph.D.
Isabelle Valadian, M.D., M.P.H.
Henry W. Vaillant, M.D., M.S.Hyg.
J. William Vinson, D.S.Hyg.
Philip Zelazo, Ph.D.

Jean Mayer, Ph.D., D.Sc., M.D. (hon.), is Professor of Nutrition,
Lecturer on the History of Public Health, and Master of Dudley House
at Harvard University. A consultant in nutrition at Boston Children's
Hospital, he is also a member of the Milbank Commission on the
Teaching of Health Sciences and the Council of the American Institute
of Nutrition and president-elect of the Society for Nutrition Education.
Professor Mayer served as first chairman of the National Council
on Hunger and Malnutrition in the United States, Special Consultant
to the President of the United States and chairman of the White House
Conference on Food, Nutrition and Health. He also served as chairman
of the Nutrition Division of the White House Conference on Aging,
and is chairman of the Health and Nutrition Committee of the
President's Consumer Advisory Council. He has served the United
Nations as a consultant to the Food and Agriculture Organization, World
Health Organization, United Nations Children's Fund, and the United
Nations Economic and Social Council and is presently a member of
the Protein Advisory Group of the United Nations and chairman of the
United Nations Task Force on Child Nutrition.

HEALTH

Jean Mayer

HARVARD SCHOOL OF PUBLIC HEALTH

D. VAN NOSTRAND COMPANY
New York Cincinnati Toronto London Melbourne

D. Van Nostrand Company Regional Offices:
New York   Cincinnati   Millbrae

D. Van Nostrand Company International Offices:
London   Toronto   Melbourne

Copyright © 1974 by Litton Educational Publishing, Inc.

Library of Congress Catalog Card Number 73-21368
ISBN: 0-442-25183-1

Published by D. Van Nostrand Company
450 West 33rd Street, New York, N. Y. 10001

Published simultaneously in Canada by
Van Nostrand Reinhold Ltd.

10   9   8   7   6   5   4

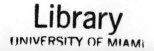

Preface

No one can be counted as educated if he or she is ignorant of the basic facts of health. These facts contribute to our understanding of ourselves, history, and society. Without sufficient knowledge of the science of health, a person cannot prevent disease or make full use of our system of medical care. Furthermore, at a time when the nation expends close to ten percent of its gross national income on the costs of medicine and citizens are called upon to make major political decisions on the structure of the health system, we need to ensure that all those admitted to establishments of higher education have an opportunity to study health. In some states, a basic course in health is compulsory in colleges and community colleges. In others, such a requirement does not exist, but throughout the country many colleges, community colleges, and junior colleges now offer a survey course in health. The most recent estimate is that as many as a million students are studying health every year. Some take it as an introduction to one of the many careers in the health fields; others because they realize that as parents, teachers, or employers they will not discharge their responsibilities properly without an understanding of health; others yet, out of a general interest in the field.

Interest in health is sufficiently widespread among present-day students who understand the benefits of studying the sciences basic to the practice of medicine and public health. They are equally interested in problems of population control and of preservation of the environment. The students of the seventies are ready to be exposed to the most contemporary view of the field and to contemplate not only what is known and what is done but also what should be investigated and what should be done. In response to the interest and demands of students and after surveying the texts currently available for introductory college courses in health, I became convinced that a more comprehensive and authoritative book was needed.

To this end, I invited a number of distinguished researchers and practitioners in the health field, who also have an intense interest in the teaching of undergraduates, to join me in attempting to bridge the distance between research and practice and students. All of them my colleagues at Harvard University, most of them associated with the Harvard School of Public Health, others with the Harvard Medical School, the Harvard Dental School, Harvard hospitals and clinics, the Harvard Law School, and Harvard College, they labored hard and with good humor to bring their expertise to bear on the four interrelated subjects of this book: human biology, medicine and preventive medicine, public health, and human ecology. For the first time, the student has available a general text covering the major fields of health written by experts who are leaders in their professions. It is our belief that this book will contribute to the coming of age of health as an essential course for all college undergraduates.

We have set out to bring to the student a greater knowledge and understanding of the biological and medical sciences and of research in those fields. This book presents yet unsolved organizational dilemmas in the health area as seen by experienced and innovative thinkers. Finally, explicitly in the chapters on history and law and implicitly through the common spirit of the authors, we hope that this book also teaches that each generation has to decide collectively that the time has come to eliminate ills which humanity has had to bear too long.

A project of this scope requires the efforts of many people. In particular I wish to express deep appreciation to Mr. Peter Thomson who served as Associate Editor and whose help was indispensible in coordinating and editing the chapters of this book. I also want to express my gratitude to Stephen Kraham, Helen McInnis, and Charity Scott of D. Van Nostrand Company. Thanks to them we were able to go from concept to publication in a relatively short period of time. What is more, we did so in a calm and pleasant atmosphere.

Jean Mayer

Contents

Introduction

The Concept of Health

Health information is nowadays conveniently packaged and publicly displayed in drugstores and supermarkets throughout the United States. Even in the privacy of your home, a well-groomed man or woman of indeterminate age coaxes you from the television set to purchase a product to ward off the ills occasioned by "iron deficiency anemia" or declares that no material wealth is as precious as health. "When you've got your health you've got it all," we are assured.

Across the Atlantic, the Spanish physician and scholar Pedro Lain Entralgo writes that he has no difficulty comprehending the meaning of health—unless someone asks him to explain his understanding in a few words. The reason for his difficulty is two-fold: ". . . first, the idea of health has a complex structure, and second, the idea of health has a variable structure." And in the British Isles, forty out of fifty men and women polled see health as a more desirable personal goal than wealth for the 1970s.

The Introduction was contributed by Barbara Gutmann Rosenkrantz, Ph.D., Associate Professor of the History of Science in the Faculty of Arts and Sciences and the School of Public Health of Harvard University.

Health is both commonplace and special, individual and social, desirable for its own sake and for what it enables us to enjoy and accomplish. However much a definition of health takes into account common-sense, philosophy, and science, we are generally accustomed to defining it on our own terms. Seldom confounded by the routine question on applications for college admission or employment asking "Do you enjoy good health?" we answer in the affirmative without pausing to wonder how to measure the difference between "good" health and just plain health. Even the qualification "corrective lenses worn for reading" is not considered an admission of disease. For most of us living in the United States at the end of the twentieth century, health is accepted as the rule rather than the exception. The inconsistency contained in the phrase "poor health" appears as a paradox only when we make the mildly entertaining observation that someone "enjoys poor health."

In other equally casual ways, we assume that health is not a fixed state identified by some absolute standard of well-being. We accept minor discomforts and major assaults on our physical integrity ranging from dental caries to fractured limbs without feeling that good health is significantly threatened. We would be amazed and amused if the customary inquiry "How are you?" were answered with a detailed description of aches and pains; we would consider the response bizarre if it included a report on blood pressure, body temperature, and pulse, or an estimate of life expectancy based on comparative age and sex-specific calculations.

If there are ambiguities in the terms we traditionally use to evaluate and communicate information about our personal health, there is profound irony in the way we customarily assess the health of whole populations. Political philosophers, historians, economists, and demographers; statisticians, sanitarians, and physicians; ministers of state and boards of health from the seventeenth century to the present have measured the health of communities and nations in terms of death. Centuries before the causes of specific diseases could be identified and before epidemics could be prevented or alleviated, death was the clearly defined event that served to measure life.

Throughout England and Europe, and in the colonies, births and deaths were recorded as early as the fifteenth century. But much as we might want to search documents of the past for a forecast of the social concerns we hold today, there is little evidence that these early records were used to assess or improve the health of individuals. Nor was the practice of marking down vital events more than minimally associated, until the end of the seventeenth century, with the need to maintain community stability.

In the seventeenth century, John Graunt, an Englishman, gathered together parish records of christenings, burials, and the Bills of Mortality published in London between 1629 and 1658 to write his *Natural and Political Observations . . . Upon the Bills of Mortality* in 1665. Graunt advertised his pamphlet with the recommendation that the study of birth and death records made it possible to preserve "Peace and Plenty." Following the four decades of social and economic disruption accompanying the Puritan Revolution and Commonwealth, Graunt anticipated reestablishment of political stability under the monarchy. Knowledge of the health of London as revealed in the vital statistics of the people might, he suggested, establish order on a firmer foundation. Graunt, however, sought first to promote social tranquillity rather than the health and long life of individuals.

During the next three centuries, people ordered their lives in ways which altered the significance of death, the length of life, and the conception of health. Over much of this stretch of time, however, mere survival and health were inseparable. Looking back, it seems that people lived at the edge of a precipice; there were no social or technical resources to serve as buffers against the natural hazards which threaten all living organisms even today. Length of life, used as the sole measure of health, suggested a perilous existence in which people's lives were at risk from the moment of conception. Sickness, health, and death had different meaning when few persons grew to adult life without experiencing the loss of a parent, sister, or brother. Yet if the expectation of health was diminished by the imminence of death, perhaps the close bonds established by mutual grief also enhanced the health and lives of those who survived. Freedom from disease was in some respects a more adequate description of health in the past, and longevity was a noteworthy accomplishment.

In the second half of the twentieth century, the unlikelihood that contagious disease will have a fatal outcome casts doubt upon the value of traditional methods of measuring health and dealing with sickness and death. Our expectations for personal health require new roles and social commitments. Physicians now have the responsibility of preserving health rather than merely curtailing disease, and the informed layman bears responsibilities for both personal health and public health policy. Yet, although most of us may expect to live beyond the age of 70, mortality rates remain the standard against which we measure national health progress. While death is depersonalized when it takes place in the aseptic atmosphere of the hospital, the threat of death from accidents and wars requires social and political involvements and personal commitments which make our present criteria of health inadequate. In a world in which we feel assured that long life is the rule, we continue to use the data of death to illustrate the advantages of health; however, because death is so distant from our daily concerns, we need to have more meaningful parameters of personal and public health.

The definition of health offered by the World Health Organization poses both the aspiration and the dilemma of contemporary achievement: "Health is a state of complete physical, mental, and social well-being and not merely the absence of disease or infirmity." The expectation that life will be long is now so much taken for granted that longevity can be entirely omitted from the definition. Yet life expectancy is the critical measure which marks off the present from the past and differentiates our health from the health of our forebears. When the struggle to maintain life beyond infancy seemed inaccessible and adults rarely lived beyond the years we now describe as middle age, were men and women less convinced that health brought happiness? When premature mortality meant death from cholera or tuberculosis rather than violent death from a car accident or bullet, were expectations for the course of life fundamentally altered? These are questions that we must ask if we are to make sense of the platitudes of the television commercial and the exhortations of the World Health Organization, for between the seventeenth and the twentieth centuries attention has shifted from personal death and the individual's record of longevity to the life expectancy of populations. Buried in the population data are experiences with disease and attitudes toward health which reflect our tolerance of certain hazards to health and our determination to eliminate other points of destruction. The pursuit of health in the past has prompted a wide range of prescriptions and proposals: special brews and diets of "natural" food, the restriction of the "noisome odors" of slaughterhouses and the elimination of open sewers, quarantine in pest houses and advocacy of life on the open range. And, in spite of the threats of disease and the inevitability of death, the quest for longevity has remained a constant inspiration.

For most of the recorded past, old age was venerated. Frequently, as in the case of Thomas Parr, who had reputedly reached the age of 152 when he died in 1635, great age was associated with sustained physical vigor. William Harvey, the renowned English physician whose experiments and observations first described the function of the heart and circulation of the blood in living organisms, was called upon to perform an autopsy on Parr. After a detailed examination of the old man's frame and organs, he announced, "All the internal parts . . . appeared so healthy, that had nothing happened to interfere with the . . . habits of life, he might have escaped paying the debt due to nature for some little time longer."

Old Parr had been summoned to Royal Court so that the king might ask him the reasons for his prolonged life. According to the tale told in a long poem published at the time of Parr's death, he replied that the cause of his longevity was that he "did penance when he was a hundred years old." The story continues that Parr, unaccustomed to the excitement, crowds, and rich food he encountered in London, simply passed away. Harvey's autopsy report corroborates this story.

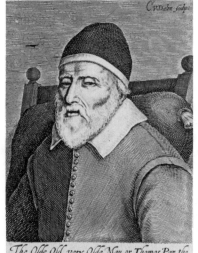

Thomas Parr, Englishman who reputedly reached the age of 152 when he died in 1635.

The causes of death seem fairly referrible to a sudden change in the non-naturals, the chief mischief being connected with the change of air, which through the course of life had been inhaled of perfect purity,—light, cool,

and mobile—whereby the praecordia and lungs were more freely venti-
lated and cooled; but in this great advantage, in this grand cherisher of
life, this city is especially destitute . . . And then for one hitherto used to
live on food unvaried in kind, and very simple in its nature, to be set at a
table loaded with a variety of viands, and tempted not only to eat more
than wont, but to partake of strong drink, it must needs fall out that the
functions of all the natural organs would become deranged. Whence the
stomach at length failing, and the excretions long retained, the work of
concoction proceeding languidly, the liver getting loaded, the blood stag-
nating in the veins, the spirits frozen, the heart, the source of life, op-
pressed, the lungs infarcted, and made impervious to the ambient air, the
general habit rendered more compact, so that it could not longer exhale or
perspire—no wonder that the soul, little content with such a prison, took
its flight.

At that time, mixing supernatural and scientific observations—Parr's
explanation of retained health and Harvey's autopsy report—was not
questioned. Both William Harvey and John Graunt witnessed the transition from a world in which supernatural factors were thought to control man's destiny, to one in which social conditions were held to influence health and well-being. In the past, the mystery of long life was
sought in the habits of individual centenarians, while magic elixirs,
natural fountains, and special abodes were sought in an effort to prolong
youth. The gift of life was linked to special qualities or potions: "the
breath of a young virgin" or, it was thought, the *aqua vitae* of the
alchemist which would perhaps restore natural powers that had been
lost.

As students of health we should examine the different elements that
have contributed to improved health and note especially two factors
that have enabled men to live longer and healthier lives. Systematic
evaluation of the relative importance of each of these factors can contribute to our knowledge of how they improved health in the past.

The first factor concentrates on the ecology of health, the biological
and environmental elements which have affected the life and growth of
organisms over a period of time. Here the epidemiologist and physiologist describe the complex interrelationships which support life on this
planet and investigate the consequence of long and short term changes
in patterns of growth and development.

The second factor in changing health and life rests in the practices
men adopt and the institutions they construct and support. The observation of these developments begins with the historian. Understanding the
social processes that have evolved requires historical perspective and
recognition of the choices which reflect attitudes often only indirectly
associated with health.

For instance, the provision of public water supplies which accompanied the growth of cities in the nineteenth century at first had contradictory consequences for health. Abundant water improved hygiene, but,

in the absence of arrangements for disposal of sewage, water supplies were often contaminated, spreading disease. However, demand for public sewers and the banning of outdoor privies frequently gained impetus as much from esthetic as hygienic considerations. The decision to allocate public money for the construction of sewers also reflected attitudes toward the persons living in the affected areas, so that often the most densely populated neighborhoods were the last to gain public waste disposal. In the past as now, ignorance has been identified as a danger to health. Attitudes toward certain groups—the poor, the immigrant, and the black—have stemmed from social values, and measures to improve personal and public health have reflected these attitudes as much as scientific knowledge about the causes of disease. Changing experience with disease and health, whatever its source, has in turn affected both personal and social expectations.

One of the benefits of recent studies in historical demography is that there is now much more information about the birth, marriage, and death rates of specific communities in England and Wales, the European continent, and North America. Fragmentary as these records are, they open up the possibility of learning more about the habits and health of persons long since dead. No clear and definitive statements can yet be made, but much that is new and illuminating has already inspired investigations which hold hope for greater clarity in the future. There is agreement that the great surge of population over the past two and a half centuries is the consequence primarily of decreased mortality rather than of increased births, while the importance of improved nutrition, sanitary reform, personal hygiene, and specific medical intervention remains at issue.

Within each of these categories there is a need for more exploration. For instance, were increased food supplies resulting from change in land ownership and agricultural productivity the single most important factor in reducing death rates throughout the eighteenth and nineteenth centuries, as the epidemiologist-physician Thomas McKeown has argued persuasively? Or, as a number of economic historians have suggested, were a multiplicity of changes associated with the economic development initiated by the Industrial Revolution responsible for a generally improved standard of living and a new social outlook that resulted in better health?

Data on population growth cannot be transformed into knowledge about attitudes toward health or reactions to the threat of disease. Age-specific mortality rates will indicate what stages of life were most perilous—how many children survived beyond the first year, how many adults succumbed in what nineteenth-century statisticians referred to as the "productive years" of 16 to 35. Age-specific fertility data—the number of children born in relation to a woman's age—will help fill out the picture. Where once most children had suffered the death of one parent before reaching the age of 14, a child today can expect to have this loss postponed until the age of 55. When experience with death is postponed, how much of a force for health is information on mortality rates? In what ways does the reduction of the death experience in childhood affect the plans and expectations of adults? To better understand what health meant in history, this sort of information must be integrated with knowledge about personal habits, attitudes toward childbirth and child rearing, acquaintance with popular health manuals, and with remedies available for staving off disease.

Until the end of the nineteenth century, only one specifically medical measure to combat infectious disease was available: inoculation with the pus from smallpox scabs in hopes of producing a milder form of that disease. After 1801, vaccination with cowpox immunized against the far more fatal smallpox virus. It is difficult to assess the positive consequences of even this measure on large class-differentiated populations across time. Some epidemiologists and demographers believe that medicine played no significant role in controlling infectious disease, the major cause of death throughout the eighteenth and nineteenth centuries, until after the introduction of sulfanilamides (sulfa drugs) around 1935. But in the mid-eighteenth century, the Overseers of the Poor in Boston, Massachusetts, demonstrated to their own satisfaction the effectiveness of inoculation, and the absence of smallpox epidemics in the first decades of the nineteenth century is evidence of the success of vaccination.

Furthermore, the laboratory scientists and physicians who identified numerous specific agents of contagion in the late nineteenth and early twentieth centuries clearly believed that medical and sanitary measures to restrict the spread of infectious diseases such as typhoid, tuberculosis, and diphtheria contributed substantially to health. It is difficult for us to describe the processes whereby knowledge about the bacteriologic causes of the most common contagious sicknesses was translated into better health, since in most instances no specific therapy was available. Even when an immunizing agent was developed, as in the case of diphtheria antitoxin, very little of what we would today consider effective treatment could be incorporated into medical practice. Nonetheless, optimism arising from the rapid growth of scientific information gave support to public health measures and led to the acceptance of social intervention where earlier attempts to arrest the spread of disease had foundered. As haphazard efforts to quarantine and disinfect were replaced by both more direct medical intervention and registration of contagious disease, the incidence of disease became an important new measure of health.

Since the turn of the century, the rate of mortality has declined dramatically at both ends of the life span. While the death rate for infants born in 1900 in the United States was 162 per 1,000, by 1960 the rate had declined to about 29 per 1,000. In the same period the comparative figure for those over 85 was reduced from 260 per 1,000 to 209 per 1,000, a less impressive decline in relative terms, but an even more substantial improvement if measured against the total population of persons over 85. While infancy remains the most hazardous period of life today, as it was throughout the past two and a half centuries, adult mortality rates have declined sharply during the first half of this century with at least one advantage for children—living grandparents. Although the age at marriage and the age of parents at the time of the birth of their first child have not changed over the past fifty years, the chance of the first child born to American white parents having four grandparents alive when he or she reaches the tenth birthday are about 1 in 14 today, while in 1920 the chances were about 1 in 90.

Encouraging as these figures may be, they tend to obscure the disparities which continue to exist. At least two important problems are not uncovered by these figures: first, the chances of a black child having the same good fortune are substantially less than those for the white child; second, it is more likely that the first grandparent to die will be the grandfather even when the grandmother is exactly the same age.

Questions about life expectancy and expectations for health must be separated, for although length of life has increased for both sexes, the excess of male mortality rates over female rates has increased from 8 percent in 1900 to about 36 percent at present. At the beginning of this century, when contagious disease was still the primary cause of death in the United States, women lived from two to three years longer than men; now that death from the chronic and degenerative diseases stands at the head of the list, women live from five to six years longer than men. Figures published by the World Health Organization in 1972 from an investigation of mortality in 34 developed countries show the same widening gap, while a recent insurance study comparing mortality among females aged 65 and over shows that this gap is the same whether women are occupied in the traditional role of housewife or employed outside the home as college teachers.

The persistence with which this type of information is cited continues to underscore the tendency to think of health first in terms of length of life. Just as William Harvey more than 300 years ago assumed that Tom Parr's reported age fixed and circumscribed his task, so today we tend, perhaps mistakenly, to think of improved health in terms of measures to prolong life. Certainly the assumptions which we bring to the consideration of health today are rooted in the past, but, if there is a lesson to be learned from history, it is that the past and present are quite different. When we measure today's experience by the experience of what has gone before, we find assuring evidence of progress.

The historians' contribution to our knowledge about and understanding of health only begins with the attempt to identify and measure the various forces which determined health in the past. Today the study of history must also consider the processes of social change through which people have gained a measure of control over the course and conclusion of their lives. In a society marked by rapid change of experience and expectation, such as ours, the study of history helps us separate and reassemble the natural and social resources of the past in order to better understand our present circumstances.

If the old measures of health are inadequate for today's health, then we must incorporate new data into our definition. We need, for instance, new biological information about the relationship between nutrition and health, and more sophisticated evaluation of the role of social values in stimulating and constraining our widening expectations.

As you study various aspects of health in the chapters to follow, you will be able to observe the vital data of the natural and social sciences. If you decide that mortality rates are no longer the single adequate criterion for health, you will also have to recognize that the choice of what is to be measured, and how it is to be assessed, is part of the social process which defines and validates the criteria of health and determines at what cost and at whose expense personal and public health can be achieved.

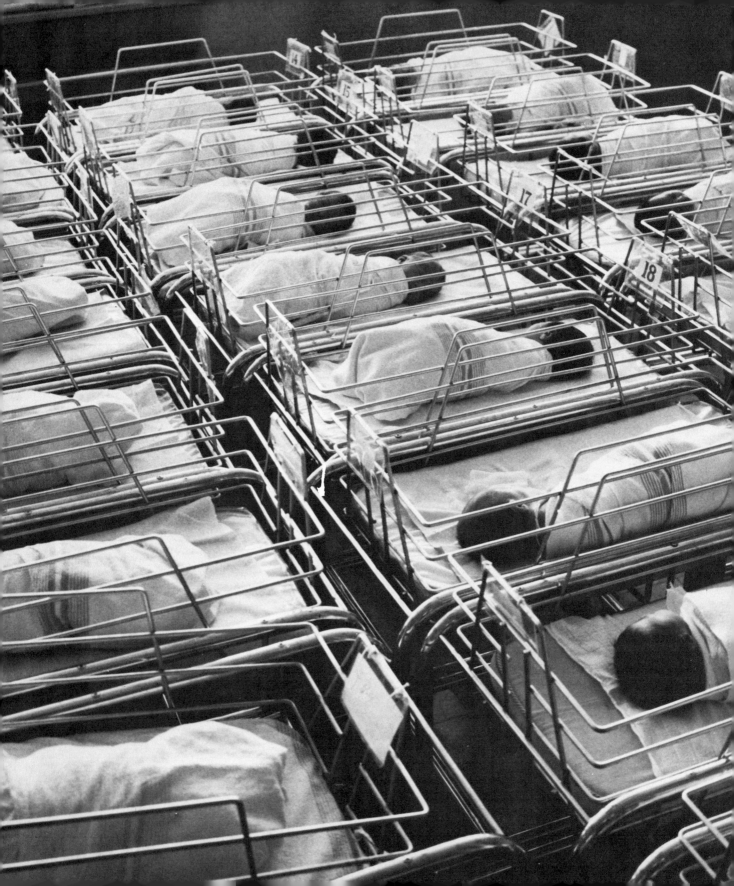

Part I

HEALTH AND THE PATTERNS OF LIFE

Chapter 1

The Human Body

Man is unique. Of the millions of species that occupy the thin film on the surface of the earth where life is found, man stands alone. He walks upright and, unlike the great apes and most other primates, his legs are longer than his arms. His feet, although not much good for grabbing branches, are well adapted for walking or running. Man has a large brain but a peculiar lack of hair. He has unusual facility in making sounds and has developed the gift of speech. He writes; he farms; he cooks with fire; he makes and uses machines. His social behavior is highly developed and his culture is complex.

For all his unique characteristics, man is also an animal. The organs of man, his heart, intestines, kidneys, and lungs, differ in few respects from the corresponding organs of monkeys, rats, or sheep. Muscle contractions, nervous or hormonal control, respiration, and digestion follow the same kinds of processes and the same chemical and physical relationships in man that are common to all other mammals and to many other living creatures. Man's uniqueness depends not on his anatomy and

This chapter was contributed by Joseph D. Brain, Sc.D., Associate Professor of Physiology, Harvard School of Public Health.

physiology but on his behavior and accomplishment. Man knows love, hope, guilt, and hate. Man reflects on his past and anticipates his future. Unlike most living things, he does not falter on the thin edge of NOW: to a greater extent than most animals, he can control his own destiny.

Physiology is the science which studies how the human body functions. The present form and function of the human body is the result of a long evolutionary process. The human body incorporates a number of properties that have demonstrated survival value throughout hundreds of thousands of years, and it shares most of these properties with other animals. Let us consider some of the major themes which are evident in the design of your body.

Redundancy of design

The human body possesses a reserve capacity for functioning. Many organs exist in duplicate. Loss of one eye, ear, kidney, or lung does not necessarily endanger life. Within the single organs of the body, there is usually a reserve capacity not used by healthy individuals. Large parts of the small and large intestine can be removed, and life goes on. The amount of blood pumped by the heart and the volume of air moving in and out of the lungs can be increased by a factor of ten or more, as occurs during extreme exercise. Consistent training can increase the limits of the body's performance. In addition to reserve capacity for function, the body has multiple control systems. Heart functioning, for example, is affected by nervous control, hormonal influences, and the amount of blood returned to the heart. Loss of any one of these controls does not immobilize the heart.

Form and function

Another constant theme of physiology is the inseparable relationship between form and function. Anatomy and physiology are two of the earliest medical sciences; they developed together. Although the structure of the organs in the body varies widely, each architecture reflects a specific physiological role. The lungs, the heart, and the bones have distinctive appearances and mechanical properties by virtue of their divergent callings. Function dictates form, and form is the machinery that makes function possible. This principle extends to all levels of organization—from whole organisms down to molecules.

Maintenance and repair

The human body is characterized by a number of systems which can prevent and repair many different kinds of injury. Minor injury, infection, and blood loss are not unusual features of everyday life. The body has its own physical barriers which prevent invasion by hostile intruders. When these fail, immunological systems immobilize, neutralize, and destroy germs or toxins which may enter and cause disease. Another element in this response to mild injury is a program of replacing failing cells. This system of preventive maintenance operates throughout life to ensure a continuous supply of new cells where they are needed. The body recycles most components of obsolete cells.

Adaptability and flexibility

The body also has enduring adaptability and flexibility in widely varying environments. It can not only survive in great extremes of temperature and humidity but also adapt to a variety of diets. Both the amount and the composition of food and liquid intake can be altered. Individual cells in the body are also flexible and can utilize a number of different energy sources. Such flexibility and inherent stability in changing environmental conditions are made possible by multiple control systems. As in most other organisms, the human endocrine and nervous systems monitor changing environments and make appropriate responses to them.

THE CELL The cell is the smallest independent unit in the body containing all of the essential properties of life. Many types of human cells can be grown in test tubes after being taken from the body. Cells which are functionally specialized are often grouped together and operate in concert as a

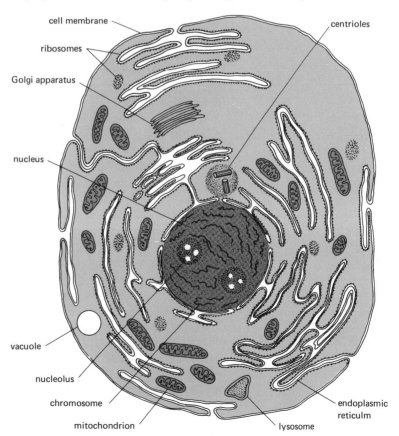

Figure 1.1. Diagram of the major organelles in a typical cell.

Figure 1.2. A cell in culture showing most of the major organelles: (a) endoplasmic reticulum, (b) Golgi complex, (c) nucleus, (d) vacuole, (e) cell membrane, and (f) mitochondria. (Courtesy of Dr. S. P. Sorokin, Harvard University)

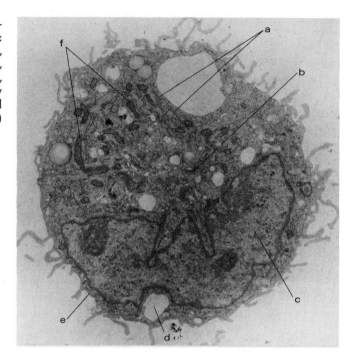

tissue, such as muscle tissue or nervous tissue. Various tissues may be arranged together to form a unit called an organ, such as the kidney, liver, heart, or lungs. Organs often function in groups called organ systems. Thus the mouth, esophogus, stomach, pancreas, liver, and intestines constitute the digestive system. If we are to understand the working of the body, we must take a close look at cells, the essential unit of these systems.

Cells are characterized by a high degree of complexity and order in both structure and function. The cell contains a number of diverse structures called cell *organelles* (small organs). These are responsible for carrying out the specialized biochemical reactions that characterize each cell. The many chemical reactions that take place in a cell require the establishment of varied chemical microenvironments. Carefully controlled transport mechanisms along with highly effective barriers—the cell membranes—ensure that chemicals are present in the proper region of the cell in appropriate concentrations.

The cell membranes, composed of a mixture of protein and lipid (a compound soluble in fat solvents), form the outer border of the cell, separating it from its surroundings. Membranes are an essential component of almost all cell organelles. Although the membrane is only 10 millionths of a millimeter thick, it is selectively permeable, allowing only certain molecules to pass through it. Thus it acts as a selective gateway for the transport of substances and specifies both the form and activities of the cell. Transport of molecules across membranes may be either passive or active. When passive, materials move from high concentration to low concentration. When active, materials move against the concentration gradient, and energy must be supplied by the cell to move the substance "uphill." Cells also can bring substances inside by the processes of *phagocytosis* or *pinocytosis* (literally "cell eating" and "cell drinking"). In these processes, the cell membrane forms a pocket that encloses material near the cell surface. The membrane gradually surrounds this material; a "bubble" containing the substance to be ingested pinches off from the rest of the cell membrane and then appears as a *vacuole* inside the cell.

Cells are not only organized but also highly miniaturized. Red blood cells, which carry oxygen in the blood, have a diameter of only 7 microns; 5 billion of them are suspended in a cubic centimeter of blood. More than 5 trillion are contained in a quart of blood. Storage of information in the cell is also highly miniaturized. All of the genetic information in a human cell can be found in only 6 billionths of a milligram of DNA (see below). In fact, enough DNA to code all the information specifying the characteristics of all the people in the world (3 billion) would only be 18 milligrams, about 0.00063 ounces.

To explore the contents of the cell in greater detail, we begin with the most important molecules found in the cell. More than 80 percent of the cell is water. Water is a nearly universal solvent for biological molecules and thus is the perfect fluid for chemical reactions in the cell. It also plays an essential part in transporting materials among and within cells and in the circulatory system. Although water is the dominant molecule in the body, a more interesting group of molecules is the organic compounds—all molecules which contain the atom carbon. Carbon atoms can combine with atoms of hydrogen, oxygen, nitrogen, and sometimes sulfur and phosphorous in various arrangements. The result is four major classes of organic compounds—nucleic acids, proteins, carbohydrates, and lipids.

The most visible and essential organelle in a cell is the nucleus; it contains genetic material and regulates the activities of the entire cell. Genetic information is coded in two long chains of DNA (deoxyribonucleic acid) which are wound about one another to form a double helix. This double-helix structure of DNA accounts for its unique ability to store, duplicate, and transfer information. Prior to cell division, or *mitosis*, DNA replicates to ensure that each new daughter cell will have a complete set of genetic information.

The area outside of the nucleus is called the *cytoplasm*. Cytoplasm contains a variety of organelles that have different appearances and different functions. An elaborate system of membranes and small granules, called *ribosomes*, makes up the rough *endoplasmic reticulum*, where proteins are synthesized.

Proteins are long chains of nitrogen-containing organic acids called *amino acids*. Proteins serve as carriers of oxygen and carbon dioxide, as

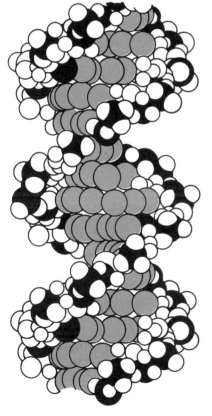

Figure 1.3. Two strands of DNA wound about each other in a double helix.

Figure 1.4. A protein manufacturing and secreting cell. This cell has a great deal of endoplasmic reticulum which reflects its function. (a) nucleus, (b) mitochondria, (c) protein droplets, (d) endoplasmic reticulum. (Courtesy of Dr. S. P. Sorokin, Harvard University)

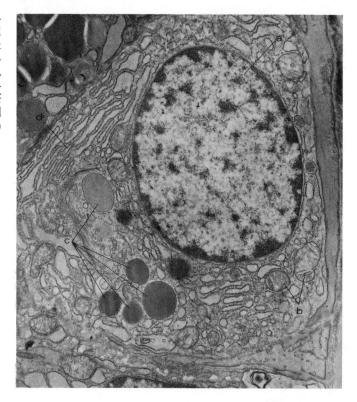

antibodies, and as some hormones. There are about 20 different amino acids, which can be assembled into an almost infinite array of different protein molecules containing hundreds of amino acids. The information specifying the form, and hence the function, of the protein is carried from the DNA in the nucleus to the endoplasmic reticulum in the cytoplasm by messenger RNA, another kind of nucleic acid similar to DNA. The messenger RNA arranges the amino acids in proper sequence prior to their linkage into protein chains.

Proteins have important structural responsibilities and are essential to bone, muscle, skin, hair, and fingernails. They also act as biological catalysts called *enzymes* and control the rate at which metabolic reactions take place inside the cell. Most enzymes are highly specific, that is, they control specific reactions.

The *mitochondria* are rod-shaped organelles which are the major sites of energy production in the cell. Molecules that can liberate energy, such as glucose, are broken down into carbon dioxide and water by enzyme-catalyzed reactions. The energy produced is mainly stored in the bond energy of a special molecule called adenosine triphosphate (ATP). This energy can then be used for any of the body's energy-requiring processes. ATP enables skeletal muscle to shorten, and this contraction can be used for external work such as lifting objects or mountain climbing or for internal work such as that performed by heart muscles as they propel the blood. Internal work finally appears as heat. Energy from ATP can also be used in the synthesis of new molecules as well as for active transport of molecules or ions against a concentration gradient.

Proteins synthesized by the cell are sometimes collected in the *Golgi apparatus*, wrapped in a membrane, and later secreted from the cell. *Lysosomes* are membrane-bound packages of enzymes which form an intracellular digestive system. The enzymes break down ingested material brought into the cell by phagocytosis. Lysosomes also digest "worn out" cellular components.

All living cells share certain housekeeping functions: energy transfer, the flow of genetic information from DNA through RNA to protein, and the formation of certain basic cellular organelles. Superimposed on these basic cell functions are other specialized functions, such as excitability (nerve cells), contractility (muscle cells), secretion of enzymes and hormones, or the production of antibodies. In a multicellular organism like man, cells differentiate and take on specific cell functions not shared by their neighbors. A division of labor takes place as cells become specialized. The result is increased efficiency for the organism.

Figures 1.5 and 1.6 show electron micrographs of different cell types.

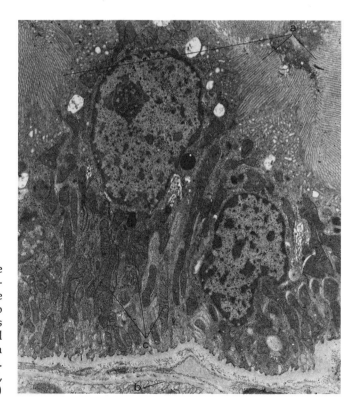

Figure 1.5. Kidney proximal tubule cell. This cell transports electrolytes from the tubular urine, above surrounding the microvilli (a) to the capillary (b). This requires much energy, and thus the cell has large amounts of mitochondria (c) to synthesize the needed ATP. (Courtesy of Dr. S. P. Sorokin, Harvard University)

Figure 1.6. Heart muscle showing mitochondria (a) and the contractile filaments (b). A single unit is shown between each pair of dark bands. The muscle has been fixed in the contracted state. (Courtesy of Dr. S. P. Sorokin, Harvard University)

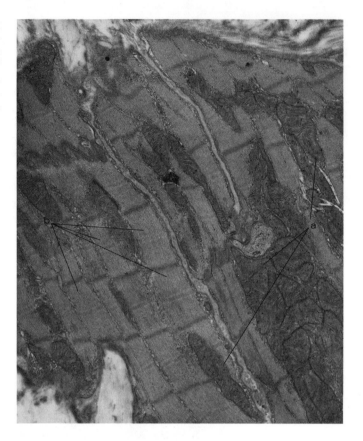

Each has a strikingly different appearance and a correspondingly different function. It is remarkable that each cell has or at least had the genetic information to carry out all specialized functions. Somehow clues in the physical and chemical environment direct the cell in developing those capabilities that are appropriate. Thus each cell has large amounts of DNA that are never read and expressed; other areas are read continuously and serve to control the specialized role the cell has in the economy of the body. Along with this control of organs, the cell itself and organelles within the cell are controlled by highly responsive systems.

THE INTERNAL ENVIRONMENT

A single-celled organism, such as an amoeba, is totally dependent on the fluid that surrounds it. Oxygen and nutrients must all enter the cell from its immediate environment. Unwanted materials, such as carbon dioxide, nitrogenous wastes (unusable parts of proteins), or excess heat, can only be excreted into the fluid outside the cell. Like the amoeba, every living cell in the human body is also bathed in fluid called *extracellular fluid.* It is similar in composition to blood plasma, except for a lower protein content.

This fluid is the only environment of a cell, and the metabolism and continued survival of the cell depend on the constant composition of the extracellular fluid. The temperature, acidity, oxygen and glucose content, and the concentration of many other molecules and ions must be maintained at appropriate levels. Almost 100 years ago the great French physiologist Claude Bernard recognized this fundamental principle and stated that ". . . it is the fixity of the internal environment which is the condition of the free and independent life."

In contrast to the carefully controlled internal environment, the external environment varies. Humans can survive a wide range of conditions. Temperature and humidity can vary from arctic to tropical environments. One can bathe in distilled water or in the Great Salt Lake in Utah. The outside world is contaminated with bacteria, allergens, carcinogens, and dusts and is very different from the immediate environment of the living cell.

How is the internal environment maintained in the narrow range that is compatible with life? We have discussed how individual cells make up tissues and organs. Their physiological role is to serve as functional units of the organs. We now turn to the physiological role of the organs themselves. Their diverse activities help to maintain the constancy of the internal environment. Claude Bernard wrote: "All the vital mechanisms, however varied they may be, have only one object, that of preserving constant the conditions of life in the internal environment." Such organs as the lungs, kidneys, and gastrointestinal tract represent an interface between the external and internal environment; these are organs of exchange. Other systems, such as the nervous and hormonal systems, measure and control the quality of the internal and external environments. This information about the body is relayed, stored, and interpreted, and commands are sent to the appropriate organs in order to ensure continued stability. Thus each cell of the body, as part of an organ, contributes to the welfare of the whole organism by maintaining the stable conditions required for life.

We shall now consider the nature of the barriers which exist between the outside and the inside worlds. Energy (such as heat) and materials from the external environment are of no consequence to the living cell and, therefore, to the human body until they cross one of the body surfaces. The elements of the external world have no impact on the body's cells for good or for ill until they penetrate these physical barriers.

One of these barriers, the skin, has a relatively simple job. It must effectively block the outside from the inside world. A relatively germ-proof and water-proof barrier, it cannot be penetrated by very large or highly charged molecules. Since the skin is composed of lipids, only molecules which are lipid-soluble can penetrate this barrier.

The skin of the average adult has a surface area of about one and a half square yards. The outermost portion of the skin is actually dead. Many layers of very thin flattened cells form this outer layer of the skin and vary in thickness from 0.05 to 0.5 millimeters. Beneath these dead cells are areas of active cell renewal where new cells are being produced to replace the cells on the body surface.

Two other body surfaces with much more surface area than the skin have conflicting physiological roles. A topologist will quickly recognize that these other surfaces are continuous with the outside skin and separate the contaminated outside world from the body's interior. One such surface is the tube that runs from the mouth to the anus, called the *gastrointestinal tract.* This body surface has hundreds of square yards of surface area. The other is the *respiratory tract* which has a surface area of approximately 70 square yards. These two surfaces, in addition to their protective functions, are designed for efficient exchange. It is essential that humans be able to absorb all kinds of nutrients and oxygen and excrete carbon dioxide. Thus, the lungs and the gastrointestinal tract have unusual problems. They must create a protective barrier which effectively excludes unwanted, harmful agents. At the same time, they must accept necessary materials from the outside world.

The gastrointestinal system

The function of the gastrointestinal system is to accept food and water from the external environment, process the food, and absorb the breakdown products and water. The substances absorbed in the gastrointestinal tract provide the source of chemical energy for bodily processes and supply the building blocks for the body's synthetic operations. Vitamins and minerals are also absorbed in the gastrointestinal system. Food enters the system in pieces too large to be absorbed across the wall of the intestines. Absorption must, therefore, be preceded by digestion. Digestion is the process of breaking down pieces of food into molecules and of changing the complex molecules into simpler forms which can be readily absorbed. It is achieved by mechanical mixing movements of the stomach as well as by the action of stomach acid and special enzymes secreted from the pancreas and from the small intestine.

A diagram of the gastrointestinal system is shown in Figure 1.7. The teeth bite off and grind down pieces of food so that they are small enough to be swallowed. In the process of chewing, the food is mixed with saliva. Saliva lubricates the food to facilitate swallowing and contains some enzymes which begin digesting carbohydrates. The food then passes through the esophagus and is stored in the stomach, where food and saliva are mixed with hydrochloric acid and the digestive enzyme pepsin. The resulting substance, called chyme, is gradually admitted into the small intestine, where most absorption occurs. In the small intestine, the stomach acid is neutralized by an alkaline secretion from the pancreas. The mass, or bolus, of chyme is then mixed with bile from the gall bladder and digestive enzymes from the pancreas and the intestinal cells. Bile acts as an emulsifying agent decreasing the size of fat droplets and thus increasing the surface area available for enzymatic attack. Pancreatic juice is the most important source of digestive enzymes.

Figure 1.7. The gastrointestinal system.

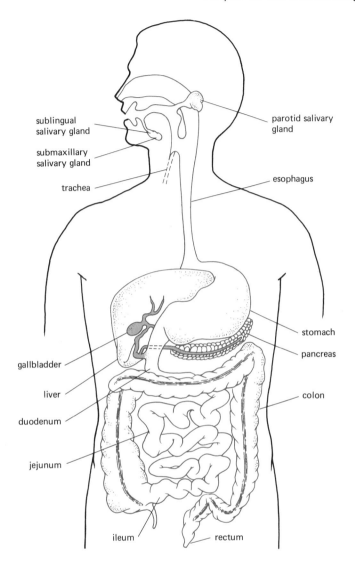

The predominant carbohydrate we eat is starch. Starch in its polymeric form (a large molecule consisting of many smaller, repeated, and connected units) is split into the less complex disaccharides by enzymes from the saliva and pancreas. Most of these are then split into the monosaccharide glucose by enzymes in the small intestine and are transported across the intestinal cells into the blood. Proteins are broken down by enzymes in the small intestine into individual amino acids which are also actively transported. The breakdown of fat into fatty acids and glycerol depends not only on pancreatic enzymes but also on bile salts secreted by the liver.

The small intestine is structured to absorb nutrients. It has an elaborate folded surface to make the total area very large. Large amounts

What are the most easily digested foods?

This raises the question of what criteria one used to measure *ease* of digestion. Easily digested and quickly digested are not synonymous phrases in a technical sense. For example, sugars are rather quickly absorbed, while fats remain in the digestive tract for many hours; yet, the normal human digestive tract is remarkably efficient in handling fats. Complex carbohydrates and proteins are digested at a different pace (somewhere in between sugars and fats).

To imply that the digestion of the more complex nutrients is difficult is to underestimate the sophistication of the enzyme systems and the cooperation of organs such as the liver and pancreas, as well as the sophistication of the digestive tract itself.

There are components of foods which are, of course, indigestible—cellulose, for example. However, the very fact that cellulose is indigestible makes it important to the diet as it is one form of roughage, or bulk.

Many negative attitudes, which may be completely unwarranted on the part of the average person, have resulted in branding foods as "hard to digest," "acidic," or "heavy." (Frequently, the appropriate direction for the criticism would be toward the *amount* eaten.)

From *Today's Health*, Vol. 51, No. 2 (February, 1973), p. 6.

of blood flow through its walls to carry away the absorbed materials. Most of the absorbed fluid is from the body itself. The average intake of liquids in adults is approximately 1.2 quarts per day. The body adds about 1.5 quarts of saliva from the mouth, about 2 quarts of acid solution from the stomach, about 2 quarts of secretion from the pancreas and liver and 1.5 quarts of fluid from the intestines. Most of the fluids (about 8.5 quarts per day) are absorbed and only a half a quart passes into the large intestine.

Some of the absorbed nutrients also come from the body itself. The small intestine is an area of very active cell renewal. The lining cells of the small intestine are replaced every one and a half days, having been exposed to a great deal of mechanical wear and tear and to contact with pathogens. They are continuously shed and replaced by new cells. As a consequence, there is no such thing as a vegetarian. We are all auto-cannibals eating about a half a pound of human flesh every day. This amount represents the cells that fall off the lining of our small intestine: they are digested and reabsorbed.

The function of the large intestine is primarily that of storage, although some water and sodium are absorbed from it. Feces are composed primarily of the indigestible remnants of food and of bacteria. These are retained in the large intestine until defecation occurs. There is no absorption of toxic materials contained in the feces, and there is no physiological significance to the frequency of bowel movements.

With the exception of the lipids, substances absorbed in the intestines are taken into the blood and then passed through the liver. After some processing by the liver, the nutrients are distributed to the rest of the body. Since they can penetrate membranes easily, the lipids pass through the intestinal wall and enter the lymph channels or lymphatics. The lymph channels contain lymph, a body fluid similar to blood but containing less protein.

As mentioned above, the inside of the intestinal tract is really part of the outside world and is thoroughly contaminated with all kinds of bacteria and other toxic materials. Despite such contamination, toxic materials entering the gastrointestinal tract and passing through without being absorbed or affecting absorption or secretion of other materials normally cause no harm. Almost everyone has swallowed an indigestible object (a corn or pit) at some time in his life. Although the object may contain toxic materials, it is of little impact because the materials do not dissolve and are not absorbed. Similarly, the lower portion of the intestinal tract contains millions of living bacteria, most of which cause no harm. In fact, their presence may prevent more dangerous bacteria from taking over.

The respiratory system

Producing sufficient energy is one of the nonnegotiable demands of life. Energy is produced by burning or oxidizing the organic molecules in

Figure 1.8. The respiratory system.

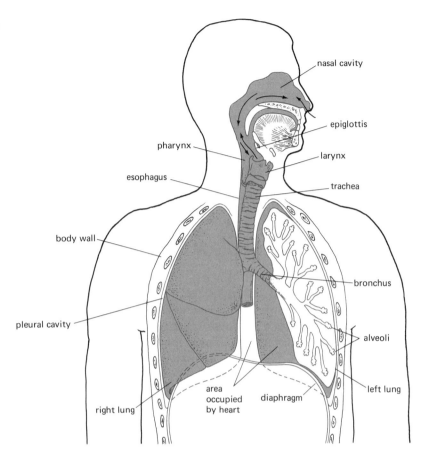

food. Oxidation is similar to burning in that it results in atoms of carbon and hydrogen being combined with oxygen to form carbon dioxide and water. Thus the consumption of oxygen and the production of carbon dioxide, a waste product of ATP synthesis, are indispensable to life. It follows that the human body must have an organ designed to exchange carbon dioxide and oxygen between the circulating blood and the atmosphere in sufficient volumes to sustain life. Within the chest lie the spongelike lungs which are compartmentalized into hundreds of millions of small air sacs called *alveoli*. Together they form a surface of approximately 70 square yards, where blood flowing through the lungs comes very close to gas contained in the alveoli. The lung provides an efficient interface with the environment, so that oxygen can enter the body and carbon dioxide can leave it.

About 6 quarts of air per minute are brought into the lungs, and about 3/10 of a quart of oxygen is transferred from the gas in the alveoli to the blood. At the same time, carbon dioxide moves from the blood to the alveolar gas and is exhaled. During exercise, however, it is possible to take in 100 quarts of air per minute and extract 5 quarts of oxygen. The rate at which oxygen enters the body is one useful measure of the total amount of energy expended by the body.

An essential link between the atmosphere containing oxygen and the cell which consumes it is the circulation. Oxygen delivery to the mitochondria within the cell depends not only on the lung but also on the ability of the blood to contain oxygen and on the ability of the circulation to transport it throughout the body. There are three processes essential for the transfer of oxygen from outside air to the blood flowing through the lung: (1) ventilation, (2) perfusion, and (3) diffusion through the air-blood barrier. *Ventilation* is the tidal process in which air is moved in bulk between the atmosphere and the lung. *Perfusion* is the action of the cardiovascular system in pumping blood throughout the lungs. *Diffusion* is the passive movement of gases down a concentration gradient between the alveolar gas and pulmonary capillary blood.

VENTILATION In order to deliver the inhaled gas to the alveolar surface uniformly, the lung has an elaborate distribution system. After moving through the nostrils and nasal cavity or through the mouth, air reaches the throat or *pharynx*. The *epiglottis* is a flap of tissue which folds over the opening of the larynx during swallowing and thus prevents any food or water from entering the respiratory tract. The *larynx* (voice box, adam's apple) is involved in sound production. It contains folds of stretched tissue, the *vocal chords*, which vibrate as air passes over and through them producing sound. In the absence of swallowing, the epiglottis does not cover the larynx, and the gas passes through the larynx into the wind pipe or *trachea*. The trachea branches into a left and right bronchus, which branch repeatedly until the alveoli are reached.

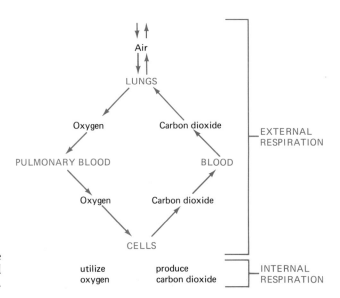

Figure 1.9. Respiration: the exchange of oxygen and carbon dioxide.

Hyperventilation

Some people will do anything for kicks, especially in a group. There isn't a law against hyperventilation—taking very deep breaths in rapid succession—and if some people have a compelling urge to freak out, it's better than taking LSD. But fooling around with your physiology until you pass out isn't sensible, even if your body can take it, and under some circumstances hyperventilation is downright dangerous. For instance, after becoming dizzy or unconscious you can injure yourself falling to the ground or hitting a sharp edge. Swimmers who want to stay under water a long time sometimes hyperventilate before diving in because they think they can pump more oxygen into the blood stream. But even with normal breathing, blood is almost completely saturated with oxygen all the time. What actually happens is that hyperventilation empties the lungs of carbon dioxide and thus removes the normal danger signal that cries "breathe" when you can't hold out any longer. Swimmers who perform this trick run out of oxygen without feeling the need to breathe and can easily drown.

From *Today's Health*, Vol. 49, No. 9 (September, 1971), p. 5.

Movement of air into the lungs is caused by the action of the respiratory muscles which expand the chest wall in such a way that the lungs fill passively. Even at the end of a normal breath, a large amount of gas remains in the lungs. Both the rate at which breathing occurs (respiratory frequency) and the amount of air coming in with each breath (tidal volume) are variable and can be altered to match metabolic demands. The ventilation rate is adjusted by the brain to keep the concentration of oxygen and carbon dioxide in the alveoli quite constant. In this way oxygen supply neatly meets oxygen demand. During increased exercise, more oxygen is consumed and more carbon dioxide is produced. Slightly increased levels of carbon dioxide make the blood more acid and stimulate the respiratory centers in the brain to increase ventilation. Other factors, such as the concentration of oxygen in the blood, may also influence ventilation, but they are less important than carbon dioxide.

PERFUSION AND DIFFUSION   Although ventilation is essential, gas exchange does not occur unless blood is uniformly distributed throughout the lungs. The right side of the heart pumps venous blood which is high in carbon dioxide and low in oxygen. The pulmonary blood vessels are highly branched, and a thin film of blood is spread just beneath the alveolar surface.

The third requirement for gas exchange in the lungs is diffusion. Diffusion is very effective if the distances to be traveled are small. In the alveoli, the blood is separated from the air by two specialized layers of cells, which together are less than 1 micrometer (.001 millimeter) thick. The concentration of oxygen is much higher in the gas inside the alveoli than in the pulmonary capillary blood. On the other hand, the concentration of carbon dioxide is higher in the pulmonary capillary blood than in the alveolar gas. Since the distance for gas to diffuse is small and since the total surface area is very large, oxygen and carbon dioxide rapidly move down their concentration gradients. In some types of disease this barrier may become thickened and gas exchange may be slowed.

The gas-exchange capability of the lungs must be linked to the needs

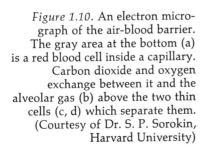
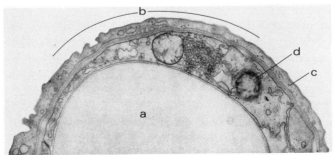

Figure 1.10. An electron micrograph of the air-blood barrier. The gray area at the bottom (a) is a red blood cell inside a capillary. Carbon dioxide and oxygen exchange between it and the alveolar gas (b) above the two thin cells (c, d) which separate them. (Courtesy of Dr. S. P. Sorokin, Harvard University)

Figure 1.11. Ciliated cells from the respiratory tract. These cells have small projectiles which contain muscle filaments. They beat about 1,000 times per minute and propel the mucus up the airways. (a) cilia, (b) cross section of cilia, (c) mitochondria, (d) nuclei of two cells, (e) border between adjacent cells. (Courtesy of Dr. S. P. Sorokin, Harvard University)

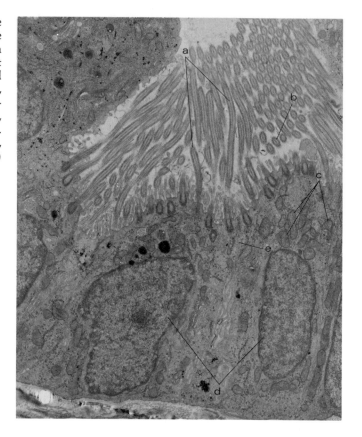

of the whole body by means of the circulatory system and by the unique properties of the blood. Oxygen and carbon dioxide can dissolve in blood, but the amount of gas carried in solution is totally inadequate for the body's needs. Fortunately, blood contains a special protein called *hemoglobin* which can carry large amounts of oxygen. Hemoglobin combines with oxygen, picking up large quantities in the lungs and then gradually releasing the oxygen in the tissues of the body. Blood containing normal amounts of red blood cells can carry about 20 cubic centimeters of oxygen per 100 cubic centimeters of blood. Hemoglobin facilitates the carrying of carbon dioxide as well.

Since the respiratory tract is an extensive area of contact between the environment and the body, it is essential to protect it and keep it clean. The nose not only removes large particles and soluble pollutant gases from the air but also warms and moistens the air entering the body. Dust particles and bacteria deposited in the respiratory tract are rapidly removed. The airways are covered with a mucous lining which is moved toward the mouth by tiny hairlike muscles called *cilia* (Fig. 1.11). There are approximately 180 million cilia per square centimeter of airway surface, and the cilia beat continuously about 1000 times per minute. As a result, the mucus containing particles and bacteria is swept toward the mouth, where it is usually swallowed, and enters the gastro-intestinal tract.

On the alveolar surface, where gas exchange occurs, no mucus or cilia exist. There, "garbage-collector" cells called alveolar *macrophages* recognize and ingest foreign particles and bacteria. Microorganisms which could cause disease are killed by macrophages, and insoluble particles are moved to the mucus carpet, where they are eventually cleared from the lungs. Thus the respiratory tract has produced an effective compromise between the requirements of protection and those of gas exchange.

The kidneys

The kidney represents another interface between the inside and the outside of the body. Its primary role is to regulate the volume and composition of the body's extracellular fluid by excreting varied urines. It is essential that the levels of such electrolytes as hydrogen, sodium, potassium, calcium, and magnesium ions be maintained strictly within narrow limits. (Electrolytes are charged particles that are involved in essential cellular processes but are not sources of energy.) Similarly, nitrogenous products of amino-acid metabolism must be eliminated before they reach toxic levels, and the volume of body water must be regulated. The body's kidneys perform these functions.

The first step in the kidney's function is filtration of the blood plasma. Although the kidneys represent less than 1 percent of the body weight, approximately one-fifth of the heart's output of blood percolates through them. Blood enters through the *renal* artery and passes through successively smaller branching blood vessels. It finally enters a capillary tuft, the *glomerulus*, through which the plasma filters into a surrounding space, *Bowman's capsule*. The blood entering the glomerulus is under pressure created by the heart. The walls of the capillaries in the glomerulus are permeable to water and small molecules, so that all the components of plasma except proteins and red blood cells pass through the capillary walls. The volume of this initial glomerular filtrate is very large, about 180 quarts every day. This fluid contains not only materials to be excreted but also many valuable substances, including glucose and amino acids. It would be disastrous if this large volume of fluid and these valuable substances were discarded. Fortunately, most of the water and other desirable materials are reabsorbed as the filtrate flows down the kidney tubule from Bowman's capsule.

As the fluid moves along the kidney tubule, some substances are reabsorbed by an active process, some are actively secreted from the capillaries back into the tubule, and others leave or enter the tubular fluid passively driven by concentration gradients. Sodium ions, glucose, and bicarbonate ions are actively reabsorbed by powerful cellular pumps in the tubule walls which can transport these substances against a concentration gradient back into the blood. Penicillin is an example of a

Figure 1.12. The kidney.

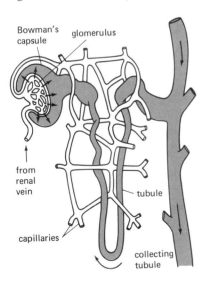

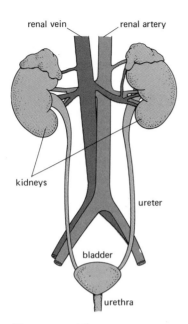

Figure 1.13. The urinary system.

substance secreted into the tubular fluid by a cellular pump. Water, chloride ions, and urea transport are controlled by passive forces.

Urea is the waste product formed by the breakdown of protein. The body is able to oxidize carbon and hydrogen, but it cannot oxidize nitrogen. Nitrogen is an important constituent of amino acids which in turn make up proteins. When we digest protein, therefore, we create unusable nitrogen wastes which are mostly excreted in the form of urea.

The level of kidney activity must be variable since its purpose is to maintain a constant internal environment in the face of variable intake of fluid and foods. The reabsorption of some materials is controlled by hormones. Sodium reabsorption is partially controlled by aldosterone, a hormone from the adrenal cortex (the outer portion of the adrenal gland and site of hormonal synthesis). The output of water from the kidneys can also be varied depending on the requirements of the body. Certain regions of the brain measure the water content of the blood; if the water content is low, antidiuretic hormone (ADH or Vasopressin) is synthesized in the hypothalamus and released from the posterior pituitary gland. The ADH reaches the kidney via the blood stream and then alters the cells in the kidney tubule so that more water is reabsorbed. Normally all the filtered glucose is returned to the blood, but the active transport of glucose can be overloaded if the concentration of glucose in the blood is too high. This sometimes occurs in a disease called diabetes mellitus, and some of the excess sugar appears in the urine.

The kidney occupies a central position in an exquisite regulatory system which monitors and controls the balance of water and many ions. If both kidneys are damaged by disease and not functioning, prompt corrective action must be taken. The diet must be carefully controlled, the blood must be regularly monitored, and elaborate, man-made machines must be used to remove waste products from the blood. Thus the humble kidneys are more than a physiological sewer for the elimination of waste products; they are superbly functioning guardians which monitor and maintain the internal environment.

The cardiovascular system

The cardiovascular or circulatory system is an elaborate distribution system which links each cell in the body with the organs of exchange and with hormonal control systems. It is composed of the heart and blood vessels and the blood contained in these organs. All of the organs of exchange and the elaborate control systems would accomplish nothing if the circulatory systems were unable to transport materials to and from individual cells.

The blood consists of a special liquid, the *plasma*, and a number of specialized cells. The cells are the red blood cells, or *erythrocytes*, which function as oxygen carriers, the white blood cells, or *leucocytes*, which defend against infection, and the *platelets*, which control the coagulation of blood. The constant movement of the blood keeps the cells suspended throughout the plasma. Approximately 45 percent of the total blood volume is composed of cells. The total blood volume is approximately 5 or 6 quarts in an adult. The plasma itself is composed of water and the important electrolytes, such as sodium, chloride, bicarbonate, potassium, and calcium. It also contains glucose and other energy sources as well as a number of plasma proteins. According to their physical properties, the plasma proteins can be divided into two broad groups, the albumins and the globulins. These proteins are synthesized by the liver, with the exception of the gamma globulins (involved in immunity), which are formed in the spleen and lymph nodes.

The cardiovascular system includes a pump, the heart, which produces blood flow, and a set of tubes through which blood flows, the blood vessels. More than 300 years ago, a great advance was made by William Harvey when he demonstrated that the cardiovascular system forms a closed system in which blood pumped away from the heart returns through another set of vessels. In actuality, the system is composed of two separate circuits, both beginning and ending in the heart, which is divided into two functional halves. The right side of the heart pumps oxygen-poor blood to the lungs (the pulmonary circulation), while the left side pumps oxygenated blood throughout the entire body (the systemic circulation). In both the systemic and pulmonary circulation, the vessels carrying blood away from the heart are called *arteries*, and the vessels carrying blood back to the heart are called *veins*. In between are much smaller vessels, including a huge number of very small, thin vessels called *capillaries*. It is at the level of the capillaries where actual exchange between the blood and the fluid surrounding individual cells occurs. The total cross-sectional area of capillaries is more than 600 times the area of the aorta, the largest artery. This greatly increased cross-section reduces the speed at which blood flows to about 0.05 centimeters per second. The low velocity and large area allow nearly complete exchange of nutrients, oxygen, and carbon dioxide across capillary walls by diffusion.

The heart is a muscular organ located in the chest and is responsible for pumping blood through the pulmonary and systemic circuits. This pumping is caused by the contraction of heart (*cardiac*) muscle. The initiation of the heart beat comes from electrical generators within the heart. It has a natural or intrinsic rate, but the rate can be influenced by both nervous and chemical pathways. The brain can slow or speed up the heart beat. Hormones or drugs carried by the blood can have similar effects. At rest, each side of the heart pumps about 5 quarts of blood per minute. This rate, however, can increase by a factor of 5 or 6 during heavy exercise. The increase in the amount of blood pumped by the heart each minute involves both an increase in the number of heart beats per minute (heart rate) and an increase in the volume of blood pumped with each stroke (stroke volume). An intrinsic property of heart muscle is its ability to contract with greater force when it is stretched to a

Figure 1.14. The cardiovascular system.

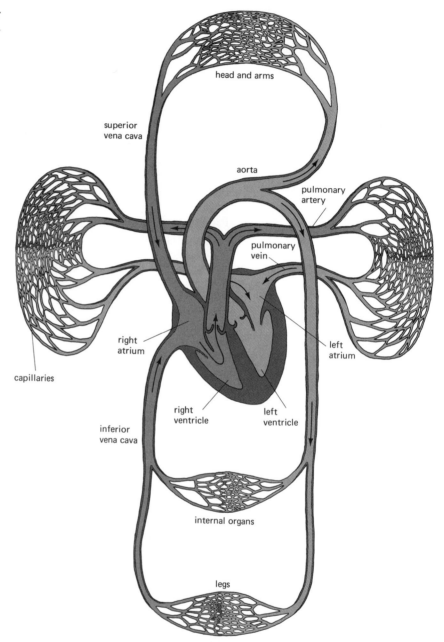

greater degree. Thus, when more blood returns from the veins and fills the heart more completely, the force of contraction will automatically increase, enabling the heart to pump the increased quantity of blood back into the arterial system.

The properties of the arteries are very important. Their elasticity enables them to accept pulses of blood from the beating heart, acting as a high-pressure reservoir which smoothes out the flow of blood into a continuous but uneven pattern. This elastic reservoir empties through the smaller arteries which have a high resistance to flow; thus the blood pressure and flow are maintained between heart beats. Moreover, the resistance of the arterioles (the small arteries) can be adjusted in order to adjust the blood pressure. With aging or with arteriosclerosis, the arterial walls may become stiffened and blood pressure may become excessively high. On a local level, control of the diameters of the small arteries can redirect blood flow to where it is most needed. For example, when a particular muscle is exercising, the arterioles supplying that muscle will expand and thus allow a greater blood flow to the muscle.

The veins have a larger diameter and, therefore, a much lower resistance to flow than corresponding arteries. They serve as a reservoir for the blood. More than 50 percent of the total blood volume is contained at any one time in the veins. The veins, like the arteries, are surrounded by smooth muscle, and their diameters can be adjusted in response to changes in blood volume.

The lymphatics form a network of thin-walled tubes that converge and finally empty into the large veins. Blood is not pumped into the lymphatic capillaries; rather, the lymphatics originate in tissue spaces where they pick up excess fluid and protein which have filtered through the walls of the capillaries. In the digestive system the lymphatics are involved in transport of fat droplets which are absorbed by the cells lining the small intestine. The lymphatic system also protects the circulation against various kinds of bacteria and other toxic agents. Lymph nodes are spaced along the lymphatics and act as filters for the lymph as it travels to its connections with the veinous system.

The circulatory system has many valves which close automatically and prevent blood from flowing in the wrong direction. Veins, lymphatics, and especially the heart itself have valves which ensure that contracting muscles will propel the blood in the proper direction. Except for the aortic valve, arteries do not have valves.

CONTROL SYSTEMS As we have indicated, the major role of the organs and systems is to stabilize the internal environment. The activities of these organs must also be regulated and integrated with each other to ensure this stability. Survival of all living things is dependent upon their ability to adapt to a changing and occasionally threatening environment. This adaptability requires a sensory system which can receive incoming information in an organized way. Incoming information, however, must be properly understood by means of a perceptual system. Finally, on the basis of that understanding, an appropriate response must occur. An effector, or response system, is therefore essential. It is not enough to see danger (sensory reception). It is also necessary to understand that it is danger (perception). Finally, to survive, the organism must avoid the dangerous part of his environment (response).

The human organism is characterized by highly efficient control systems called *homeostatic systems.* Their function is to maintain a steady state. Homeostatic processes usually contain a feedback system. In order to maintain the steady state, the control center of the organism must pick up information about the system, just as a thermostat controlling the temperature in a house must be able to sense the temperature of the house and turn the furnace on and off.

There are control systems operating at different levels of organization. Individual cells have control systems which determine how much and what kind of protein will be synthesized. There are local responses which act in the immediate vicinity of a stimulus and influence the cells nearby. For example, exercising muscle liberates chemicals which act on neighboring blood vessels, cause them to dilate, and thus increase the supply of blood to those muscles.

For the whole organism there are two major control systems: the nervous system and the endocrine or hormonal system. The first is a vast network of independent but interconnected cells called *neurons.* The second consists of a group of glands which secrete potent chemicals, called *hormones,* into the blood.

The nervous system

The nervous system is far superior to the hormonal system in speed and selectivity and depends on a specialized system of nerve cells or neurons whose function is to initiate, receive, and give instructions by means of electrical impulses directed over well-defined pathways. The electrical impulse flowing down a neuron is called an *action potential* and represents a depolarization of the cell membrane. It results in a movement of charged ions across the membrane of the nerve cell, and the nerve cell which is normally negatively charged inside temporarily becomes positively charged. "Firing" refers to the successful initiation of this action potential. Neurons do not lie in direct apposition to each other but are separated by a tiny space called the *synapse.* Chemicals released from one nerve diffuse across the synapse and stimulate or inhibit the next nerve. Most neurons are connected to many other nerve cells; some are connected to as many as 10,000 cells via the synapses. One of the important functions of the synapse is to ensure that action potentials are conducted from nerve to nerve in only one direction. Since all the transmitter substance is stored on one side of the synapse and all the receptor sites are on the other side, information can flow in only one direction. Most drugs influencing the nervous system act at the synaptic level and modify the synthesis, storage, release, or binding of the transmitter substance.

All neurons consist of three main parts (Fig. 1.15). The cell body is the area of the neuron where the nucleus and most of the cytoplasm are located. The *axon* is the nerve fiber which carries the nerve impulse (action potential) along the nerve cell away from the cell body. The *dendrite* is the thickly branched nerve fiber which conducts the nerve

Figure 1.15. The transmission of a nerve impulse (action potential) from the axon of one neuron across the synapse to the dendrites of another neuron.

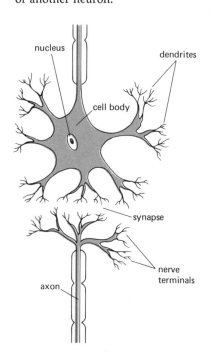

impulse toward the cell body. The axon is thus considered the transmitter of the nerve impulse, and the dendrite the receiver.

There are three main types of neurons. First, there are sensory neurons through which we gain information about the world around us and inside us. Second, motor neurons transmit electrical impulses from the brain and spinal cord to the "working" cells, which may be muscles or glands. These neurons must stimulate effector organs so that the organism can adjust and respond to the environment. Finally, there are interneurons which connect sensory and motor neurons. These cells are engaged in information transmission and processing and in decision-making. The vast majority of cells in the nervous system are interneurons which analyze and integrate the input and pass on appropriate commands to the motor system.

Sensory inputs begin in specialized cells that are designed to respond to different kinds of energy in the internal and external environments. Most are designed to respond only to a single type of stimulus. They have varied structures and locations but all have one thing in common—they convert one form of energy into another form resulting in generation of nerve impulses. Certain cells in the brain are sensitive to the temperature of the blood; other cells are pressure sensitive and monitor the blood pressure. Others measure the concentration of carbon dioxide or the pH. Thermal receptors in the skin measure only heat and cold, and the rods and cones in the eye respond only to light. Some receptors are highly sensitive: the smell receptors in the nose, for instance, can detect just a few molecules of some substances. Information about the stimulus is coded in accordance with the number of nervous impulses generated and the number of nerves stimulated simultaneously. As the strength of a particular stimulus is increased, individual nerves fire faster and more nerves fire.

That part of the nervous system which is enclosed and protected in the bony skull and the vertebral column (backbone) is called the *central nervous system*. The brain and spinal cord are contrasted with nervous tissue which lie outside the skull and vertebral column and are known as the *peripheral nervous system*. The central nervous system of man is his most complex and essential organ. It is the essence of man, the *sine qua non* of human existence. The brain and spinal cord not only preserve the internal environment and control posture and movement but also are responsible for all subjective experience such as dreams, emotions, ideas, memory, and creativity. In short, the central nervous system is responsible for all hallmarks of human activity.

The spinal cord and brain are wrapped in three sheets of connective tissue called *meninges*. (When they become infected or inflamed, the disease is called meningitis.) One of the spaces between the meninges is filled with fluid called cerebrospinal fluid, which protects the spinal cord and brain from bouncing against the bones of the skull or vertebrae during movement.

The spinal cord has two important functions. It transmits impulses to and from the brain and acts as a reflex center. Some sensory nerves are connected to motor nerves that are in the spinal cord. Commands to effector organs like skeletal muscle can, therefore, be issued without the brain's participation.

Most sensory information is relayed to the brain, which perceives and organizes the information. In addition to motor areas which control and coordinate voluntary movements, the brain also has areas concerned with involuntary functions. For example, the medulla (the most posterior part of the brain just above the spinal chord) has a number of important nerve centers that by reflex control respiration, heart rate, the diameter of the blood vessels, and such functions as swallowing and vomiting. Although one can voluntarily initiate swallowing, coughing, or vomiting, the act becomes involuntary once started and is controlled by the medulla.

Some involuntary motor commands are routed through the *autonomic nervous system* which has an important homeostatic role. This system has nerves that terminate in the heart, secretory glands, the gastrointestinal tract, and the smooth muscle of the lungs and blood vessels. The autonomic nervous system is composed of two parts, called the sympathetic and parasympathetic divisions. Generally, these two subdivisions of the autonomic system have opposing effects. Thus, parasympathetic nervous stimulation of the heart decreases heart rate; stimulation of the sympathetic nervous system increases it. Like an accelerator and brake on an automobile, this dual system provides fine control over physiological functions. In general, the sympathetic system is designed to help the body cope with challenges from the external environment such as fear, fight, and flight activities. The parasympathetic system, on the other hand, is more concerned with responses to the internal environment such as the secretion of enzymes during digestion.

The endocrine system

The endocrine system represents the second major control and communications system of the human body. In the nervous system, information was carried by nerve action potentials. With the endocrine system, chemicals called hormones are secreted into the blood by glands. They travel through the circulatory system to distant parts of the body, where they act selectively on specific tissues or "target organs." Hormones have widely varying chemical structures; some are amino-acid derivatives, some are polypeptides (small proteins), and some are steroids (chemicals produced from the compound cholesterol).

As shown in Figure 1.16, the endocrine system is composed of bits of tissue scattered throughout the body. These specialized tissues are called endocrine glands. The smallest is the pineal gland, which is about the size of a period in this book. Add to it the other endocrine glands and the total weight of the system is only 4 to 7 ounces. Yet they control growth and development. They help determine height, weight, and

Figure 1.16. The major endocrine glands.

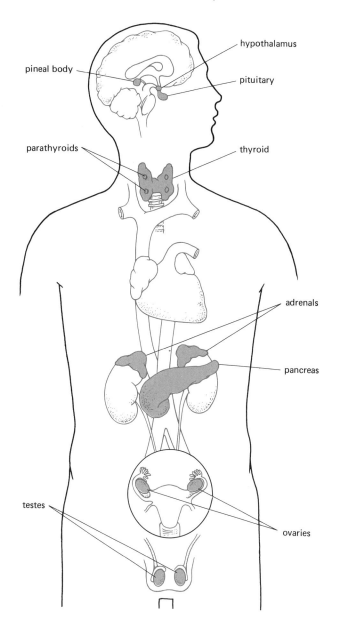

appearance. They regulate metabolism. They control the onset of puberty, regulate the menstrual cycle and ovulation, and control some of the events occuring during pregnancy and birth. They affect mental and emotional development and mobilize vital defenses. When they function in perfect concert, one is well and healthy. When they do not, one may be miserable, suffer from diseases, and look and act in bizarre ways. These effects are all expressed through the action of small amounts of hormones. In an entire lifetime, the average woman produces only 1/5 of an ounce of the female sex hormones estrogen and progesterone. Yet the continuation of her femininity and of the human race depends on the proper release of these hormones.

The concept of a hormone as a chemical messenger traveling through the blood and acting on a distant organ is a relatively new one. Castration (removal of the testes) has been used for thousands of years to alter the behavior and appearance of male animals (including man). When a rooster is castrated, it becomes a capon. In 1848 Arnold Berthold transplanted the testes of a rooster into its abdominal cavity. He noted that the rooster developed normally and not as a capon. He concluded that "... the testes act upon the blood and the blood correspondingly acts upon the entire organism."

In the earlier part of this century, investigators worked hard to identify hormones and isolate them from biological products. It was not always easy. In order to recover 1/100 of an ounce of testosterone, one investigator processed a ton of bull's testicles. In order to get 1/12,000 of a gram of estradiol (a hormone with estrogenlike activity), another investigator began with 80,000 pig ovaries. In the 1940s and 1950s, the structures of hormones were determined so that it became possible to make synthetic hormones, some of which even outdid nature in their biologic activity. Today synthetic and purified natural hormones are used to compensate for the failure of human glands. They are also used as an effective means of birth control.

As can be seen in Table 1.1, hormones have diverse actions. They share certain common characteristics, however. Their main function is to regulate the rates of existing bodily process, not to initiate new functions. They are not the raw materials for reactions, nor are they enzymes, although they exert their effects in minute catalytic concentrations. Hormones may activate enzymes, increase enzyme production, or influence membrane transport. Insulin, for example, facilitates the transport of glucose into cells. It also influences the activity of enzymes, which convert glucose to glycogen, its storage form in liver and skeletal muscle. Another characteristic of hormones is their specificity. Only certain tissues or cells are influenced by these hormones. Such susceptible cells have receptor sites which can bind the hormone.

The concentration of hormones in the blood is controlled by the balance between production, storage, and elimination of each. Elimination results from conversion of a hormone to an inactive form, largely in the blood or in the liver, or excretion of the unchanged hormone, mainly via the kidney. In some cases a hormone may also be activated in the blood.

The rate of secretion of a hormone can be controlled by a number of factors. No hormone is secreted at a precisely uniform rate. Some, for example, cortisol from the adrenal cortex, are secreted in synchrony with the body's 24-hour biological clock and correlate with periods of activity and inactivity. Such a circadian (literally, "about the day") rhythm can

Table 1.1 *Human hormones and their effects*

Hormone	Source Organ	Target Organ	Effect
Insulin	Pancreas, Islets-Beta cells	Many body tissues	Increases glucose uptake and utilization in body; net decrease in blood glucose level
Glucagon	Pancreas, Islets-Alpha cells	Many body tissues	Net increase in blood glucose level
Growth hormone	Anterior pituitary	Many body tissues	Stimulates bone growth, enlargement of soft tissue; affects metabolism
Thyrotropin	Anterior pituitary	Thyroid	Stimulates production of thyroid hormone and growth of thyroid gland
Adrenocorticotrophic hormone (ACTH)	Anterior pituitary	Adrenal cortex	Stimulates growth of adrenal cortex and production of cortical hormones
Follicle-stimulating hormone (FSH)	Anterior pituitary	Ovary	Stimulates development of ovum (egg)
		Testes	Maintains production of sperm
Luteinizing hormone (LH, ICSH)	Anterior pituitary	Ovary	Stimulates ovulation and estrogen secretion
		Testes	Stimulates secretion of androgens
Prolactin	Anterior pituitary	Mammary gland, ovary	Stimulates milk production
Oxytocin	Posterior pituitary	Smooth muscle in breast and uterus	Milk ejection in female breast, contraction of uterus
Vasopressin (Antidiuretic hormone)	Posterior pituitary	Kidney, vasculature	Causes reabsorption of water in kidney, contraction of vascular smooth muscle
Mineralocorticoids (e.g., Aldosterone)	Adrenal cortex	Kidney, sweat glands	Conservation of sodium
Glucocorticoids (e.g., Cortisol)	Adrenal cortex	Many body tissues	Affects metabolism of protein, glucose, fat; suppression of inflammation
Epinephrine (Adrenaline)	Adrenal medulla	Many body tissues	Mobilization of body's resources to meet stress
Norepinephrine (Noradrenaline)	Adrenal medulla Sympathetic nerves	Many body tissues	Similar to epinephrine; neural transmitter in some sympathetic nerves

Table 1.1 Human hormones and their effects (Continued)

Hormone	Source Organ	Target Organ	Effect
Androgens	Adrenal cortex, Testes	Many body tissues	Maintains male sex characteristics
Estrogens	Adrenal cortex, Ovary	Many body tissues	Maintains female sex characteristics
Progesterone	Adrenal cortex, Ovary, Placenta	Many body tissues	Regulation of female sex cycles
Thyroid hormone (T_3, T_4)	Thyroid gland (Follicles)	Many body tissues	Increase basal metabolic rate
Calcitonin	Thyroid gland (Interstitial cells)	Bone, kidney	Lowers blood calcium levels
Parathyroid hormone	Parathyroid gland	Bone, kidney, intestine	Raises blood calcium levels

be disturbed on long international flights or whenever outside clocks get badly out of phase with the body's biological clocks. This disturbance is responsible for some of the fatigue that travelers experience. Reproductive rhythms also play a part in endocrine function, and most of the hormones having to do with sex have complicated cycles of production that correlate with ovulation, menstruation, pregnancy, parturition (birth), and lactation (Table 1.1).

The secretion of some hormones is under nervous control. An example is the release of epinephrine by the adrenal medulla. Other endocrine glands respond to their local environment. Vasopressin (an antidiuretic hormone) is released in response to changes in the total concentration of all molecules and ions in the blood; as the blood becomes more concentrated, the body retains more water to dilute the blood, and conversely the body excretes water when the blood is too dilute. Insulin is released by the pancreas in response to high blood-glucose levels, and aldosterone is released in response to low sodium levels in the blood.

As can be seen from Table 1.1, the pituitary gland secretes eight hormones, some of which control the secretion of other endocrine glands. Until recently, the pituitary gland was regarded as the master gland of the body; it was viewed as an independent structure orchestrating many of the hormonal rhythms. Research has now shown that it was a mistake to regard the pituitary as being independent of the central nervous system. Anatomically, the pituitary is located just beneath part of the brain called the *hypothalamus*. In fact, the hypothalamus controls the production and secretion of anterior pituitary hormones by various "releasing factors," hormones manufactured in the hypothalamus. Tiny amounts of these chemicals are released into the blood flowing through the hypothalamus. This blood goes directly to the anterior pituitary gland to control the release of hormones from it. Thus the activity of the

The potential of the body

It is taken for granted that the human body can meet the demands of everyday life without difficulty. What most people do not appreciate is the tremendous reserve capacities for performance that their bodies have. Those who have trained and/or tested their bodies to their limits help give us some idea of the capabilities that humans have.

How much deprivation can one endure? Bertha Van Der Merwe of South Africa went without sleep for 11 days, 18 hours and 55 minutes. Angus Barbieri of Scotland fasted for 382 days and drank only tea, coffee, soda water, and water. The world's breath-holding record is 13 minutes, 42½

seconds; Robert L. Foster of California set it in a swimming pool.

The world of athletics provides ample opportunity for men and women to test the limits of their bodies. In 24 hours Wally H. Hayward of South Africa ran 159 miles, 562 yards. John V. Sigmund of Missouri swam 292 miles down the Mississippi River in 89 hours, 48 minutes. A half-dozen men have run 100 yards in 9.1 seconds. A weight greater than the heaviest Rolls Royce, 6,270 pounds, was lifted by Paul Anderson, an American. Mrs. Josephine Blatt lifted 3,564 pounds at the Bijou Theatre in Hoboken, New Jersey.

Is man's capacity still increasing? Is the human race getting

smarter, stronger, and better able to meet life's challenges? Could anyone be "smarter" than John Stuart Mill or Johann Wolfgang von Goethe, both believed to have had IQ's of over 200? It is doubtful that anyone will top the confirmed record of a Russian lady of the nineteenth century who had 69 children in 27 confinements. And yet, world records are constantly being surpassed.

Adapted from Norris and Ross McWhirter, *Guinness Book of World Records* (New York: Bantam Books, 1970).

anterior pituitary gland and, therefore, the activity of many other glands throughout the body (such as the testis, adrenal cortex, and thyroid glands) are all controlled by the hypothalamus and the central nervous system. The concentrations of circulating hormones controlled by pituitary activity feed back to the hypothalamus and thus determine directly or indirectly the secretions of the hypothalamus.

The release of posterior pituitary hormones oxytocin and vasopressin is also controlled by the hypothalamus. These substances are synthesized in the hypothalamus. The existence of these physiological pathways between parts of the brain and the pituitary gland make it abundantly clear that mental state and attitudes can influence physiological function. Here is an authentic basis for psychosomatic disease, which can result in physical symptoms.

There is also increasing interest in man's ability to control various visceral functions which were once thought to be under the exclusive control of the autonomic nervous system. The ability of certain Eastern holy men to control their heart rate, blood pressure, and metabolism now becomes plausible. Practically, it suggests a new form of medical therapy, in which persons suffering from high blood pressure can learn to lower it. Philosophically, it helps bury the traditional dualism that mind and body are separate.

DEFENSE MECHANISMS

The human body is skilled at preserving a carefully controlled internal environment that provides an excellent place for human cells to reproduce, grow, and function. Unfortunately, this environment is also attractive to other organisms, and the body must wage a continuing battle to prevent the invasion of harmful organisms.

The skin forms one level of defense, representing a barrier which keeps out many kinds of pathogens. Another defense directed against viruses is a protein called interferon. It is a nonspecific substance whose production is stimulated by viral infections, and it confers some protection against viral diseases. Many other body tissues secrete another kind of protein, lysozyme, which can destroy some kinds of bacteria. In addition, there is the elaborate immune defense system which is discussed in Chapter 9.

Mechanical injury and breaks in the circulation occur continuously in all humans. This damage is dealt with by mechanisms which prevent blood loss and repair the damage. Blood loss is prevented by overlapping mechanisms. Following injury, blood vessels constrict and, as they become smaller, blood flow decreases. Platelets in the circulating blood attach to the injured areas and gradually form a plug in the vessel wall. Finally, the clump of platelets releases a substance which triggers the clotting mechanisms. Clotting takes place when a soluble protein in the plasma, fibrinogen, gradually polymerizes to form an insoluble plug of fibrin which remains until the damage is repaired by wound-healing mechanisms.

Another kind of injury, whether or not it involves breaks in blood vessel walls, is followed by an inflammatory response. This response is characterized by swelling, a sensation of heat, pain, and redness. Blood vessels dilate, blood flow to the injured area increases, and phagocytic cells leave the blood and enter the damaged region. Depending on the degree of injury, repair may be complete or a scar may remain. For many kinds of injury, the inflammatory response is a healthy one since it causes an accumulation in the injured area of phagocytic cells which are available to ingest bacteria.

BIOLOGICAL BACKFIRE

Homeostatic mechanisms are usually characterized by automatic, stereotyped responses to certain stimuli. In the long run, these adaptive changes have survival value. Usually they are beneficial to man and perpetuate him; that is why they have persisted. In some instances, however, these responses can be inappropriate, leading to injury and death. This is called biological backfire.

The gastrointestinal mucosa, red and white cells suspended in the blood, and the skin are examples of areas of rapid cell turnover. These cells must be replaced continuously by cell division throughout life. At the same time cell renewal systems capable of rapid division (especially when damage requires repair) make cancer possible. Cell division can become unregulated and lead to tumor formation.

Clotting is an absolutely essential attribute of blood if excessive blood loss is to be prevented. In some pathologic states, however, clotting is excessive and the result may be blood clots blocking blood vessels. When these clots prevent adequate blood flow to parts of the brain or heart muscle, death can result. In any location, they can lead to tissue death (see Chap. 12).

The bactericidal activity of the alveolar macrophages in the lung represents another example of biological backfire. These macrophages have evolved mainly to combat bacterial challenges and thus are well specialized for ingesting and killing bacteria. If any material enters the lungs, alveolar macrophages ingest (phagocytose) the material, enclose the material in a membrane-bound sac, and inject digestive enzymes into the sac. This response can backfire, however, if the macrophage has ingested a toxic and nondigestible substance. Following the internalization of silica, asbestos, or cigarette smoke, the activation of the enzyme systems may lead to the release of enzymes from the macrophage and to macrophage death.

In each of these cases, modern science and medicine are attempting to control biological backfire by a better understanding of the response. As we come to understand the factors that control cell renewal, clotting, immunity, and the killing of microorganisms by macrophages, we gain insight into how these mechanisms can malfunction and cause damage. Such understanding can lead to a strategy of control. For example, as the mysteries of the clotting mechanism are being unraveled, the clotting activity of the blood and the tendency to form damaging clots can be controlled more precisely by using anticoagulants—drugs which interfere with clotting.

Biological backfire also applies to human behavior. Sexual drive and the desire for children, for example, has enormous survival value in perpetuating the human race. In modern times, however, we have begun to approach the limits of our environment, and overpopulation has become one of the most important areas of human concern. In order to avoid biological backfire, priorities must be redefined in order to ensure the continuation of life on our planet. Similarly, some kinds of aggressive behavior offered an evolutionary advantage to certain tribes of early man. Now that nuclear weapons have replaced bones and fists, these aggressive urges must be redirected; otherwise the biological backfire could be fatal for human survival.

Questions

1. Describe the structures and functions of the major cell organelles.
2. What are the basic processes that facilitate digestion and absorption? What are the control mechanisms affecting these processes?
3. Discuss the characteristics and importance of enzymes.
4. Oxygen can dissolve in plasma. Why is hemoglobin necessary for the transport of oxygen in the blood? What function does oxygen serve in the body?
5. What physiological mechanisms bring about an increase in the rate and depth of breathing?
6. Identify and discuss the three major processes involved in the production of urine. What structures are involved and what major chemicals are moved by each process?

Key Concepts

ATP – adenosine triphosphate; the universal energy currency in the body which can be used for external work, in the synthesis of new molecules, and by cellular transport mechanisms

Enzyme – a kind of protein that controls the rate at which metabolic reactions take place inside the body cell but does not take part in those reactions

Hormone – a potent body chemical secreted by endocrine glands that circulates through the blood to distant sites where it acts selectively on specific tissues or organs

Neuron – the fundamental cellular unit of the nervous system which consists of a nerve fiber (dendrite) to receive a nerve impulse and another nerve fiber (axon) to carry the nerve impulse once past the cell body to the next neuron

Organelle – "small organ"; a specialized structure within the cell that is responsible for carrying out specific biochemical reactions

Selected Readings   Comroe, Julius H., Jr. "The Lung," *Scientific American*, 214(1966), 56–66+.

Lowey, A. G., and P. Siekevitz. *Cell Structure and Function.* New York: Holt, Rinehart, and Winston, 1969.

Tepperman, J. *Metabolic and Endocrine Physiology: An Introductory Text.* Chicago: Year Book Medical Publishers, Inc., 1962.

Vander, A. J., J. H. Sherman, and D. S. Luciano. *Human Physiology: The Mechanisms of Body Functions.* New York: McGraw-Hill Book Co., 1970.

Villee, C. A. *Biology,* 6th ed. Philadelphia: W. B. Saunders, 1972.

Wiggers, C. J. "The Heart," *Scientific American*, 196(1957), 74–78+.

Chapter 2

The Cycle of Life

Reproduction is a universal property of living things. Single-celled organisms as well as complex multicellular animals all have the ability to replicate themselves. Immortality would make reproduction unnecessary. But, death, too, is a universal property of living things. Thus reproduction and death are forever related.

Between conception and death are growth, development, and aging. Each event or process is significant psychologically as well as physiologically. The structures, processes, physiology, and behavior of living things change through time and thus with age. Until adulthood is reached, these gradual changes are called *maturation*. Maturation consists of two processes: growth and development. Growth means an increase in length, width, and weight. In the process of growth, the cells of the body increase both in number (as a result of cell multiplication) and in size (as a result of cell hypertrophy). Development, on the other hand, is the

This chapter was contributed by Isabelle Valadian, M.D., M.P.H., Associate Professor of Maternal and Child Health, and Joseph D. Brain, Sc.D., Associate Professor of Physiology, Harvard School of Public Health.

result of cell differentiation. As they grow, cells differ from each other in order to perform different jobs: a white blood cell performs a function different from that of a red blood cell, and it differs accordingly in structure. Development refers to qualitative changes, whereas growth indicates quantitative changes. Although distinguishable as processes, growth and development are nonetheless inseparable in function: both contribute to the process of maturation. As different systems and structures within the body grow, they also develop and mature. At each age, different structures and systems show spurts of growth and development as the changing needs of the human organism are met and new needs emerge.

Growth, development, and aging start at conception and are continuous and changing processes throughout life; moreover, what happens in one stage carries over and influences the next. However, being continuous does not mean that change occurs at a constant rate—growth, for example, is far from uniform at each stage. On the other hand, change is not haphazard. These changes follow an orderly and predictable sequence, meeting needs as they arise and creating other needs which in turn will be met by further growth and development. Thus we all pass through well-defined stages of maturation and aging whose duration and speed may differ from individual to individual, but whose sequence will be similar for everyone. The different parts of the body do not all grow and change simultaneously. Different structures and systems show growth spurts at different ages, both determined by and determining the changing needs of the body. Growth occurs in two general spurts or cycles: the first cycle is from conception through infancy, the second is during adolescence. Between infancy and adolescence, growth is relatively slower. Once maturation is achieved, growth stops but aging continues. This pattern of two rapid growth cycles separated by a relatively slow growth is characteristic of growth in height and body weight. This same pattern is followed by certain tissues such as bone and muscle and by certain organs of the digestive, excretory, respiratory, and circulatory systems.

Other systems are characterized by a different pattern of growth. Growth in the central nervous system and the organs of vision and hearing, for example, is rapid in the prenatal period and in early infancy and then slows down except for a slight spurt in late adolescence after which growth ceases to occur. The brain grows fastest in the months just preceding birth. At the time of birth, the infant brain weighs 20 percent of the weight of the adult brain, whereas the infant weighs only 5 percent of the weight of an adult. By the time the child is one year old, the brain has reached 75 percent of its mature weight (Fig. 2.1). The reproductive system grows and develops in a pattern diametrically opposed to that of the central nervous system. There is little genital growth during early and middle childhood, but a rapid growth period of the uterus and ovaries in the female and of the testes and prostate in the

Figure 2.1. Drawing illustrating the relative size of the head and trunk in persons of various ages. (From *Growth by Robbins, Brody, Hogan, Jackson, and Greene,* Copyright 1928, Yale University Press)

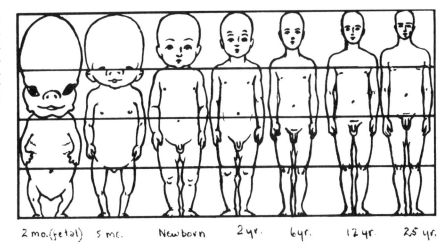

2 mo. (fetal)   5 mo.   Newborn   2 yr.   6 yr.   12 yr.   25 yr.

male begins just before puberty and continues through puberty until early adolescence. During middle adulthood in the female, there is a rapid decline in the ability of the ovaries to produce eggs and female hormones.

The thymus, tonsils, follicles of the spleen, and lymph tissues of the intestines grow rapidly in childhood until by late childhood they are proportionately nearly double the adult size. Their growth, referred to as lymphoid growth, slows down and ceases by puberty. Enlarged tonsils and adenoids are characteristic in middle and late childhood, but these actually shrink in size before adolescence. Thus each organ system or process has its own cycle of life with its individual pattern of growth and degeneration, development and deterioration.

THE REPRODUCTIVE SYSTEM

Because man ages and because he exists in an environment which is sometimes threatening and destructive, reproduction is essential for the survival of man as a species. In this chapter we will discuss the physiology of the reproductive system; many important and related aspects of human sexuality will be dealt with in Chapter 4.

The *gonads,* the testes in the male and the ovaries in the female, are the most important reproductive organs in the body. In each sex, they have a dual responsibility. The first is to produce sex cells—the sperm and the egg. The second is to secrete hormones which control the secondary sex characteristics. In the female, estrogens are secreted which have a feminizing influence. In the male, androgens (mainly testosterone) are secreted which have a masculinizing influence.

Male reproductive physiology

Figure 2.2 shows a diagram of the male reproductive tract. The testis shown is composed of many hundreds of feet of tightly coiled tubes, called the *seminiferous* ("seed-bearing") *tubules,* where the spermatozoa

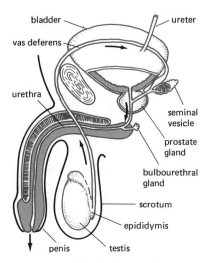

Figure 2.2. The male reproductive tract.

or sperm are produced. These tubes are lined with special cells which continually divide and gradually mature into sperm. Once fully developed, the sperm are stored in the epididymis and vas deferens until erection and ejaculation occur.

Erection is the enlargement and stiffening of the penis which occurs during sexual excitement; it facilitates penetration of the penis into the female vagina. The penis is composed of three cords of vascular tissue which are potential spaces that can be filled with blood. When stimulated, the arterioles supplying the penis increase in size, and the penis becomes filled with blood and hence more rigid. The genital ducts automatically contract, mixing the sperm with secretions from the seminal vesicles and the prostate gland. This mixture is called *semen*. If stimulation is sufficient, ejaculation (the rapid expelling of seminal fluid) occurs. The average volume of the semen is about 3 milliliters and contains hundreds of millions of living sperm. The release of semen from the penis is accompanied by intense pleasurable sensations, and the entire event is called an *orgasm*.

Both the production of sperm and the continuation of the secondary sex characteristics depend on *testosterone* and the *gonadotropic hormones* (hormones that stimulate or act on the gonads). Testosterone is produced by special endocrine cells in the testes, called the interstitial cells, which lie between the seminiferous tubules. Not only is testosterone essential for production of sperm, but it is also responsible for all physical characteristics of masculinity. Facial, armpit, and pubic hair, the deepening of the voice, the coarsening of skin texture, and the characteristic male distribution of muscle and fat tissue are all dependent on testosterone secretion by the testes. Castration (surgical removal of the testes) prevents the development of these characteristics.

The gonadotropic hormones are hormones that are released from the anterior pituitary gland which is controlled by the hypothalamus. The anterior pituitary hormones travel in the blood and act on the testes. FSH, or follicle-stimulating hormone, is also essential for the production of sperm. LH, or luteinizing hormone, acts on the interstitial cells to promote the production of testosterone.

Female reproductive physiology

The ovaries, like the testes, are responsible for producing sex hormones and sex cells. Also as in the male, the hypothalamus in the female regulates the production of gonadotropic hormones from the anterior pituitary gland. The gonadotropins stimulate the ovary to secrete *estrogen* and *progesterone*. These two hormones in turn cause anatomical changes in the lining of the uterus (called the *endometrium*), the mouth of the uterus (called the *cervix*), the fallopian tubes, vagina, and breast. There are, of course, marked differences between the functioning of the testes and that of the ovaries. Although sperm are produced continuously and more than 300,000,000 active spermatozoa are contained in each cubic

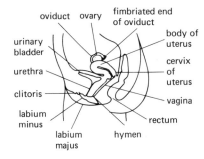

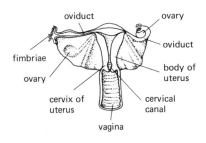

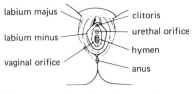

Figure 2.3. The female reproductive tract.

centimeter of semen produced by a mature healthy man, only one egg per month is released from the ovaries. One sperm is required to fertilize an egg, but many hundreds of millions of sperm are required to make that event possible. The mature human ovum is only 1/175 of an inch in diameter and weighs about 1/20 of a millionth of an ounce. By comparison with the sperm, however, the ovum is gigantic. The sperm is only about 1/500 of an inch long, and its mass is only 1/90,000 of the egg. Figure 2.3 diagrams the important features of the female reproductive tract. In contrast to those of the male, most of the important female sexual organs are internal rather than external. Only the *vulva*, the area surrounding the opening of the vagina, is easily visible. The external female genitalia include two protective layers of flesh called the *labia majora*. These moistened outer lips cover the smaller and more delicate inner lips called the *labia minora*, the urethral orifice which leads to the bladder, and the *clitoris*. The clitoris, like the male penis, is composed of erectile tissue which stiffens and enlarges during sexual excitement. It ranges in size from 1/4 to 1 inch in length and plays an important role during the female orgasm. The *hymen* is a thin membrane located at the opening of the vagina. Stretched and broken by sexual intercourse, it may be incomplete, perforated, or absent even in virgins. The *vagina*, or birth canal, extends from the external genetalia to the cervix. It is a strong, elastic structure which not only surrounds the penis during sexual intercourse but can expand to serve as the pathway through which a baby enters the world.

The ovaries are paired, bean-shaped structures 2.5 to 3 centimeters long and 1.5 to 2 centimeters in diameter. At birth the ovaries contain about 2,000,000 follicles, each of which has the potential of developing into an ovum or egg. During childhood, however, many of these disappear, and approximately 300,000 remain at puberty. During a woman's reproductive years, only about 300 to 400 ova mature and are released. When ovulation occurs, the egg and some accompanying supporting cells are released directly into the abdominal cavity. Fortunately the *fallopian tubes*, or oviducts, have a funnel-shaped ending which quickly collects the released egg. Each tube is about 10 to 12 centimeters in length and about 0.5 to 1 centimeter in diameter. These tubes guide the egg to the *uterus*, or womb, a pear-shaped structure which connects with both the tubes and the cervix. In nonpregnant women, the longest dimension of the uterus is only 6.5 to 8 centimeters; it grows considerably during pregnancy. The cervix connects the uterine cavity with the vagina.

The endometrial lining of the uterus can be thought as a bed of nutritious earth into which the fertilized egg can be planted. If no fertilized egg appears, the endometrial lining is discarded and the body starts all over again by preparing a new ovum for release and by slowly relining the uterus. The growth, secretion, and finally degeneration and release of the endometrial lining of the uterus is a sequence known as

The homunculus

With the development of the microscope in the 1600s, men of learning were able to examine many things microscopically. Male semen was one substance looked at under the crude microscope of the day. Sperm cells were visible, but it is surprising how accurately early microscopists could draw and describe the tiny cells with their crude optical equipment.

As a result of the discovery of sperm cells, two schools of thought developed on the subject of human reproduction. "Ovists" believed that humans developed from the female egg, independently of male sperm. "Animalculists" held to the theory that the sperm were the seeds from which babies grew in the uterus. It was believed that within each sperm cell was a tiny, preformed, and perfectly shaped man called a "homunculus." The growth of the fetus and later the child was considered to be just an enlargement of these miniature men. Microscopists claimed to be able to see the little homunculi in sperm cells.

In the nineteenth century, optical microscopes improved, and scientists were able to describe sperm cells accurately. By the end of the century, the true functions of the egg and sperm were understood by biologists.

the *menstrual cycle* (Fig. 2.4). Interestingly, only primates menstruate, although many other species exhibit cyclic ovarian activity.

A complex of hormonal interrelationships among the hypothalamus, the anterior pituitary, and the ovaries controls the events of ovulation and menstruation. The first day of bleeding is usually referred to as "day one" of the menstrual cycle. Following the four or five days of menstruation, the ovarian *follicles* gradually mature under the influence of follicle-stimulating hormone from the anterior pituitary gland. An ovarian follicle is a small, spherical sac containing the maturing egg,

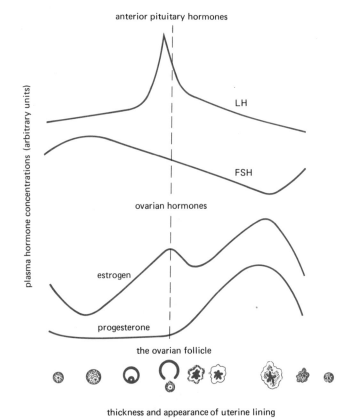

Figure 2.4. Summary of the physiological, hormonal, and anatomical changes during the menstrual cycle. (From A. J. Vander *et al., Human Physiology: The Mechanisms of Body Function,* New York: McGraw-Hill Book Co., 1970, p. 457)

some fluid, and supporting cells. The follicle gradually appears on the surface of the ovary as a tiny blister; *ovulation* occurs when a blister or follicle ruptures and the egg is released. Under the influence of the luteinizing hormone (which helps trigger ovulation), the ruptured follicle is converted into a structure called the *corpus luteum* which is the source of progesterone, a hormone necessary for the maintenance of pregnancy. The corpus luteum will stop functioning in about two weeks after ovulation unless it is supported by a special gonadotropin which is secreted from the developing embryo. If conception has occurred, the corpus luteum continues to develop and release progesterone. This encourages the lining of the uterus to prepare itself for the implantation of the developing embryo. If conception does not occur, the corpus luteum gradually disappears. The lack of progesterone secretion from the corpus luteum triggers menstruation.

Thus alterations in hormone secretions by the ovary help control the structural changes in the endometrium. Estrogens are the major hormones secreted prior to ovulation, while progesterone is the major product after ovulation. The endometrium is initially stimulated to grow by the estrogen hormones and then prepared by progesterone to receive the embryo. If implantation fails to occur, progesterone secretion stops, reducing the blood supply to the endometrium and resulting in its loss. Each month the entire sequence is repeated.

THE BEGINNING OF LIFE

For thousands of years, the beginning of life was a mystery and the existence and contents of the fertilized egg, or *zygote*, unknown. Hundreds of years ago when it became possible to see cells with primitive microscopes, many embryologists believed that the human form was contained in miniature in the fertilized egg. Some early scientists believed that the sperm contained a miniature man, or *homunculus*. During pregnancy this preformed individual expanded. We now know, however, that the human exists in the zygote only symbolically, in the form of coded information necessary to make and maintain the human being.

Fertilization

Fertilization of the egg usually occurs in the fallopian tubes and occasionally in the uterus. Sperm are deposited in the vagina at the time of ejaculation. The mechanisms by which sperm are transported from the vagina to the fallopian tube are not completely understood. The sperm reach the beginning of the tubes in a matter of minutes, a speed far too fast to be accounted for on the basis of sperm swimming rates. It is likely that both the uterus and oviducts have muscular contractions which assist in the transport of sperm.

Both the sperm and the eggs have only twenty-three chromosomes each, one half of the normal number (see Chap. 7). When the sperm and egg combine at conception, the full compliment of twenty-three pairs of chromosomes or a total of forty-six is created. Sperm cells have an average life of about forty-eight hours following ejaculation.

The egg is released approximately fourteen days plus or minus two before the onset of the next menstrual period. Fertilization usually occurs within twelve hours of the release of the egg. Therefore there is a maximum range of approximately sixty hours each month when conception is possible. Unfortunately the exact period of those sixty hours is often difficult to determine.

Embryonic and fetal development

Once the sperm penetrates the egg and their genetic information fuses, the nine month process of embryonic and fetal development begins. Figure 2.5 shows some of the events that occur following sperm penetration of the newly released egg. Without increasing in mass, the fertilized egg divides repeatedly while simultaneously continuing its movement down the oviduct toward the uterus. By the time it reaches the uterus, it consists of many cells. This ball of cells is called a *morula*. Gradually, the morula develops an inner cavity with a cluster of cells on one side. This structure, now called a *blastula*, attaches to the wall of the uterus, an event called *implantation*. Soon the placenta will develop to better supply the developing embryo's nutritional needs.

The *placenta* is a superbly designed device optimized for the exchange of materials between the mother and the fetus through their circulatory systems. Because there are many square yards of surface available for exchange, it is the vital link between the unborn baby and the mother. By the time of the infant's birth, the placenta weighs almost

Figure 2.5. Egg development and early embryonic growth. (From Robert Rugh and Landrum B. Shettles, *From Conception to Birth—The Drama of Life's Beginnings,* New York: Harper and Row, 1971, p. 26)

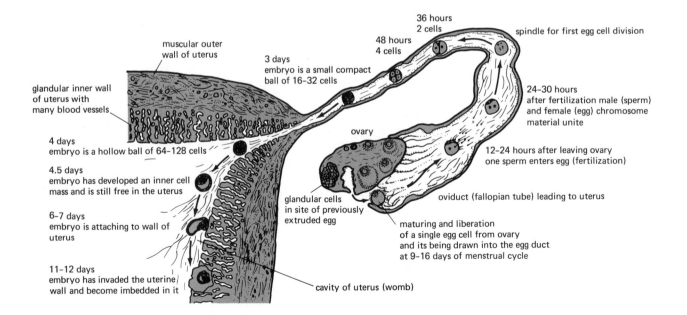

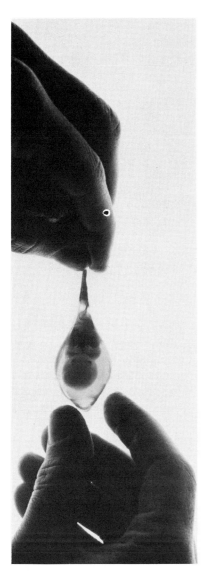

Figure 2.6. Unruptured ectopic pregnancy in left fallopian tube. Fetus aged 6 to 7 weeks. (Courtesy of Robert L. Wolfe, Biomedical Graphic Communications, University of Minnesota Hospital)

1½ pounds. It is connected to the fetus by the *umbilical cord* which is composed of one fetal vein and two fetal arteries. Substances are transferred from one circulation to the other by passive diffusion as well as active transport. The fetus is essentially a parasite of the mother, and its environment depends on her habits and nutrition. The fetus depends on the mother through the placenta for nutrition, respiration, and excretion.

Although initially the embryo is simply a cluster of undifferentiated cells, all the major organs are laid down during the first three months of pregnancy. During embryonic development, the genes contained in each cell will, in response to clues in the chemical and physical environment, either trigger or suppress the production of enzymes. By altering the speed of specific chemical reactions, the enzymes will cause individual cells to become specialized. The basic structure of the arms, legs, eyes, ears, and other vital organs is laid down between the second and tenth weeks of pregnancy. By the end of the first three months, although the fetus is very small (about three inches long weighing approximately half an ounce), it already has a human appearance and the basic architecture of the body has been laid down.

The nervous and cardiovascular systems are among the first to become functional. By the third week after conception when the fetus is only 1/16 of an inch long, the heart has already begun to beat. By the twentieth week, the beat is of sufficient intensity to be easily detected with a stethoscope from the outside. Modern techniques permit detection as early as the tenth week. The circulation of the fetus is dramatically different from that of the newborn. Approximately 50 percent of the cardiac output is circulated through the placenta while the lungs receive only 10 percent. After birth, there is no placental circulation and 100 percent of the cardiac output from the right heart passes through the lungs on its way to the left heart and the rest of the body.

The respiratory system is one of the most critical systems for the survival of the newborn. Breathing air is impossible inside the uterus, but the unborn baby does move fluid in and out of its lungs. If babies are born prematurely, the alveoli may tend to collapse and respiratory distress syndrome may result. Swallowing is another essential function being practiced by the fourth month. Just prior to delivery the fetus may swallow approximately 500 milliliters of fluid per day.

Forty weeks after conception, about 800 milliliters of amniotic fluid surrounds, protects, and cushions the unborn baby. Through a variety of new techniques and equipment, this fluid environment is now accessible for study, and it is possible from it to identify at an early stage the sex and genetic makeup of the fetus. A physician can sample some of the fluid in which the fetus is bathed by inserting a needle through the mother's abdomen—a process called *amniocentesis*. By analyzing the fluid, it is possible to detect the sex of the fetus, Rh disease, and the presence of certain birth defects (see Chap. 7).

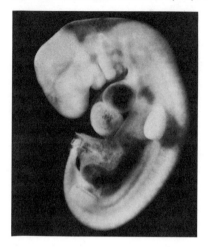

Figure 2.7a. 29-day human embryo, magnified 9 times.

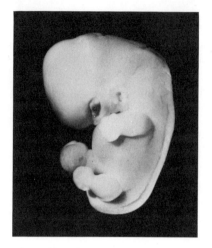

Figure 2.7b. 37-day embryo, magnified 4 times.

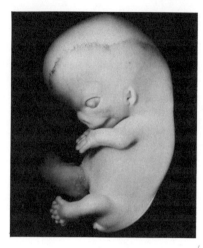

Figure 2.7c. 42-day embryo, magnified 3.5 times.

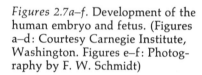

Figures 2.7a–f. Development of the human embryo and fetus. (Figures a–d: Courtesy Carnegie Institute, Washington. Figures e–f: Photography by F. W. Schmidt)

Embryonic and fetal development is characterized by growth. The most rapid and crucial period of growth in a person's life takes place within the cloistered setting of the uterus. Rapid cell multiplication and differentiation causes the ovum, microscopic at the time of fertilization, to develop in the first three months of pregnancy into a fetus of about 10 centimeters in length and 15 grams in weight. The fetus at this stage has acquired 10,000 times the quantity of new tissue it had at the time of conception and has also acquired most of the gross anatomical features of the human body.

The fetus grows in length most rapidly in the second trimester and in weight most rapidly in the third trimester. In these two periods, therefore, factors such as malnutrition may result in stunted growth or low birth weight. Premature infants are usually shorter and always lighter than full term babies.

The second trimester also shows rapid development of the organs which were grossly formed in the first trimester. By the end of the second trimester, the fetus has a chance of survival outside the uterus, although without the additional three months of maturation in the uterus, this chance is small even with great care and attention.

The third trimester is one of tremendous weight gain through an increase in fat and muscular tissues which pad and protect the inner organs after birth and will cushion the fetus's body during the arduous birth process. Premature infants lack much of this protective padding.

What is most remarkable about this embryonic and fetal development is the absolute necessity for all systems to be operative during growth. Even as organs are being formed and cells are differentiating,

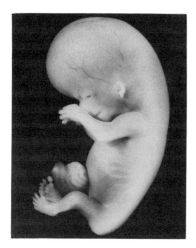

Figure 2.7d. 56-day embryo, magnified 2 times.

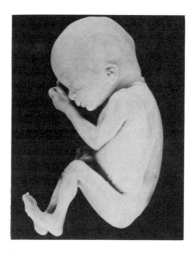

Figure 2.7e. 4-month fetus, reduced to about one-half its actual size. Note disproportionate head size.

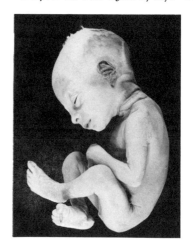

Figure 2.7f. 6-month fetus between one-half and one-third its actual size. Body is now more proportionate to head.

the major systems of the body must continue to function. It is like asking a mechanic gradually to change a Volkswagen into a Mack truck. A difficult task in itself, but added to it is the requirement that the vehicle must continue to run reliably down the highway at sixty miles per hour as it changes. At no time must any of the systems stop functioning. Thus as growth occurs, physiological systems must be synchronized and operating effectively.

Pregnancy

We have emphasized the vast changes which occur in the developing baby, but equally dramatic alterations are present in the mother. During pregnancy, almost all organs and systems are altered. Early pregnancy has its characteristic signs. Menstruation stops, urinary frequency increases, and there is increased excretion of a hormone called chorionic gonadotropin in the urine. It is the measurement of this hormone which is used as a common laboratory test to verify pregnancy. Also characteristic is the persistence of the corpus luteum and its continued secretion of progesterone. The uterus enlarges; its inner capacity gradually increases one thousandfold. The amount of smooth muscle in the uterus also increases. The depth and rate of ventilation increases. The cardiac output increases as does the blood volume. The body begins to prepare for *lactation* (milk production); the breasts enlarge and become more vascular, and the sensitivity of the nipples is increased. Nausea is a common symptom during the first three months although it may persist longer; sensitivity to odors is heightened. Recently scientists have become curious about why the fetus is immunologically tolerated within

Table 2.1 Growth of human embryo and fetus*

Post conception age	Length		Weight	
	inches	millimeters	ounces	grams
19 days	1/50	0.7		
20 days	1/25	1.5		
21 days	1/16	2.0–2.3		
22 days	1/8	2.5–3.0		
3–4 weeks	1/8 +	2.8–3.8		
4 weeks	3/16	4–5	0.0007	0.02
5 weeks	5/16	7–8		
6 weeks	1/2	12–13		
7 weeks	11/16	16–20		
8 weeks	1 1/8	22–30	0.035	1.0
9 weeks	1 1/2	35–45		
10 weeks	2 1/8	48–55		
11 weeks	2 1/2	64–66		
12 weeks	3	75–80	0.5–0.70	14–20
13 weeks	3 5/8	91–93		
14 weeks	4 3/16	105–107		
15 weeks	4 3/4	119–121		
16 weeks	5 1/4	132–134		
17 weeks	5 3/4	147±	3.7–4.2	
18 weeks	6 1/4	160±		
19 weeks	6 3/4	173±		
20 weeks	7 1/4	185±		
21 weeks	7 3/4	197±	7.0–10.9	200–310
22 weeks	8 3/16	208±		
23 weeks	8 1/4	219±		
24 weeks	9 1/4	236±	1 lb. 6. oz.	635–650
28 weeks	10 5/8	270±		
32 weeks	11 3/4	310±	2 lbs. 10 oz.	1,080–1,225
36 weeks	13 5/8	346±	3 lbs. 10 oz.–4 lbs.	1,670–1,700
38 weeks	14 1/2	362±	4 lbs. 12 oz.–5 lbs.	2,240–2,400

* After Robert Rugh and Landrum B. Shettles, *From Conception to Birth—The Drama of Life's Beginnings* (New York: Harper & Row, 1971), Appendix A.

the mother's body; for unknown reasons the immune mechanisms are not activated (see Chap. 9), and the presence of foreign fetal protein within the mother's body is accepted.

Adequate prenatal care will increase the probability of having a healthy, normal baby. The mother's health and the health of her developing baby should be monitored by a qualified obstetrician. It has already been pointed out that the first months of development are most critical. They are characterized by rapid growth and the organization of the major organ systems and skeletal structures. The fetus is therefore very vulnerable to outside influences during the first three months of pregnancy. Any organ may be affected by lack of oxygen, infection, radiation, trauma, nutritional deficiencies, drugs, and chemicals. Thus death of the fetus or malformation is most likely to occur in the first trimester. Both animal experiments and unfortunate natural occurrences in humans (such as the thalidomide disaster, see Chap. 17) affirm this statement. All prospective mothers should understand these hazards to the fetus in the first months of pregnancy when the vital organs are being formed. This understanding is important because women are not always aware that they are pregnant until after the first few weeks, and they may inadvertently expose their babies to risks of medications and other hazards.

New evidence suggests that severe malnutrition of the mother during early pregnancy can actually reduce fetal brain weight by hindering cell growth both in size and number. Differentiating between malnutrition and other conditions is seldom easily or consistently possible. Malnutrition as a sole cause of brain damage is therefore difficult to establish. However, enough evidence exists to indicate the importance of prenatal and postnatal services and the necessity of good nutrition at these times.

Even with the best of maternal habits, approximately 10 percent of all pregnancies terminate in spontaneous abortions called *miscarriages*. A large percentage of these spontaneous or natural abortions occurs for good reasons. Almost one-fourth of aborted fetuses studied have severe chromosomal abnormalities. In many cases, these abnormalities were incompatible wtih continued survival of the fetus.

Birth

The baby will be born approximately 266 days after conception, or 280 days after the beginning of the last menstrual period. Approximately 35 percent of all babies will arrive within fifteen days ahead or behind the scheduled date. Prematurity, a hazardous condition with higher mortality rates, is correlated with smoking, diabetes, poor nutrition, excessive physical or emotional stress, and other environmental factors. Two weeks to ten days before the birth of the infant, the fetus and uterus descend into the pelvic basin. This "lightening" or "dropping" can usually be sensed by the mother since it reduces pressure on the diaphragm and lungs and makes breathing easier. Also during this period there are occasional uterine contractions, for the muscles involved in birth are warming up.

Birth, or *parturition*, consists of a complex series of events which result in the movement of the fetus from the uterus through the pelvis and vagina to the outside world. There are three main stages of labor. The first stage begins with the onset of regular contractions of the uterine muscles and lasts until the cervix is completely dilated (usually

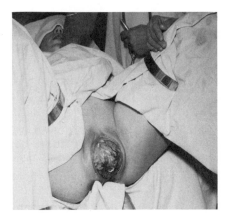

Figures 2.8a–f. Birth and delivery. (Photography by Robert A. Kolvoord) (*a*) The second stage of the birth of the child. The baby has passed through the fully dilated birth canal (uterine cervix) and is now in the vagina. The top part of the infant's head is just beginning to appear.

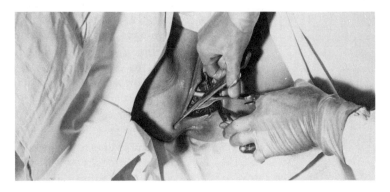

Figure 2.8b. Frequently the vulva is not sufficiently large to permit the passage of the baby without some tearing of the tissues of the mother. In order to prevent such a tear that might be difficult to repair, the attending obstetrician may make a medical or lateral incision of the vulva to enlarge the opening. This is called an episiotomy, and the clean incision heals in a short time, leaving no unpleasant aftereffects.

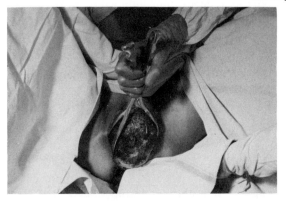

Figure 2.8c. In many cases the natural forces of the mother's bearing down and the contractions of her uterus are not sufficient to expel the head of the child in an expeditious manner, and forceps may be used to assist in the process. Only a gentle wrist action is necessary in the use of the forceps, and no force that might injure the baby is employed.

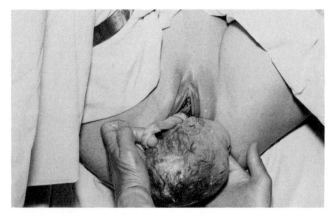

Figure 2.8d. The stage of birth just following delivery of the head of the baby. A portion of the umbilical cord may be seen in the obstetrician's finger. The baby has now turned around (rotated). Several rotations are performed in such a manner to facilitate the passage of the various parts of the body through the birth canal and out from the vulva with a minimum of strain on the child and mother.

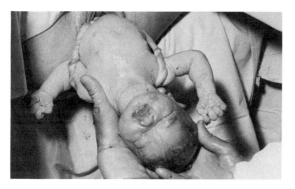

Figure 2.8e. A short period of time elapses after the birth of the head of the baby before the contractions commence again. When this happens, the trunk, legs, and arms of the baby are delivered. Once the baby is completely out of the mother's body, the second stage of the birth process is ended.

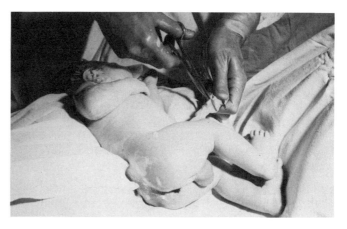

Figure 2.8f. Following the delivery of the baby, attention is turned to the infant. If respiration has not already started, this may be stimulated by stroking the baby's back or gently slapping the buttocks. The baby must then be carefully cleaned off after the physician has completed tying and cutting the umbilical cord, which is no longer necessary to sustain the infant's life.

about 10 centimeters). During the second stage of labor, the fetus descends through the cervix, passes through the birth canal or vagina, and is delivered. During the third stage, the placenta separates and is also delivered. These are not three distinct stages but a continuous progression of events. The first stage of labor averages 13.5 hours in women having their first baby and 7.5 hours in women who have already given birth to children. The second and third stages of labor are much shorter, usually less than an hour. During and shortly after birth, many important changes take place. The blood vessels in the umbilical cord close tightly to prevent bleeding. Much of the fluid contained in the lungs is expelled during the passage of the baby through the birth canal, and the rest of the fluid is absorbed into the baby's circulation. The blood stops bypassing the lungs and instead flows through the pulmonary circuit.

Immediately after birth, the umbilical cord, which attached the fetus to the placenta while in the uterus, is cut. The infant is no longer supported by the mother's systems and must quickly begin to breathe in order to obtain essential oxygen. Crying occurs spontaneously as an important means of expanding and activating the lungs. Establishment of respiration usually occurs in less than a few seconds after birth; delay of more than a few minutes may lead to death or to brain damage.

The first breath

According to Stanley James of Babies Hospital in New York City, ... pressure changes [in the chest cavity] may play a major part in causing the infant to take his first breath. While the baby is still in the womb, his lungs are crumpled up and deflated, although they contain some fluid. When the baby passes through the birth canal, his chest cavity is subjected to considerable pressure. This forces the fluid out through the nostrils and mouth. Immediately after birth, when the constriction has been removed, the chest expands the way a sponge does after being squeezed, and air rushes into the lungs to fill the vacuum. The baby's first sound may not be the traditional cry, but a cough, designed to expel the last remaining fluid in the lungs.

If Dr. James is correct, the baby's first intake of air is a passive process. Thereafter, he must actively breathe for himself. And the effort this involves is sometimes Herculean. The first independent breath may take as much as 10 times the inhalation force required of an adult. The first few breaths expand the baby's lungs up to three quarters of their total capacity, but the healthy newborn does not seem to find this too much of a strain. His lungs expand this much every time he cries in anger.

From J. M. Tanner and G. R. Taylor, *Growth* (New York: Time Inc., 1965), pp. 60–61.

Other adaptive anatomical and physiological changes happen more gradually. Circulation is satisfactorily established over a two to four week period, depending upon individual differences. At times, breathing is almost imperceptibly shallow in the newborn; at other times it may be very rapid. Variations in heart rate and respiration patterns within the first few weeks of life are normal and should not cause alarm. The infant's mechanisms for regulating body temperature may also be partially ineffective at birth. Care must be taken to maintain his environmental temperature so that it is adjusted to his needs until his own built-in mechanisms begin to function well.

Other major adaptations for ingesting, absorbing, and utilizing necessary foods and for eliminating residues through urination and bowel movements occur promptly and spontaneously in the healthy newborn, although establishing regularity in these functions takes longer.

GROWTH AND DEVELOPMENT

The infant

By the time of birth, growth rate is already decelerating. Although the infant is still growing at a rapid pace, the increments per unit of time both in length and weight diminish. The infant will double his birth weight in five months, triple it in one year, and quadruple it in three years. The growth rate of length follows a similar pattern, reducing its speed during the second year of life by about one half. Growth of the head is particularly rapid, reflecting the rapid growth of the brain during early infancy.

Neuromuscular function develops with the growth of the central nervous system. The movements of the newborn are reflex responses, uncoordinated and involving the whole body. Coordination comes with development of the neuromuscular structures, and thus the child is able to exercise his ability to reach with his hand, grasp objects, raise his head, roll over, sit, creep, stand, and walk. Testing the child's development against developmental norms is useful for assessing both his motor development and his mental functioning, since one cannot be distinguished from the other at this time.

The abilities to move, to control the body, and to relate to and manipulate objects are all determined by the stage of development of the neuromuscular system. Feeding and toilet-training as well as other expectations of infant behavior should be based on his developmental readiness rather than his chronological age. Careful health and developmental examinations made periodically will allow the child's own unique maturation pattern to be observed and charted, permitting observation of his progress. Pediatricians recommend these regular checkups to see whether a child is adhering to his own schedule for growth and development. Advice to parents can be based upon observation at regular intervals of the child's growth and development over a period of time. Such observation ensures prompt attention to any abnormality and helps parents provide appropriate care at each age for each individual child.

The preschool child

The deceleration in weight and length growth rates continues, although the decline in the rate of weight gain is more rapid. Consequently, the child of this age (two to six years old) not only looks thinner but is in fact thinner, with far less fat under the skin than the infant has. This normal occurrence sometimes causes anxiety on the part of parents, especially since children of this age tend to show less interest in food compared with the avidity for eating shown in infancy. Yet in a healthy child, a decrease in appetite indicates that his developmental priorities are shifting to areas related to his increased curiosity about the world around him and to his abilities to explore and function in it. He is increasingly concerned with learning how to coordinate the many abilities and functions acquired during his first two years of life, including walking and running, throwing and catching a ball, climbing stairs, and jumping.

Mastery of these functions is achieved through repetition. A child's environment, therefore, should provide ample opportunities for such activities as walking, running and jumping; it should include toys which help coordinate eye and hand movements with reasoning faculties; and it should expose him to interaction with other children. Through play, he expends the tremendous amounts of energy which in earlier years were utilized in weight and height gains. As the child grows older, his development of motor skills reflects the kind of opportunities and environment to which he has been exposed.

At this age, care must be taken to insure that the child receives proper nourishment, since his own attention is focused elsewhere. This means not forcing an unwilling child to consume large amounts of food, but rather presenting small amounts of food which are high in protein, essential vitamins and minerals, and tempting to a small or finicky appetite.

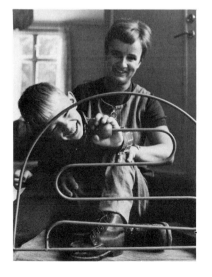

Figure 2.9. The mind develops as the hand learns. (Courtesy of the World Health Organization)

During this period of exploration and learning, care must also be taken to protect the child from excessive fatigue which his constant physical activity can cause. Periods of rest should be included routinely in his day. While inactivity cannot be imposed on a child, changes in activity to simpler, quieter forms of play such as being read to or singing can be restful. Also important for the conservation and restoration of energy needed for growth and repair is sleep. On the average, total sleeping time is fourteen to sixteen hours in infancy and decreases to twelve to fourteen hours in early childhood. Some children concentrate their sleeping in the night and resist daytime naps; others will spread out their sleeping over several naps; still others will resist sleep even when most tired.

Accidents are common in early childhood. They are caused by the child's insatiable curiosity, overactivity and fatigue, and his clumsiness due to instability of newly acquired motor skills. Accidents stand first among the causes of death of preschool age children, and certain kinds of accidents are especially common at certain ages when the child is trying to master a new skill. With increasing ability to use his hands, for example, a child begins trying to open doors in cars and houses, to turn on stoves, to take things apart, and to stick objects into holes, such as hairpins into electric outlets. By age three, when he can climb and run, stairs and wide streets are attractive but dangerous playgrounds.

The school age child

With no sharp demarcation from the preceding years, the slowly decelerating growth rate merges into a pattern of stable, slow growth. There is an increasing reversal of the relationship between the growth rate in height and that in weight: the rate of gain in height still declines or remains constant, while the rate of gain in weight increases slowly, so that children tend to look stockier. They appear and are in fact heavier in proportion to height. They do not seem much taller.

Growth at this age is primarily in the dimension of breadth. The bones become thicker, the trunk broadens and deepens while changing only moderately in length; shoulders and hips develop similarly in boys and girls. The muscle masses develop more fully as greater coordination is achieved. From the simple activities of the preschool age such as running and jumping, the motor activities of the school age child are becoming more efficient, strenuous, prolonged, and complex, demanding precise and large scale muscular coordination. The school age child learns to consolidate and refine skills acquired in the preschool years. When a child is two or three years old, for example, he may begin throwing balls; a school age child will learn to throw it well and accurately. Moreover, all other movements need not cease for him to concentrate on ball-throwing: he can displace his body, reach, throw, and use his increasingly accurate sense of static and dynamic balance. He now has the skills for participation in team play and has generally developed a wide range of abilities for vigorous activities. As with the younger child, playing is an essential part of learning, but the older child usually learns about muscle use, nerve coordination, and timing through group games.

Identifying the appropriate amount of such play and the ideal sports for each individual is difficult sometimes but important. While inactivity leads to inadequate physical development, intensive effort or overtraining may result in harmful fatigue. The differences among healthy children in size, appearance, and ability increase with age and begin to have a practical significance. For example, the stocky, muscular child is likely to be strong and successful in sports that emphasize body contact and strength, whereas a small, thin child may be average in certain sports but excellent in track or gymnastics.

There are increasing discrepancies not only in physical appearances and abilities among children of the same age but also in the expectations adults have for them. Frequently undue pressure is placed upon a child who appears taller, stronger, and older.

As school age children mature, differences between girls and boys become more apparent. Boys tend to excel in skills requiring muscular strength, speed, and coordination of large body movements, whereas girls generally possess greater manual dexterity. Increasing evidence suggests that cultural conditioning and parental expectations may account for many of these differences. Perhaps changing attitudes towards the role of women and increasing support for female athletes will lead to a blurring of these differences. Important differences in development due to sex will always remain, however. For example, girls sexually mature about two years before boys do.

Puberty to adulthood

During this second period of rapid growth and development, the child becomes a mature man or woman with an adult physique and capable of reproducing. This second stage of growth is characterized by profoundly complex, interrelated changes which affect the adolescent physically, psychologically, emotionally, and socially. Duration is hard to establish accurately, but the process begins with changes in hormonal activity and ends with the last stages of reproductive system and body maturation. It covers over half of the entire growth and development period, extending through almost the entire second decade of life.

The end of the second growth cycle is more difficult to pinpoint from the psychological, emotional, and social standpoints than from the physical, since cultural and social mores are directly related to them and can vary greatly from culture to culture. Adulthood depends upon societal definitions and expectations. However, the major recognizable physical events occur within a shorter, more well defined period called *puberty*. *Adolescence* is the term used to describe the period immediately before, during, and immediately after puberty.

Prepubescence includes early, invisible changes relating to the beginning of altered hormonal activity, starting at about age eight in girls, and about age ten in boys. The sharp change in hormonal functioning which marks the onset of the second growth cycle is triggered by the hypothalamus. The hypothalamus stimulates the pituatary gland to produce hormones which in turn cause increased hormonal activity in the testes or ovaries and in the adrenals. The ovaries secrete estrogen, and the testes excrete testosterone.

Puberty starts abruptly and is characterized by great change. Girls generally enter puberty at about ages ten to twelve; boys, at about ages twelve to fourteen. The changes which take place in this period are so complex that puberty is often viewed as a time of disorderly and unharmonious growth. There is, however, as definite a pattern at this time as at any other, but because of the wide individual variation in growth at this age and the tremendous scope of the changes taking place, it is difficult to follow the process clearly. Physical changes which take place during adolescence can be organized into the following broad categories: height and weight growth spurt, segmental growth, growth of body components, and physiological changes.

GROWTH SPURT IN HEIGHT AND WEIGHT Weight gain begins earlier than height gain and is more variable. Height changes are more abrupt: a child who has been growing 2 or 3 centimeters per year will suddenly grow 5 or 6 centimeters per year for a couple of years and may then grow as much as 9 to 11 centimeters in one year—his year of maximum growth—after which his rate of growth will decelerate increasingly each year until it ceases at maturity. Boys tend to have later growth spurts than girls, but even among members of the same sex there are great individual differences.

SEGMENTAL GROWTH Body proportions undergo many changes during adolescence. Although the head undergoes very little change in size, the face (particularly the nose and the lower jaw) does change. These changes do not increase the circumference of the head, but they do affect the facial configuration and expression by straightening the profile and causing the chin to protrude.

Rapid growth of the other parts of the body follows a predictable sequence: first the chest, then arms and legs, and last the trunk, which begins its growth spurt after all other parts of the body have stopped growing. There is about a year between the time of peak growth of the legs and that of the trunk. This lag in growth of the trunk changes the relationship between the length of the extremities and the total body height and accounts for the familiar picture of the awkward, clumsy adolescent and the description of him as "all legs and arms."

GROWTH OF BODY COMPONENTS Bones and muscles participate fully in the growth spurt, and their maximum growth period coincides with the

Figure 2.10. Growth charts of girls and boys from birth through age 18, showing increase in height and rate of growth. The sharp peaks indicate the adolescent growth spurts.

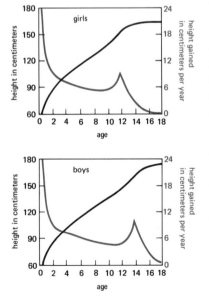

maximum growth in height and weight of the whole body. Fat tissue, on the other hand, follows a different schedule for growth. After rapid accumulation of fatty tissue in the last trimester of prenatal life and the first 6 to 8 months following birth, the rate of accumulation decreases until about ages 6 to 8. At this time, fat gradually accumulates again in both sexes until the rapid growth period of adolescence when the rate of fat accumulation decelerates. This pattern during adolescent growth is more marked in boys than in girls: boys actually lose fat. In boys, the amount of fat decreases in absolute terms as well as relative to the rapid growth of bone and muscle tissue. In girls, the rate of fat accumulation decreases and appears less relative to growth of other body components, but there is no significant loss of fat in absolute amounts. After the period of maximum growth of bones and muscle tissues, fat accumulation again increases—more so in girls than in boys.

Many organs grow faster during the adolescent growth spurt, such as the larynx which contributes to the noticeable voice changes of the male, the heart, and most strikingly the reproductive organs (Tables 2.2 and 2.3). Some of the reproductive organs are not visible: the ovaries and uterus of the female, the prostate of the male. Others are visible and/or palpable: the testes, the scrotum, the penis, and the breasts. These visible reproductive organs, together with the pubic, axillary, facial, and body hair, are commonly referred to as the secondary sex characteristics. The changes in appearance of the secondary sex characteristics have

Table 2.2 Sexual development—boys

Sequence	Age*, yrs. Ave. (range)
1. Growth of testes	12 (9.5–13.5)
2. Pubic hair	12.3 (9.5–15)
3. Growth of penis, prostate and seminal vesicles	12.5 (11.5–14.5)
4. Axillary and facial hair, subareolar, breast tissue	14 (12–17)
5. Full growth of the penis and voice change	15 (13.5–16.5)
6. Full growth of the testes and maturation of spermatogenesis	16 (14.5–18)

* Onset unless otherwise stated

Table 2.3 Sexual development—girls

Sequence	Age*, yrs. Ave. (range)
1. Enlargement of areola and budding of breast	11 (8–13.5)
2. Pubic hair	11 (8–14)
3. Development of breast, pigmentation of areola, axillary hair, uterine enlargement	13 (10–16)
4. Menarche	13 (10–16.5)
5. Ovulation	14 (11–18)

* Onset unless otherwise stated

been standardized and charted; although they take place in a continuous sequence, it has been possible to define the stages of maturation represented by development of each of the secondary sex characteristics.

In boys, the first observable change is the sudden increase in the size of the testes accompanied by increased pigmentation of the scrotum and closely followed by an increase in length and thickness of the penis. The growth of the pubic hair follows a well-defined sequence. At first it appears sparsely and is downy, pale in color, and confined to the base of the penis. Within a year it becomes darker, coarser, and increasingly curly, spreading over a wider area until it covers the entire pubic area. Axillary and facial hair appears about two years after pubic hair.

About one year after the initial growth of the testes, nocturnal emissions, or wet dreams, begin to occur. These are caused by ejaculation during sleep; some boys may experience them quite frequently, others very seldom.

The ability of the male to discharge semen does not necessarily indicate fertility. The point in the maturation process at which fertility is established in the male has not been determined, and evidence indicates that there is wide variation among individuals.

In girls, the first sign of puberty is the change in the appearance of the breasts. The *areola* (the dark ring around the nipple) enlarges and darkens; both the areola and the nipple protrude noticeably on the flat chest. This process is referred to as *budding*. After the budding of the breasts, fat tissue begins accumulating under the areola. As the breasts begin to enlarge slightly, they are referred to as primary breasts. Finally the development of glandular tissue begins, and the areola recedes into the rounded contour of the developed breast, leaving only the nipple protruding. Budding and primary breast development may also occur in boys, but this is temporary, attributable to fat accumulation, and recedes after a short time.

Pubic hair growth follows a similar pattern with girls as with boys. The color, texture, and density are initially very light; hair appears sparsely first above the vulva and spreads gradually over the entire triangular pubic area, darkening, coarsening, and becoming increasingly curly within a year's time.

Unlike boys, girls experience a definite event which indicates their approaching maturity: the onset of *menarche,* the establishment of their menstrual period. At first, menstrual periods tend to be irregular and are usually anovulatory (without a mature egg produced by the ovaries). Just as the first appearance of semen in boys does not necessarily indicate fertility, so do the first menstrual periods of girls seldom indicate consistent production of ova. Fertility is established when the menstrual flow becomes ovulatory. It takes months, and sometimes one or two years, for all menstrual periods to be consistently ovulatory.

The skeletal system experiences growth during the overall growth spurt. In addition to growing in length and thickness, bones also change

Menstrual cramps

Menstrual cramps are especially common in teenagers. The severity of the pain is variable but for some girls it can be so severe as to be disabling.

Although there are numerous theories about the causes of the pain, none has sufficient evidence to support it over the others. What is known, however, is important: First, in the overwhelming majority of cases the girl is healthy and has no disease of the reproductive organs. Second, the painful periods only follow menstrual cycles in which ovulation has occurred. If ovulation does not occur during a cycle, the next period will be painless.

In most cases the recommended treatment is to use simple painkillers, such as aspirin. Stronger painkillers are undesirable when used month after month because they can be habit forming.

The girl should be encouraged to carry on her normal daily activities. Excessive restriction of activity during menstruation is unhealthy and can actually make the pain worse.

When the pain causes major incapacities, a physician may prescribe further treatment.

From *Today's Health*, Vol. 51, No. 2 (February, 1973), p. 13.

from flexible cartilage to true bone, becoming much harder and less resilient. This process is called *ossification*. The size, shape, and outline of the areas where true bone is forming can be determined with X-ray film. The standard of development is based upon age-specific descriptions for the average healthy child. By comparing the film of an individual child with the standard film which it most closely matches, the individual skeletal age can be determined, and the amount of deviation from the expected level for his chronological age can be ascertained. There are standards established for different segments of the body, including the knee and foot, but the standard of the hand and wrist is the most practical for comparison because there are many ossification centers in this region and it can be safely exposed to X rays. Maturation of the skeleton is complete when it reaches the expected stages of development for an eighteen year old, regardless of chronological age.

Some physiological capacities are closely related to the amount and rate of overall body growth and reach peak growth rate during adolescence. Blood volume, number of red blood cells, hemoglobin, total lung capacity, muscle strength, and sex hormones are some examples. Some of these which increase significantly in adolescence continue to increase well into mature adult life; they are blood pressure, total lung capacity, and muscle strength. Other functions reach maximum growth values early in childhood and do not increase at all during the second growth cycle.

The two types of sweat glands in the skin increase their activity during the adolescent growth spurt. The activity of the *apocrine glands* is related to emotional stress. These glands secrete a white, fatty fluid which reacts upon contact with bacteria on the skin to cause body odor. The *sebaceous* glands respond to heat and physical activity and secrete an oily substance called *sebum*, which inhibits the evaporation of water on the skin, thus helping to cool the body and maintain stable body temperature. A heavy secretion of sebum can clog skin pores and contribute to the formation of acne.

The adolescent growth spurt in height can be correlated with the stages of development attained by the different systems and organs. At the onset of the height spurt among girls, for example, breasts are at the budding stage, and the first, downy pubic hair is beginning to come in sparsely. The year of maximum growth is followed within one year by the onset of menarche. Similarly among boys, height growth is a good indication of sexual maturation, and when sequential height measurements are available, it is possible to detect the beginning of the spurt, to predict the course of further development, and offer much needed guidance and counseling to the adolescent.

Behavioral changes in adolescence

In addition to the profound physical changes described above, the maturing child experiences tremendous psychological and behavioral changes. This period more than any other demonstrates the interrelationships between biological and behavioral development.

The physical changes happen bewilderingly quickly and create major tasks of adjustment for the adolescent. His first job is to accept these changes without fear, discomfort, or shame. Next he must learn to deal with the new emotional and physical demands created by the rapid development of his reproductive system: his sexual drives become as real as the urge to breathe, but not so easily handled.

Skilled counseling should be available to all young people at this stage of development and should begin with clear information about the physical changes that are taking place. Equally important in good counseling is help in interpreting the way in which these changes will affect the adolescent's day-to-day life. Counseling should help the adolescent handle the many new and sometimes contradictory expectations and demands which will confront him and which originate both from within himself and from his environment. The ability to deal with societal expectations is crucial to effectual adult functioning, and it begins with a sense of self-respect which counseling should help instill. He should be able not only to accept his new attributes but also to like the kind of adult he is becoming and to take pride in his emerging character.

The difficult job of counseling the adolescent is made easier by one emerging trait: the adolescent is interested in himself. He is trying to learn who he is and what kind of an adult he will be. The description of the teenager spending hours in front of the bathroom mirror, peering anxiously at his suddenly different and momentously important face is a symbol of this newly awakened self-interest. Healthy and normal, this introspection can lead the adolescent toward consideration of realistic goals for himself.

With self-interest comes an increased desire for the admiration and liking of his peer group. The adolescent does not want to be different from others his own age whom he likes, admires, and competes with. "Different" is often considered as "abnormal" by the adolescent, and parental pressure to conform to a different set of standards from those espoused by his friends and peer group can cause real unhappiness and rebellion.

Delayed or early maturation are chief among the causes for anxiety; both are usually physiological, but they lead to entirely different problems. There may normally be as much as six years between early and late maturation. The late maturer, however, is often justifiably unhappy, since the school systems in this country generally group children by chronological age rather than by developmental stage. The late maturer therefore finds himself among children who are taller, heavier, stronger, and more obviously developed than he. He shows a weaker performance in sports which require strength and endurance and is consequently apt to be left out of activities in which his classmates participate. He may be so self-conscious about his body that to dress and undress in the school gym causes anxiety. Physically he is probably normal; the late maturer is simply adhering to his own schedule for development. The problem is emotional and can become so intense that even after physical maturation, the harmful effects of his poor adolescent adjustment may continue to hinder healthy adult functioning.

Late maturation may be more painful for boys than for girls in our society. For girls, the major concerns in late maturation relate to breast development and menstruation. For boys, slow height growth causes the most acute concern. This concern may be due to societal expectations which consider a couple mismatched if the girl is taller than the boy.

Early maturation creates other, perhaps less troublesome, problems. An early maturing boy is stronger physically and is thus more likely to possess greater ability and self-confidence in sports than his peers. Because of his more mature appearance, however, adults tend to expect more mature performances in other areas such as school work and social situations. If his biological development is not matched by his emotional, social, or intellectual development, he may experience excessive stress and pressure. The early maturing girl may also suffer from isolation from her classmates. She attracts and is attracted to older boys, and her behavior, normal for her stage of maturation, may be considered promiscuous by her less mature classmates and even by adults who compare her with children of her own chronological age.

Many other sources of anxiety for adolescents are exaggerations of temporary problems such as acne, menstrual irregularity and accompanying discomfort, problems of appetite and weight gain, and swelling of male breasts, all of which fall within the range of normal phenomena.

Adolescents vary in their capacity to adapt, but since most of these problems are temporary, counseling can be very effective. The lasting effect of such problems depends largely upon how successfully the individual adapts to them when they occur.

Factors affecting growth and development

There are two determining factors in the process of maturation: heredity (genetic makeup) and environment (the natural and social surroundings). Individual differences in the timing and magnitude of maturation are many and represent the combination of inborn characteristics and the traits developed from environmental influence.

Eye color and texture and color of hair are genetically determined; they are controlled by a small number of genes and respond little, if at all, to environmental influences. Other attributes, such as the general pattern of growth, the rate of growth, and the body build, are also primarily genetically determined, but the number of controlling genes is relatively large, and the environment has a greater opportunity for influencing development. But to state that genes determine growth potential and that environmental influences determine the development of inborn potential is an oversimplification of a complex process. Genetic and environmental factors are rarely so clearly distinguished from each other.

Illness may permanently affect the course of maturation if it is prolonged or chronic, and if it interferes with the metabolism. Short term illness, such as the common childhood illnesses, do not permanently retard growth. They cause instead a deceleration in growth rate, after which there is a limited period of especially rapid, "catch-up" growth. The components of growth differ from each other in their response to illness: weight is more responsive and height is significantly more resistant to environmental influence. Whether the child can be restored to his healthy pattern of growth depends upon the duration and timing of the illness and whether it was an isolated or a recurring event. The drive to grow is strong, and usually only an intensive, strong, and prolonged illness causes permanent deviation from the established patterns of growth.

Nutrition, housing, clothing, and warmth are environmental factors which greatly affect growth and development and which are frequently influenced by family income. It has been shown that children of unskilled workers with low incomes are smaller and less developed than children of the same race and age from a higher income bracket. Lack of education is a significant factor influencing growth and development, since it is often correlated with ignorance of nutrition, of the necessary components of health care, and of the importance of prenatal care.

In general, improved standards of living, improved nutrition, and freedom from many of the previously common major infectious diseases are factors which account in large part for each successive generation's greater overall growth. Moreover, adolescence begins earlier with each successive generation. The earlier maturation of the reproductive system has implications for earlier sexual activity and childbearing capacity. More rapid maturation means that adolescents attain adult size, physique, and sexual maturity at a chronological age far below that at which society permits the assumption of adult roles and status. This may be an important factor in the increase of out-of-wedlock births from 38 per 1000 in 1940 to 67 per 1000 in 1968 for girls 15 to 17 years of age. These children attain physical maturity and size at a chronological age at which they are still expected to be emotionally and financially dependent upon their parents and perhaps have years of education to complete before they may take an active role in society. Some of the problems of youth in contemporary society may result from society's position that the adolescent, though physically mature, is not yet culturally or legally mature and independent.

AGING Gradual change is characteristic of all stages of life. Even after maturity and full adulthood is achieved, all physiological systems continue to change. Blood pressure gradually increases and the ability of the respiratory system to exchange oxygen and carbon dioxide gradually declines

Figure 2.11. Old people, many of them over 80, taking jazz ballet lessons. Group dancing is one of the best ways of stimulating both physical and social activity. (Courtesy of the World Health Organization)

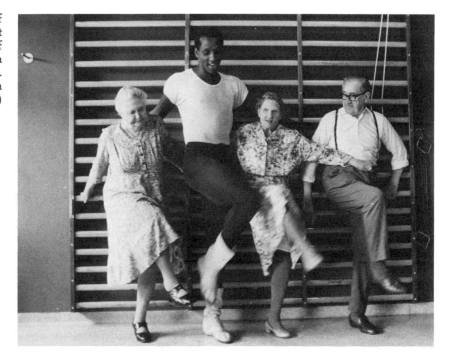

with advancing age. Irreplaceable cells in the central nervous system gradually disappear.

In women, the reproductive system undergoes important changes sometime between age forty and fifty-five. Menstruation and ovulation stop, and the levels of circulating female hormones are reduced. These events are called menopause or "change of life." Many women are relieved at their loss of fertility, but the sudden changes in hormone levels may cause other problems. The skin may become drier and more wrinkled. The vagina may have a slightly thinner lining, and the quantity of lubricating secretions is reduced. In some women menopause may cause sudden sensations of heat, called "hot flashes," as well as emotional problems. Many of these changes can be prevented or reversed by administration of estrogens. Even when the loss of ovarian hormones is overcome by taking a pill, the menopausal woman must adjust to and accept her new status. Often menopause coincides with the time children leave home, causing further stress. For women who do not define themselves only as mothers, however, middle age represents new freedom and opportunities. Loss of fertility should not be equated with loss of sexuality. For many women, freedom from worry about conception leaves them with renewed interest in sexual activity.

Although men may experience some reduction in sexual drive as they enter middle and old age, their reproductive systems undergo no abrupt changes similar to those of menopause. Most men remain fertile and sexually active even in the later decades of life. Middle age holds many psychological hazards for men, however. Many men find that they will not advance much further in their careers and that some goals will never be realized. Others have difficulty accepting their declining physical abilities and their changing physical appearance.

For both men and women, advancing age means an increased probability of sickness and disease. Although older persons may be immune to many infectious diseases, they are more vulnerable to noninfectious diseases such as arthritis, cancer, cardiovascular, and respiratory diseases (see Chap. 11).

Everyone dies eventually. Yet although death is inevitable, it is often difficult to understand and accept for ourselves and for those near us. Not only is death difficult to comprehend psychologically, but also the physiology of death is not fully understood. In the past, death was defined by physicians as the stopping of vital functions such as circulation and respiration. Recently great improvements in medical care have complicated the criteria for death and have raised a number of moral and legal issues. Consider an individual whose brain is totally and irreversibly damaged. He responds to no stimuli and exhibits no reflexes; there is no measurable electrical activity in his brain, and he is not capable of breathing on his own. Some patients in this condition, however, can be kept "alive" on a mechanical respirator which will breathe for him. Such a person is hopelessly damaged and has suffered total brain death. The legal and ethical considerations in the definition of death are discussed in Chapter 17.

Questions
1. Discuss the roles of the sex hormones in terms of ovulation, fertilization, and menstruation.
2. Which are the first organs and systems to become functional in the fetus? When do they develop? Why do you think they are the first?
3. What are possible effects of malnutrition on the fetus? How do the effects differ according to the stage of fetal development at which malnutrition occurs?
4. Which is the first observable sign of puberty in boys in most cases? In girls? What are other physical changes which occur during puberty?
5. Were you a late or an early maturer? How do you think your physical development may have affected your psychological and social development?

Key Concepts
Estrogen – the hormone secreted by the ovaries which initially stimulates the growth of the endometrial lining of the uterus at the start of the menstrual cycle

Gonads – the primary sex organs: the ovaries in the female and the testes in the male; the gonads produce the sex cells (egg and sperm) and secrete the sex hormones

Maturation – the combination of the processes of growth (an increase in size) and development (a change in structure according to function)

Progesterone – the hormone secreted by the ovaries which continues to stimulate the growth of the endometrial lining of the uterus, particularly after ovulation, in preparation for implantation of the fertilized egg

Puberty – the second period of rapid growth and development in an individual's life, resulting from dramatic changes in hormone levels

Selected Readings Cutright, P. "The Teenage Sexual Revolution," *Family Planning Perspectives*, 4(1972), 24.

Day, B., and H. N. I. Liley. *Modern Motherhood: Pregnancy, Childbirth, and the Newborn Baby*. New York: Random House, 1967.

Lowrey, George H. *Growth and Development of Children*, 6th ed. Chicago: Year Book Medical Publishers, Inc., 1973.

Odell, W. D. and B. L. Moyer. *Physiology of Reproduction*. St. Louis: Mosby Co. ,1971.

Rugh, Robert and L. B. Shettles. *From Conception to Birth—The Drama of Life's Beginnings*. New York: Harper and Row, 1971.

Stuart, Harold C. and Dane G. Prugh. *The Healthy Child*. Cambridge, Mass.: Harvard University Press, 1962.

Chapter 3

Psychological Development

THE DEVELOPMENT OF PSYCHOLOGY: AN OVERVIEW

Man's physical health is often intricately linked to his psychological well-being. Even the earliest psychologists recognized this. In fact, the theories of Sigmund Freud, the Viennese physician and neurologist who founded psychoanalysis, were stimulated largely by his attempt to understand and treat a case of hysteria (a physical disability that has no physiological basis). People have become blind, deaf, and unable to walk even though there was nothing organically wrong with them. A hysterical patient torn between a compulsion to masturbate and his guilt over the act may resolve the conflict by developing a paralyzed hand.

Since those early days a great deal of evidence has shown that psychological factors are often the basis for physical ailments known as psychosomatic (mind-body) illnesses. Mental stress, conflict, and anxiety frequently produce ulcers, colitis, hypertension, and even common hives. The more severe psychological disturbances known as psychosis are often accompanied by physical disability. Psychotic patients may experience a

This chapter was contributed by Philip R. Zelazo, Ph.D., Lecturer in the Department of Psychology and Social Relations, Harvard University.

paralysis known as catatonia in which they remain "frozen" in a particular posture for years. Another physical manifestation typical of psychotics is hallucinations. They experience visual, auditory, and tactual "visions" even though there is no corresponding external stimulation. A patient with 20/20 vision whose sense of touch is intact may see —even feel—animals or large insects crawling on a blank wall. To him, they are real and threatening.

The study of abnormal behavior, like the study of disease, depends on a sound understanding of normal functioning. The relics of even early civilizations suggest that man has long been preoccupied with understanding his thoughts and actions. Skulls dating from ancient Egypt show evidence of trepanning, an operation in which priest-physicians cut holes in the skull to release "evil spirits" thought to be the cause of abnormal behavior.

Until very recently in history, the only sources of psychological knowledge were poets, philosophers, judges, and village elders. Although these men were often capable of remarkable insights into behavior, their approach was not very scientific. The paradox of the nonscientific study of psychological development is that, for every wise and careful observation, there seems to be an equally insightful but contradictory one. Intuition is fallible all too often. Thus science has created procedures, rules, and tools (such as statistics), to help us determine what is and what is not true with greater reliability and validity.

Psychology's transition from philosophy to science occurred during the latter half of the nineteenth century when a number of intellectual forces converged. Freud began publishing his theory of psychoanalysis in the 1880s. As Charles Darwin's work on evolution became known among scientists, it carried implications for the evolution of behavior. Discoveries about the physiology of the eye, ear, and brain added more knowledge that was helpful to the study of behavioral development. Then, in 1879, a popular German lecturer of psychology, Wilhelm Wundt, established the first laboratory of experimental psychology. Wundt is now regarded as the father of modern psychology.

Even though nearly a century has passed since Wundt set up his laboratory, the science of psychology is still in its infancy. It is so new that 90 percent of all the individuals who have earned a Ph.D. in psychology are alive today. The branch of psychology dealing with the development of human behavior has, by now, built up considerable knowledge about the growth of social and emotional responsiveness and thinking, reasoning, and problem-solving abilities. The last three are often called "mental" powers, but, in psychological circles, they are grouped under the heading "cognition" or "cognitive capacities." But, for all that is known about these abilities, much research remains to be done.

While experimental psychology has produced a sound methodology and a rapidly expanding list of stimulating facts, it has brought forth only a few principles of behavior. There is a long way to go to match the body of laws that are the foundation of such physical sciences as chemistry and physics.

Nevertheless, there are three tentative principles (that is, potential laws) of psychological development which are generally accepted, grounded in reasonably good research, and serve as a sound beginning for the study of psychological development. These are: *operant conditioning, classical conditioning*, and *discrepancy*. The purpose of this chapter will be to define and discuss each, and, since growth is a continuous process, to examine how these principles operate at each stage of human development: infancy, the preschool years, early school years, adolescence, and adulthood.

It should be emphasized that psychologists are not in full agreement about principles of behavior, but the importance of the three to be discussed is rarely disputed. Acting singly or in combination, they seem to account for many of our habits as well as intellectual and emotional reactions. There is no single blueprint for psychological development. The growth of cognitive powers, for instance, is a particularly tangled and largely uncharted journey influenced by multiple factors. Helpful as these three tentative principles are to our study of development, they cannot be held responsible for all of man's complex behavior.

OPERANT CONDITIONING

Learning through pleasure or pain

It has long been claimed that man is hedonistic—that is, he seeks pleasure and avoids pain. If this is so, the point seems to have been missed by the many rulers and societies throughout history who have favored the use of punishment to control man's actions. Our penal system is an excellent illustration of the widespread conviction that punishment can effectively change behavior. Yet the system, at least as it is operated, indicates the glaring inadequacies of punishment as a corrective. Too few convicts mend their ways in prison, and there are more second offenders than any such system should tolerate. Even the death penalty has failed as a deterrent to serious crimes.

B. F. Skinner, the American psychologist and controversial author of *Beyond Freedom and Dignity* and the utopian novel *Walden Two*, believes that society has its priorities backward. He contends that reward, which psychologists call positive reinforcement, is a far more desirable and effective means of controlling behavior than punishment, or negative reinforcement. In Skinner's view, punishment is inherently unpleasant: it produces undesirable anxiety and avoidance reactions that make the control of behavior more difficult. What is more, punishment often breeds resentment and hostility from the recipient. If the tables are turned, he may assume a punitive attitude and seek revenge through an even more antisocial act than he was punished for in the first place. In any case, both reward and punishment are often used in our society to control behavior by the process known as conditioning.

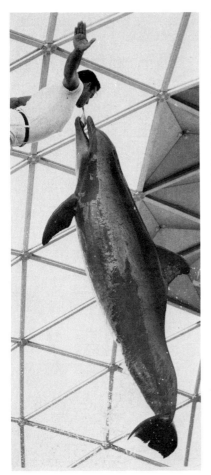

Figure 3.1. Operant conditioning. Dolphins can be trained to perform difficult acts by reinforcing a successful performance with a reward. Here the dolphin leaps 15 feet into the air to take a small fish from the trainer's mouth; a tiny slip by the dolphin could mean serious injury to the trainer. (Photo courtesy of Aquatarium and Zoological Gardens, St. Petersburg Beach, Florida)

Reinforcement by reward

Hardly a moment goes by in our lifetimes when we are not subjected to some kind of stimulus—something, such as a word, a voice, an object, a color, or a sound, that provokes a physical, mental, or emotional reaction, called a response. A given stimulus can elicit any number of responses. But when a particular stimulus becomes paired with a specific response, the result is called *conditioned behavior*. A new link or association has been formed—in a sense, programmed—that was not previously there. Once the association has been made, the response is regular and automatic: the ring of a telephone (stimulus) prompts us to pick up the receiver (conditioned response).

A stimulus often has more than one possible response, and it takes another person to sort out the "right" one. Thus, a parent seeking to establish a desirable behavior pattern in a child provides a reward whenever the child responds in the desired manner. This is called *contingent positive reinforcement*: reward depends upon response. With repetition a desired response followed by reward eventually becomes a habit and will persist even if the reward is administered less often. The use of contingent reinforcement to change behavior is known as *operant conditioning* (a concept developed by Skinner). The child always has a choice of responses—his act is willful, not a reflex—and it is his "correct" response that operates to gain the reward.

Anyone who has trained a dog has used operant conditioning: the reward of praise or a "dog yummie" depends on whether the pet performs according to his master's wishes. On a slightly more sophisticated level, circuses use the same technique to train animal acts.

The same principle applies to human development. A mother who wishes to toilet-train her two-year-old child can do so easily by giving the child soda, ice cream, cookies, praise, or any other reward that the youngster values each time he has a toilet success. Whenever the child has the urge to urinate he has a choice of responses: he can wet his pants, or he can head for the bathroom and earn himself a reward. For proper reinforcement, the reward should be immediate. A random (noncontingent) reward is ineffective.

Even though it is possible to toilet-train a child using only the reward system, it would be foolish not to explain and illustrate the behavior to the child. He is quite capable of imitating complex acts. Moreover, the child should be rewarded for partial as well as total successes. If the aim is to get the child to brush his teeth regularly, any serious effort on his part merits parental approval. His attempts may not be as thorough as adult standards of oral hygiene demand, and he may be a bit messy about it; but, over a period of time, the parent can demand that he upgrade his performance. With repeated contingent reinforcement, the child will show improvement until eventually he brushes his teeth thoroughly and without prompting.

REWARD ON SCHEDULE Once a desired behavior has been established by rewarding each success, it can be maintained longer if it is subsequently reinforced on a partial schedule. Rewarding every second success then every third or fourth will build a more persistent habit. Eventually success becomes its own reward, and surveillance by parents is unnecessary.

There are many possible schedules of reinforcement but two seem to be most applicable to human behavior: fixed ratio and variable ratio. A *fixed ratio schedule* requires a specific number of desired responses to earn a single reward. To take the toilet-training example, one reward may be given for every fourth successful trip to the bathroom. In a *variable ratio schedule*, a reward may be given on the average of every fourth response. Three rewards are earned for every twelve responses, but reinforcement may be given randomly: the third, fifth, and eleventh responses, for example. Variable ratio scheduling is what stimulates gamblers to remain at slot machines, winning less but enjoying it more.

The elimination of a response is simply a matter of withholding rewards. If responses are allowed to occur over a long period without reinforcement, the desired behavior will diminish.

Reinforcement by punishment

The use of punishment to control behavior by parents and society at large seems to be far more widespread than the evidence of its effectiveness would warrant. Psychologists agree that it has extreme limitations, but they are exploring its capabilities and consequences. In recent years, punishment has been employed for smoker therapy. As the smoker puffs on a cigarette, he is periodically jarred by severe electric shock. Punishment is applied on a random basis so the patient never knows on which puff to expect it. Therapists claim some success, though there is undoubtedly a considerable amount of backsliding.

Other research indicates that punishment alone does not change the probability of a response unless the means of punishment is present. In other words, the punished response is not weakened but merely suppressed. However, some psychologists argue that punishment can be useful to suppress an undesirable response while an alternative desired response is strengthened. This viewpoint is the basis for psychotherapy used with homosexuals who desire a switch to heterosexual orientation. If the patient is male, the therapist presents him with erotic photos of males and simultaneously administers electric shock. Punishment is terminated only by the presentation of erotic photos of women, thereby creating a positive association with females. This method has successfully conditioned homosexual patients so that they have been able to enjoy relationships—even marriage—with members of the opposite sex. Whether or not it serves as a long-range corrective remains to be seen.

CLASSICAL CONDITIONING

As you enter a movie theater, the smells and sounds coming from the popcorn machine can make your mouth water. You may not even see the machine, much less taste the popcorn, but your salivary glands are turned on as if it were the real thing. Why? You have been conditioned; in this case, it is called *classical conditioning.*

Classical conditioning involves a stimulus that automatically triggers a reflex action (unlike the voluntary response of operant conditioning). The original stimulus is presented simultaneously with a second, neutral stimulus that has no inborn relation to the reflexive response. After many paired stimulus presentations, the stimulus with the inborn relation is withdrawn and the neutral stimulus alone elicits the reflex. A new association has been conditioned.

The "classical" aspect comes from the early days of psychology when it was the first learning process to gain attention. It is also known as Pavlovian conditioning after the Russian physiologist Ivan Pavlov whose laboratory discoveries led to the principles and techniques of the process. In his classic experiment, Pavlov sounded a buzzer (neutral or conditioned stimulus) immediately before placing meat powder (un-learned stimulus) in a dog's mouth. The powder naturally caused the dog to salivate (unlearned reflex response). After repeated pairings, the buzzer alone produced saliva in the dog's mouth (conditioned response). The same sort of learning has taken place when the sound from the popcorn machine starts saliva flowing in your mouth.

Conditioned emotions

Some emotions, such as fear and anxiety, seem to develop as a result of classical conditioning. There is considerable evidence that the association of a harmless stimulus with an intensely painful experience can produce a phobia (irrational fear of a neutral stimulus). The so-called Albert

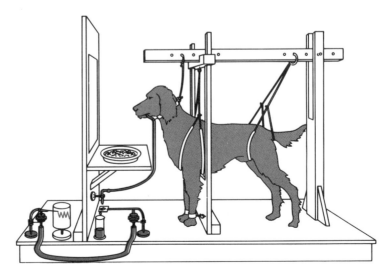

Figure 3.2. Classical conditioning: Pavlov's dog. At first the meat powder which caused the dog to salivate was accompanied by the sound of a buzzer; eventually the sound of the buzzer alone caused the dog to salivate. The saliva was collected in a tube attached to the dog's salivary gland.

experiment suggests how this may occur. Albert, an eleven-month-old infant, was presented with a white rat. The boy showed no fear and tried to play with the animal. The next time the rat was presented, the researcher set off a loud noise behind Albert's head, frightening him. This stimulus pairing was repeated several times until the appearance of the rat by itself was enough to make Albert cry. The boy also generalized his fear to anything that was furry like the rat: a dog, a rabbit, even a Santa Claus mask. Fortunately for Albert, classical conditioning must be reinforced regularly or it will dissipate. His fear of furriness disappeared after little more than a month.

To take the matter out of the lab and into everyday life, the painful experience of a near drowning may precipitate a deep-seated hydrophobia (irrational fear of water). If the associations are intense enough, a single pairing of them may be sufficient to establish them in an individual's emotional makeup. Often such phobias are extremely persistent because avoidance of the feared stimulus reduces anxiety and is, therefore, rewarding. Eliminating the fear is a matter of repeatedly encountering the conditioned stimulus (water) without the pain-producing unconditioned stimulus (near drowning).

THE DISCREPANCY HYPOTHESIS

Conditioning can shape and control behavior, but it does not explain how people acquire knowledge or process information. The development of thinking, reasoning, and problem solving—as well as components of those capacities such as concepts, symbols, images, and principles— seems to follow a different set of rules.

One theory about these types of learning first appeared in the 1940s but only recently gained sound research backing. This is the *discrepancy hypothesis*, the work of several cognitive theorists including the Swiss psychologist Jean Piaget. According to the hypothesis, events that are moderately different from what we already know are more likely to attract and hold our attention than events that are either too familiar or too novel.

One of the more convincing experimental demonstrations of the discrepancy hypothesis involved 40 infant boys who were divided into 5 groups of 8 each. The boys were shown that if they pressed a bar in front of them, a panel would light up. The stimulus appearing on the panel was a colorful geometric shape. At first all of them saw the same thing.

Three groups were then introduced to objects that differed in shape but remained identical in color and total area. A novel stimulus presented to the fourth group varied in shape. color and brightness but was similar in area. The fifth (control) group saw no change. Preference (measured by the number of times the bar was pressed to light up the panel) was strongest and lasted longer among the groups receiving a stimulus that was only moderately different from what they had origi-

Figure 3.3. Conditioned emotion: fear. (A) Albert was not initially afraid to play with a white rat. (B) A loud noise set off the next time Albert was presented with a rat startled and frightened him. (C) After repeated pairings of the rat and noise, Albert became frightened at the appearance alone of the rat. (D) Albert generalized his fear to anything furry like a rat, such as a beard.

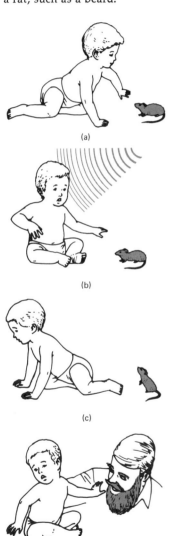

nally seen. Those viewing the novel object were initially attentive, then lost interest. The group that saw the standard repeated over and over became bored and fretted the most.

A moderately discrepant stimulus probably generates the most interest because it is sufficiently different from what is already known to demand some thoughtful effort. Novelty, on the other hand, is too unrelated to what has been established; it requires too much effort to be mastered. And, since no real effort is required by repetition, it evokes boredom. Experiments such as this one imply that attention to information that is moderately different from what is already known may be a biological characteristic of humanity. That is, it appears that we are innately "programmed" to prefer moderately different stimuli, as Piaget contends.

Observational learning

The discrepancy factor seems to be one of the most important ingredients in the developmental phenomenon known as observational learning. Children acquire much of their behavior by watching parents and peers. Often they imitate behavior new to them following only brief exposure to it. Reward or punishment seems to be unnecessary for such learning to take place. But it follows from the earlier discussion that moderately discrepant events attract and sustain attention longer than either familiar or completely novel events, and it should also determine which events children imitate. This pursuit of moderate variation seems to form the basis for the child's "natural curiosity."

Long before children have the advantage of formal schooling, they learn a wide variety of complex actions including aggressive and dependent behaviors, group games, tricycle and bicycle riding, and sophisticated sentence structure. First and second grade children watching a filmed sequence of adult aggression can instantly develop new forms of aggressive behavior.

Observational learning is a lifelong process. Adults continue to acquire complex skills such as skiing and tennis largely through direct observation. Even adult reliance on written instructions may be regarded as a symbolic form of observation when the action to be learned is described rather than demonstrated.

Emotional reactions

Why do we experience fear and anxiety, pleasure and laughter, sadness and grief? There is growing evidence that many of man's emotional reactions are a part of cognitive learning and that discrepancy is at work here, too. Events that are very different from our usual experience and, therefore, difficult to comprehend often produce uncertainty and fear. A visit to a dark, strange neighborhood can have this effect. Yet the

Learning vs. performance

An important distinction between learning (the acquisition of knowledge) through observation and performance as influenced by anticipated positive and negative reinforcement is illustrated in an experiment by Albert Bandura. Each child in three groups of nursery school children individually observed a televised presentation of an aggressive adult model receiving reward, punishment, or no consequences for his aggressive behavior. The model's behavior was similar in each of the three conditions: he approached an adult-size Bobo doll, ordered the doll out of the way, and, when receiving no reaction, displayed four novel aggressive behaviors, each accompanied by a different verbal response. For example, he would push the doll on its side, sit on it, and punch it in the nose saying, "Pow, right in the nose, boom, boom." In the model-rewarded condition, a second adult appeared at the end of the aggressive sequence, liberally praised the model, and gave him chocolate, a soft drink, and popcorn. In the model-punished condition, the second adult sharply scolded the model and called him a big bully. The model tripped while withdrawing from the second adult, who proceeded to sit on him and spank him with a rolled-up magazine. In the no-consequence condition, the model received neither reward nor punishment.

Immediately after each child observed one of the sequences, he was brought into a room containing a number of attractive toys (those used in the presentation and new ones). The child was left alone with the toys and permitted to play for ten minutes while observers recorded the occurrence of imitative aggressive behaviors from behind a one-way mirror. The number of imitative responses in each of the three groups was used as a measure of the relative influence of punishment, reward, and no consequence on a child's performance—on what a child did, not necessarily on what he learned, from watching a model. The ingenious feature of this study followed the free-play session. Fruit juice and sticker-pictures were offered to the children as incentives for reproducing each of the aggressive physical and verbal responses performed by the model.

The free-play session indicated that the children who had seen the model punished displayed significantly fewer matching responses than the children who either had seen the model rewarded or had seen him receive no consequence for his aggression. More importantly, when the children were given rewards contingent upon each imitative aggressive response, all differences were eliminated; the children who observed the model being punished learned as many aggressive behaviors as the other children even though punishment seemed to have inhibited the expression of aggression during free-play. The children in all groups learned an equal number of aggressive responses from simply watching a televised sequence; what they imitated, however, seems to have been influenced by the anticipated positive and negative consequences.

From A. Bandura, *Journal of Personality*, 1(1965): 589–95.

fantasy terror produced by reading a murder mystery in the security of one's home may actually be pleasurable. Humor often stems from the resolution of incongruous circumstances. Both adults and children laugh at the solution of a problem that follows a misleading implication (mild uncertainty). Mildly different experiences tend to be resolvable and even funny whereas very different ones may not be.

INFANCY Cognitive development

ATTENTION Psychologists have identified four qualities that attract and hold attention during this period. The two that most affect the newborn infant are biologically based: high contrast and movement. High contrast stimuli that capture a newborn's attention include the hairline around a face, the light and dark borders of the wallpaper around his crib, and changes in his mother's voice. The addition of movement to any such stimulus makes it even more compelling.

It has also been observed that during the first few months of life, sounds evoke more response (in the form of looking, smiling, and vocalization) than visual stimuli. A baby responds only to his mother's voice at first, later to both her voice and her moving face, and, at about three months of age, he will respond to her face alone. Three months is also the age when most infants smile a great deal at all faces, strangers' included.

It is believed that at about the age of two months, discrepancy is added to contrast and movement as a major attention claimer. The infant is held by slight variations of familiar stimuli: changing content in the mother's speech or the addition of glasses to her face, for example. These differences in stimuli continue to be important throughout the first year.

Some psychologists claim that a fourth process—the ability to generate hypotheses or explanations of unfamiliar events—develops around the end of the first year. Evidence suggests that when an infant has a greater density of associations to a particular stimulus, he pays attention longer. As he matures, the stimulus does not become less compelling as might be expected with increased familiarity. Rather, there is a decline from high interest to low interest followed by a return to high interest. Researchers speculate that this renewed interest is the result of cognitive changes within the child; that is, the child begins to formulate hypotheses and develop associations to each stimulus sequence about the time he reaches his first birthday.

Two facts support this contention. Research data show that the rate of infant heart beats accelerates as they become aware of stimulus discrepancies. Well-controlled experiments with adults also show a correlation between mental effort and increases in heart rate: the more difficult the task, the greater the acceleration. Secondly, twelve-month-old infants who become less upset when their parents leave them with strangers exhibit greater attentiveness to a sequence of moderate differences than do children who become very distressed over parental departure. This attentiveness—the willingness to look longer at new stimuli—in laboratory studies and the absence of distress upon parental departures may reflect the beginning of thinking and understanding at that stage of life.

OBSERVATIONAL LEARNING   About the end of his first year, the child develops one of his most important means of acquiring information: he begins to imitate others more frequently. An infant observing an event new to him automatically stores much of the information. In line with the discrepancy hypothesis, moderately different stimuli attract and sustain his attention longer than either familiar or completely novel events.

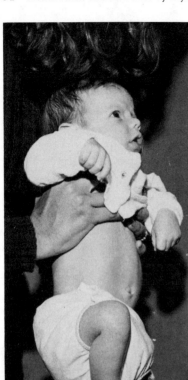

Figure 3.4. If the newborn infant is held under his arms and the soles of his feet are allowed to touch a flat surface, walking steps much like those of an adult will be elicited. With daily exercise of the walking reflex, infants increase the number of steps they take. Here a six-week-old infant demonstrates a strong walking response after several weeks of training.

One example of interaction between parent and child, the "peek-a-boo" game, illustrates the use of both imitation and moderate discrepancy in learning. The adult, usually the mother, repeats a sequence such as hiding behind the crib, then popping up and exclaiming, "Peek-a-boo!"—an act which usually evokes laughter from the baby. She continues this until the child's delight (and her own) begins to wane. Then she intuitively changes the game (creates a moderate discrepancy), an act which renews the child's interest and eventually induces him to laugh again. This apparently simple game helps the infant to acquire new actions (a process called accommodation) and to exercise his existing knowledge (assimilation). Thus a baby experiences the joys of learning by exercising his "biologically programmed" capacity to attend to and master moderate changes in his world.

When infants watch the behavior of others, they display patterns of smiling, looking, and vocalizing. These patterns indicate that babies are able to mentally process the behavior they observe long before they are physically capable of imitating it. As their motor systems mature, they develop the capacity to copy the actions of others. Significantly, no direct positive or negative reinforcement is necessary for observational learning. One psychologist, Albert Bandura, calls it "a case of no-trial learning."

Motor development

As the child acquires each important motor skill—be it sitting, crawling, standing, or walking alone—he is temporarily consumed by the experience. He practices fairly incessantly until he masters the ability, then almost immediately moves on to the next plateau. Standing alone usually precedes walking alone by only two weeks. The child seems to waste no time resting on his achievements; he is constantly extending his capacities.

Motor skills, like other developmental capacities, seem to be propelled, in part, by the pursuit of moderate discrepancy. Although newborn babies cannot walk alone, research studies have shown that given the opportunity to practice the walking reflex, these infants can show a sharp increase in the number of steps they produce by eight weeks of age (Fig. 3.4). This learned behavior apparently demonstrates the presence of reflex behavior that is programmed into the infant from the moment of birth.

There also appears to be a correlation between early walking and later mental development. Mobility offers greater freedom for exploration. Whether the child is crawling, using an infant walker, or toddling under his own power, he can make contact with a much larger and richer environment than when he was confined to his crib.

Social and emotional development

During the first year of life, an infant reveals virtually none of the complex social behavior exhibited by adults. There is little reason to believe that he loves or hates, is cooperative or competitive, is acquiescent or power-driven. He lacks language, has minimal mobility, and is largely incapable of group interaction. He is totally dependent on others for survival and will remain so for years to come. Yet this seemingly helpless child is immensely powerful. Through his very helplessness, he can strongly influence others and control his environment.

Nature equipped the infant with social responses that elicit biased results. Some are as much a reflex as the newborn walking response. If the child has gas pains, is hungry, falls, feels cold, or experiences any discomfort, he cries. That response, in turn, motivates an adult to remove the source of distress, even at 3:00 o'clock in the morning. The adult response is not only one of empathy but a strong desire to eliminate the abrasive, annoying sound.

VOCALIZATION There is little pattern to vocalization under the age of about three months. Deaf children and even children of deaf parents show no systematic difference in the sounds they make from children whose hearing is normal. However, researchers have demonstrated that social responses from adults can increase vocalization by three-month-old infants. When adults smiled, vocalized, or touched in response to each infant vocalization, there was a consistent rise in the number of responses from the children. Clearly, positive social reinforcement can shape the disposition to vocalize.

SOCIAL SMILING Several studies show that smiling can also be controlled by operant conditioning. Three-month-old infants tend to smile at everyone, even strangers. Social reinforcement from adults can stimulate a smiling infant to smile more. However, research also indicates that discrepancy enters in. As an adult's face becomes more familiar to a child, less effort to recognize and assimilate the face is required of the child and smiling declines.

FEAR OF STRANGERS Around the age of 6 to 7 months, infants stop smiling indiscriminately at any adult who appears on the scene and become more sober. At about 12 months (sometimes as early as 8 or 9), babies become fearful and start crying at the sight of a stranger. Even then, research has shown that they behave this way only when separated from the mother by some distance (four feet or more). By this age the child's mental capacity has developed to where he can sharply sort out differences between familiar and unfamiliar persons. A stranger's face, although recognizable now as a face, may be too unfamiliar (the discrepancy factor) to be assimilated and is thus frightening to a baby. The presence of a familiar person can buffer that fear.

Many theorists assume that when an infant protests over being separated from his mother, he is demonstrating his attachment or love for his mother. However, experiments in which mothers left their babies in an unfamiliar room with a familiar or unfamiliar person contradict that belief. Most crying occurred when the stranger remained alone with the child. Crying did not occur when the mother departed and the father (a familiar person) remained. When fathers were used in these studies, distress over the father's departure was virtually identical to the reaction when the mother left, even though fathers are usually less available to their children than mothers. Fathers who normally spent more time with their children had babies who protested less. The same studies repeated at home showed that about three times more distress occurs in the unfamiliar laboratory. These findings imply that fear, not love, is the major motivation behind separation protest, but they do not deny that the infant comes to love and be attached to his mother.

THE PRESCHOOL YEARS

Cognitive development

The transition from age two to three is characterized by remarkable advances. Perhaps the most striking is in the area of language. A three-year-old has a vocabulary of approximately 900 words and adds about 50 new words per month. He can easily group things according to class. If in a laboratory situation the child is asked to pick out animals from a variety of objects, he readily identifies and retrieves dog, kitten, cow, elephant, and so on.

Sustained involvement is another new development. Activities that interest a three-year-old, such as modeling clay or watching "Sesame Street," can hold his attention for as long as thirty minutes. The preschool child also acquires the ability to assume the perspective of another person for the first time. Children pretend to be Daddy or Mommy driving the car or cooking dinner.

The three-year-old is physically coordinated. He can run and negotiate turns while running. He can leap, jump, climb, somersault, and ride

The preschooler's capacity for reading and writing

A research psychologist named Omar Khayyam Moore created an extremely responsive and favorable linguistic environment and showed that preschool children could learn to read and write, listen and speak effectively, and to integrate their skills in a cooperative group effort. This environment contains an interacting computer that listens and responds to the child and is programmed to teach reading and writing efficiently. Children are introduced to the environment by an older child, and rules for its use are explained. The computer is available to each child for only thirty minutes each day, and if he chooses to leave before thirty minutes he loses his turn until the next day. The child is never forced to use the facility; he chooses to do so.

The computer looks like a large typewriter, and children are usually eager to play with it. The child's fingers and the typewriter keys are color coded to facilitate identification of the letters. Above the keyboard is a panel on which letters, words, or sentences appear for the child to match. In the beginning only the correct key matching the letter on the panel will depress and activate the next instruction. Later, only the correct word or sentence will activate the next task. The child's speech is recorded, and the computer asks only words and sentences the child gives it. Each of the tasks is graduated in difficulty (moderately discrepant) and programmed so that mastery at one level is a precondition for the next; immediate knowledge of success is its own reward (contingent positive reinforcement).

From Omar K. Moore, "The Preschool Child Learns to Read and Write," Y. Brackbill and G. Thompson, *Behavior in Infancy and Early Childhood* (N. Y.: The Free Press, 1967).

a tricycle. The child is curious, exploring, usually in motion and often underfoot.

LANGUAGE Reinforcement plays a major role in the way a child develops his ability to use language, though it is certainly not the only force at work. His early linguistic environment, especially the models supplied by parents, strongly influences the rate at which a child acquires this capacity. Children living in institutions where they receive less verbal interaction and mental stimulation from adults exhibit depressed verbal and cognitive development. On the other hand, single children living with their families and receiving abundant adult verbal interaction and instruction are generally the most advanced in language ability.

Social and emotional development

Until about two years of age, most children encounter relatively few parental prohibitions. Parents place valued objects out of the infant's reach. They usually assume that the child is too young to comprehend and avoid dangers, so they either supervise him closely or place him in safe locations. But, by the toddler stage, few objects are unreachable for the mobile and curious child, and there are few safe locations that will contain him for long. Restraints are inevitable.

Unfortunately, parents too often emphasize prohibitions. The development of social behavior becomes synonymous with inhibitions, and punishment in some form seems necessary to inhibit exploration and aggression. Punishment also fosters the development of a conscience. Independence and achievement, on the other hand, seem more readily acquired when parents employ positive reinforcement, serve as good models (observational learning), and use reasoning.

AGGRESSIONS Konrad Lorenz and other theorists in the behavioral science called ethology insist that aggression is instinctive in mankind. Some claim that frustration is all that is necessary to trigger human aggression. Two sources of frustration leading to aggressive behavior have been identified: (1) external and internal barriers that prevent or delay the achievement of an important goal; and (2) internal conflicts between incompatible responses.

Others, however, have demonstrated experimentally that mere observation of aggressive models is a sufficient stimulus for aggression. Children imitated aggressive adults and peers (in "real life" as well as on television). Goal blockage and frustration are not required.

Contrary to popular belief, aggression and hostility are not synonymous. Professional football players block and tackle one another with great vigor, but their aggressive behavior is "part of the game." It is not hostile even though it sometimes causes injury. But "clotheslining" (throwing up an arm to catch a running opponent across the neck) is a deliberately hostile act designed to inflict pain or injury.

Language and culture

Some psychologists believe there is a strong correlation between linguistic development and socioeconomic class. According to their studies, the children of middle-class parents perform much better than lower-class children on tests involving linguistic and cognitive abilities. Further studies indicate that poorer performances occur because of the linguistic limitations of lower-class parents.

Recently, other researchers have begun to question the validity of these findings. While they do not deny the influence of parental models, they argue that other environmental factors are also instrumental in shaping the poor language skills of lower-class children.

Linguistic weakness at the bottom of the socioeconomic scale also suggests at least a partial reason why those children achieve lower scores on standard intelligence tests. Those examinations rely heavily on verbal ability. Efforts are currently underway to devise testing procedures that are less verbal. Other tests are being phrased in language that is more akin to what the child hears in his own environment (Black English, for instance). Hopefully, such revisions will provide a less biased intelligence quotient for lower socioeconomic children.

Figure 3.5. Although sometimes professional football players block and tackle with enough force to cause injury, their behavior is aggressive, not hostile. (Courtesy of the New York Jets)

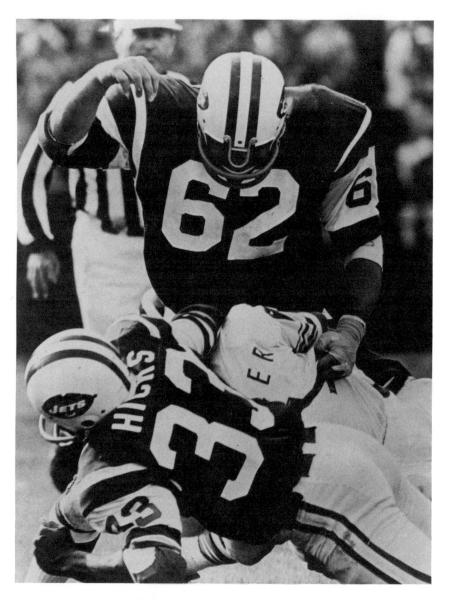

Paid aggression

If Dick Butkus could have his way, combat would never be over. "Football is what I am," he says bluntly. "I love the hitting."

Since joining the Chicago Bears in 1965, the former University of Illinois All-American has come to epitomize violence on the football field. A perennial All-Star, he plays with reckless abandon. "You can see the intensity in his eyes," says former teammate Ed O'Bradovich. "He has complete and total desire to win. I don't give a damn if we're 40 points down with a minute to go, he just has to get in there and hit. Even at practice."

After one Sunday of Dick's punishing forearms and brain-fogging tackles, the Baltimore Colts took a bus to O'Hare Airport. When it stopped for a red light, a trailing car hit the rear bumper. "There's Butkus again," said one of the bruised Colts.

He works himself up to such a competitive pitch that on the day of a game he won't answer a direct question. "He'll just grunt," adds Mike Ditka of the Dallas Cowboys. "With the highest respect, I've got to say Dick is an 'animal'."

From *Today's Health*, Vol. 51, No. 7 (July 1973), p. 62.

Studies have also shown that aggressive behavior can be maintained by reward and punishment. In one experiment, nursery school children verbally punished for aggression in doll play showed decreased aggression in a subsequent doll play session. Children in another group who received no punishment actually increased aggressive behavior.

CONSCIENCE During the preschool years, the first seeds of conscience are planted. Explaining why a particular behavior is undesirable may be the most effective form of discipline. Reasoning helps the child to internalize values. And, once he accepts the values, he takes his standards wherever he goes.

Moral behavior must be learned; it is not instinctive. The development of a conscience (or "super-ego" as Freud called it) is closely connected to the techniques for instilling inhibitions. When a parent relies solely on punishment to enforce prohibitions concerning aggression, sex play, lying, or stealing, he generates anxiety. But, if he establishes rules based on reasons the child understands, he may produce a healthy sense of guilt in the child. A child who is physically punished need not accept an "I must not steal" dictum as his own. He only knows he must not get caught by his parents. Furthermore, negative reinforcement can often backfire. The child who was punished for touching an "untouchable" object comes to regard it as "forbidden fruit," and that may be even more irresistible.

A preschool child has few internalized values and experiences little guilt. The parent must convince the child that stealing can be harmful to others, that he would not want his own valued possessions stolen, and that society agrees to abide by this rule for the good of everyone. Once the child accepts these ideas he will be more likely to experience guilt if he violates them. The anticipation of "doing wrong" will provoke fear which, if strong enough, will short circuit the transgression.

INDEPENDENCE To a large extent, child-rearing in our society is a matter of developing independence and self-sufficiency—values that have especially deep roots in the American culture. On the other side of that coin, the causes of emotional dependency remain somewhat of a mystery. It may be that social fears formed during the toddler period surface later as emotional dependency.

Investigations of emotional dependence during the preschool and early school years often include conditions of social isolation and physical threat, conditions similar to those that elicit separation protest during the toddler period. This similarity implies that children who have difficulty assimilating the stranger in the unfamiliar (discrepant) laboratory during the toddler period may also have greater difficulty assimilating isolation in the unfamiliar laboratory during the preschool period. In other words, the fearful toddler who shows persistent separation protest may become the fearful preschooler who is labeled emotionally dependent.

Emotional dependence should be distinguished from instrumental dependency. This highly desirable social skill is nurtured when a child seeks help from an adult to complete a task rather than give up or waste his time brooding over failure. The orientation is toward the task rather than the person. The adult can reinforce this positive aspect of dependence by providing just enough assistance for the child to accomplish goals on his own. Instrumental dependence may assist the child in developing a sense of achievement and independence.

Identification

One psychological viewpoint states that identification is facilitated by a combination of desirable qualities possessed by parents (competence and love, for example) plus an awareness of similarity to the parents (in name, appearance, or ability). To be similar is to share envied qualities.

That view is not universally accepted. Psychologists agree only that identification is a complex and important process in early socialization. Many characteristics attributed to identification can be acquired through observational learning alone. Nevertheless, it seems reasonable to assume that a child's attachment to his parents eventually leads to internalization of their values and behavior. Parents are more a source of nourishment to the child's development than more distant adults and are, therefore, more likely to serve as effective models for identification.

Psychologists also seem to have overlooked the fact that parents identify with their children. They tend to reinforce behavior that increases similarity to themselves. A son is often given the same first name as his father. Pride in an infant's first smile or first steps appears long before the child himself is capable of experiencing pride and perceiving similarity. Identification is a two-way process.

COMPETENCE A child who experiences many successes followed by liberal praise and rewards acquires a feeling of confidence in his own ability to solve problems. Psychologists believe that this sense of competence begins to grow with the child's very first achievements.

A child's belief in his own competence seems to be largely a product of his social environment. If he is given problems matched to his level of development and reinforced by recognition for his problem-solving successes, he will approach new challenges with vigor. But, if he encounters problems beyond his level and is criticized for his failure to solve them, fear and anxiety may result. The child may begin to avoid future challenges. The competent child is better equipped to be independent because independence reflects, to a large extent, the capacity to solve problems with one's own ability.

IDENTIFICATION When a child thinks, feels, and behaves as though the characteristics of another person belong to him, he is said to be "identified" with that person. The other person is known as a "model," and most often it is a parent. An eight-year-old boy may feel proud and important when his father takes his school class on an outing. The child may behave as if he has incorporated some of his father's leadership qualities.

Sex-typing refers to the adoption of behavior, values, attitudes, and interests appropriate to one's own sex. It is a major contributor to the identification process and a strong influence on adult sexual and social behavior. Our society strictly reinforces "sex-appropriate" behavior.

The key, and controversial, word in the definition is "appropriate." Sex-typing is one of the issues most passionately denounced by the women's liberation movement. Preschool boys are encouraged to explore and be aggressive. They are discouraged from crying and doll play. But, with preschool girls, dependence is tolerated, cooperation and social poise are encouraged, and rough-house activities are discouraged. Until recently, children's books depicted women as nurses, never as doctors. Only men could be doctors. Television commercials generally relegate Mommy to playing her traditional role in the kitchen or dispensing expertise on such vital matters as floor wax, diapers, and detergents. Television Daddies drive cars, play sports, and serve as all-around authorities, making decisions on matters like life insurance.

There can be no denying that this Victorian bias is a pervasive and powerful one in our culture. Yet there is little reliable research and too often there are more conjectures than data.

THE EARLY SCHOOL YEARS

Cognitive development

Numerous skills appear between the ages of five and seven that imply the emergence of a new cognitive capacity. It is as though the child develops a central organizing ability. He can evaluate his thoughts and inhibit his first impulse, allowing him to consider alternate modes of action. Five-year-olds tend to be impulsive. They seldom contemplate their actions before drawing pictures. The seven-year-old child does more planning.

Jean Piaget, perhaps the most influential developmental psychologist to date, has identified several new capacities at this stage. The child, says Piaget, is able to comprehend a variety of dimensions simultaneously and understands that liquids and solids can be transformed in shape without altering their mass, volume, or continuous quantity. In a laboratory demonstration of continuous quantity, the child sees that two identical, short, wide beakers contain the same amount of water. The water is then poured from one beaker into a tall, thin container. The child must judge whether the amounts are the same or different. Five-year-old subjects believe that the taller beaker contains a larger amount of water. Seven-year-olds realize that they contain the same amount.

The seven-year-old, according to the Swiss theorist, understands relational terms. He recognizes that bigger is a relative notion, whereas five-year-olds seem to regard bigger as absolute. Shown a pair of objects, the younger child would properly identify the larger as "bigger"; but he would continue to regard it as bigger even when it is paired with a new and larger object. Seven-year-olds can make the distinction.

Piaget believes that preschoolers cannot relate objects in series along a single dimension. They are incapable, he states, of arranging sticks from small to large in increasing steps. By age seven, such a task is possible.

Social and emotional growth

Throughout early school years, children make significant strides toward emotional independence. They require less supervision, stay away from home for longer periods of time, accept responsibility for minor duties, and are increasingly responsive to their peers.

Emotionally, it is time to develop the ability to delay gratification. The child must realize that his immediate wishes can no longer be fulfilled on demand. He must begin to work for long-term goals—saving money to buy a bicycle, for instance. Learning how to delay gratification provides practice in tolerating mild stress, an experience that seems very important for achievement in our pressurized society. Clinical evidence indicates that adolescents and adults who are unable to cope with stress and who experience neurotic or psychotic episodes often come from environments that have been overprotective or overindulgent.

Studies have revealed a correlation between mental ability and impulsive and reflective temperaments. In the Matching Familiar Figure Test, reflective children tend to take more time before matching the correct picture to the standard. They are more often correct than impulsive children. Contrary to the popular myth that a quick response means a "bright" child, the impulsive youngster who makes a quick decision is more often wrong.

Closely related to delay of gratification is the notion of assigning responsibility to a child. Once he is given duties, he must exercise his intellect and moral character. Responsibility in measured doses, such as emptying the trash, walking the dog, and cutting the grass, helps give him a head start in preparing for his eventual independence.

CONSCIENCE   By the early school years children seem to view moral behavior mostly in terms of conformity to a rule, approval of others, and the dictates of authorities. By preadolescence they make moral decisions based on principles adopted for themselves. Punishment and self-satisfaction continue as major motivators of morality, but they are somewhat less important than during the preschool years.

Throughout the early school years, especially around preadolescence (ages 10–12), a child is more likely to be troubled by internal conflict. If he violates a closely held value, he experiences guilt. A ten-year-old boy may accept the idea that stealing is bad yet still succumb to the temptation to steal a handsome pocket knife. Aside from the guilt he experiences for breaking his own moral code, he may be beset by a variety of fears: getting caught, punishment, loss of esteem in the eyes of parents and friends. If this anxiety is strong enough, he may resolve the conflict by returning the stolen knife.

The survival of a democratic society depends, to a considerable degree, on the development of conscience and the control of behavior through healthy doses of guilt feelings. A community without a sense of right and wrong is a chaotic one; each individual regards his own survival as paramount, and the rest be damned.

At the other extreme, severe prohibitions can lead to neurotic and psychotic turmoil within adolescents and adults. Excess guilt and anxiety can suffocate a person emotionally, socially, and intellectually. In the course of life it is virtually impossible to always avoid conflict over one's own standards. If the conflict is not to be damaging, parents trying to develop a conscience in their children must create a fine balance between too many and too few restrictions, too much and too little guilt.

ADOLESCENCE

Cognitive development

While the preadolescent is capable of generating hypotheses about a particular problem, the adolescent is able to take a problem which has multiple factors operating simultaneously and consider all possible solutions in a logical manner. Given the letters ABCD, most adolescents could arrange them in all 16 possible combinations (A, B, C, D, AB, AC, AD, BC, BD, CD, ABC, ABD, ACD, BCD, ABCD, NONE). Most younger children could not. The 7 to 12-year-old child tends to deal only with thoughts that occur to him spontaneously. He is less likely to exhaust all combinations systematically.

The adolescent's way of thinking is characterized by an abstract quality not seen at earlier levels. He is capable of learning that the letter *a* may represent any unknown number in algebra. He can also abstract the salient qualities from specific events and deal with the abstractions. Thus the adolescent reasons that $a + b = b + a$, and this rule may apply to any two numbers represented by a and b. The younger child seems not to generalize beyond his experiences with specific numbers: $4 + 5 = 5 + 4$ and $12 + 8 = 8 + 12$, for example.

At this stage of development, there is an inclination to test hypotheses against evidence. A younger child might be willing to accept the idea that a groundhog sighting his own shadow is a reliable indicator of future weather conditions. An adolescent is likely to be more skeptical and will check the evidence supporting this claim.

The adolescent also becomes self-conscious of his emergent capacity for rational thought. He applies this process to himself, examining his plans for the future and his objectives in life.

The capacity for rational thought makes the adolescent aware of inconsistencies in his world that he would not have noticed at an earlier age. The awareness plus growing introspection sharply increase the number of inner conflicts. The adolescent questions his beliefs about family, religion, sex, and school. He becomes confused and outraged by political and religious leaders who profess one standard of morality and live by another that is quite contradictory.

Faced by inconsistency, the adolescent, for the first time, tries to establish some order. He seeks to ferret out conflicts and replace them with compatible values. This search often marks the beginning of the quest for his own identity. Attempting to become an individual separate from his parents, he often rejects everything because most of his ideas and behavior were instilled before he was capable of introspection.

But a person without beliefs—at least in himself—is a person without direction, and he cannot endure in aimless search forever. Inevitably, the adolescent must adopt a number of beliefs if he is to emerge from this sort of mental limbo.

Social and emotional growth

CONFLICT Aimlessness has many emotional correlates. Without goals and direction, it is difficult to complete tasks, to master challenges, and to derive a sense of accomplishment. An adolescent who lacks direction is more likely to encounter conflict and anxiety. Conflict seems to greet the adolescent at every turn. The capacity for introspection and for examination of consistency among beliefs makes it inevitable.

UNCERTAINTY Uncertainty is another source of fear and anxiety and a consequence of a young person's capacity to question his own beliefs. His rejection of authority and acceptance of the view that things can be relatively good or bad also contributes to doubts. The adolescent no longer accepts the proposition that it is categorically bad not to tell the whole truth. He can appreciate that half-truths may be more desirable in order to avoid hurting someone's feelings. The price of this relativistic view is greater uncertainty, and the consequence of uncertainty is greater anxiety.

YOUNG ADULTHOOD

Cognitive status

As thinking, reasoning, and problem-solving capacities develop and expand from infancy to adolescence, discrepancy seems to play a major role in their evolution. Moderately different stimuli command more attention than novelty or repetition because they can be easily integrated with what we already know, yet they also demand some mental effort. There is every reason to believe that discrepancy continues to be important to the cognitive functioning of adults.

Repetition of stimuli bores all of us eventually. We seek extensions and variations of what we already know whether it involves studying the subtle relationships between the works of several composers, learning a new chess strategy, attempting a slightly more difficult ski slope, or experimenting with a different form of sexual foreplay. A totally novel experience—an unprepared introduction to calculus or chemistry, for example—may not sustain a young adult's interest because he does not have the background to understand it. The gap between old knowledge and new is simply too great. Similarly, a first date or a first attempt at public speaking may be such a novel experience that it is actually frightening.

Another aspect of adult mental development begins to emerge during adolescence: the capability to systematically examine a problem and consider all possible solutions. It has been argued that with the attainment of this ability, man also gains the capacity for self-evaluation. As he does, he continually strives for mental consistency and seeks to resolve conflict and uncertainty—a never-ending process that characterizes the adult years. Man is also equipped from infancy to pursue moderate variations of what he already knows; he seems biologically predisposed to search continuously for new knowledge (or seems dissatisfied with the status quo, depending on one's viewpoint). Cognitive restlessness appears to be an innate characteristic of humanity. In other words, our cognitive apparatus is a positive feedback unit: the more knowledge we get, the more we seek. That probably explains why some men feel compelled to climb Mount Everest or to walk on the moon or to decipher inscriptions in pre-Columbian Mayan tombs.

Social and emotional status

By the time a person reaches adolescence he has developed a personal moral code which has a built-in potential for anxiety (whenever he violates his own rules). Since the adolescent can examine inconsistency and conflict between newly acquired thoughts and feelings and his established value system, he is confronted by the likelihood of increased anxiety. The transition from adolescence to adulthood is marked by increased responsibility, and therein lies another source of stress. Emotional maturity is a much-talked-about but ill-defined notion that involves many qualities. One of the most important is the ability to tolerate stress—to cope with fear, conflict, and anxiety.

FEAR   Adult fears, in general, center on acquiring a satisfying job with a comfortable income; achieving a successful marriage; providing for a family; and preserving the ideologies that a person has identified as his own. The last covers a broad spectrum: for example, the United States Constitution, the free enterprise system, religious doctrines, and the principles of a political party. When these and other closely valued beliefs are threatened, the adult experiences uncertainty followed by fear.

LOVE AND SEXUALITY   Adolescence and early adulthood in our culture are characterized by increased interaction with members of the opposite sex, sexuality, and emotional attachment. The components of romantic love become integrated as adults grow able to extend empathy, trust, and affection to one another.

The capacity for heterosexual love is a second aspect of emotional maturity. The necessary prerequisites for heterosexual relationships seem to be the establishment of a proper sexual identity and emotional identification with admired adults. Psychoanalysts suggest that earlier parent-child relationships determine adult heterosexual experiences. Some believe that children who experience good relationships with parents of the opposite sex tend to marry individuals who resemble that parent.

The use of reinforcement to change adult behavior

Though the adult is a far more complicated individual than he was as an infant, operant conditioning is still an effective means of shaping and changing his behavior. It has frequently proven successful when other procedures have failed. Reinforcement through reward—and sometimes punishment—has been used to change smoking habits, to reduce weight, and even to lower the blood pressure of patients suffering from essential hypertension (high blood pressure having no specifiable cause).

Reinforcement through reward is also gaining popularity as a teaching technique in the nation's universities. Programmed instruction, especially programmed workbooks and manuals to accompany introductory textbooks, are being used with increasing regularity at the college level. Another form of programming involves a simple teaching machine. The machine presents new material to students who are required to reproduce the information immediately after presentation. The student's correct response permits access to the next question. Each "right answer" seems

Reinforcement and essential hypertension

The effectiveness of contingent reinforcement as a means of reducing high blood pressure was demonstrated in an experiment performed by a research team at Harvard University Medical School. Though the number of individuals involved was small, the results suggest that the technique may be valid on a larger scale. Using special equipment, the researchers monitored the blood pressure of each of seven patients constantly during the period of the experiment. When systolic pressure dropped below a prescribed level for each patient, a tone sounded briefly and a light flashed. The patient's task was to produce as many tones and lights as possible by repeating the physiological conditions that led to their onset. The light and tone signals were, in effect, a reward signaling patient success. Every series of 20 tones and lights produced additional rewards: a photographic slide of scenic views and a token amount of money (five cents) that was allowed to accumulate over trials. By the completion of the experiment, five of the seven patients showed significant decreases in systolic blood pressure. It remains to be seen whether these individuals will maintain lower blood pressure levels outside laboratory conditions. If they do, contingent reward may serve as a relatively simple behavioral corrective for essential hypertension and a reliable alternative to pharmacological and surgical treatment.

From H. Benson, D. Shapiro, B. Tursky, and G. Schwartz, *Science*, 173 (1971), 740–2.

to increase the probability that it will be repeated in the future—in other words, learned. Immediate feedback from the machine about the correctness of the answer combined with a common human desire to be correct serves as reward that strengthens the student's learning.

Recent research on college teaching suggests additional possibilities for the contingent reward approach. Researchers at Georgia State University conducted an experiment to test the effect of rewards on three different, precisely defined levels of performance in an abnormal psychology course. The course was divided into weekly seminars with the instructor that included discussion periods and film showings and a performance session during which students were tested on questions chosen at random from each weekly unit.

As the students responded orally to the instructor's questions, he recorded the number of correct and incorrect answers per minute during testing. Students in the experimental groups were told that they would receive an A grade whenever they gave a specified number of correct answers for each minute of testing. During the semester, the instructor varied his criteria of performance from high to medium to low levels. Regardless of the level demanded, each student was rewarded with an A if he met the instructor's criteria.

A control group of students had an equivalent amount of interaction with the instructor, but those students were not given any teacher-defined criteria for performance. They were instructed to do their very best in the course and told that they would be graded on a curve.

By the end of the semester, performance of the experimental groups during medium and high criterion sessions was markedly higher than that of the control group. Those students who set their own standards of performance averaged scores that were equivalent to the teacher-defined low criterion condition. The results also revealed more uniform performance among students when criteria were specified for them. The most important finding, however, was that when high criterion levels of achievement are precisely defined and rewarded, student performance reaches a correspondingly higher level. It appears that if teachers expect more and can define that expectation with precision, they will get more. Results such as these indicate that positive reinforcement holds considerable potential as a teaching tool on the college level, and its use is likely to increase in coming years.

Questions

1. Do you think positive reinforcement (rewards) or negative reinforcement (punishments) more effectively changes behavior? Do you think effectiveness can vary at different stages of development and for different types of behavior? Why or why not?

2. Experiments indicate that aggression displayed on television shows can influence aggressive behavior in children. Would you recommend restrictions on the amount of violence and hostile behavior permitted on television? Why or why not?

3. What are various ways in which moderate discrepancies influence learning during infancy?
4. Describe various changes in cognitive development that take place from the preschool years through adolescence.
5. Describe various changes in social and emotional growth that take place from the preschool years through young adulthood, particularly in regard to conscience. Why is the internalization of values important for society as well as for the individual?

Key Concepts   *Classical conditioning* – the process of creating an association between a stimulus that automatically elicits a reflexive response and a second, neutral stimulus (unrelated to the reflexive response) until eventually this neutral stimulus alone automatically elicits the response

Cognition – the act or process by which knowledge is gained through perception, judgment, and the powers of thinking, reasoning, and problem-solving

Conditioned behavior – behavior that is regulated by an association between a particular stimulus and the specific response that is elicited by the stimulus

Discrepancy hypothesis – a theory of cognition which states that people are more attentive to information and events that are moderately different from what is already known than to those that are either too familiar or too novel

Operant conditioning – the use of contingent positive reinforcement (giving a reward following a certain desired response) in order to change behavior

Selected Readings   Elkind, David. *Children and Adolescents.* New York: Oxford University Press, 1970.

Ginsberg, H., and S. Opper. *Piaget's Theory of Intellectual Development: An Introduction.* Englewood Cliffs, N. J.: Prentice-Hall, 1969.

Mussen, P., J. Conger, and J. Kagan. *Child Development and Personality,* 3rd ed. New York: Harper and Row, 1969.

Parke, Ross. *Readings in Social Development.* New York: Holt, Rinehart and Winston, 1969.

Skinner, B. F. *Beyond Freedom and Dignity.* New York: Alfred A. Knopf, 1971.

Chapter 4

Human Sexuality

The contemporary American social scene includes an unprecedented emphasis on human sexuality. A decade or two ago the sexual content of advertising, entertainment, and literature was subtle and muted. Today it booms forth brashly and explicitly. Nudity has become commonplace in magazines with a wide general circulation. Modern films depict lovemaking in detail. Sexual techniques have become a matter for open discussion. More and more schools are offering courses in sex education. In short, sex is no longer a secret subject. Although the views that various people have about sex are probably as divergent as ever, it is clear that American attitudes and behavior in sexual matters have undergone substantial change. Laws concerning sex are also being revised; those concerning abortion, contraception, and homosexuality are recent examples. If social attitudes about sexual activity continue to

This chapter was contributed by Robert H. Holtrop, M.D., Associate Professor in Obstetrics and Gynecology, Boston University School of Medicine, and Research Associate and Lecturer in Population Studies, Harvard School of Public Health.

Sexual difficulties arising from prudery

Dread or disgust are readily linked to sexuality in our culture. Young people may be kept in ignorance about the facts of life, or the facts may have been misrepresented to them. They may have heard noisy, fully enjoyed sex play on the part of their parents as part of what Freud called the "primal scene," and misinterpreted the mother's ecstatic groans during climax as evidence of the father's brutality and the mother's agony. Or, the mother may have silently, with martyred air, implied to her daughter what pigs men are and what a cross women have to carry. The father may have warned his son about venereal disease and the horrible ease of making girls pregnant. The daughter may have been shielded from the baser facts of life—though how this is possible today is hard to fathom. Let it suffice to say there is more opportunity for a daughter to grow up associating sexual love with guilt, pain, danger, filth, or disgust than to view it as fun.

From Sidney M. Jourard, *The Transparent Self* (New York: D. Van Nostrand Co., 1971), p. 44.

change, more legal modifications may follow. Such changes are not unlikely and should be anticipated.

There is a lamentable level of sexual ignorance in today's society, however. Uninformed adults fail to teach the young about sex, and fear and guilt may distort sexual expression. The current emphasis on eroticism results in the development of unrealistic expectations and a great deal of confusion about sexual values. An understanding of sexuality is basic to the prevention of sexual unhappiness, and in spite of the recent emergence of sexual matters as acceptable topics for public discussion, many—perhaps most—people in our society are not adequately informed about sex.

Human sexuality is much more than gender difference—it represents a very complex set of interactions between human individuals. Sex may have its primal origin in the hormones, but it is channeled, directed, and modified by social, moral, and psychological factors into an intricate pattern of expression. Its biological purpose may be procreation, but its dynamic reaches into every area of human activity. This dynamic is sometimes called *libido*.

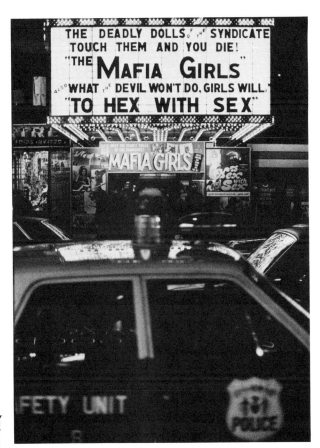

Figure 4.1. Today the sexual content of advertising, entertainment, and literature booms forth brashly and explicitly. (Peter Martens, Nancy Palmer Photo Agency)

THE DEVELOPMENT
OF LIBIDO

Libido is frequently defined simply as "sex drive." Its significance is much broader in range than this definition suggests, however. Libido has primitive beginnings very early in childhood within the mother-child relationship. Experiencing the love of its mother, the child acquires the capacity to love—to form creative, positive relationships with other persons. The psychic energy which stimulates the formation of these interpersonal relationships can be called libido. As the individual matures, the libidinal expression changes, as does its target. The child's affections are directed first toward the mother, later toward the father and the siblings and peers in a variety of patterns. During the evolution of the libido the erotic component of love becomes increasingly prominent, and libido acquires the "sex drive" connotation. But libido also includes love in the broader sense and can be considered to be the drive behind all sorts of distinctly human pursuits. Libido includes both a creative and an aggressive, erotic component.

With very rare and unfortunate exceptions, a child is born distinctly either male or female, and the determination of biological gender is quite simple. Thereafter, the parents, by their example and teachings, impart to the child his or her *gender identity*, the culturally defined role that is to be played by members of each sex. He or she is taught how to feel and behave in a masculine or feminine manner. Gender identification is made easier by the presence of a parent of the same and of the opposite sex, allowing the child the opportunity for identification with the parent of the same sex and interaction with the parent of the opposite sex.

The development of the secondary sex characteristics (genital en-

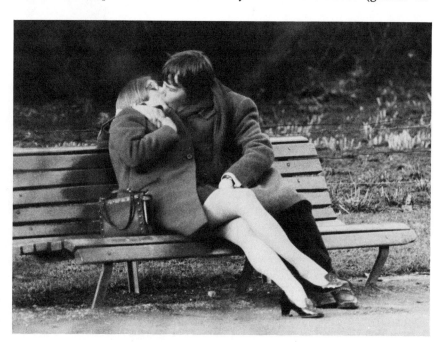

Figure 4.2. "Love—the most important creative act." (Courtesy of World Health Organization)

largement, pubic hair, axillary and facial hair, and breast development) at the onset of adolescence is due to hormonal changes that affect sex during role differentiation to an appreciable degree. This development occurs during *pubescence,* or time of puberty, and is associated with profound changes in both physical and psychological spheres for boys and girls. The reproductive organs become functionally operative, and gender identification, which was established earlier in childhood, is now subjected to remarkable endocrine adaptation as the steroid hormones of sexual maturity are secreted in significant amounts. The muscular, angular body of the male becomes sharply differentiated from the soft, curvaceous body of the female. Thus, the differences between the sexes—differences taught since early childhood as part of gender identities—become apparent in the increased physical differentiation that occurs during puberty. These physiological differences, and their social significance, are a matter of great preoccupation for the adolescent.

During and after pubescence the libidinal impulses of both the male and the female human reach out for sexual fulfillment. For some in adolescence and adulthood, this fulfillment finds expression only in the erotic and self-asserting aspects of sexuality. Such sexual expression can simply be called lust. It carries no concern for one's partner and treats the partner purely as a sex object, without other value. Lust precludes any consideration for the sexual needs of the partner.

More usually, the primal libidinal sex drive is modified by human feelings of affection and mutual concern. Erotic fulfillment is achieved in a love relationship. The definition of love is elusive. In most simple and practical terms it can be described as a positive emotional attachment to another person. Thus, love is a variable quality which comes in a great many forms. It may have one or many objects. It may be weak or strong. Its essential characteristics are that it is positive, it is interpersonal, it is caring.

Social control of libidinal expression

Society has been concerned with the expression of libidinal drives since the dawn of history. Since parenthood is an essential building block of the family, and since sexual activity is essential to reproduction, it is not at all surprising that there have always been social controls on sexual expression. Some of these controls are legal; incest (sexual intercourse between persons who are closely related by blood, such as a father and daughter) has been prohibited by law in many cultures of the world, for example. Most social control of sexual expression has an even more compelling power than the force of law, however. Cultures control sexual behavior through the establishment of ethical *norms,* social notions of what is right and good. These norms, which are taught to us almost from the time we are born, are a powerful means of controlling behavior. It is worthy of note that cultural norms with regard to sexual behavior vary a great deal.

Traditionally, American society has sanctioned the fulfillment of libidinal impulses in sexual expression only within certain rather narrow limits. Sexual intercourse has been approved only in monogamous marriage (marriage between one man and one woman). It is assumed that love exists between the partners in such a marriage. Thus, good or right or approved fulfillment of the libidinal drive is socially defined as sexual expression within the context of a deep interpersonal commitment.

This norm has always been violated by some individuals of both sexes in American society. Recently, it appears that more people are engaging in sexual expression, including sexual intercourse, outside of marriage.[1] People also seem increasingly willing to be open about this sexual expression and to approve of it in others. However, the norm still shows its influence in that more people approve of sexual relationships in which love or strong affection exists between the partners than of relationships which are simply expressions of lust (Table 4.1). Social approval for libidinal expression continues to have a strong influence on our notions of what is right and good in sexual behavior.

*Table 4.1 Approval of petting and full sexual relations**

	Adults		Students	
	For males	*For females*	*For males*	*For females*
Petting				
When engaged	60.8%	56.1%	85.0%	81.8%
In love	59.4	52.6	80.4	75.2
Strong affection	54.3	45.6	67.0	56.7
No affection	28.6	20.3	34.3	18.0
Full sex relations				
When engaged	19.5	16.9	52.2	44.0
In love	17.6	14.2	47.6	38.7
Strong affection	16.3	12.5	36.9	27.2
No affection	11.9	7.4	20.8	10.8
N	(1390)	(1411)	(811)	(806)

* From I. L. Reiss, *Premarital Sexual Standards in America* (Glencoe, Ill.: Free Press, 1960).

Western social attitudes toward the erotic have long been confused and inconsistent. In times when sexual expression was not an approved topic for public discussion, the erotic has taken on connotations of secrecy and shame. It has also been effectively separated from expressions of love, which were thought to be much more noble and pure than expressions of sexual desire. Thus, literary reference to sexuality in Victorian times dwelt almost exclusively with the nonerotic expression of libido. In contrast, some contemporary authors refer to sex and sexual activity in purely erotic terms, to the exclusion of the interpersonal relationships involved. These changes in literary style are indicative of

[1] K. E. Davis, "Sex on Campus: Is There a Revolution?" *Medical Aspects of Human Sexuality* (January, 1971), pp. 128–42.

Sexual enjoyment

Although good sex grows out of a good relationship, that is not to say that you can't enjoy sex with someone you only recently met. You can, and those who say you can't are still under the influence of those Victorian myths.... The idea that sex without love is destructive, alienating and unpleasurable is a purely cultural evaluation much akin to the idea that sex is dirty. Anyone knows that sex with love is best, but that doesn't necessarily mean that any other kind or degree of sexual involvement is wrong, debasing, or the result of neuroses. Sex can be, and is, enjoyed with varying amounts of affection, warmth, comradeship. It may not be as rewarding, fulfilling or rich an experience as sex with love but it can still be enjoyable, exciting and generally life-enhancing....

Yet sex need not always be a profound experience. There are many other dimensions to sex, and all can be enjoyed. It can be fun or serious, exploratory or comfortably humdrum, it can be creative and tender, or casual and teasing; it can be passionate, exotic, erotic or just plain lustfully abandoned. And above all it can be playful, as (Abraham) Maslow here describes it: "It is quite characteristic of self-actualizing people that they can enjoy themselves in love and sex. Sex very frequently becomes a kind of game in which laughter is quite as common as panting ... It is not the welfare of the species, or the task of reproduction, or the future development of mankind that attracts people to each other. The sex life of healthy people, in spite of the fact that it frequently reaches great peaks of ecstasy, is nevertheless also easily compared to the games of children and puppies. It is cheerful, humorous and playful."

Nena and George O'Neill, *Open Marriage: A New Life Style for Couples* (New York: Avon Books, 1972), pp. 249–51.

changes in social attitudes toward eroticism. Neither represents a desirable balance, and each mirrors some confusion in sexual values, a confusion that has prevailed in spite of our current openness about sexual matters.

In today's society there can be no doubt that sex, and in particular the erotic component of sex, is exploited in literature, in theater, in commerce, and even in politics. The contemporary view seems to be that erotic pleasure is good and should be enjoyed. The enjoyment of eroticism takes a variety of forms in contemporary culture. It includes the voyeuristic pleasure of watching explicitly sexual cinema. It also includes new understanding of healthy patterns of sexual arousal and response in both men and women. The fact that patterns of sexual arousal and response can be studied and discussed today represents in itself a profound degree of social change.

HUMAN SEXUAL RESPONSE

Arousal

The sex drive in males and females is equal. Contrary to nineteenth-century Victorian opinion, women have a libido which is as powerful as that of men. The stimuli that cause sexual arousal in women may be different from those that cause arousal in men and the speed of response may be different, but the need for sexual expression and release is of equal potency in both sexes.

Frequency of sexual arousal has great individual variability and is age and gender related. A pubescent boy has a very short or nonexistent refractory period (the state of temporary resistance to sexual stimulation following orgasm) and is capable of almost instantaneous erection. He may experience very frequent arousal leading to several orgasms a day. These are usually achieved by masturbation or nocturnal emission. A middle-aged man typically has a refractory period of hours and a much slower response to sexual stimulus. He may have much less frequent arousal, perhaps only a few times a month. In women the pattern is quite different. Response to sexual stimulus is much slower to develop in young women than in young men. It becomes quicker, more intense, and more frequent in most women as they approach middle age and after they have borne children.

Arousal derives from many sources in both males and females. The social conditioning of boys and girls does much to determine what the adult individual finds sexually arousing. Psychological factors such as the presence or absence of affection or guilt are important, as are such physical factors as fatigue and state of health. Many other conditions operate to modify arousal stimuli, including time of day, place, weather, odors, and the physical appearance of the sexual partner.

The initial arousal usually derives from a look, a gesture, or a word. It typically begins in a subtle and nonvolitional way and progresses to more direct expression of desire and affection. Such expression may be verbal or nonverbal and takes as many forms as there are couples. Successful arousal techniques include a whole range of behaviors through which lovers express their mutual endearment, desire, and pleasure.

Arousal stimuli, if sufficiently potent and not inhibited, lead to sexual excitation, the first stage of physiological sexual response. While the experience of sexual intercourse will be described here primarily in physiological terms, it should be recognized that the sex act is far more than a physiological event. It is an event which involves the whole individual, psychologically as well as physically.

The events of the sexual response cycle are analogous (parallel) in the male and the female, although certain physiological changes occur somewhat differently. In both sexes, the response can be divided into four phases: *excitement, plateau, orgasmic,* and *resolution.*

The sexual response cycle

EXCITEMENT PHASE Depending on the type of stimulus causing arousal, the first, or excitement, phase of sexual response may be quite brief or prolonged. Sexual excitation may be lost because of interruption, fear, or anxiety during this phase, or it may be partially lost and then regained. The initial stimulus may be simply a thought, a visual image, or direct stimulation of sensitive tissues.

The most obvious feature of this phase in the male is the erection of the penis. Penile erectile tissue becomes engorged with blood, causing the organ to stiffen and rise upward from its pendulous position. It greatly increases both in length and diameter. The testes are elevated toward the perineum as the excitement stage progresses. The scrotal sac tightens and wrinkles at first; if the excitement phase is prolonged, it later relaxes and then tightens again.

Figure 4.3. The male pelvic region during the sexual response cycle. The figure on the left shows the genitalia in an unexcited state, with the size and position of organs and tissues in the excitement and plateau phases indicated by dotted lines. The figure on the right shows the genitalia in the orgasmic phase, with changes in the resolution phase indicated by dotted lines.

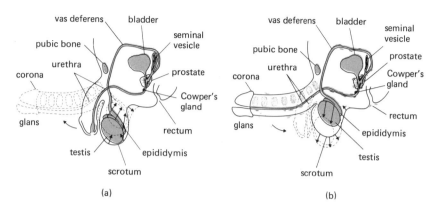

Parallel physiological responses occur in the female almost immediately after the onset of the excitement stage, usually within thirty seconds after the stimulus has begun. The vagina shows evidence of the accumulation of thin mucoid substance on its walls and a color change from red to purple. The clitoris, containing erectile tissue, becomes engorged with blood and slightly swollen, although this is not always obvious to the observer. The labia minora become congested, and the labia majora flatten and separate slightly.

Figure 4.4. The female pelvic region during the sexual response cycle. The figure on the left shows organs and tissues in an unexcited state. The figure on the right shows changes in the size and position of organs and tissue during the excitement and plateau phases, with organ positions during orgasm indicated by dotted lines.

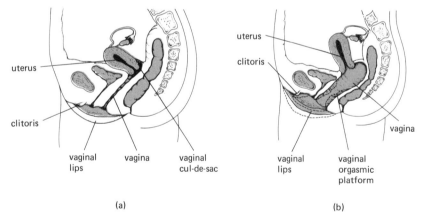

In addition to these genital changes, a number of other responses occur in the excitement phase that are common to men and women. The sex flush, a transient measleslike rash, may begin to appear, especially over the abdomen but sometimes on the neck, face, and chest as well. It is usually more prominent and more extensive in women than in men, but certainly not universal or consistent in either sex. Nipple erection may occur in both sexes although it is usually prominent in the female and occurs early. Later in the excitement phase the pigmented area around the nipple of the female (the areola) also becomes engorged, and the breasts themselves become larger because of engorgement. Blood pressure and pulse increase in both sexes, and there is a general increase in muscle tension as the phase progresses.

PLATEAU PHASE In the plateau phase, many of the excitement stage reactions progress to a more pronounced degree. In the male, the penis undergoes further minor changes with the outer edge of the glans becoming somewhat more engorged. Small glands along the urethra secrete a few drops of clear mucus. The testes also become engorged and may increase their size by half late in the plateau phase. They are also drawn up close to the perineum (preparatory for orgasm) by further increases in the general muscular tone late in this phase.

In the female, the vaginal color becomes a deeper purple. The expansion of the upper portions of the vagina progresses as its lower third shrinks remarkably in diameter. The congestion in this lower third of the vagina, combined with progressive congestion in the labia minora and contraction of vaginal muscles, has been called the orgasmic platform. The Bartholin glands may secrete a small amount of mucoid fluid during the plateau phase. The clitoris at this phase exhibits a constant and unusual phenomenon: it retracts under the clitoral hood, withdrawing from its usual overhanging position until, in some cases, it is reduced to less than half its normal length. The vagina lengthens and expands, and while this is happening the uterus is pulled upward into the abdomen by slowly increasing vascular congestion, causing a ballooning effect in the inner (upper) two-thirds of the vagina.

Restless body movements are associated with a gradually increasing muscular tension. As the muscular tension mounts in both sexes there may be strong muscular contractions in the face around the mouth, the muscles of the neck, and the abdomen. It is not unusual for muscle cramps, called carpo-pedal spasm, to occur in the hands and feet. The blood pressure and the pulse may persist in their previous elevations or be a bit more intense. Late in the plateau phase an increased rate of respiration (hyperventilation) begins. If the level of excitement is high, thrusting movements of the pelvis become involuntary, and the hands may undergo involuntary grasping and clutching motions. In those who have it, the sex flush progresses and reaches its peak.

ORGASMIC PHASE Orgasm in the male is associated with ejaculation, the involuntary expulsion of semen through the urethra. The increased muscular tension of the late plateau phase is but slightly exaggerated. A sudden increase in the diameter of the urethral bulb is the signal that orgasm is about to occur. Smooth muscle contractions occur in the vas deferens, the seminal vesicles, and in the prostate, emptying those organs of their products and secretions. The involuntary thrusting becomes associated with strong contractions of the muscles of the pelvic floor which propel the ejaculate. These contractions occur at intervals of about 0.8 seconds. The first few are very forceful, but the vigor of them rapidly decreases. The muscles of the rectal sphincter likewise undergo a few involuntary contractions at a similar interval.

The orgasmic phase in the female is characterized by a series of strong involuntary contractions in the lower third of the vagina. These occur at intervals of 0.8 seconds at the inception of orgasm, but the later contractions of the series may be somewhat further apart. There may be a few to a dozen such contractions. Uterine contractions also occur.

Abdomen, hands, feet, arms, legs, face, and neck may all be involved in intense contractions. (Some people in whom orgasmic reaction is unusually intense complain of subsequent muscular aches and pains.) The sex flush (if it was present in the previous phase) persists through orgasm; its intensity is said to be greatest when orgasmic sensation is greatest. Blood pressure, pulse, and respiration increase greatly.

RESOLUTION PHASE Immediately following orgasm, the penis undergoes a partial decrease in size and rigidity very rapidly. Then it decreases more slowly, the length of time needed to return to pre-excitational softness depending on several variables such as the type and duration of excitational and plateau stimulation and the persistence or absence of resolution phase stimulation. Maintaining postorgasmic coital contact will delay penile softening; engaging in nonsexual activity such as reading or watching television will hasten it.

The resolution phase in the male is associated with a refractory period during which the individual is incapable of responding to further or renewed sexual stimulation. This refractory period is of indeterminate length and shows a great deal of variability. It may last from a few minutes to a few hours in normal individuals, and increases with age.

Unlike the male, the female has no definable refractory period. Many women can, with continued stimulation, have multiple orgasms, moving from orgasm to plateau without an intervening phase of resolution or excitation. During the resolution phase the labia minora and majora quickly return to their normal state. The vagina resumes its resting shape, and the uterus resumes its normal size and position, usually within half an hour. The areolae, then the nipples, and next the breasts lose their congestion. The breasts usually return to normal within ten minutes. The clitoris resumes its normal position within a few seconds of the time of the last orgasmic contraction, although it may maintain vasocongestion for many minutes.

PATTERNS OF SEXUAL ACTIVITY

There is no one, single, normal form of sexual activity. Although some sex behaviors are unusual, this does not mean that they are abnormal, nor does it imply that they are wrong. Ethical judgments vary, as noted above, according to cultural and individual norms. Any sex behavior that is mutually enjoyable, expresses affection, hurts no one, and is not offensive to an unwilling observer could be considered "normal."[2] There

[2] James Leslie McCary, *Human Sexuality*, 2d ed. (New York: D. Van Nostrand, 1973), p. 162.

simply are no objective criteria that are accepted by all cultures for determining whether a given sexual behavior is normal or abnormal. What is usual in one period of time or in one society may be quite unusual in another. The fact that many people are ready to brand any sexual behavior that is unfamiliar to them as "perverted" simply indicates their ignorance and, perhaps, the intensity of their feelings about this subject.

At the same time, there are some sexual practices that are felt to be unhealthy by most people in our culture. One criterion that can be applied to determine whether a sexual behavior is healthy or not is the degree to which the behavior is motivated by feelings of affection, as suggested by Judd Marmor:

> In our culture, a key distinguishing factor between what is regarded as healthy or unhealthy sexual behavior is whether such behavior is motivated by feelings of love or whether it becomes a vehicle for the discharge of anxiety, hostility, or guilt. Healthy sexuality seeks erotic pleasure in the context of tenderness and affection; pathologic sexuality is motivated by needs for reassurance or relief from nonsexual sources of tension. Healthy sexuality seeks both to give and to receive pleasure; neurotic forms are unbalanced toward excessive giving or taking. Healthy sexuality is discriminating as to partner; neurotic patterns often tend to be nondiscriminating.[3]

Sexual activity is a peculiarly benign and pleasurable form of human recreation. Healthy sexual behavior includes an almost infinite variety of activities, and there is no danger of excessive activity since sexual behavior is effectively limited by fatigue in both sexes, by vaginal and sometimes muscular soreness in the female, and by the refractory period in the male. Although monogamous marriage is the socially legitimatized vehicle for sexual expression and heterosexual marital coitus the most accepted method of achieving sexual gratification in our culture, these are not by any means exclusive ways of satisfying sexual needs. Several alternative styles of sexual activity exist and are widely practiced.

Heterosexual activity

COITAL Sexual intercourse between a man and a woman, which is called *heterosexual coitus*, remains the most universally practiced method of sexual expression. There seems to be no immediate prospect of a change in the popularity of this activity; contemporary men and women still show as great an interest in it as did the last several generations of humans. Indeed, our species' survival depends on its enduring popularity.

Heterosexual coitus includes a wide range of possible techniques and positions which are subject to multiple variations. Serious students

[3] Judd Marmor, " 'Normal' and 'Deviant' Sexual Behavior," *Journal of the American Medical Association* 217 (1971): 165–70.

Sexual myths (and the facts)

A large penis is necessary to a woman's sexual gratification.
(Since the vagina has very few nerve endings, penile size has no physiological bearing on a woman's satisfaction in intercourse.)

Sexual intercourse should be avoided during pregnancy and menstruation.
(There is no physiological reason to avoid intercourse until the last weeks of pregnancy; intercourse during menstruation may be beneficial in relieving menstrual cramping and is, in any case, not harmful.)

The amount of hair on a man's body is an indication of his virility.
(Sexual performance in both men and women depends more upon psychological factors than it does on anything physiological.)

Abortion, whether legal or criminal, is always dangerous.
(Abortion under sterile surgical conditions is statistically safer than childbirth.)

Masturbation is a habit of immature young men that may lead to acne, warts on the hands, lunacy, or impotence.
(Masturbation is commonly practiced by both men and women all of their lives and is quite harmless.)

People suffering from sexual problems such as impotence or frigidity can expect little help with their problems.
(Most people who seek counseling for sexual problems achieve relief of those problems.)

Today's young people are going wild sexually.
(Adults have been complaining about the sexual permissiveness of young people for at least two thousand years.)

of the subject have cataloged hundreds of ways to copulate. We will make no effort here to duplicate such a list or to provide an illustrative catalog. The intercourse techniques a couple develops are largely dependent upon personality, social standards, emotional maturity, and physical characteristics. Whatever forms their expression may take should be enjoyed, not subjected to laboratory analysis. However, when difficulties are encountered in achieving sexual satisfaction in intercourse, counseling should be sought.

NONCOITAL Noncoital heterosexual activity, sexually oriented physical contact between a man and a woman that does not involve actual copulation, is the traditional rite of mate selection in our culture. Parenthetically, there seems to be no reason to place more confidence in this method of mate selection than in other methods which are used by other cultures, although it is a ritual greatly enjoyed by the participants. The rite usually begins in heterosexual dating, where it progresses through such intermediate steps as hand-holding, kissing, necking, petting, "heavy" petting, and even mutual masturbation or extragenital coitus. The pattern is usually a progressive one with limits determined by such factors as the age of the couple, the degree of their interpersonal commitment, their personal standards of conduct, and the norms of the community. Noncoital activity often develops gradually into coital activity as the individuals and their relationship mature. It is sometimes difficult to define the exact division between noncoital and coital activity. Within marriage, noncoital sexual stimulation, such as orogenital or manual manipulation, is now recognized to be widely (and by many happily) practiced. Such activity is not considered perverse or abnormal so long as it is pleasurable and inoffensive to both participants.

Premarital coitus may or may not be more common today than it was ten years ago, but it is certainly more admissible and more discussable. There is less social censure associated with it, and there is remarkably less fear of undesired pregnancy because of the widespread availability of effective contraceptives (see Chap. 20).

Nevertheless, a very significant case for chastity is still present today. Premarital sexual intimacies carry with them a significant risk of infection with venereal disease (see Chap. 10). The risk is directly proportional to the degree of promiscuity prevalent in a social group. While most venereal disease is easily treated, its consequences are sometimes devastating to future fertility and to self-esteem. In many individuals premarital sexual intercourse is also a violation of learned patterns of ethical behavior and carries the penalty of anxiety and guilt. Personal, parental, religious, and social standards cannot be violated with impunity. The cost is often much greater than the reward.

It is certainly not true that advanced levels of noncoital heterosexual expression, such as mutual masturbation, or premarital coitus are universally approved in our culture. There is a great deal of variety in

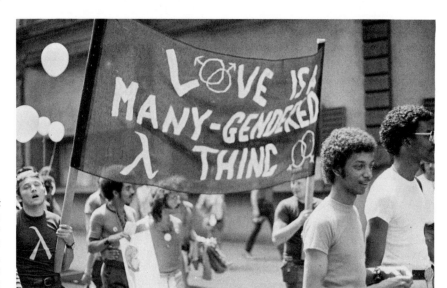

Figure 4.5. Some laws against homosexuality have recently been repealed, and repressive law enforcement against homosexuals has been relaxed in some areas. (Howard Petrick, Nancy Palmer Photo Agency)

norms within different communities and among different individuals. In spite of our openness about sex, individuals must still take responsibility for deciding what levels of sexual expression are appropriate and healthy for them in any given relationship.

Homosexual activity

Homosexuality is defined as a fixed pattern of adult sexual activity with a person of the same sex. Relatively few adults, approximately 4 percent

Sigmund Freud: letter to an American mother

April 9, 1935

Dear Mrs. X

I gather from your letter that your son is a homosexual. I am most impressed by the fact that you do not mention this term yourself in your information about him. May I question you, why do you avoid it? Homosexuality is assuredly no advantage, but it is nothing to be ashamed of, no vice, no degradation, it cannot be classified as an illness; we consider it to be a variation of the sexual function produced by a certain arrest of sexual development. Many highly respectable individuals of ancient and modern times have been homosexuals, several of the greatest men among them (Plato, Michelangelo, Leonardo da Vinci,

etc.). It is a great injustice to persecute homosexuality as a crime, and cruelty too. If you do not believe me, read the books of Havelock Ellis.

By asking me if I can help, you mean, I suppose, if I can abolish homosexuality and make normal heterosexuality take its place. The answer is, in a general way, we cannot promise to achieve it. In a certain number of cases we succeed in developing the blighted germs of heterosexual tendencies which are present in every homosexual, in the majority of cases it is no more possible. It is a question of the quality and the age of the individual. The result of the treatment cannot be predicted.

What analysis can do for your son runs in a different line. If he is unhappy, neurotic, torn by con-

flicts, inhibited in social life, analysis may bring him harmony, peace of mind, full efficiency, whether he remains a homosexual or gets changed. If you make up your mind he should have analysis with me (I don't expect you will!!) he has to come over to Vienna. I have no intention of leaving here. However, don't neglect to give me your answer.

Sincerely   yours   with   kind wishes,   Freud

P.S. I did not find it difficult to read your handwriting. Hope you will not find my writing and my English a harder task.

Sigmund Freud, "Letter to an American Mother," *American Journal of Psychiatry* 107 (1951), pp. 786–87. Copyright 1951 by the American Psychiatric Association.

of males and 3 percent of females, remain exclusively homosexual all of their adult lives, but many persons have had at least some degree of homosexual interest or activity at one or more times in their lives (Table 4.2). In some this behavior has been a transient adolescent activity. Others show an alternating pattern of sexual preference in their adult lives, engaging in both heterosexual and homosexual behavior; this is called *bisexuality.*

Table 4.2 Percentages of homosexual and heterosexual experience in young adults, ages 20–35*

Experience	In females	In males
Entirely heterosexual experience		
Single	61–72%	53–78%
Married	89–90	90–92
At least some homosexual experience	11–20	18–42
More than incidental homosexual experience	6–14	13–38
As much or more homosexual experience		
than heterosexual experience	4–11	9–32
Mostly homosexual experience	3–8	7–26
Almost exclusively homosexual experience	2–6	5–22
Exclusively homosexual experience	1–3	3–16

* From data in A. C. Kinsey *et al, Sexual Behavior in the Human Female* (Philadelphia: Saunders, 1953), p. 488.

Homosexuality is variance from what is usually accepted as normal sexual behavior in our culture. While not considered socially normal, homosexuality cannot be clearly defined as an illness. Its causes are obscure, and it is frequently associated with unhappy lives. Homosexuals are often subjected to cruel social discrimination and unkind ridicule.

Sexual gratification among homosexuals is derived from embrace, body contact, manual stimulation, and orogenital or anogenital copulation. The sexual relationships established by male homosexuals often are of short duration; this implies a degree of promiscuity and increases the danger of venereal infection. Female homosexuals, on the other hand, tend to develop relationships of somewhat longer duration.

Society has in the recent past treated homosexuals rather severely, but it has not always been so. In ancient Greece, for example, homosexuality was considered quite acceptable. Currently some laws against homosexuality have been repealed, and repressive law enforcement against homosexuals has been relaxed in some areas. With greater understanding of the nature of homosexuality, further progress along these lines can be anticipated.

Autosexual activity

When sexual arousal occurs in a solitary individual, the event is described as *autosexual.* No other person is involved, and there are no considerations of interpersonal commitment or affection. Autosexuality is an erotic event that is directed at the self. Such events are common and perfectly normal in most circumstances for both sexes at all ages. They are almost universal in occurrence.

MASTURBATION *Masturbation* is any type of autostimulation which is applied to evoke a sexual response in one's self. In males this is usually accomplished by manual stroking of the shaft of the penis with or without lubrication. Women may use a variety of techniques including manual or digital manipulation to stimulate the clitoris directly or indirectly, rhythmic motion of the thighs, and insertion of a finger or foreign body into the vagina with rhythmic motion. Whatever the method, the stimulation can be carried forward to a satisfactory orgasm.

Masturbation is frequently practiced by most adolescent boys. It is also common in young girls, although perhaps not as frequent as in boys. This sexual behavior is clearly harmless despite much that has been written by theologians and physicians of a generation or two ago. It may indeed be of some value psychologically in helping one to learn about his or her own likes and dislikes in sexual stimulation. It can be considered a symptom of disturbance only if it becomes a compulsive form of behavior that interferes with normal activities.

Sexual fantasy usually accompanies masturbation. It is perfectly normal so long as it does not inhibit an individual from also seeking interpersonal forms of sexual expression.

NOCTURNAL ORGASM When other forms of sexual expression are denied or when the need for erotic expression is great, most people, young and old, have dreams of intense erotic content. These sometimes terminate in orgasm. In males, the orgasm produces ejaculation of seminal fluid, thus the common name for noctural orgasm—"wet dream." Women as well as men have this sort of dream. Since there is no ejaculatory evidence, many women forget the noctural orgasm in a relatively short time. The lower incidence of reported erotic dreams leading to nocturnal orgasm in women is therefore somewhat suspect. Perhaps unfortunately, these dreams have a tendency to terminate just short of orgasm for both men and women.

Nocturnal orgasm like the dream process itself is entirely involuntary. Adolescents in whom this phenomenon may be very frequent sometimes feel guilt, anxiety, or shame after experiencing erotic dreams. This is indeed unfortunate. Such individuals should be reassured that the event is physiologically and psychologically healthy.

SEXUAL HYGIENE For both males and females, normal bathing at reasonable intervals is all that is required for the maintenance of genital hygiene under usual circumstances. In our culture sexual attractiveness has been so popularized that we all think of it as essential and many of us suffer from some anxiety about our sexual desirability. It is highly dependent on personal cleanliness and the freedom from offensive odors, which are likely to accumulate with any prolonged abstention from soap and water. It is not dependent on the substitution of aromas in spite of all the advertisements designed to play on our anxieties. Cosmetics, perfumes, perineal sprays, and powders do little if anything to substitute for bathing; in the genital area they may do harm.

Males

Circumcision of infant males is and has been widely practiced in our culture for the last quarter of a century. This surgical procedure involves the removal of the foreskin, the prepuce, of the penis. While the universal desirability of infant circumcision is doubtful, it must be said that it simplifies the maintenance of cleanliness in the male. Smegma, a white cheesy substance which is a waste product of genital skin, accumulates under the prepuce and behind the glans on the penis of uncircumcised males (Fig. 4.6). Such men must retract the prepuce at each bathing and carefully wash the accumulated smegma away. Circumcision obviates the need for this special care, since the smegma does not accumulate behind the circumcised glans. In some uncircumcised men the retraction of the prepuce may be difficult or impossible and may require the attention of a physician.

A slight amount of clear mucoid discharge from the penis after sexual excitation is usual and normal. This glandular secretion is not accompanied by pain. The occurrence of urethral pain, pain on urination, or a cloudy discharge is abnormal and requires a doctor's attention, as does any sore on the genitalia.

Men should perform self-examination of the testicles from time to time, in order to detect any abnormal swellings or tumors. The testicles are smooth, relatively firm, and should be of nearly equal size. Because of a peculiarity of human anatomy, the left testicle almost always hangs somewhat lower than the right; this should cause no alarm. A marked disparity of size or an increased hardness of one testicle signals the need for a physician.

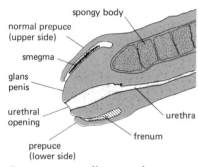

Figure 4.6. A collection of smegma under the prepuce of the penis.

Females

Unless special attention is applied to remove it, smegma may accumulate under the clitoral margins or between the labia minora and majora. It is best removed by careful bathing of the external genitalia, paying attention to the fold between the labia and very gently retracting the prepuce to bathe the clitoris.

There is normally a small amount of clean white discharge from the vagina each day. This is a natural mechanism of vaginal cleansing. It should simply be bathed away from the external genitalia.

Douching is a washing of the vagina with a quantity of liquid delivered by a very low pressure stream into the upper vagina. If properly done, douching is not harmful and in some women enhances a feeling of security about personal cleanliness. Under ordinary circumstances, however, douching is simply not necessary. Unless there is a vaginal infection present, the vaginal secretions do not cause any odor until they have accumulated on the external genitalia for several hours, and external bathing solves that problem adequately.

A variety of non-venereal vaginal infections can occur. They require special attention and a prescription (see Chap. 10). One of these is an infestation with a very common protozoan organism, *Trichomonas vaginalis*. This is a benign but bothersome infection which causes a profuse thin discharge, sometimes slightly itchy, with a bad odor. Another is infection with *Candida albicans*, a yeast. This organism causes little discharge, but it produces an intense itching and burning of the vagina and vulva. It is characterized by a yeasty odor. Both of these illnesses are easily treated and need not cause prolonged suffering. Since the organisms that cause these infections may be transmitted to and carried by the male, it is essential that men who have had sexual intercourse with infected women also be treated.

Questions
1. Describe the development of libidinal expression from early childhood to adulthood.
2. What are the traditional American norms with regard to sexual expression?
3. Briefly outline the major physiological changes that occur in the male and in the female during each of the four phases of the sexual response cyle.
4. List and briefly describe the common forms of sexual activity.
5. Name two symptoms of the male genitalia and two symptoms of the female genitalia that require a doctor's attention.

Key Concepts
Heterosexuality – sexual attraction to, or sexual activity with, members of the opposite sex

Homosexuality – sexual attraction to, or sexual activity with, members of the same sex

Libido – the erotic and creative drive in the human species

Norm – a social standard of right behavior

Refractory period – the state of temporary resistance to sexual stimulation following orgasm

Sexual response cycle – the four stages of human response to sexual stimulation: the excitement phase, the plateau phase, the orgasmic phase, and the resolution phase

Selected Readings
Comfort, Alex, *The Joy of Sex*. New York: Crown, 1972.

Hettlinger, Richard F., *Living With Sex: The Student's Dilemma*. London: Seabury, 1967.

Masters, W. H. and V. E. Johnson, *Human Sexual Response*. Boston: Little, Brown, 1966.

McCary, James Leslie, *Human Sexuality*, 2d ed. New York: D. Van Nostrand, 1973.

O'Neill, Nena and George O'Neill. *Open Marriage: A New Life Style for Couples*. New York: Avon Books, 1972.

Chapter 5

Nutrition

Nutrition is the science that deals with the effects of food on the body. Because good food is necessary not only for survival but also for health and because a diet low or missing in certain components, such as vitamins, can cause grave diseases, nutrition is an important component of public health. The science of nutrition deals with the study and treatment of diseases due to deficiencies and as such it is a part of medicine. Inasmuch as it deals with the digestion of food, the excretion of the residues, and the role of nutrients, it is also part of physiology. The study of the chemical reactions in the body through which food is utilized makes nutrition close to biochemistry.

Nutrition has progressed considerably since the French chemist and physiologist Antoine Lavoisier first started measuring the needs of the body for chemical (food) energy in the 1770s. We now know not only how much food the body needs (as we shall see, this need is usually expressed in calories) but how much of several types of nutrients is needed or usable. Yet nutrition is not a "finished" science. We are constantly discovering new facts, such as the need for additional *trace minerals* (elements needed in tiny amounts) or additional roles in the chemistry of the body—called its *metabolism*—for those nutrients which we do know to be required.

Nutrition is a science central to human life, and one which in turn is very close to a number of other professions. Nutritionists are interested in community food programs for feeding patients in hospitals, elderly people in nursing homes or "golden age" programs, and children in schools and orphanages. They are interested in new foods, such as those used in space exploration, those derived from algae, and chemically synthesized foods. In their endeavors, nutritionists are close to food technologists (those interested in the processing of foods), home economists (those interested in the management and preparation of foods), chemists (those who make new foods from oil and other raw material), dietitians (those who feed special groups such as hospital patients), and nutrition educators (those who teach sound food habits).

NUTRITIONAL NEEDS

We need to eat for three general purposes: (1) to obtain the energy necessary to keep our bodies warm and our organs functioning and to enable us to move and work; (2) to obtain the substances needed to extract energy out of foods and to utilize these foods; and (3) to obtain the materials necessary to replace parts of the body and to permit growth. *Nutrients* are the components of foods which the body uses to fulfill these three purposes.

From the moment food enters the mouth, digestion, which converts the food into products that can be assimilated by the body, begins. The act of chewing itself begins the breakdown. Saliva starts the conversion by changing starch into maltose, a form of sugar. The process is continued in the stomach by gastric juice which begins to digest the food proteins. Through the small and large intestines the digestion of sugars, starches, fats, and proteins continues as the body, by an exceedingly complex series of activities, separates out from the food usable and unusable substances, transferring the usable ones to the intestinal cells and from there to the blood and the lymph vessels. Unusable products are sent to the colon to be excreted.

Metabolism, however, does not take place solely in the gastrointestinal tract. It goes on throughout the body, involving every cell of the body at every moment of the day.

Important in the digestive process are organic compounds, called *enzymes*, that exist in all parts of the body. There are thousands of different enzymes, and each one has a specific function to perform. All enzymes are proteins or combinations of proteins, vitamins, and minerals, and they all act as *catalysts:* they make a chemical reaction happen that would not happen at all, or would happen very slowly, without them. While the enzymes facilitate such reactions, they are not changed by them. But a certain amount of each enzyme is destroyed every day, and new ones must be formed from newly ingested nutrients.

The total amounts of energy and the various types of nutrients each individual needs depend on a number of factors:

SIZE Other things being equal, a large person requires more food than a small person. For some nutrients, such as vitamin A, the need is proportional to the body size: if one person is twice as large as another, the need for the nutrient will be twice as great. In other cases, as with total food energy (measured in Calories), the need increases with body size but not proportionately. If a person is twice as large as another, he will need close to one and a half times as much food, not twice as much.

TEMPERATURE More food is needed when the outside temperature is low because more energy is then required to keep the body at a constant temperature. The requirement for nutrients needed to utilize this extra food to produce the extra energy will also be increased.

WORK When a person does physical work or exercises, he or she expends more energy (considerably more energy if the work or the exercise is hard) than when he or she is resting.

GROWTH Pound for pound, children need more energy and more of the vitamins needed to free this energy from food than adults. They also need more protein (for new tissues), more iron (for new blood), more calcium (for new bones), and generally more of every nutrient than do grown-ups. Pregnant women as well need more energy, more proteins, more vitamins, and more minerals to provide nourishment for the baby growing inside the womb. Similarly, once the baby is born, more food and nutrients are needed for the mother's body to manufacture milk.

Energy

In order to maintain our body structure and temperature, to digest our food and keep our heart pumping and, in general, to keep all the body functions going, and to work, play, grow, and reproduce we need energy. Energy is provided by the oxidation (combination with the oxygen of air) of our foods and specifically of three kinds of nutrients: carbohydrates, fats, and proteins.

The energy contained in foods is measured in units known as *Calories*. Throughout this chapter the word *calorie* is written two ways. When a lowercase *c* is used, the word is simply a noun of general reference, like protein or carbohydrate. When Calorie appears with a capital *C*, it represents a precise metabolic measurement: a kilocalorie. A Calorie is the amount of energy equivalent to the heat needed to elevate the temperature of one liter of water (approximately one quart) by one degree centigrade (1.8 degrees Fahrenheit). One gram (one ounce is approximately 28 grams) of carbohydrate yields four Calories when utilized by the body. One gram of fat yields nine Calories. One gram of protein yields four Calories. Examples of calorie requirements for persons of various sizes, ages, sexes, and occupations are given in Tables 5.1 and 5.2.

*Table 5.1 Samples of caloric requirements per day for people of different sexes, ages, and activities living in different climates**

1. A twenty-five-year-old, 154-pound house painter in Minneapolis (mean annual temperature is 50° F.)

Activity	Calories
Working Activity (10 hours)	
8 hours standing and painting (3 Cal./min.)	1,450
2 hours gardening or sports (5 Cal./min.)	600
Non-occupational Activity (6 hours)	
1 hour washing, dressing, etc. (2.5 Cal./min.)	150
4 hours driving, sitting, etc. (1.7 Cal./min.)	400
1 hour domestic work (3.5 Cal./min.)	200
Rest in Bed	500
Total	3,300

2. A fifty-three-year-old, 132-pound housewife in Minneapolis

Working Activity (8 hours)	
Domestic work (1.9 Cal./min.)	910
Non-occupational Activity (8 hours)	
1 hour washing, dressing, etc. (2 Cal./min.)	120
1 hour shopping and driving (1.8 Cal./min.)	100
6 hours sitting (1.3 Cal./min.)	470
Rest in Bed	400
Total	2,000

3. A 21-year-old, 121-pound woman with a newborn baby in northern California (mean annual temperature is 68° F)

Working Activity (10 hours)	
Domestic work, care of baby, etc. (2 Cal./min.)	1,200
Non-occupational Activity (6 hours)	
1 hour washing, dressing, etc. (2 Cal./min.)	120
1 hour walking at 3 mph. and shopping (3.2 Cal./min.)	200
2 hours playing golf or gardening (3.0 Cal./min.)	360
2 hours sitting (1.2 Cal./min.)	140
Rest in Bed	400
Lactation allowances (600–700 cc. milk)	800
Total	3,220

* Jean Mayer, *Overweight: Causes, Cost, and Control,* © 1968. By permission of Prentice-Hall, Inc., Englewood Cliffs, N. J.

Table 5.2 Caloric cost of various activities*
(Over and above resting metabolism)

Activity	Calories per Hour
A. Domestic Occupations	
(WOMEN, 120 LBS.)	
Sitting at rest	15
Standing relaxed	20
Mental work	5–8
Writing	10–20
B. Physical Exercise	
(MEN, 150 LBS.)	
Walking slowly (2.6 mph)	115
Walking moderately fast (3.75 mph)	215
Walking very fast (5.3 mph)	565
Running ⎫	800–1,300
Swimming ⎪	300–1,000
Rowing ⎬ dependent on speed	1,000–1,300
Cycling ⎭	150–600
Wrestling	600–1,000

* Mayer, *Overweight*, © 1968. By permission of Prentice-Hall, Inc., Englewood Cliffs, N. J.

THE NUTRIENTS   There are six categories of nutrients that the body needs: water, carbohydrates, fats, proteins, vitamins, and minerals. Sometimes water is separated from other nutrients; we then say that the body needs water and nutrients.

Water

Water is the most important constituent of the body (55 to 70 percent by weight). Blood, which consists primarily of water, carries food and oxygen to the tissues. Cells not only contain water, *intracellular fluid*, but also exist in a liquid environment, *extracellular fluid*, a sort of internal sea not very different in composition from sea water. Food is digested with the help of many digestive fluids—saliva in the mouth, gastric juice in the stomach, pancreatic juice, bile and intestinal juice in the intestine—representing a secretion of several quarts per day. We eliminate those by-products of food utilization that our body cannot use as a liquid (urine). Finally, we keep cool in the summer through evaporation of water from the lungs and through sweating. Generous amounts of drinking fluid are necessary if all these needs are to be satisfied. Obviously, we need more water in the summer, in hot countries, or if we exercise vigorously. Even at rest in a temperate environment an adult can stay alive only for about one week without water, as compared to about five weeks without food. If the temperature is high, survival time is much shorter.

Carbohydrates

The carbohydrates are the sugars and starches. They are usually the main source of energy in the diet and, in the United States, represent about 45 percent of the diet's calories. In poor countries they may represent up to 80 percent of the calories because they are found in cheaper and more abundant foods.

The main sugar in the American diet today is sucrose, the ordinary white or, if unrefined, brown sugar. Sucrose is a *disaccharide*, that is, it is made up of two "simple" sugars (*monosaccharides*): fructose, found in fruits, and glucose. Lactose is the disaccharide found in milk; it is made up of the monosaccharides glucose and galactose. Milk and fruits obviously have more to offer than just sugar. The foods in which sucrose is the main ingredient often provide little else than calories. Starches are found in particular in cereals (bread, flour, and breakfast cereals) and in potatoes. The starches are more complex nutritionally, in that the foods which contain them also have a number of other nutrients. Their structure is more complex as well. They may contain hundreds of glucose (or exceptionally fructose) units and are thus called the *polysaccharides*.

Regardless of their initial structure, all the carbohydrates are broken down in digestion to monosaccharides; by far the most important to body metabolism is glucose. Glucose is the "blood sugar" which is absorbed from the intestine or released by the liver from the "storage" polysaccharide, glycogen. Glucose, carried by the blood to all parts of the body, is our primary source of energy. Since it is used for fuel each day, it must be replaced by the breaking down of more dietary carbohydrates. It can also be made from protein if dietary carbohydrate is not available. Glucose imparts fuels to every cell of the body and is stored as glycogen in the liver and in all the muscles including, of course, the heart. But it is even more important to the central nervous system which has a lower storage capacity. Glucose is essentially the only form of energy available to the brain. As a result, a long period of low blood sugar can cause permanent brain damage.

Fats

Fats and oils (fats which are liquid at room temperature) are another main source of energy in the American diet and represent a little more than 40 percent of its calories. Fats are often divided into visible fats, those fats and oils which we add to food, such as butter, shortenings of various types, corn oil, peanut oil, and other cooking or salad oils, and invisible fats, those that are already contained in foods, such as butterfat in nonskim milk, and the fat in meats, eggs, fish, and nuts. Except for one oil, coconut oil, fats that are liquid at room temperature seem to have a different effect inside the body than fats that are solid at about 70 degrees Fahrenheit.

Fats are made of three long molecules of fatty acids, which are made up of hydrogen, oxygen, and carbon atoms on a long chain that is attached to a molecule of glycerol (better known to many of us as glycerin). Glycerol is a short molecule with only three carbon atoms in a row, so that the structure looks rather like the prongs of a fork attached to the broad part of the fork.

The total number of hydrogen atoms the different fatty acids hold determines their appearance at room temperature. *Saturated* fatty acids contain as many hydrogen atoms as the molecule has room for; *unsaturated* fatty acids hold two less; and *polyunsaturated* fatty acids lack at least four atoms of hydrogen. The saturated fatty acids are found in the hard fats of land animals, in dairy products from these animals, and in hydrogenated vegetable fats.

The latter are originally liquid vegetable oils to which food manufacturers add hydrogen atoms to keep the product solid at room temperature. If you examine the labels of margarine and shortening, you will see that many of these products are composed of hydrogenated vegetable fats or a mixture of hydrogenated fats and vegetable oils; unsaturated and polyunsaturated fatty acids are found in vegetable oils and fish oils. The body can manufacture many of the fatty acids from carbohydrates, proteins, and other fatty acids, but the polyunsaturated fatty acids must be provided ready-made by foods, and hence they are often called *essential* fatty acids.

These facts are important because it has been established that the saturated fats we consume in foods have a marked effect on the level in our blood of a substance called *cholesterol.* Cholesterol is white, wax-like, and solid at body temperature. It is manufactured by the body and is also consumed in some foods. As we mature and age, particularly if we are physically inactive, cholesterol begins to be deposited in the arteries, narrowing them so that eventually they may be completely blocked (see Chap. 11). We do not yet understand why this happens, but we do know that dietary fats that are saturated appear to raise the blood cholesterol level and speed this process. The unsaturated fats seem to have no effect on blood cholesterol levels, while polyunsaturated fats lower cholesterol and thus retard its deposition.

Proteins

The American diet usually contains about 15 percent proteins which, as we have seen, are one of the sources of energy. Proteins are important primarily because after water they are the main constituents of all body structures—muscles, tendons, skin, and the other tissues. While an adult's body often contains more fat than proteins, proteins contribute much more to make the body what it is, for only proteins can do the essential work of repair, maintenance, and growth. There are thousands of kinds of proteins which are all made of the same twenty building blocks, the amino acids, much as the thousands of words in our language are made of the same twenty-six letters. Of the amino acids, about half can be manufactured by the body (the *nonessential* amino acids). Half are essential for animals and man because their bodies do not know how to make them. Proteins are called complete if they contain enough of all the essential amino acids so that the body can utilize them. The absence or an inadequate amount of any one of the essential amino acids (for man, there are eight) makes it impossible for the body to use the others properly. The absent or most inadequately present one is said to be "limiting." We can get complete proteins from animal sources, since the animals have already manufactured the essential amino acids for us.

Animal proteins are found in meats, fish, eggs, milk, and cheese. Vegetable proteins, those found in beans, nuts, cereals, vegetables, and fruits, are usually incomplete—that is, they have less of one or more of the essential amino acids than we need. The proteins in vegetables can be combined, however, either with small amounts of animal protein or with each other (as beans with seeds, cereals with nuts) to give a complete protein. This is done particularly in baby foods formulated for underdeveloped nations to replace milk when the infants are weaned.

Need for protein and other nutrients is usually expressed as Recommended Dietary Allowance (RDA): it is the amount which will cover requirements not just for the average individual but with a large enough margin of safety for 99 percent of all normal subjects. The RDAs for a mixture of animal and vegetable proteins typical of the American diet, for both sexes and various ages, are given in Table 5.3 (p. 124–25).

Vitamins

The body is a good chemist. It makes thousands of different kinds of substances. We have already seen that it is not a perfect chemist: it cannot manufacture some of the fatty acids nor can it make some of the amino acids. Similarly, there are some complex substances which are needed in milligrams, or even micrograms, that the body is unable to make. These are called the vitamins. Because vitamins are an essential part of many enzymes, the body has a daily requirement for them. They have to be provided by the foods we eat or by vitamin supplements for our body to function at its peak of efficiency. If there is a serious shortage of one or several vitamins, we are said to be deficient in that vitamin or vitamins and suffering from a *deficiency disease*. Extreme deficiencies are fatal. To be declared essential, a nutrient must meet two requirements: (1) a deficiency of that nutrient in an otherwise adequate diet must produce a recognizable deficiency state, and (2) supplementing the diet with that specific nutrient must cure the deficiency and bring about renewed health and growth.

Most vitamins are designated by letters of the alphabet because at one time we did not know their chemical structures and could not give them proper scientific names. Some vitamins have proved to be two or more related substances which have a similar role in the body. There are several D vitamins, for example. In some cases, a food contains a substance called a *provitamin*, which can be transformed into the vitamin itself by the body. Various carotenes—red and yellow pigments found in such foods as carrots, tomatoes, and leafy vegetables—are provitamins which are transformed into vitamin A in the body. The vitamins are usually divided into water-soluble vitamins, found in the watery parts of cells and foods, and fat-soluble vitamins, which are dissolved in fat or in the fat part of cells in foods. Because they are soluble in fat and not water, the fat-soluble vitamins can be stored in such cells as liver cells. Water-soluble vitamins, however, are either utilized within a short period or flushed out of the body in excreted fluids, principally the urine. A person who has been well-fed but for some reason is not getting enough of all vitamins will thus be depleted more rapidly of water-soluble than of fat-soluble vitamins.

The fat-soluble vitamins are A, D, E, and K. The water-soluble vitamins are the vitamins B—in particular vitamin B_1, vitamin B_2, niacin, pyridoxine, vitamin B_{12}, and folic acid—and vitamin C.

VITAMIN A Vitamin A is found in nature as the provitamin carotene in green and yellow plants and as two forms of the vitamin itself, one in fresh-water fish and land animals and the other in salt-water fish and animals. Vitamin A has a number of functions. It is essential in the growth and maintenance of epithelial tissue which comprises the skin and the covering of internal cavities (mucosa). It is also important in the harmonious development of the bones. Finally, it helps to maintain the outside of the eye, and when made into a pigment in the retina of the eye enables us to see by becoming discolored when the light strikes the retina.

VITAMIN D Fish liver oil, liver, eggs, summer butter, and milk are sources of vitamin D, which is also formed when the skin is exposed to the sun. Vitamin D is necessary for the utilization of calcium. It acts in the intestine to help the body absorb calcium and in the bones (including the teeth) to facilitate the action of both calcium and phosphorus which must cooperate to form new bone. Rickets, seldom seen in the United States, is a disease caused by a deficiency of vitamin D, which results in a fragile and malformed skeleton.

VITAMIN E A number of the important roles of vitamin E have been described in experimental animals. However, this has only been done by first producing a clear-cut vitamin E deficiency. Animals who have been made vitamin E deficient become sterile if they are males, and cannot conceive or else abort the fetuses if they are females. Vitamin E defi-

Rickets (vitamin D deficiency)

Rickets, in its severe form, is a disease which affects the whole child, not just the bones. The rachitic infant is restless and unhappy. He is usually suffering from digestive disorders; his stomach is distended, in part because his chest is deformed, in part because his abdominal muscles are flabby. This flabbiness, together with the laxness of the ligaments of the joints, often causes the limbs to be twisted into unusual postures.

Bone changes are characteristic. The earliest observed is craniotabes and skull deformities. Round or oval unossified areas are found in the skull; these yield like parchment when pressure is applied by the finger. The skull is often enlarged.

The chest also shows changes in early infancy as the ribs grow rapidly without hardening up: the sides are pulled in while the sternum is pushed out in front, striking forward like the keel of a ship or a "pigeon chest." After the age of six months, the ribs develop a beaded appearance at the junction of the bone and the cartilage ("rickety rosary"). As the child starts to crawl and stand, his arms and legs become deformed as well: the arm is bowed and enlarged at the wrist. The legs may be curved outward (bow-legs) or inward (knock-knees).

Table 5.3 Recommended daily dietary allowances[a] of the Food and Nutrition Board, National Academy of Sciences, National Research Council, Revised 1973

	Age (years) from – up to	Weight kg	lbs	Height cm	in	Energy Calories	Protein gm	Fat-soluble vitamins Vitamin A activity (IU)	Vitamin D (IU)	Vitamin E activity (IU)
Infants	0.0–0.5	6	14	60	24	kg × 117	kg × 2.2[b]	1400	400	4
	0.5–1.0	9	20	71	28	kg × 108	kg × 2.0[b]	2000	400	5
Children	1–3	13	28	86	34	1300	23	2000	400	7
	4–6	20	44	110	44	1800	30	2500	400	9
	7–10	30	66	135	54	2400	36	3300	400	10
Males	11–14	44	97	158	63	2800	44	5000	400	12
	15–18	61	134	172	69	3000	54	5000	400	15
	19–22	67	147	172	69	3000	52	5000	400	15
	23–50	70	154	172	69	2700	56	5000	—	15
	51 +	70	154	172	69	2400	56	5000	—	15
Females	11–14	44	97	155	62	2400	44	4000	400	10
	15–18	54	119	162	65	2100	48	4000	400	11
	19–22	58	128	162	65	2100	46	4000	400	12
	23–50	58	128	162	65	2000	46	4000	—	12
	51 +	58	128	162	65	1800	46	4000	—	12
Pregnancy						+ 300	+ 30	5000	400	15
Lactation						+ 500	+ 20	6000	400	15

[a] The allowance levels are intended to cover individual variations among most normal persons as they live in the United States under usual environmental stresses. The recommended allowances can be attained with a variety of common foods, providing other nutrients for which human requirements have been less well defined.

[b] Assumes protein equivalent to human milk. For proteins not 100 percent utilized factors should be increased proportionately.

ciency, if it is severe, will cause a form of muscle-wasting in these animals that is not unlike muscular dystrophy in man (though muscular dystrophy is not caused by vitamin E deficiency). These animals also show heart abnormalities. Animals on unbalanced diets very high in polyunsaturated fats, like cats fed nothing but red meat tuna, develop a painful "yellow-fat" disease that can be reversed by feeding them vitamin E.

But vitamin E deficiency is rare in Americans on an average diet. It is almost impossible to avoid getting an adequate amount of vitamin E if you eat vegetable oils, whole grain cereals, meats (especially liver),

Water-soluble vitamins							Minerals				
Ascorbic acid (mg)	Folacin[c] (µg)	Niacin[d] (mg)	Riboflavin (mg)	Thiamin (mg)	Vitamin B_6 (mg)	Vitamin B_{12} (µg)	Calcium (mg)	Phosphorus (mg)	Iodine (µg)	Iron (mg)	Magnesium (mg)
35	50	5	0.4	0.3	0.3	0.3	360	240	35	10	60
35	50	8	0.6	0.5	0.4	0.3	540	400	45	15	70
40	100	9	0.8	0.7	0.6	1.0	800	800	60	15	150
40	200	12	1.1	0.9	0.9	1.5	800	800	80	10	200
40	300	16	1.2	1.2	1.2	2.0	800	800	110	10	250
45	400	18	1.5	1.4	1.6	3.0	1200	1200	130	18	350
45	400	20	1.8	1.5	1.8	3.0	1200	1200	150	18	400
45	400	20	1.8	1.5	2.0	3.0	800	800	140	10	350
45	400	18	1.6	1.4	2.0	3.0	800	800	130	10	350
45	400	16	1.5	1.2	2.0	3.0	800	800	110	10	350
45	400	16	1.3	1.2	1.6	3.0	1200	1200	115	18	300
45	400	14	1.4	1.1	2.0	3.0	1200	1200	115	18	300
45	400	14	1.4	1.1	2.0	3.0	800	800	100	18	300
45	400	13	1.2	1.0	2.0	3.0	800	800	100	18	300
45	400	12	1.1	1.0	2.0	3.0	800	800	80	10	300
60	800	+ 2	+ 0.3	+ 0.3	2.5	4.0	1200	1200	125	18 +	450
60	600	+ 4	+ 0.5	+ 0.3	2.5	4.0	1200	1200	150	18	450

[c] The folacin allowances refer to dietary sources as determined by *Lactobacillus casei* assay. Pure forms of folacin may be effective in doses less than ¼ of the RDA.

[d] Niacin equivalents include dietary sources of the vitamin itself plus 1 mg equivalent for each 60 mg of dietary tryptophan.

fish, poultry, milk, eggs, beans, fruits, nuts, or green leafy vegetables. The conditions seen in the experimental animals develop only over a long period of severe deficiency, and there is so far no indication that vitamin E has any special effect except under those conditions. It is present in the human body and therefore probably required by man, but its specific role is unknown.

VITAMIN K This vitamin is essential for the formation in the liver of a form of protein called *prothrombin*. The prothrombin, when it enters the plasma, makes it possible for blood to clot normally. It is not certain why vitamin K is indispensible to this process. Vitamin K is found in nature in rich supply in green, leafy vegetables. However, it is probable that normal adults get all the vitamin K they need from a peculiar source: it is synthesized from nutrients in the large intestine by a bacteria: Escherichia coli. E. coli then shares the vitamin with its host. Only newborn babies, whose intestinal flora of microorganisms has not yet developed, and adults who have a defect in fat absorbtion need a vitamin K supplement.

VITAMIN B₁   Vitamin B_1 is also called thiamine. It is found in foods that are also good sources of protein, like pork, fish, eggs, poultry, beans, and whole grain cereals. Like the next five B vitamins listed, it is a component of enzymes that perform the complicated but vital cellular process called oxidation, which in a series of steps progressively combines oxygen with carbohydrates, fats, and protein in such a way that at each major step, energy is released for maintenance, exercise, and growth.

Each of these vitamins has a different role, and acts in a different stage, but each must be present. Thiamine is particularly essential in breaking down carbohydrates for use as energy. Because the central nervous system and the heart are especially dependent on the utilization of carbohydrates, the deficiency of thiamine (beriberi) is accompanied by disturbances in both the central nervous system and the heart (beriberi heart disease).

VITAMIN B₂   Riboflavin is another name for vitamin B_2 which is found in milk, whole grain cereals, green vegetables, and liver and is important in carbohydrate, fat, and protein metabolism. Like other B vitamins, it is necessary for growth. Surveys done in the last five years have shown that the American diet tends to be low in riboflavin.

NIACIN   Niacin, or nicotinic acid, has been called vitamin P or PP because it prevents pellagra. Niacin has an interesting relationship with protein. Not only is its presence essential for the proper utilization of protein, but some of our needed niacin can be produced in the body by the conversion of tryptophan, an essential amino acid, into the vitamin. Good sources of niacin are meats, dairy products, and whole grain cereals.

VITAMIN B₆   Vitamin B_6 is made up of four closely related compounds: pyridoxine, pyridoxal, pyridoxamine, and pyridoxal phosphate. Each has a slightly different molecular structure. Vitamin B_6 plays an essential part in the metabolism of amino acids, fats, and carbohydrates. In particular, it takes part in the process that enables the body to synthesize nonessential amino acids, and it is also needed in the process that

Beriberi (vitamin B₁ deficiency)

The adult form of beriberi is usually insidious in onset. It is characterized by a triad of symptoms: cardiovascular disturbances, neurological disturbances, and edema. Depending on the predominant feature, it is termed cardiac, neuritic, or wet beriberi. Neuritis is the most frequent symptom and progresses from fatigue, headaches, and insomnia, to heaviness and stiffness of the legs with areas of paresthesia (lack of sensation) or tenderness and lack of appetite. Eventually, neuritic beriberi becomes dry or paraplegic beriberi with the whole nervous system affected: walking is impaired, reflexes disappear, burning, numbness, and loss of power are experienced in arms and legs, and the patient becomes unable to move.

Cardiovascular symptoms include enlargement of the heart (beriberi heart), changes in electrocardiogram, and circulatory failure which may end in sudden death.

Edema is conspicuous in wet beriberi, beginning in feet and legs and ascending to the abdomen, the chest, and in particular the pericardium.

Infantile beriberi is characterized by edema followed by wasting, sudden paroxysms of pain, a cyanosed face, and eventually death in heart failure.

converts tryptophan to niacin. It has a key role in the normal functioning of blood cells and many tissues, particularly the nervous system. Vitamin B₆ can be obtained from meats, cereals, and some vegetables and fruits—especially dried fruits.

PANTOTHENIC ACID This vitamin is found in all living things (hence the Greek root of its name). It would be almost impossible to develop a deficiency unless you were eating a diet of highly processed foods from which the vitamin had been removed. Experimental pantothenic acid deficiencies produced (with some effort) in human beings have resulted in symptoms of fatigue, headache, sleep disturbances, nausea, and gastric distress.

BIOTIN Another vitamin also present in almost all foods is biotin. A few people on strange diets that called for a large consumption of raw eggs have succeeded in making themselves deficient in biotin, which is inactivated by a protein in the egg whites. Enzymes containing biotin function in protein metabolism and help the body to synthesize fatty acids and to utilize glucose. Biotin also has a part in the utilization of vitamin B₁₂ and folic acid. These last two B vitamins are both vital for the formation of the red blood cells.

FOLIC ACID Folic acid is so named because it was first extracted from leaves. It is also widely available in other foods, but green, leafy vegetables, liver, and yeast are the richest sources. Folic acid is needed to prevent one form of anemia in which the red cells in the blood and bone marrow become much larger than normal. This form of anemia is caused by malnutrition and can appear during pregnancy if the mother has been eating a generally inadequate diet that will not provide for both her and the fetus. Folic acid is important in the metabolism of certain amino acids.

VITAMIN B₁₂ Vitamin B₁₂ is an important part of the enzymes that catalyze protein, fat, and carbohydrate metabolism. It is essential in the prevention of pernicious anemia, another form of anemia. One variety of pernicious anemia is brought on by changes in the gastric juices that prevent a patient from absorbing nutrients properly. It can be cured only by injections of B₁₂ under a doctor's supervision.

Another variety of pernicious anemia can be caused by a dietary deficiency of B₁₂. Unlike any of the other B vitamins, B₁₂ is found only in foods of animal origin, and thus it is essential even for vegetarians to have some form of animal food (such as milk) or else to have regular supplements of the vitamin. The dietary anemia develops slowly, but a deficiency eventually brings about changes not only in the blood but in the nervous system as well.

VITAMIN C Vitamin C, or ascorbic acid, is found in fruit (especially oranges and lemons) and potatoes. Though the juices of citrus fruits have long been recognized as preventatives of scurvy, a disease caused by vitamin C deficiency, we still do not have a complete picture of how the vitamin acts in the body. It is important in the oxidation of a number of amino acids and in some reactions involving folic acid. It is known to be important to the maintenance of connective tissue which holds the various body organs and structures together. Without ascorbic acid in the diet, there may be internal bleeding, and wounds will not heal properly.

Minerals

Of all the nutrients, the minerals are the least understood. We are now in about the same stage in the understanding of mineral nutrition as we were in the early decades of this century in understanding the vitamins.

Minerals perform a number of functions in the body: they maintain the rigidity of the skeletal structure; they promote homeostasis by regulating the acid-base balance of the extracellular fluids and helping to maintain osmotic pressure (the balance of solutions on either side of a membrane); they are essential parts of hormones or vitamins; and they are part of metal-enzyme complexes, binding the enzymes to proteins. Some of the minerals essential to human life and health have been known for some time. Their chief functions are at least recognized if not always completely understood, and a recommended daily allowance has been established for them, although this could be subject to change with new discoveries. Most of the minerals that fall into this category are needed in fairly large amounts and thus are more easily measured and traced in the body by current methods of determination. Those minerals which we need in substantial amounts are called *macro elements*. As our biochemical techniques become more precise, we can detect the presence and eventually define the roles of smaller and smaller amounts of other minerals—the so-called trace elements. For a summary of what is known so far about a number of minerals in normal nutrition, see Table 5.4 (p. 130–31).

The macro elements

CALCIUM, MAGNESIUM, AND PHOSPHORUS These three minerals are essential components of the skeleton, including the teeth. They work together in bone formation and maintenance, and a deficiency of one affects the metabolism of the others. Of all the minerals, calcium is present in the body in the greatest amount—almost 2 percent of total body weight. Ninety-nine percent of that is in the skeleton, but calcium is also necessary for blood clotting, muscle contraction, and transmission of messages along the nerves. The best single dietary source of calcium is milk.

Phosphorus makes up about 1 percent of body weight, and most of it also is in the skeleton. Phosphorus is involved in the metabolism of protein, fat, and carbohydrate. It helps produce energy and build new tissues. Phosphorus is present in milk, lean meats, fish, green and yellow vegetables, eggs, beans, nuts, and whole grains. Foods that contain the most calcium and protein are also high in phosphorus, so it is safe to assume that a diet adequate in calcium and protein will also contain an adequate supply of phosphorus.

The body contains about one ounce of magnesium. Much of it is combined with calcium and phosphorus in the bone, and the rest is distributed in red blood cells and body fluids. Magnesium, like phosphorus, is needed to utilize carbohydrates for energy, to make protein, and to maintain muscles. There is quite a bit of magnesium in beans (including soybeans), peas, whole grains, nuts, and seafood.

SODIUM   About 30 to 40 percent of the total 3 to 4 ounces of sodium in an adult's body is present in bone. Sodium is found in blood, lymph, digestive juices, and the fluid that bathes the cells. It is one of the two components of table salt, which is taken much too liberally in the American diet—10 to 15 times as much as the body needs. Since high salt intake is a factor in hypertension (high blood pressure) which in turn is a factor in heart disease and stroke (see Chap. 11), it would be better to satisfy our daily need for sodium by eating reasonable amounts of milk, meat, eggs, and vegetables such as carrots, beets, spinach and other leafy greens, celery, artichokes, and asparagus without adding salt from the shaker.

CHLORINE   One reason for using table salt at all is for its other component, chlorine. Less than two ounces of chlorine are found in the fluids outside the cells, particularly in the fluid in the brain and spinal cord. It is also in blood fluid (serum) and in the digestive acid of the stomach. Chlorine helps sodium to balance the acid-base ratio of the intracellular fluid.

SULFUR   Sulfur is obtained mainly from dietary protein. It is found in hair, nails, bones, tendons, and the fluids that lubricate the joints. It is an element in the complicated process by which the body eliminates common poisonous substances and in energy release during cellular metabolism. Sulfur is found in lean meats, fish, fruits, and vegetables.

The major trace minerals

IRON   Iron is an essential component of hemoglobin, the pigment of red blood cells which loosely combines with oxygen in the lungs and carries it to all the body tissues. The amount of iron present in the adult human body varies from about 2 grams in a small woman to as much as 6 grams in a large man. The amount needed from food varies, since

Iron deficiency anemia

Iron deficiency results from one or a combination of the following: inadequate diet, impaired absorption, blood loss (including excessive menstrual bleeding), or repeated pregnancies. Some patients with iron deficiency anemia have no sense of ill health. Others complain of vague symptoms such as weakness, fatigue, or lassitude. More severe anemia may be accompanied by pallor, dyspnea on exertion, palpitation, and a sense of dead tiredness. The patient's hands and feet may feel cold. Appetite is often capricious; epigastric pain, constipation or diarrhea, and nausea are not uncommon. The fingernails and toenails may be lusterless, thin, brittle, and spoon-shaped. Eventually, as the blood hemoglobin falls below 8 grams per 100 milliliters (normal 13 to 15 grams), the heart may become dilated, murmurs may be heard, the spleen may be enlarged, and stomach acid secretion is impaired.

Table 5.4 Summary of functions of minerals and manifestations of mineral deficiencies

Mineral	Function	Characteristics of the deficiency state
calcium	formation of bones and teeth regulation of muscle contraction, nerve irritability and the rhythm of the heartbeat activation of some enzymes blood clotting	rickets osteomalacia osteoporosis tetany
phosphorus	formation of bones and teeth constituent of high-energy compounds nucleoproteins, phospholipids, enzyme systems and buffer salts	emaciation fragile bones rickets
magnesium	activation of phosphatases and oxidative phosphorylation enzymes relaxation of nerve impulses and muscle contraction a constituent of chlorophyll	vasodilation soft tissue calcification atherosclerosis tetany
sodium	regulation of pH, osmotic pressure and water balance transmission of nerve impulses active transport of glucose and amino acids	nausea anorexia muscular weakness and cramps
potassium	regulation of osmotic pressure and acid-base balance activation of a number of intracellular enzymes regulation of nerve and muscle irritability	weakness, anorexia, abdominal distention tachycardia pulmonary edema adrenal hypertrophy
chlorine	activation of amylase a constituent of hydrochloric acid regulation of osmotic pressure and acid-base balance	poor growth in rats
sulfur	part of some amino acids, some vitamins, some hormones, bile, melanin synthesis of sulfomucopolysaccharides detoxifying agents	not found

Potassium

Potassium is the most important element in the fluids contained inside the cells (intracellular fluids), just as sodium is the characteristic element in the fluids outside the cells (extracellular fluids). The red and white blood cells contain about twenty times as much potassium as sodium, while skeletal muscle contains about six times as much potassium. Besides ensuring proper osmotic pressure of cells, potassium is involved in many biochemical reactions. It is necessary to maintain at the right level the contractility of skeletal and smooth muscles and of that particularly crucial muscle, the heart. Potassium deficiency is unlikely ever to occur in a healthy individual fed anything like a normal diet, but it can result from protracted diarrhea, prolonged vomiting, diabetic acidosis, or kidney disease. It can also accompany drug therapy for hypertension if the patient's diet is not supplemented with large amounts of potassium-containing foods (such as fruit juices, bananas, dried fruit) or potassium supplements. Potassium deficiency causes muscular weakness, nervous irritability, mental disorientation, and abnormalities in cardiac function. Excessive concentration of potassium in the body fluids (usually resulting from kidney disease or dehydration) is toxic and may cause serious disturbances in heart beats and even cardiac arrest.

the body stores are lost mainly from the blood during hemorrhaging and menstruation and drawn on during pregnancy and growth. Iron deficiency produces an anemia in which the red cells grow smaller than normal. This anemia is not uncommon, even in the United States; it causes few deaths but leaves the body weakened and open to illness and infection. Milder degrees of iron deficiency are quite common among children and young women of child-bearing age. Iron is one of the trace minerals for which a daily requirement has been set: 10 milligrams for

Mineral	Function	Characteristics of the deficiency state
iron	part of hemoglobin, myoglobin and heme enzymes	anemia
copper	hemopoiesis, metabolism of vitamin C and energy, formation of melanin, phospholipids and elastin	anemia depigmentation of hair (in animals) demyelination of nerve bone disorders
manganese	synthesis of chondroitin sulfates, bone formation, urea formation, amino acid transport, lipotropic agent, cholesterol synthesis, oxidative phosphorylation	ataxia infertility (in animals)
zinc	activation of carbonic anhydrase and several dehydrogenases alkaline phosphatase, carboxypeptidase wound healing, metabolism of nucleic acids associated with insulin	hepatosplenomegaly dwarfism hypogonadism
iodine	constituent of thyroxine which regulates metabolism	goiter cretinism
fluorine	imparts greater resistance to tooth decay stimulates new bone formation	dental caries
cobalt	constituent of vitamin B_{12}	anemia wasting disease (in ruminants)
chromium	increases effectiveness of insulin	impaired glucose tolerance curve
molybdenum	activation of xanthine oxidase	poor growth malformed young (in rats)
selenium	maintaining stability of membranes increasing retention of vitamin E	growth retardation

From J. R. K. Robson, F. A. Larkin, A. M. Sandretto, and B. Tadayyon, *Malnutrition: Its Causation and Control* (New York: Gordon and Breach, 1972), Vol. 1, Table 29.

men, 18 for women. It can be obtained from liver, the prime source, as well as fish, egg yolk, whole wheat bread, green leafy vegetables, peas, and beans.

IODINE The mineral iodine is part of the hormone secreted by the thyroid, a gland situated at the base of the neck. Thyroid hormone is essential in combining oxygen with digesting food, a process which in turn is essential to basic metabolism. Severe iodine deficiency causes goiter and, at its worst, cretinism—permanent brain damage and arrested physical development. Iodine can be obtained from seafood, the best source, from other foods grown near salt water, where the soil is rich in iodine, or from iodized table salt in moderate amounts.

FLUORINE A great deal has been said about the possible toxicity of fluorine, yet every nutrient, even water, is toxic in large enough doses. At the recommended level in the water supply, however, fluorine not only promotes solid tooth formation in children but may aid retention of calcium in adult bones, helping to prevent or retard the development of porous or brittle bones in old age. If it is not present in the water supply, it should come from supplements.

NUTRITIONAL DISEASES

The state of nutrition of an individual can be poor because: (a) he does not have enough food to eat (he is said to suffer from undernutrition or starvation in extreme cases); (b) he lacks one or more nutrients in his diet (he is then said to suffer from a deficiency disease, or primary malnutrition); (c) he is suffering from a disease which prevents him from properly digesting or absorbing his food (he is said to suffer from secondary malnutrition); or (d) he is eating a diet which, while not deficient, is faulty because it is too much for his needs or too high in saturated fat and cholesterol or sugar, and contributes to degenerative diseases, which are caused by organs aging and becoming defective.

Scurvy (vitamin C deficiency)

The adult suffering from scurvy typically complains of weakness and pain in the limbs. Multiple small hemorrhages occur all over the body, particularly in the gums and about the tender hair follicles of the lower extremities. As the disease progresses, inflammation and hemorrhage of the gums become more marked; infection occurs at the base of the teeth; the breath becomes fetid. Eventually the alveoli (the sockets that grip the roots of the teeth) in the jawbones are resorbed and teeth are loosened and fall out. Hemorrhages become increasingly widespread. Wounds do not heal and may reopen. Resistance to infection is low. Death may result.

Scurvy in children used to be known as Barlow's disease. The child afflicted with scurvy is usually wasted, pale, and fretful and howls when his limbs are touched. His gums usually bleed. His legs are flexed and externally rotated. He stays in this position because of the extreme pain caused by hemorrhages, which are most likely to occur around the bones of the legs.

Undernutrition

Undernutrition occurs when a person does not have enough to eat. Undernourished children are thin and stop growing and tend to be quiet because they do not have enough energy to run and play. Undernourished adults similarly lose weight. Undernourished persons of all ages are prone to disease. If food is seriously lacking, weight loss is extreme and we speak of starvation. If many persons are starving, there is a famine. Famines occur periodically throughout the world as a result of three types of causes: natural disasters (especially droughts), plant and animal diseases, and wars and civil conflicts.

Deficiency diseases—primary malnutrition

Lack of protein causes a disease known by its African name, *kwashiorkor*, and characterized by swelling (edema), changes in color and texture of the skin and hair, and damage to the liver, the pancreas, and the intestine. The disease attacks mainly young children and is fatal unless the patient is given protein. An extreme lack of calories and/or protein has been shown to cause mental retardation in very young infants.

Vitamin A deficiency causes night blindness, a lack of vision in dim light and a blinding by sudden exposure to light. The skin and mucosa are abnormal. Extreme deficiency causes total blindness and eventually death. In vitamin D deficiency, or *rickets*, the calcium is not properly

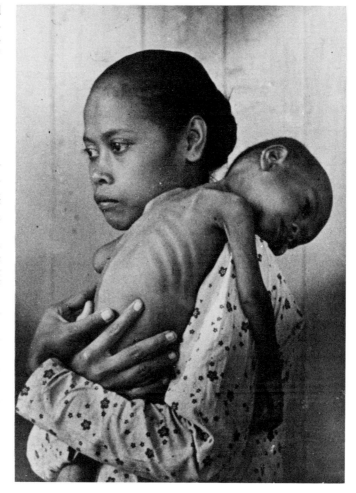

Figure 5.1. An Indonesian child suffering from malnutrition. (Courtesy of the World Health Organization)

Vitamin A deficiency

Vitamin A is an essential component of a retinal pigment called *visual purple,* or *rhodopsin,* which is bleached in the presence of light; the bleaching process acts as a stimulus to the rods of the retina. The bleaching of visual purple is the important element in night vision. Poor night vision (night blindness) is often the first sign of vitamin A deficiency.

Elsewhere in the body, deficiency of vitamin A results in several morphological changes, particularly in the epithelial tissues. Epithelial cells in the skin and mucosae multiply excessively, become flattened and heaped upon one another. The sweat glands of the skin and the tear glands of the eye are blocked by plugs of *keratin,* the hard constituent of skin and nails. The lack of tears and the accumulation of flattened epithelial cells cause changes in the cornea, first in spots (Bitot spots), later as blindness. Ultimately the whole cornea softens, and the condition known as *keratomalacia* occurs. Usually accompanied by infection, it leads to perforation and loss of the eye. Typically the skin becomes thick, with raised papulae, which gives it the appearance of toadskin. The digestive tract, gums and teeth, urinary system, and genital duct are also affected. In animals it also causes irregular development in the skeleton, including the skull and vertebral column, with secondary damage to the brain and spinal cord.

deposited in the bones, leading to a deformed skeleton. Vitamin B_1 deficiency is called *beriberi.* It is widespread in many areas of the world, particularly in areas of Asia where polished rice (from which vitamin B_1 has been removed by milling) is the main food. Vitamin B_1 deficiency causes damage to nerves, edema, and a certain type of heart disease. In the United States, flour is enriched with vitamin B_1 (as well as with B_2, niacin, and iron). Vitamin B_2 deficiency causes cracking at the corners of the lips and itching. The deficiency disease *pellagra,* characterized by skin disease, diarrhea, and insanity, occurs when the diet is low in protein containing the amino acid tryptophan as well as low in niacin. Corn is low in niacin and tryptophan, and persons in some parts of the United States who ate primarily corn with little or no animal protein used to develop pellagra. Corn is now enriched in the United States, and the number of persons with pellagra has been drastically reduced. Lack of

Pellagra

The pellagrin is characterized, in order of development of the syndrom, by loss of weight, strength, and appetite and by insomnia, vertigo, headache, dyspepsia, loss of appetite, and diarrhea. He may also complain of irritability, loss of memory, and depression. His pupils may be dilated, and there is often observed a characteristic dull lifeless stare. Pigmentation may develop in the face. As the disease progresses, the triad, the "three D" signs, become more and more manifest: diarrhea, dermatitis, and dementia (ending in death, if unrelieved). Diarrhea becomes acute and is accompanied by foul and bulky stools, vomiting, abdominal pain, and lack of appetite (all of which make the dietary deficiency self-accelerating). Those parts of the skin which are exposed to light or pressed upon by tight clothing show a characteristic dermatitis: the face and neck darken ("Casal's necklace"), as do the dorsal surfaces of the hands and lower forearms, elbows, and the dorsal parts of the feet in barefooted persons. The skin often becomes scaly and looks like cracked enamel or a "crazy pavement." Sometimes it is dark, smooth, and shiny. The tongue becomes scarlet, smooth, and beefy looking, and sometimes has the appearance of a map ("geographical tongue"). Mental symptoms become more and more severe, with tenseness and emotional instability going on to insanity, sometimes permanent.

vitamin B_6 causes convulsions in infants. Lack of folic acid and vitamin B_{12} causes blood disorders in which abnormal red cells are formed. Vitamin C deficiency or scurvy causes bleeding gums and generally causes very small blood vessels (capillaries) to break easily. It also causes joints to become very painful. Scurvy used to be very common among sailors and others who were deprived of fresh fruits for long periods.

There are a number of mineral deficiencies which cause diseases. Lack of sufficient iron in the diet causes the most common form of anemia, iron deficiency anemia: the red blood cells are normal in shape but are small and pale because they lack hemoglobin. Anemic persons are given "iron pills" or liquid preparations in addition to a diet rich in iron.

Lack of fluoride in the water causes an increase in dental caries. Lack of iodine causes the thyroid gland to become bigger and to form a bump on the front part of the neck, a condition known as goiter. The patient with this condition has little energy and a body temperature that is often lower than normal. Iodine deficiency can cause retardation of the growth of the body and the mind. Adding iodine to salt ("iodized salt") has decreased drastically the number of persons with goiter in the United States.

Lack of zinc causes a decreased rate of growth and maturation. It has been identified in some American children, including middle class children on poor diets. In its Western form, as evidenced in the Middle East, it causes dwarfism and lack of sexual maturation.

Secondary malnutrition

In a number of diseases such as sprue, celiac disease, and cystic fibrosis of the pancreas, food is improperly digested and absorbed. A person with such a disease may have to be put on a special diet. Similarly, with diseases in which food cannot be eaten or digested at all, the patient may have to be fed through tubes leading either into the stomach or, using special nutritional preparations, into the blood.

Degenerative diseases

Finally, there are diseases associated with too much food or too much of certain foods. Eating more than is needed for growth and maintenance leads to overweight. Increasing exercise and/or dieting may then be prescribed. Excessive amounts of sugar in the diet increase the chance of dental caries. Excessive amounts of dietary fat, especially saturated fats and cholesterol, lead to an increase in the level of blood cholesterol. As cholesterol rises, so do the chances of heart attacks, strokes, and other diseases of blood vessels (see Chap. 11). Adult men are particularly prone to heart attacks in the United States, in part because our diet is high in saturated fats. For this reason an adult man or even an adolescent boy would be well advised not to continue to consume a diet as high in saturated fats and cholesterol as that of children. This is particularly so if the adult man leads a sedentary mode of life, as most Americans now do.

FOOD AND HEALTH

Source of nutrients

The key to good nutrition is a varied diet containing as high a proportion as possible of fresh, unprocessed, or minimally processed (canned and frozen) foods; the greater the diversity of such foods, the fewer the chances that any nutrients will be missing. To facilitate thinking about the different types of foods and their contributions to good nutrition, foods have often been grouped into certain categories. The "basic seven" classification was popularized during World War II. More recently a "basic four" classification has been introduced: the milk group, the meat group, the bread-cereal group, and the vegetable-fruit group. The basic four system is not satisfactory. There is no reason, for example, to classify potatoes and spinach together. It would make more sense to group together the main sources of animal protein and good quality vegetable proteins (milk, meat, fish, eggs, peas, and beans), and separate starchy fruits (bananas) and roots (potatoes) from green, leafy vegetables and other fruits. We will use the "basic seven" classification to describe foods because it gives a much more satisfactory grouping of foods that contain similar nutrients. It must be noted, however, that even the "basic seven" do not cover "fabricated foods" like cocktail cheese puffs, imitation cream, vegetable-protein "bacon" chips, or the complex convenience foods like TV dinners and frozen or canned, completely prepared main dishes, such as stews, lasagna, or pizza, which have become so popular in the past decade. The only way in which these can be described adequately is through comprehensive nutritional labeling which will be discussed later.

The basic seven

The seven food groups are: (1) leafy, green, and yellow vegetables; (2) citrus fruits, tomatoes, raw cabbage, and salad greens; (3) potatoes and other vegetables and fruits; (4) milk and milk products; (5) meat, poultry, fish, eggs, dried beans and peas, and nuts; (6) bread, flour, and cereals; and (7) butter and fortified margarine.

Nutritionists generally recommend that a person eat one serving of food from each of the basic seven groups every day. Other foods may be added to the seven as desired, depending on eating habits and activity. For example, a teen-age boy and a man doing hard work may require several average servings because of rapid growth and vigorous activity. A young child may need only about half the adult serving.

GROUP 1. LEAFY, GREEN, AND YELLOW VEGETABLES This important food group includes: string beans, spinach, green peas, broccoli, kale, and asparagus. It also includes carrots, squash, pumpkins, sweet potatoes, wax beans, and rutabagas. These vegetables may be eaten raw, cooked, canned, or frozen. They supply large amounts of vitamin A, and many also provide iron, calcium, thiamine, riboflavin, niacin, and vitamin C. They also supply fiber which helps regulate the intestines. One or more daily servings are suggested for this group.

GROUP 2. CITRUS FRUITS, TOMATOES, RAW CABBAGE, AND SALAD GREENS This group includes all citrus fruits and their juices: lemons, limes, oranges, and grapefruit. Fresh berries and crisp salad greens are good sources of vitamin C. The foods in this group furnish vitamin A, iron, and calcium. One or more daily servings are recommended for Group 2.

GROUP 3. POTATOES AND OTHER VEGETABLES AND FRUITS This group includes all the fruits and vegetables not in Groups 1 and 2. These include beets, onions, celery, eggplant, corn, parsnips, cucumbers, and white turnips. At least one potato a day is suggested for active children and adults. Potatoes are a source of vitamin C if eaten baked or boiled. A second serving from Group 3 is also recommended. Fruits in the group include apples, grapes, peaches, pears, pineapples, figs, prunes, raisins, plums, and bananas. This group supplies many of the carbohydrates needed by the body. Fruits furnish sugar, and some of the vegetables such as potatoes, corn, and parsnips are a source of starch. The foods in this group also provide generous amounts of vitamins and minerals.

GROUP 4. MILK AND MILK PRODUCTS Milk in any form belongs in this group. It may be fresh, dried, evaporated, or made into cheese or ice cream. A child should have from three to four cups of milk a day. An adult needs at least two cups daily. Cheese can replace milk for an adult consuming an otherwise varied diet who does not like or cannot tolerate milk. Milk and cheese serve as valuable sources of calcium, vitamin A, riboflavin, and high-quality proteins. Skim milk is as good a source of nutrients as whole milk except for vitamin A; it is preferable to whole milk for adults and others who have to cut down on calories and saturated fats.

GROUP 5. MEAT, POULTRY, FISH, DRIED BEANS AND PEAS, AND NUTS This group is the chief source of protein in the diet as well as a source of energy (from the protein and fat). It is also a rich source of iron, phosphorus, thiamine, and niacin. Nuts and dried beans and peas furnish some starch and include lentils, soybeans, and peanut butter. Legumes and nuts can be substituted for other foods in this group. But when this is done, milk or cheese should be added to the diet at the same meal to supply essential amino acids. Eggs are an excellent source of a variety of nutrients which are particularly useful to children and young women, but they are not recommended for adult men because they are high in cholesterol. The diet should provide one to two daily servings from the foods in this group.

GROUP 6. BREAD, FLOUR, AND CEREALS This group includes breads, biscuits, crackers, and cereals. All of these should consist of whole grain or enriched flour or cereal. The enriching process is important if flours and cereals are milled because milling removes much of the outer coat of the grain. This outer coat is rich in minerals and vitamins. Undermilled cereals not only are rich in nutrients but also provide fiber which is useful in preventing constipation and possibly diverticulitis and cancer of the large bowel. The diet should provide at least two daily servings of bread or cereals. Foods in this group are valuable energy sources and also provide protein.

GROUP 7. BUTTER AND FORTIFIED MARGARINE Fortified margarine has enough vitamin A added to equal the amount normally found in butter. These foods are chiefly energy producers and excellent sources of vitamin A. Their consumption should be restricted for persons watching their weight and for adult men and older women who have been told to modify their diet in order to lower their blood cholesterol level. Such persons are usually advised to lower their overall intake of fat and to replace butter and "hard" margarines with polyunsaturated vegetable fats. (They are also advised to eat no more than two eggs a week and to replace part of the beef and pork in their diet by lower fat poultry and fish.) In such diets, vitamin A will come from yellow and green vegetables, fruits, liver, and/or dietary supplements.

Finally, it should be noted that the seven food groups omit mention of sugar and sugar-based foods such as candy and soft drinks. These make no contribution to the diet except in the form of calories. They can be termed "empty calories" to denote their lack of nutrients.

Nutritional labeling

The First White House Conference on Food, Nutrition and Health which met in 1969 to consider ways of improving the nutrition of all Americans recommended that all foods, and particularly complex, processed foods, be labeled in such a way that consumers could understand what contribution these foods make to their nutrition. Labeling is done at present on a voluntary basis (except for fortified foods, foods that purport to be whole meals, or foods that make any nutrition claims). The nutrient panels on the labels give the number of calories per portion, the grams of protein, calories and fat per portion, and the percent of Recommended Dietary Allowances for adults (baby foods have their own scale) for a number of key nutrients contributed by one common portion.

Selecting foods

Meals should be planned several days in advance to make sure that the daily diet includes foods from each of the basic seven groups. A wise shopper buys foods that are as fresh as possible. Many foods, especially fruits and vegetables, lose vitamins A and C as they become stale and wilt. Canned and frozen products add variety to meals by making most foods available throughout the year. Modern food processing methods try to ensure that canned and frozen foods retain their nutritional values. High-quality processed products may compare favorably with cooked fresh foods in vitamin content and other nutrient qualities, particularly if the fresh foods were harvested before maturity or were kept for long periods of time before being used. Such treatment decreases their nutritional value.

Cooking and preparation

It is important not to add unnecessary calories, saturated fats, and sugar to foods. For example, frying foods considerably increases their caloric and saturated fat content. Broiling meat (cooking it on a grill) actually decreases its fat content: the fat drips out and is not consumed.

Food must be kept and cooked carefully in order to conserve nutritional values. Most foods should be preserved in the refrigerator. Food should be cooked for the shortest possible time in as little liquid as possible. Some vitamins and minerals dissolve in the cooking liquid. For this reason, cooking liquids should be eaten along with the food. The liquids often contain vitamin C, riboflavin, thiamine, niacin, and some minerals.

Crusty or well-browned baked goods may be lower in thiamine content because of overbaking. Milk in glass containers should not be exposed to light for long periods of time because light destroys riboflavin. Fatty foods that become rancid lose vitamin A and polyunsaturated fatty acids.

Production and planning social food programs

Food in a country is provided through agriculture and imports. It is processed by food manufacturers and distributed through a complex retailing system. Food programs for schools, industry, and poor people are designed to make sure that the population is well fed. In our country, it is the responsibility of the United States Department of Agriculture to ensure that the American people are properly fed. The Department of Agriculture operates the Food Stamp program which provides $126 worth of food stamps a month for a family of four. (More food stamps are given to a larger family, fewer to a smaller family.) There were 14 million recipients in 1973. The stamps are free for the very poor and are paid for on a progressive scale by those a little more fortunate but still eligible. The USDA also operates the donated commodity programs (22 foods of which 18, on the average, are available once a month in bags and cans). These go to 3.5 million recipients, particularly to those in areas where food stamps could not be redeemed in supermarkets because of the lack of retail establishments (in Alaska or on Indian reservations, for example). Finally, the USDA operates the subsidized school lunch program (free for 9.5 million poor children in

1973), which includes free breakfasts and summer food programs for 1 million children below the poverty line.

The Food and Agriculture Organization (FAO) of the United Nations was created at the end of World War II to improve the nutrition of the world as a whole. The World Health Organization (WHO) and more specifically the United Nations Children's Fund (UNICEF) also have responsibilities in world nutrition.

Questions

1. What bodily needs do the nutrients fill? Having read this chapter, can you put together a list of the different needs and the nutrients that meet them?
2. What factors determine how much energy and what kind of nutrients are needed by an individual?
3. How do fats differ in their long-term effect on health?
4. Describe the roles of several minerals in the body. What are the sources of these minerals?
5. You're a healthy, normal, young adult living in the United States. You do a lot of eating out, including in drug stores and at hamburger stands. What nutrients do you think you should watch to make sure your intake is adequate?

Key Concepts

Calorie – the amount of energy equivalent to the heat needed to elevate the temperature of one liter of water by one degree centigrade

Carbohydrates – complex substances which during digestion are broken down into simple sugars (monosaccharides), especially glucose, for absorption by the body cells; primarily sugars and starches, carbohydrates are usually the main source of energy in the diet

Fats – complex substances which provide energy and are composed of fatty acids and glycerol; saturated fatty acids are associated with an increase in the amount of cholesterol that is deposited in arterial walls

Proteins – complex substances which provide energy and are composed of amino acids; the main constituent in the body after water, proteins do the necessary work of repair and growth

Vitamin – a complex substance needed in minute amounts which helps to regulate body metabolism but which does not supply energy; the body is unable to make vitamins, and so it relies on food or vitamin supplements to provide them

Selected Readings

Bogert, L. J., G. M. Briggs and D. H. Calloway. *Nutrition and Physical Fitness.* Philadelphia: W. B. Saunders Company, 1973.

Goodhart, R. S. and M. E. Shils. *Modern Nutrition in Health and Disease.* Philadelphia: Lea & Febiger, 1973.

Mayer, J. *Human Nutrition: Its Physiological, Medical, and Social Aspects.* Springfield, Ill.: Charles C Thomas, 1972.

Mayer, J., ed. *United States Nutrition Policies in the Seventies.* San Francisco: W. H. Freeman and Company, 1973.

National Academy of Sciences. *Recommended Dietary Allowances,* 8th ed. Washington, D.C.: U.S. Government Printing Office, 1974.

Stare, F. J. and M. McWilliams. *Living Nutrition.* New York: John Wiley & Sons, Inc., 1973.

Chapter 6

Weight Control

There is little doubt that the ability to store large amounts of fat was necessary for survival in the long periods of human history when the availability of food was seasonal and when man had to endure prolonged deprivation of food. There are still populations, those living in the Southern Rim of the Sahara for example, who endure yearly, predictable periods of food shortages and live then on stored foods and on their fat reserves.

In the United States and other developed countries, and among the wealthy classes in poor countries, the accumulation of fat is no longer necessary for survival and instead has serious drawbacks from the viewpoints of health, mobility, aesthetics, and enjoyment of life and social acceptance. As a result, weight control has become a matter of intense interest, not only among medical and public health workers but also among the public. Out of this concern for weight control has grown an industry, much of it impregnated with quackery, which produces sensational books (many of them touting "cures" based on pretended suspension of all laws of nature), pills of various colors and potencies (some useless, some only temporarily effective, some highly dangerous), belts, weights, corsets, steam baths, and so on, which are peddled to a desperate and credulous clientele.

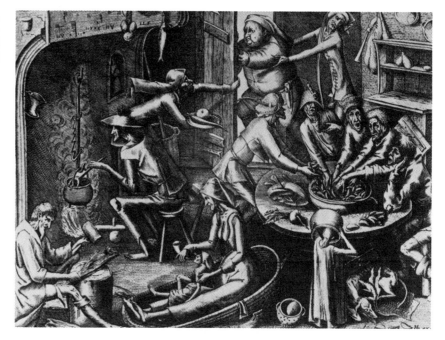

Figure 6.1. The fat and the lean. Sixteenth-century Flemish engraving. (Courtesy of the World Health Organization)

DEFINITION AND DIAGNOSIS

The terms *overweight* and *obesity* are often used indiscriminately. Overweight, strictly speaking, is a weight in excess of normal or desirable norms. Obesity is properly defined as a body condition in which fat content is well in excess of normal or desirable norms. In general, overweight individuals are obese, but an extremely muscular man, such as a professional, highly-trained athlete, with a large skeletal frame can be overweight according to tables of desirable weight without being obese. Conversely, a sedentary individual with poorly developed muscles and an excessive proportion of fat can be obese without being overweight. In this chapter, we will use the scientifically correct term *obesity* even though we recognize that it is often associated in the public mind with a more extreme degree of fatness than is meant here. When we use the term *overweight*, it will be as a synonym for obesity.

The diagnosis of a very obese person is obvious from appearance alone. A more moderate amount of obesity is identified by measuring subcutaneous fat through skinfold measurement: half of the body fat is situated under the skin, and pinching a double skinfold with a caliper and reading the thickness recorded gives a good estimate of total body fat. The instrument used is a "constant pressure" caliper which pinches with the same pressure no matter how thick the skinfold is. Measurements from the triceps skinfold—on the back of the arm (Fig. 6.2)—and the subscapular skinfold—on the back and below the scapula, the flat triangular bone in the back of the shoulder—correlate particularly well with results of other methods of determining total body fat. These include measurement of body density (based on the fact that fat is lighter than water whereas other body tissues are heavier), measurement of total body water (adipose tissue—the tissues which contain fat cells—contains very little water), and of total body potassium (adipose tissue contains very little potassium).

Skinfold determinations are particularly useful in children: while in healthy adults weight loss means loss of fat and weight gain means gain of fat, children are expected to gain weight as part of the normal process of growth. The composition of the weight gain is the crucial variable.

MEDICAL SIGNIFICANCE

The medical significance of obesity was originally derived from insurance companies' studies (Table 6.1). These studies have sometimes been criticized for being based on weight and not on fatness, and for failing to take into account the different human body types. Nevertheless, no one denies the general conclusion that marked overweight shortens life and has a significant effect on mortality from diseases of the heart and blood vessels, diabetes, kidney and liver diseases, and from accidents.

The initial studies of insurance companies were confirmed in 1959 by the large scale "Build and Blood Pressure Study" of the Society of Actuaries which was a long term follow up of 5,000,000 insured persons. As compared to the rate of mortality among men with the best risk, the mortality among men 15 to 69 years old who were 20 percent or more overweight was 50 percent greater; that of men 10 percent overweight was 30 percent greater. While the effect on women was less marked, the trend was the same.

In addition to its effect on mortality, obesity has both physiological and psychological effects. A number of chronic illnesses are made worse by overweight. The combination of arthritis and overweight, for example, leads to a much greater degree of immobilization than would one of the conditions alone, and immobilization, in turn, is bad for each condition. Whatever the complex nature of the interaction between adult diabetes (*maturity-onset* diabetes) and obesity, there is little doubt that the condition of the middle-aged diabetic is often dramatically improved by weight reduction. Obese people are accident-prone, more likely to hurt themselves badly when they fall, and poorer surgical risks after an accident.

Obesity is a complicating factor in *atherosclerosis*—a disease in which the arteries fill up with the fatty substance cholesterol. The extra blood vessels in the fatty tissue must be supplied by an overworked heart; the obesity limits exercise drastically, and exercise is important in controlling atherosclerosis. Obese people are also prone to hypertension —high blood pressure—which can cause strokes or contribute to heart attacks (see Chap. 11).

There are also serious psychological hazards to obesity. The "psychology of being obese" is a subject which has received much attention. In the affluent Western world, and particularly in the United States where emphasis is placed on active youth, the obese are truly a minority

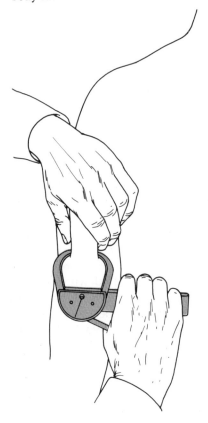

Figure 6.2. By measuring the thickness of an arm skinfold, the caliper is able to estimate total body fat.

Exercise and weight control

There are two fallacies often encountered when the relation of exercise to weight control is discussed. The first is the erroneous belief that exercise consumes few calories. It is wrongly assumed that it will help little in establishing the caloric deficit necessary to lose weight. In fact, exercise is the major variable in energy output. For a 150-pound person, walking slowly (2.6 miles per hour) consumes 115 calories per hour; walking moderately fast (3.75 miles per hour) consumes 215 calories per hour; walking very fast (5.3 miles per hour) consumes 565 calories per hour. Running, swimming, or rowing can mean expenditures of up to 1200 calories per minute.

The second fallacy is the belief that if you exercise more you will automatically eat more. Actually, an increase in food intake follows an increase in exercise only if you are already fairly active. Then your appetite will in fact regulate your food intake so as to equate caloric intake with caloric expenditure. The proper function of this mechanism is limited, however, to a range which we can term the "normal range of activity," a broad zone which goes from moderate activity to heavy work. Outside this range, we reach the limits of adaptation.

Table 6.1 Desirable weights for men and women aged 25 and over* (in pounds according to height and frame, in indoor clothing)

Height		Small frame	Medium frame	Large frame
Men				
Feet	**Inches**			
5	2	112–120	118–129	126–141
5	3	115–123	121–133	129–144
5	4	118–126	124–136	132–148
5	5	121–129	127–139	135–152
5	6	124–133	130–143	138–156
5	7	128–137	134–147	142–161
5	8	132–141	138–152	147–166
5	9	136–145	142–156	151–170
5	10	140–150	146–160	155–174
5	11	144–154	150–165	159–179
6	0	148–158	154–170	164–184
6	1	152–162	158–175	168–189
6	2	156–167	162–180	173–194
6	3	160–171	167–185	178–199
6	4	164–175	172–190	182–204
Women				
4	10	92– 98	96–107	104–119
4	11	94–101	98–110	106–122
5	0	96–104	101–113	109–125
5	1	99–107	104–116	112–128
5	2	102–110	107–119	115–131
5	3	105–113	110–122	118–134
5	4	108–116	113–126	121–138
5	5	111–119	116–130	125–142
5	6	114–123	120–135	129–146
5	7	118–127	124–139	133–150
5	8	122–131	128–143	137–154
5	9	126–135	132–147	141–158
5	10	130–140	136–151	145–163
5	11	134–144	140–155	149–168
6	0	138–148	144–159	153–173

* Adapted from Metropolitan Life Insurance Co., New York. New weight standards for men and women. *Statistical Bulletin* 40:3, Nov.–Dec., 1959.

group. Family, friends, insurance companies, and others may pressure the obese to lose weight, and penalize them, emotionally or financially, when they do not. Studies have shown that obese girls exhibit traits similar to those cited by social anthropologists as characteristic of

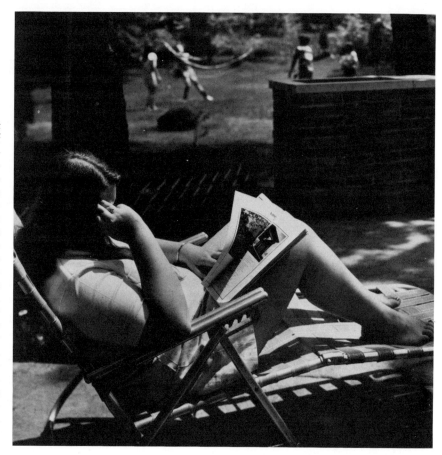

Figure 6.3. (From *Science Year. The World Book Science Annual.* © 1972 Field Enterprises Educational Corporation.)

Somatotypes

Somatotyping refers to the most useful and widely used method of relating physique to disease in general. William H. Sheldon, a well-known physical anthropologist who has tried for at least three decades to describe more precisely the various body types, has established a basic classification of human beings according to their physique as endomorphs, mesomorphs, or ectomorphs—the somatotypes. The endomorph has a more or less large body with short arms and legs, while the mesomorph is, at least for men, more aesthetically proportioned. The ectomorph has a body that is large in comparison with short arms and legs. When endomorphy predominates, abdomen mass overshadows the bulk of that section of the body above it; all regions are notable for softness and roundness. When mesomorphy predominates, the chest is massive and muscular and dominates over the abdomen; body joints are prominent. When ectomorphy prevails, the individual tends to be slender, delicate in bone structure, and stringy in muscular development.

minority persons subjected to intense prejudice: heightened sensitivity, obsessive concern (with weight in this case, rather than with color or ethnic origin), passivity, and withdrawal. And indeed, obese girls are subject to discrimination: their social interactions are often less, they are asked less frequently on dates, and one of our studies shows that there is a pattern of discrimination against them in college admission.

PREVALENCE OF OBESITY

We do not have good data on the prevalance of obesity for the population as a whole. Insurance data comparing the weights of insureds to the weights associated with lowest mortality show that half of American men between 30 and 39 years of age are at least 10 percent overweight and 25 percent are at least 20 percent overweight. The greatest prevalence is in the 50 to 59 age group where 60 percent of men are over 10 percent overweight and 33 percent are at least 20 percent overweight. For women, the percentage of overweight individuals under 40 is somewhat lower than that of men; from ages 40 to 49 the percentage is the same, while above age 49 it is greater than for men!

Data for children are sparse. Figures obtained in my study of the Boston suburbs indicate that 10 percent of the school population is obese, and up to 20 percent in certain high schools. While we do not have enough good longitudinal studies (studies where the same subject is followed during a significant portion of his life time, for example from birth to age 25), it is my impression, developed in the course of studies in children over a span of many years, that the obesity which develops before age 9 or in adolescence (approximately after age 16) is unlikely to be eliminated without a serious effort at weight control. By contrast, the obesity which develops just before the onset of puberty may be an exaggeration of the normal accumulation of fat which generally occurs at that age and is often self-correcting in the course of the next few years.

Finally, it has been noted that in the United States, obesity is much more prevalent among people in the lower socioeconomic range than in the upper-middle and upper classes. Explanations advanced for this finding are at present entirely conjectural. A different pattern is seen in poor countries, where the lower socioeconomic classes simply do not have enough food.

MECHANISM OF DEVELOPMENT

To explain obesity by ascribing it to overeating is an oversimplification which redefines the problem but does not in any way explain it. Certainly, obesity will not develop in an adult unless caloric intake is in excess of caloric expenditures. In growing children where caloric intake must be in excess of expenditures to insure growth, a reduction in intake generally reduces obesity as well, although, if marked, it may also slow growth. On the other hand, an intake in excess of expenditures, may indicate one of a number of combinations: an adolescent or adult may be normally or almost normally active, but be taking in too many calories; a person may have a caloric intake in the normal range but be very inactive; or a person's caloric intake may be slightly higher than the calorie requirement and his activity slightly decreased. All such combinations are found in individuals of both sexes and in any age group. In my studies I have found that obese men tend to be characterized by a normal to high intake and a low activity; low physical activity is now the general rule for nonrural men working in nonmanual activities. Obese women usually also show a normal to high intake and low physical activity. Obese children and adolescents often eat significantly less than their active contemporaries but show an extremely low physical activity. It should be noted that a pound of adipose tissue which contains our fat cells, on the average, is equivalent to 3,500 calories. A daily excess of 100 calories, whether arrived at by the consumption of half a sandwich or by the elimination of 20 minutes of walking will add up to 3,000 calories per month, over 35,000 calories per year—the equivalent of 10 pounds of fat!

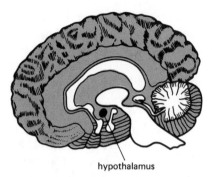

Figure 6.4. Cross-section of the brain. The hypothalamus is located approximately at the dark dot. (Copyright by *Nutrition Today*. Reproduced by permission.)

Figure 6.5. The mechanism of hunger. LA—lateral center; VM—ventromedial center. (Copyright by *Nutrition Today*. Reproduced by permission.)

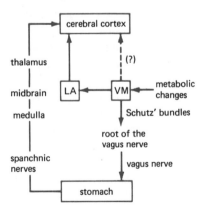

Regulation of food intake

The body mechanism regulating how much food you eat—like the mechanism regulating thirst—is a complex system which relies on components both inside and outside the brain. An essential part of the mechanism is situated in a part of the brain called the *hypothalamus* (Fig. 6.4). A pair of symmetrical centers, the *ventromedial* or *satiety centers* located at the center front of the hypothalamus, act sometimes in opposition to, sometimes in concert with, another pair of symmetrical centers, the *lateral* or *feeding centers* located farther to the sides of the hypothalamus. These lateral centers appear to be constantly active, initiating the feeding mechanism and controlling the desire to eat. The ventromedial centers act as brakes on the feeding centers in healthy persons by signalling when a point of satiety is reached. In our studies we have shown that the ventromedial centers also appear to exert some control over the "hunger contractions" which appear when an individual has not eaten for a number of hours and are felt as hunger by most persons. In periods between meals, glucose, the primary source of fuel of the central nervous system, is depleted more rapidly from the blood than either fat or protein. Cells in the ventromedial nucleus (*glucoreceptors*) that are especially sensitive to the rate of blood glucose utilization, sense the depletion. It is not certain whether the centers signal the cerebral cortex directly. They do, however, send signals along the nerves in two other directions: one is to the lateral or feeding areas, which, in turn, signal the cerebral cortex. The other is by way of nerve fibers which originate in the satiety area, through a system called the *Schutz' bundle*, to the vagus nerve, and on to the stomach, which begins hunger contractions (Fig. 6.5). (The satiety centers also control secretion of gastric acid, the digestive juice of the stomach.) The hunger contractions activate the spanchnic nerves in the stomach, which send independent signals to the cerebral cortex that more fuel is needed. When there is once again a high rate of blood glucose utilization, the satiety centers send out a signal for eating to stop, thus braking the feeding centers.

In children and adults it would appear that this fuel-sensing activity of the satiety center is one chief factor in control of hunger. *Appetite* is the term used to cover the psychological as well as physiological factors which make us desire certain types of foods. *Hunger* is the result of prolonged deprivation which makes us desire almost any food. The rate at which blood sugar is utilized is governed by a number of complex body functions, including the level of glucose available to the bloodstream and the level of insulin in the blood. In newborn animals and human infants, it seems that other factors, in particular gastric filling (whether or not the stomach is full), are more important. The role of such factors appears to decline as the hypothalamus matures; this occurs in a few months in experimental animals. In humans there is as yet no definitive evidence, but it is probably within the first three years of life. The role of other factors such as the size of body fat reserves, learning, and conditioning is currently under active investigation.

The mechanism of regulation of food intake is obviously complicated. Like all complicated mechanisms, it is vulnerable to many possible influences which can interfere with the proper functioning of any one part, and thus with the normal functioning of the whole, such as: a physical injury to the ventromedial centers of the hypothalamus; diabetes, which alters the hypothalamic reaction to blood sugar; or a psychological trauma that leads to overeating as an emotional compensation. Any of these factors and a number of others can cause a food intake temporarily or permanently increased over energy expenditures.

THE OBESITIES

Studies with experimental animals have shown over a dozen different forms of obesity in the rat and mouse alone. Among them are the *obese-hyperglycemic syndrome,* characterized by a weight of up to 100 grams or more instead of the normal 30 grams for a mouse, high blood sugar and cholesterol, resistance to the action of insulin, and many other hormonal, biochemical, and behavioral abnormalities; several forms of genetic obesity; obesity caused by destruction of the ventromedial area—surgically, electrolytically, or chemically; obesity caused by secretions of certain tumors; and two forms of obesity related to diet—one in which an animal goes on eating but is immobilized, the other brought about by carbohydrate-free, high-fat diets. Thus, genetic, traumatic, and environmental factors can all be at the origin—involved in the etiology—of obesity.

Nothing we have learned in studying obesity in humans suggests that its causes are any less varied. While classification of human obesities is in its infancy, enough data are available to show that in our species, too, genetic, traumatic, and environmental factors are involved.

Genetic factors

Human obesity has a strong familial component: in the Boston area, the proportion of normal weight parents who have obese youngsters is 7 percent; if one parent is overweight, the proportion rises to about 40 percent; if both parents are overweight, the proportion of overweight children is over 80 percent. Studies of adopted children, both in Boston and London, suggest that genetics is a dominant factor in this picture: the weight of children adopted from birth shows little association with that of their foster parents. Similarly, studies of identical twins reared in different environments, in situations where food is freely available to both twins, show that the twins tend to maintain similar weights regardless of environmental influences. Hereditary significance has also been attached to possession of certain body types. Apparently, highly ectomorphic individuals (with bodies characterized by an elongated skeleton, long and narrow hands and feet) can be quite inactive without gaining

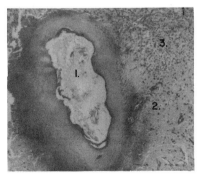

Figure 6.6. A portion of rat cortex with an electrolytic lesion. 1. At the center of the lesion is an area of dead tissue. 2. Surrounding this area is a region consisting mostly of gitter cells, the phagocytes for nervous tissue which ingest microorganisms or other cells and foreign particles. 3. Around the gitter cell area is a dense band of glia cells, which make up the supporting web of nervous tissue. Lesions made by this method are less precise and cause greater damage to the surrounding area than lesions made by gold thioglucose injections.

The glucostatic mechanism

The *glucostatic mechanism* was suggested in the early 1950s when studies with experimental animals and human subjects showed a direct relationship between a high rate of utilization of blood sugar and a feeling of satiety. The reverse was also true: when the subjects had low blood sugar they showed a desire to eat. It was already known that the ventromedial area of the hypothalamus exerted control over feeding behavior, but not how the control mechanism(s) operated.

The suggestion was made that there might be cells within the hypothalamus that were especially sensitive to the presence or absence of glucose (the body's main source of energy, and the only source of energy for the brain) which, reacting to a need for more glucose, triggered the desire to eat and, conversely, the desire to stop eating when the need for glucose was satisfied. At the time the glucostatic mechanism was postulated, there was no way of directly testing it, since the only ways of manipulating the action of the ventromedial area were by injecting anaesthetic or by destroying the cells by electrolytic lesions. It was then discovered that injections of *gold thioglucose*, a glucose linked to a sulfur-hydrogen group, which in turn is linked to gold, would selectively destroy cells in the region of the satiety center. A number of other gold thiocompounds were tried: gold thiomalate, gold thiogalactose, and so on, but only the combination of gold and glucose produced the ventromedial hypothalamic damage and the resulting obesity. It appeared that the glucose was being drawn from the blood vessels into the receptive cells, and that the gold, drawn in with the glucose, reached a toxic level and destroyed the cells, thus destroying their control over appetite regulation. The effect is specific to the ventromedial area.

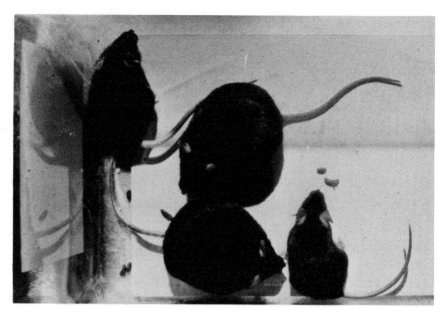

Figure 6.7. Two of the mice from this litter inherited genes that created an excess of fat cells and thus caused extreme obesity. (From Science Year. *The World Book Science Annual.* © 1972 Field Enterprises Educational Corporation.)

weight, while mesomorphic individuals (with a more robust skeleton and a much more developed muscle mass) are dependent on a relatively high exercise level to control their weight without dieting.

Traumatic factors

Experimental animals have been shown to develop obesity when subjected both to physiological and psychic trauma. Hormonal imbalances are an example of the first, punishment for not overeating an example of the second. Human beings have been said to sometimes develop obesity as a result of emotional trauma that can be traced to a particular stress period in their lives. Human obesity resulting from physiological stress has been repeatedly observed: for example, damage to the hypothalamus from tumors, infection, or physical injury produces a *hypothalamic obesity*—one resulting from damage to the feeding or satiety centers—that is hauntingly similar to that seen in experimental animals.

Environmental factors

Finally, environmental factors are important. The importance of the *nature* of the diet has probably been overemphasized: in a number of studies in Boston, we could not find any difference in the type of foods selected by overweight, normal weight, or underweight women and high school girls or in the proportion of calories from carbohydrates, fats, and protein. The *quantity* consumed is, of course, crucial. By contrast, the role of exercise in weight control is still being underemphasized. Studies conducted a number of years ago showed that in humans as in animals, while it is true that increasing physical activity in an already active subject increases appetite and food intake, the reverse is not invariably true: below a certain level of activity, a further decrease in exercise does not lead to a corresponding degree of reduction in food intake. In fact, at extremely sedentary levels of activity, food intake increases somewhat. The result, of course, is obesity.

TREATMENT OF OBESITY

There is a sound medical as well as cosmetic rationale for the weight reduction of individuals who carry an excessive amount of fat. The insurance companies' data show not only that overweight shortens life, but also that life expectancy improves for overweight individuals who lost weight and stay reduced. Furthermore, in a number of medical situations, such as maturity-onset diabetes, the Pickwickian Syndrome (where excess adiposity—the amount of adipose or fat tissue in the body —interferes with respiration), and liver disease, the condition of the patient usually is visibly improved by weight reduction.

The physician or dietitian treating an overweight person first acquires, through medical records and interviews, a thorough knowledge of the patient's weight, his dietary habits, his caloric intake, and his exercise habits. Past changes in food intake and in physical activity are identified. The family history regarding overweight, illness, and causes of death of close relatives often gives clues to the probable course of obesity, if uncorrected, as well as to the relation of obesity to future health problems and longevity. Knowing how the patient's weight reacts to various types of crises or changes in living habits and how the patient

Fad diets

The American people are constantly bombarded with advice on how to lose weight. Since anyone can lose some weight in the first flush of enthusiasm, the diet, no matter how absurd, sells for a while—and someone becomes rich. In the past year we have had a grapefruit diet, a banana diet, a hard boiled egg diet, and countless yoghurt diets. We have had low-protein diets: high-carbohydrate diets, the Duke, Kempner, or rice diet, and the so-called Rockefeller diet. The most recurrent diets, however, have been low-carbohydrate diets—called high protein diets but, in fact, mostly high-fat. The first such diet was devised in England by a Dr. William Harvey in the early 1860s and publicized in 1863 by William Banting. The diet has since reappeared as the Du Pont or Pennington diet (1953), the so-called Air Force diet (1960), the "Calories don't count" diet of Dr. Taller (1961), and the "drinking man's" diet (1964). Recently it became the Stillman diet (1967)—this time consumed with many glasses of water. Finally, in 1972, it has reappeared as "Dr. Atkins' Diet Revolution," in particularly extreme form.

In the words of a release of the Council on Foods and Nutrition of the American Medical Association: "The 'diet revolution' is neither new nor revolutionary. It is a variant of the 'familiar' low carbohydrate diet that has been promulgated for years. The rationale advanced to justify the diet is, for the most part, without scientific merit." Even more serious: "The Council is deeply concerned about any diet that advocates an 'unlimited' intake of saturated fats and cholesterol-rich foods [another aspect of the Atkins diet]." The Council concludes that individuals responding to such a diet with a rise in blood fats will have an increased risk of coronary artery disease and atherosclerosis (hardening of the arteries), ". . . particularly if the diet is maintained over a prolonged period."

The value of various types of exercise

We know that a moderate amount of daily exercise such as a one-hour walk is a useful, sometimes necessary tool in weight control. Different types of exercise have different benefits for the body. An hour of vigorous exercise, such as tennis, swimming, or jogging at a moderate clip, has been shown to have a favorable effect not only on weight and general circulation but often on blood pressure as well. A regimen of many hours of hard physical labor every day has been shown to help in maintaining a low blood cholesterol, even when the diet contains a sizable proportion of saturated fats. The style of life which includes a large amount of daily physical activity is still seen in certain "primitive" situations, but is obviously not compatible with the life-styles and work habits of most modern Americans. More feasible is the practice of three or four brief periods of intense physical activity every week (squash, running, fast swimming) which has been shown to assist in maintaining the elasticity of blood vessels, the coronary arteries in particular, and in keeping open alternative blood vessels ("collateral circulation") if some of the coronary branches are narrowed or occluded by the cholesterol-containing plaques seen in atherosclerosis. Emphasis on these types of exercise which act on the circulatory system and are thus useful for long-term survival is not meant to denigrate team sports— they are fun, teach cooperation, and some of them, such as soccer, hocky or water polo, entail highly vigorous exercise—or to diminish the satisfaction of training for strength (weight lifting), suppleness and grace (ballet dancing), or skill (golf). It simply is meant to remind us that survival should be the first priority of health-conscious persons.

has felt and behaved during past periods of dieting and weight loss indicates whether the patient should attempt to reduce and at what rate.

When the decision has been made to reduce by the patient, the practical task is to take off excess fat at a rate which will be clearly observable, yet not so extreme as to be incompatible with sound nutrition, health, or the carrying out of daily duties without excessive fatigue. A daily deficit of 1,000 calories will take off two pounds a week (more at the beginning of the reduction regimen), a rate of loss sufficient in almost all cases. Half this rate is acceptable in cases where a small and inactive person cannot tolerate a deficit of more than 500 calories per day.

This deficit can be reached by reducing intake, increasing activity, or both. Reduction of intake should be done on a diet which is nutritionally adequate, has sufficient satiety value, and provides the basis for a long-term, sound dietary regimen. Fad diets, including some recently popularized high-fat, low-carbohydrate diets should be avoided. In some persons, spacing of the allotted calories over five snacks rather than three meals is useful in preventing excessive hunger; obviously, the addition of eating occasions necessitates a particularly tight self-control.

Increasing physical activity is always desirable unless there are strong medical contraindications. It usually involves a rearrangement of the dieter's schedule so as to make enough time available for brisk walking or practicing a sport; it may mean a basic, lifelong decision to reorganize one's way of life.

Psychological support is always important during dieting. For the patient, sometimes it involves nothing more than the encouragement of family or roommates and the establishment of a satisfactory relationship with the doctor and the dietitian. For the therapist, it involves deciding who should reduce, establishing a satisfactory relationship with the patient, inducing the motivation to reduce, correcting body image (if the patient sees himself or herself as thinner or fatter than he or she is), and understanding the patient's sensations of hunger and satiety. Group therapy—either in a clinic setting or in organizations such as Weight Watchers and TOPS—has often been found helpful in supporting certain patients during weight reduction.

A proper psychological approach is especially important when dealing with children and adolescents. A punitive attitude toward obese children is inexcusable. They must feel themselves beloved and worthwhile persons who are being helped to correct a physical problem and encouraged to be fit, rather than made to feel ashamed of their appearance or guilty every time they eat. In adolescent girls, a very dangerous syndrome called *anorexia nervosa* in which the patient starves herself— not infrequently to death—can occur if the subject thinks herself an object of derision or pity because she is too fat. This disorder of self-image, if accompanied by a compulsive personality which enforces a rigorous regimen of exercise and caloric restriction, leads to a profound

12 practical rules on how to reduce

1. Keep your eye on portion size. A diet is not simply a list of permitted foods which you may eat in any amount. A diet tells you not only what courses compose the day's meals but how much of each course to eat. Learn to regulate portion size.

2. Count every calorie. That means every calorie, including small snacks. A cupful of nuts eaten in the course of an evening adds up to 800 calories!

3. Beware of "nonfattening" foods. Too many people think there are "fattening" foods (usually starchy foods whose caloric content they overestimate), and "nonfattening" foods, such as roast beef (420 calories for 5 ounces) yoghurt (150 calories for a cup of plain yoghurt made with whole milk), or orange juice (110 calories for a cup of unsweetened orange juice). All foods are fattening if you eat enough of them —except perhaps celery sticks. By contrast, a small amount of food contains few calories: 60 calories for a slice of bread, 100 calories for a banana or medium size potato.

4. Stop leaning on protein. Protein, too, contains calories (4 calories per gram—the same as carbohydrates). "Protein foods" are often high in fat and rich in calories (¾ of the calories in frankfurters are fat).

5. Remember that you can drink calories as well as eat them: there are 150 calories in a glass of beer and 160 in a martini. Two beers with the evening cashew nuts add up to 900 calories!

6. Remember that polyunsaturated oils and margarines are better for a low cholesterol level, but they contain as many calories as other oils and fat.

7. Cook lean—don't add unnecessary calories as you cook.

8. Cut down drastically on sugar. White or brown, refined or raw, it is a prime source of empty calories.

9. Cut down moderately on fat. This won't modify the caloric value of your diet, but it will keep you from retaining water as you lose weight and will thus insure a smoother weight loss. Cutting down on salt will also keep you from retaining water and will decrease your chances of developing high blood pressure.

10. Remember that expending calories by exercise is as useful as cutting down on the calories you eat.

11. Look up tables of calories both for foods and for exercise.

12. Weigh yourself frequently.

weight loss. By the time weight goes down to 60 percent of the normal, the patient's hold on life becomes precarious. A tendency to overdiet, although not to that extreme, is all too common among adolescent girls and young women, often in an attempt to be thinner than their skeleton will allow them to be.

In America today the problem of underweight is not widespread, although there is malnutrition among some underprivileged groups in our population, like migrant farm workers and residents of Indian reservations. *Kwashiorkor*, an extreme form of protein-calories malnutrition, has even been seen in some young children in these populations. This problem can be corrected by sufficient good-quality food and an income with which to buy it.

In general, it can be said that a healthy, well-nourished adult who is underweight by ten pounds or so stands a better chance of avoiding some of our most prevalent diseases, like heart disease and stroke, and of living a long and active life. Gross underweight, as in anorexia nervosa, and gross overweight, when it is obesity, are reverse sides of the same coin. In weight control, as in life, reasonableness and moderation are the best policies in the long run.

Questions

1. Is there ever any good reason (a) for putting on fat, (b) for being underweight?
2. Is there any difference between overweight and obesity? If so, what?

3. What methods are used to diagnose obesity in an individual? Are they equally useful in all cases?
4. List the various effects of obesity on an individual and give some examples of each.
5. How prevalent is obesity in the United States? In different age groups? In different economic groups?
6. Is eating too much the only way to get fat?
7. Describe the internal mechanisms that regulate food intake.
8. What factors, internal and external, influence the development of obesity?

Key Concepts

Anorexia – pathological absence of appetite or hunger when either or both are clearly appropriate

Appetite – the complex of sensations, up to a point pleasant or at least not unpleasant, by which a person is aware of the desire for and the anticipation of ingesting palatable food; specific appetites relate to desires for specific foods

Hunger – the complex of unpleasant sensations, felt after prolonged deprivation of food, which will impel a person to seek, work, or fight for immediate relief by ingestion of food; the passage from appetite to hunger is dependent on the duration of deprivation, the rate of energy expenditure, and other factors

Obesity – excessive accumulation of body fat

Overweight – weight in excess of normal range (which may, as in the case of many athletes, not involve obesity at all)

Satiety – the complex of sensations which impels a person to stop eating because hunger and appetite have been satisfied, even though food is still available

Regulation of food intake – the action of the mechanism or mechanisms whereby the body adjusts ingestion of food to requirements for maintaining health, the proper functioning of the body, and growth in the case of the young

Selected Readings

Blakeslees, A. L., and J. Stamler. *Your Heart Has Nine Lives.* Englewood Cliffs, N. J.: Prentice-Hall, 1966.

Blix, G., ed. *Occurrence, Causes and Prevention of Overnutrition*, Second Symposium of the Swedish Nutrition Foundation. Uppsala: Almqvist & Wiksells, 1964.

Mayer, J. *Overweight, Causes, Cost, and Control.* Englewood Cliffs, N. J.: Prentice-Hall, Inc., 1968.

Obesity and Health, a source book of current information for professional health workers. Publication 1485 of the U.S. Public Health Service. Washington, D. C.: U.S. Government Printing Office, 1966.

Wyden, P. *The Overweight Society.* New York: Wm. Morrow, 1965.

Chapter 7

Genetics

In recent years there has been increasing awareness of human genetics and genetic disease. Newborn babies in many states have blood tests performed to make certain they do not have certain rare but treatable genetic diseases. Newspapers have carried stories of the debate as to whether a man with two Y chromosomes (instead of the normal single Y) is more likely to commit violent crimes. As part of the trend to greater racial awareness, many realize each race has a predisposition to different genetic diseases: blacks have become concerned that genetic diseases common among blacks have not received a sufficient amount of research study and federal financial support, and Jews have learned that there are certain genetic diseases which they are much more prone to have than non-Jews. Part of the stimulus for the debate over legalizing therapeutic abortion is the fact that it has recently become possible to identify serious and untreatable genetic diseases in the fetus and allow selective abortion of abnormal fetuses.

This chapter was contributed by Lewis B. Holmes, M.D., Assistant Professor of Pediatrics, Harvard Medical School, and Associate Pediatrician and Director of the Genetics Clinic at Massachusetts General Hospital.

As public interest in genetics has increased, there have been many new developments in the scientific aspects of genetics. *Genetics* is the branch of biology concerned with heredity, the reproductive process by which physical traits and functions are passed from parents to their offspring. In recent years the chemical nature of a gene has been learned, and the means by which genes express normal and abnormal traits are now becoming clear. The total number of diseases caused by abnormal genes is not known, but many new genetic diseases are discovered each year. *Genetic diseases* are those caused by errors in the heritable material (genes) that are passed from parents to offspring.

In this chapter we will discuss human genetics in light of those problems most likely to affect our lives. The four general topics will be: chromosomal abnormalities, single mutant genes, multifactorial inheritance, and genetic counseling including prenatal diagnosis.

CHROMOSOMES   Each cell in the body contains 46 chromosomes in its nucleus, and each chromosome contains thousands of genes. The genes determine the physical traits and functions of the individual. In some individuals an entire chromosome or a portion of a chromosome containing thousands of genes may be missing or may be present in excess of the normal number. Such conditions, called *chromosome abnormalities,* occur as a result of errors in cell division.

During most phases of cell division, the individual chromosomes are a single strand of material, and it is difficult to see each one separately. However, during *metaphase,* the phase of cell division just before the cell divides, the chromosomes duplicate themselves, becoming shorter and easier to study. As can be seen in Figure 7.1, the shape of the chromosomes in metaphase depends on the location of the point where the arms come together, the *centromere.* Since about 1970, it has been possible to identify each chromosome through staining procedures. Figure 7.2 shows how it is now possible to group the 46 human chromosomes into 23 pairs: 22 nonsex pairs, called *autosomes,* plus one pair of sex chromosomes.

The only apparent chromosomal difference between males and females is in the pair of sex chromosomes. Males have one X chromosome and a much smaller Y chromosome; the chromosomal status of the normal male is thus written as 46,XY. Females have two identical X chromosomes and are referred to as 46,XX. In reproduction, one member of each of the 23 pairs of chromosomes is provided by the female and one member is provided by the male (see Chap. 2). A woman's eggs contain 23 chromosomes, one of which is an X; a man's sperm can contain either an X or a Y chromosome, so they are either 23,X or 23,Y.

MEIOSIS   There are two types of divisions of the cells in the body, and chromosome abnormalities can arise from errors in each process of division. The first type of cell division is *meiosis,* which results in the

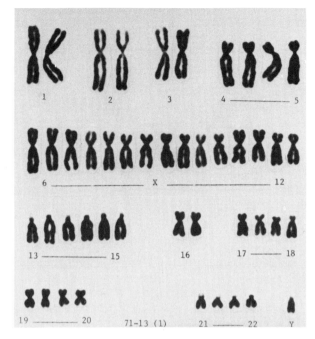

Figure 7.1. Chromosomes of a normal male, 46, XY. Notice the lack of characteristics that distinguish pair 4 from 5, 17 from 18, and 13 from 14 and 15, etc. The bent appearance of numbers 1 and 5 has no significance. Magnification ×2600. (Courtesy of Dr. L. Atkins, Boston, Mass.)

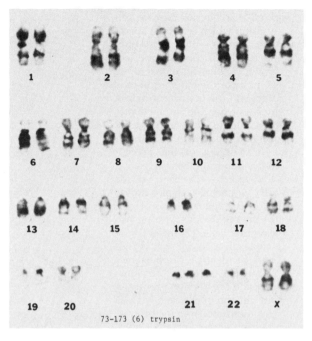

Figure 7.2. Chromosomes of a female with trisomy 21. The different banding patterns allow identification of each of the 22 pairs of autosomes, as well as the X and Y chromosomes. Note that although the 21 chromosome is small, its banding pattern is different from that of number 22. Magnification ×2600. (Courtesy of Dr. L. Atkins, Boston, Mass.)

formation of sperm in the male and ova or eggs in the female. The sperm and the ova each have only 23 single chromosomes (22 autosomes and 1 sex chromosome), because in meiosis the original number of chromosomes (46) in the germ cells of each parent is reduced by one half. One member of each pair of the parent's chromosomes goes to a daughter cell (Fig. 7.3a). The error in meoisis that leads to chromosome abnormalities occurs when one pair of chromosomes stays together rather than separating and moving to opposite ends of the cell (Fig. 7.3b). This process can affect any of the chromosomes.

MITOSIS The second type of cell division is *mitosis.* This procedure occurs in all cells except the egg and the sperm. During this type of division a single cell divides into two complete new cells (*daughter cells*) each of which has the same number of chromosomes as the original cell (Fig. 7.4a). The most common errors in this process occur when both members of a pair of chromosomes fail to separate, resulting in one daughter cell having one extra chromosome and the other daughter miss-

Figure 7.3. a. Normal meiosis, cell division which results in sperm and ova. In these illustrations only two pairs of chromosomes are shown. (1) Nucleus of cell when none of the chromosomes is visible; (2) the period just before division when the chromosomes are visible; (3) the chromosomes form pairs each with its homologous chromosome; (4) the chromosomes duplicate themselves and line up across the center of the cell; (5) one of each pair moves to the opposite ends of cell; (6) the cell divides forming two daughter cells; (7) the chromosomes in each cell split in half and the identical chromosomes move in opposite directions; (8) the cell divides, producing four daughter cells each with 23 chromosomes from the original cell with 46 chromosomes. b. Abnormal meiosis. The process is normal until the cell divides. (5) When the cell divides, one pair of chromosomes stays together rather than separating and moving to opposite ends of the cell; (6) the cells produced are unbalanced in that one contains one chromosome too many and the other one chromosome too few; (7) each chromosome splits into two and these move in opposite directions; (8) the cell divides, producing four daughter cells: two with 24 chromosomes and two with 22 chromosomes.

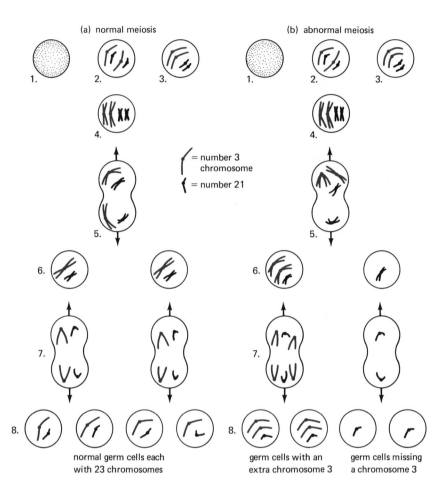

ing one chromosome (Fig. 7.4b). If the abnormal cells produced by these errors continue to develop in the fetus, the individual will develop a chromosome abnormality (*chromosome mosaicism*) with some of the individual cells having 46 chromosomes and some either 45 or 47. If the abnormal division occurs after there have been several cell divisions of the fertilized *zygote* (a fertilized ovum that results from the mating of a sperm cell and an egg cell), the resulting individual can exhibit several different chromosome abnormalities each in different cells.

CHROMOSOME ANALYSIS A laboratory test, *chromosome analysis*, can identify the presence of additional chromosomal material or the lack of the normal amount of chromosomal material. The additional material may be an entire chromosome, called *trisomy*, or only a portion of a chromosome. There may be an absence of an entire chromosome, called *monosomy*, or a piece of chromosome material.

Figure 7.4. a. Normal mitosis, the type of cell division in all but germ cells. (1) Nucleus of cell when none of the chromosomes is visible; (2) the chromosomes are visible (only two of the 46 shown in these illustrations); (3) each chromosome duplicates itself; (4) the chromosomes line up across the center of the cell; (5) the duplicated chromosomes split in half and move to opposite ends of the cells; (6) the cell divides into two daughter cells, each with the same number of chromosomes as the original cell. b. Abnormal mitosis. The process is normal until the cell divides. (5) When the cell divides, one pair of chromosomes stays together rather than separating; (6) the cell divides with one too many chromosomes going to one daughter cell and one too few to the other daughter cell.

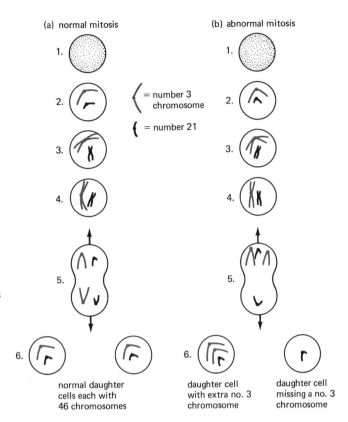

The first chromosome abnormality in man was identified in 1959. In the short time since then, we have learned that these problems are very common. About 1 in every 200 newborn infants has a significant chromosome abnormality.[1] Many more chromosomally abnormal fetuses do not survive long enough to become newborn infants. By studying cells of spontaneous abortions or miscarriages, it has been learned that about 25 percent of these are apparently due to a serious chromosome abnormality.[2] Since it is known that between 10 and 20 percent of all pregnancies end in spontaneous abortion, it is estimated that between 3 and 5 percent of all conceptions result in a major chromosome abnormality. Ninety percent of these abnormalities do not survive long enough to be born alive. To illustrate the features of the different types of chromosome abnormalities that occur in liveborn infants several specific disorders will be described.

[1] J. L. Hamerton *et al.*, "Chromosome studies in a neonatal population," *Canadian Medical Association Journal*, Vol. 106 (1972), 776–79.
[2] D. H. Carr, "Genetic Basis of Abortion," *Ann. Rev. Genetics*, Vol. 5 (1971), 65–80.

CHROMOSOME ABNORMALITIES

Chromosome analysis

There are probably over 100,000 different genes in the 46 human chromosomes. Unfortunately, many people think that these genes can be "checked" by chromosome analysis, whereas only gross excesses or deficiencies of chromosome material are visible. Human chromosomes can be studied easily from either white blood cells or skin cells, called fibroblasts, although the former is much more widely available, faster, and less complex. For testing the white blood cells a blood sample is usually obtained from a surface vein in the arm; for testing infants the blood is obtained by pricking the heel. The blood is incubated at body temperature (37°C) in a mixture of serum, antibiotics, and phytohemagglutinin (a chemical which stimulates white blood cells to divide). This mixture is kept in an atmosphere of 95 percent oxygen and 5 percent carbon dioxide for 3 to 4 days.

At the end of the incubation period a drug (colchicine) is added to the mixture that causes cell division to stop in metaphase, the stage in which the chromosomes are most appropriate for inspection because they are more compact and it is easier to identify each one individually. The chromosomes are easily seen through a light microscope at a magnification 100 times their normal size. Analysis can be done visually through the microscope. To facilitate the inspection and to make a permanent record, the chromosomes from one nucleus are photographed. Chromosome analysis is available in hospital laboratories throughout the world. In the United States the cost ranges from $75 to $150.

Nonsex chromosome abnormalities

DOWN'S SYNDROME The most common chromosomal abnormality of the autosomes (nonsex chromosomes) is Down's syndrome, formerly called *mongolism*, named for Dr. Langdon Down who first described this disorder in 1866. Unfortunately Dr. Down thought the affected individuals resembled persons from the Asian country Mongolia and as a result the terms *mongolism* and *mongoloid* came into use. The use of these terms is misleading because there is no real similarity in appearance between these groups, and Mongolians are no more prone to Down's syndrome than any other racial or national group.

Down's syndrome results from the presence of an extra chromosome 21, and thus the disease is also called *trisomy 21*. The infant with Down's syndrome has several physical abnormalities.[3] He or she is shorter than average, more prone to serious abnormalities of the heart and intestine, and has poor muscle. Most have a similar facial appearance (Fig. 7.5) and are easily recognized by this. Some of their most familiar features are a flat, round facial profile, upward slant of the eyes, extra skin folds (epicanthal folds) where the eye meets the nose, a protruding tongue, small ears with overfolding of the upper portion, incurved fifth finger of each hand, and a single crease across the palm of the hand (simian crease). An individual with Down's syndrome usually has only some of these features. Any one of these major or minor birth defects can occur in someone who is perfectly normal. However, it is the combination of so many features that makes it possible to easily recognize Down's syndrome. These individuals also have slow development in childhood. They eventually learn to walk and talk, but do so later than their normal brothers and sisters. While the early development of some infants seems close to normal, most will have an I.Q. between 25 and 50. In general, they are likable, happy, and friendly.

Down's syndrome occurs once in every 700 live births in the United States and is ten times more common than other diseases resulting from an extra chromosome such as trisomy 13 and trisomy 18 (Table 7.1). The precise reason why these trisomies occur is not known. One of the major factors is the age of the mother. The incidence of all trisomies increases markedly in older women. For example, statistics in Massachusetts[4] showed that for women between 20 and 24 years old the frequency of Down's syndrome was 1 in 1667 infants; ages 25 to 29, 1 in 1428; ages 30 to 34, 1 in 909; ages 35 to 39, 1 in 227; and over 40 years old the frequency was 1 in 77 births. The presumed reason for this greater frequency in older women is the fact that a woman's eggs are as old as she is. Ova develop in the ovary of the unborn female and

---

[3] D. W. Smith and A. A. Wilson, *The Child with Down's Syndrome (Mongolism)* (Philadelphia: W. B. Saunders Company, 1973).

[4] J. Fabia, "Illegitimacy and Down's syndrome," *Nature*, Vol. 221 (1969), 1157–58.

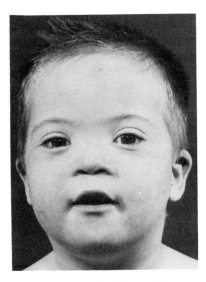

Figure 7.5. A young boy with Down's syndrome showing the flat round face, epicanthal folds, and small ears with overfolding of the upper portion.

no new ones develop after birth. As a result, when the 45-year-old woman ovulates and her egg is fertilized, this egg is 45 years old. In contrast, the sperm of an adult male is being made at all times. The age of the woman's egg is important because an older egg is more prone to undergo errors in meiosis.

Table 7.1 *The most common chromosome abnormalities*

Disease	Incidence	Clinical features
Total incidence of all chromosome abnormalities: 1 in 200 newborn infants[a]		
Autosomes		
Down's Syndrome	1 in 700[b]	mental retardation
		abnormal face and hands
		heart and intestinal defects
		poor muscle tone
		short stature
Trisomy 18	1 in 6,800[c]	heart, brain, kidney abnormalities
		liver disease
		limb deformities
		mental retardation
Trisomy 13	1 in 7,600[c]	brain, eye, heart deformities
		cleft lip and palate
		extra fingers and toes
		mental retardation
Sex chromosomes		
47,XYY	1 in 600[a]	possible tall stature
		possible abnormal behavior
47,XXY (Klinefelter's Syndrome)	1 in 900[a]	small testicles
		breast tissue
		sterility
		poor social adjustment
47,XXX	1 in 1,100[a]	mental retardation
45,X (Turner's Syndrome)	1 in 3,300[d]	short stature
		lack of normal ovaries
		short neck
		abnormal lymphatic vessels

[a] J. L. Hamerton *et al.*, "Chromosome Studies in a Neonatal Population," *Canadian Medical Association Journal*, Vol. 106 (1972), 776–79.
[b] J. Fabia, "Illegitimacy and Down's Syndrome, *Nature*, Vol. 221 (1969), 1157–58.
[c] A. I. Taylor, "Autosomal Trisomy Syndromes," *Journal of Medical Genetics*, Vol. 5 (1968), 227–52.
[d] W. M. Court Brown, Sex Chromosome Aneuploidy in Man," *Int. Rev. Exp. Pathol.*, Vol. 7 (1969), 31–97.

DOWN'S SYNDROME DUE TO TRANSLOCATION While most individuals with Down's syndrome have trisomy 21, there is one important exception. About 1 to 2 percent have Down's syndrome due to the translocation or movement of the extra 21 chromosome to another chromosome (Fig. 7.6). There are no physical differences between individuals

Figure 7.6. Chromosomes of a male with Down's syndrome due to translocation of the third number 21 onto a number 14 chromosome. Note that while the banding pattern of all chromosomes is similar to that shown in Fig. 7.2, there is variation in the clarity. This variation is common with the new staining techniques, and while it is frustrating, it also underscores the value of experience in interpreting the findings. Magnification ×2600. (Courtesy of Dr. L. Atkins, Boston, Mass.)

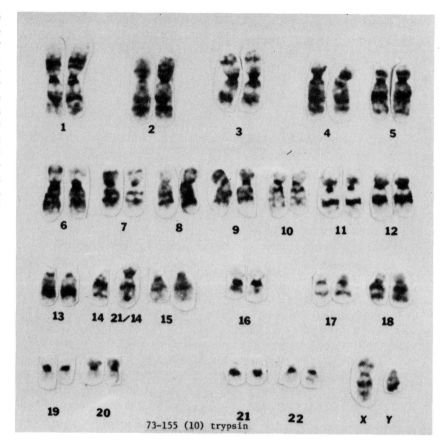

with Down's syndrome due to trisomy 21 and translocation of the extra 21 chromosome. The importance of recognizing the translocation is that often one of the parents is a carrier of this abnormality. The carrier has a total of 45 chromosomes, instead of the normal 46, with the second 21 chromosome translocated to another chromosome. If one parent is a carrier, there are several possible consequences for the child: he can have Down's syndrome due to translocation; he can be a carrier but physically normal; he can be entirely normal; or he can have one of several different lethal chromosome imbalances and die before birth. In practice, if the father is a translocation carrier, there is about a 5 percent risk his child will have Down's syndrome. If the mother is the carrier, the risk is 10 percent.

TRISOMIES 18 AND 13 The only other abnormalities resulting from extra nonsex chromosomes that occur with any appreciable frequency in newborn infants are trisomy 18 and trisomy 13. Each is much more serious than trisomy 21 both in terms of the severity of the resulting physical abnormalities and mental retardation and in terms of the length of their survival. Infants with an extra chromosome 18 usually have severe abnormalities of the brain, heart, kidney, liver, intestine, hands, and feet and almost all die in the first year of life. Infants with an extra chromosome 13 also have severe abnormalities of many internal organs. In addition, they often have more visible deformities such as cleft lip and palate, small or absent eyes, and extra fingers and toes. These infants rarely live more than a few weeks or months.

Sex chromosome abnormalities

There are several other chromosome abnormalities in humans that are almost as common as Down's syndrome. These abnormalities involve extra sex chromosomes in males and females. The incidence of these problems has been established by performing chromosome analysis on a large number of newborn infants (Table 7.1). The most remarkable aspect of the sex chromosome abnormalities is that the affected individual may show few or no physical and mental abnormalities.

IN MALES The two most common sex chromosome abnormalities in males are the presence of an extra X or an extra Y chromosome. The male with an extra X chromosome is 47,XXY, a condition which is also called *Klinefelter's syndrome*. The affected infant has no physical abnormalities. Affected adults are always sterile and often have some breast tissue, small testicles, and a more feminine distribution of body hair and fat. They often have problems in social interactions, have difficulty holding a job, and have a high divorce rate.

The male with an extra Y chromosome is 47,XYY. This condition has received a considerable amount of publicity because some of these individuals have unusually tall stature and often exhibit antisocial behavior. However, it is incorrect to assume that all 47,XYY males will be antisocial. For example, it was incorrectly reported that the man convicted of murdering several student nurses was 47,XYY. The report and diagnosis proved to be false, but the retraction received little publicity.[5] Research studies on affected males identified at birth are underway and will hopefully determine whether or not these infants are likely to have abnormal behavior when older and if so, how often this is true. It seems likely that many of these infants will be entirely normal.

IN FEMALES The most common chromosome abnormality in females is the presence of an extra X chromosome. The 47,XXX women have no associated physical abnormalities; however, they are more likely to be mentally retarded than normal 46,XX females.

Only one abnormality in men or women associated with significant physical abnormalities is due to the absence of one sex chromosome. The affected individual is 45,X and female. This condition, also called *Turner's syndrome*, is not as common as other sex chromosome abnor-

[5] E. B. Hook, "Behavioral implications of the human XYY genotype," *Science*, Vol. 179 (1973), 139–150.

malities. The reason for the low incidence in newborns is that most of the 45,X fetuses do not survive to birth. About 98 percent of the 45,X fetuses are aborted spontaneously and account for one quarter of the chromosome abnormalities in spontaneous abortions. The affected individual who does survive has several medical problems: marked shortness of stature, a lack of normal ovaries which prevents both sexual maturation and fertility, deficient lymphatic vessels in their legs, and a short neck. These females are not mentally retarded, although some have specialized learning problems.

Figure 7.7. Small deletion of the short arm of a number 5 chromosome (arrow) in a male with the cat-cry syndrome. Magnification ×2600. (Courtesy of Dr. L. Atkins, Boston, Mass.)

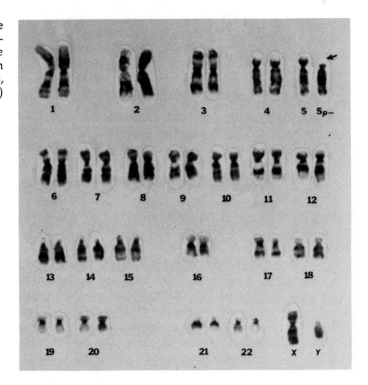

Chromosome deletions

During the past twelve years a small but significant portion of chromosome abnormalities has been shown to be due to the lack of a piece of a chromosome (a deletion). Affected individuals are almost always mentally retarded and have a variety of major and minor physical abnormalities.

Illustrative of the chromosome deletions is the *cat-cry syndrome*, which is due to a deficiency of a portion of the short arm of a number 5 chromosome (Fig. 7.7). This condition is so-named because the affected newborn infants have a high-pitched mewing cry due to abnormalities of their larynx and vocal cords. Aside from this, these infants are recog-

Screening newborn infants

Many states now require by law that a sample of blood be obtained from each newborn infant on the fourth or fifth day of life to detect genetic disorders not otherwise noticeable. The blood is obtained by making a small cut in the infant's heel. The drops of blood are soaked into small areas of filter paper and mailed to the state laboratory. There the filter paper is heated to kill all bacteria, and a small round portion is cut out and placed in an agar gel tray. In the agar is a particular kind of bacteria that grows rapidly in the presence of a specific amino acid. If after several hours there is an abnormally large area of discoloration in the agar because of the excessive growth of the bacteria the infant is retested because the test shows that he appears to have too much of a particular amino acid.

In Massachusetts this method is used to detect elevations in four amino acids: phenylalanine, tyrosine, methionine, and leucine. The abnormally high level in the blood of each amino acid means the presence of a deficiency in metabolism. Each of these metabolic defects is due to a separate autosomal recessive gene.

The overall testing program using blood and urine samples has shown that one in every 3,000 newborns has some type of amino acid disorder. The cost of the testing is $2.00 an infant. The result is early detection of many different hereditary diseases, and the treatment, dietary restriction of the specific amino acid, is much more beneficial the earlier it is begun.

nizable by their widely-spaced eyes and obvious mental retardation. As adults they are short, have small heads, are mentally retarded to a severe degree, and often have physical deformities.

No one knows the frequency of any of the chromosome deletions. They are particularly important because they often cause physical and mental abnormalities that are difficult for the physician to diagnose. Fortunately, they are usually identified promptly by chromosome analysis. Another important aspect of the chromosome deletion is that sometimes it represents a translocation that is hereditary, and thus parents and other close relatives must have chromosome analysis to see if they carry a chromosome translocation that makes them likely to have a child with a chromosome deletion.

SINGLE GENES   A human chromosome contains thousands of genes. Each chromosome consists primarily of deoxyribonucleic acid (DNA), which is two helically twisted chains of proteins and sugars held together by the pairing of four chemicals—adenine with thymidine and cytosine with guanine (see Chap. 1, Fig. 1.3). A gene is a small portion of DNA. Each gene determines the characteristics of a specific protein which influences the function of certain cells in the body.

The site of each gene on a chromosome is called a *gene locus*. Both members of a pair of autosomes have the same genes at the same locations along their structure. Therefore, the function of one gene on a specific chromosome is added to and influenced by the function of the gene at the same locus on the other chromosome in that pair of chromosomes. The two genes which occupy the same locus on a pair of chromosomes are called *alleles*. In humans, these alleles are not always identical. The state of having identical alleles at a specific locus on a pair of chromosomes is termed *homozygous*. When the alleles at a specific locus are different, this is termed *heterozygous*. The fact that peoples' genes are not always exactly the same accounts for normal human variations.

Genes can be either *dominant* or *recessive*. A gene is dominant if the presence of the gene is always apparent in the features of the person. Conversely, a recessive gene is one which is not always apparent in the person's features. If the child receives a dominant gene from either or both parents, the dominant gene will be evident in his appearance. If he receives a recessive gene from *both* parents, he will have the recessive characteristic.

Because of limitations in current medical technology, we cannot see a single normal or abnormal gene on a human chromosome. The presence of a gene can only be identified by studying the product(s) of the gene or the disease caused by the gene. For this reason, understanding the diseases due to single genes is important for understanding human genetics.

Abnormal single genes are called *mutant genes,* meaning the normal gene has been changed or mutated. The cause of this change or mutation is not known. It is known that in humans the spontaneous mutation rate remains constant in each generation. The rate in humans is estimated to be one mutation per 100,000 to 1,000,000 gene loci per generation.

The method of transmission of single mutant genes from parents to offspring is called *Mendelian inheritance.* This terminology pays tribute to Gregor Mendel, a biologist in the nineteenth century who showed the patterns of inheritance of individual factors in his work with plants. An effort has recently been made to catalog all of the single mutant genes in humans. In 1971, the third edition of *Mendelian Inheritance in Man* by V. A. McKusick listed 1,876 different genetic abnormalities. The total number of diseases listed in the first edition of this book in 1966 was 1,487. Some of the most common diseases are shown in Table 7.2. Based

Table 7.2 *Common single mutant genes*

Disease	Incidence of affected individuals	Incidence of heterozygous "carriers"
Autosomal dominant		
Type II hyperlipoproteinemia	1 in 100[a]	—
Neurofibromatosis	1 in 2,500[a]	—
Autosomal recessive		
Sickle cell anemia	1 in 500[b]	1 in 11[b]
Cystic fibrosis	1 in 2,500[a]	1 in 25[a]
Tay-Sachs disease	1 in 3,600[c]	1 in 30[c]
X-linked recessive		
Glucose-6-phosphate dehydrogenase deficiency	1 in 6 to 9 males[b]	1 in 24[b] females
Hemophilia	1 in 8,000 males[a]	1 in 5,500[a] females

[a] Incidence in white Americans
[b] Incidence in black Americans
[c] Incidence in Jews with Eastern European ancestors

on the fact that many new genetic diseases are being recognized each year, it seems likely that the process of identifying all the abnormalities has just begun.

DISEASES DUE TO SINGLE MUTANT GENES   In humans, the single abnormal gene runs in families. The ways in which mutant genes are inherited will be discussed in relation to several diseases which illustrate common problems and the many ways in which a mutant gene can affect an individual. Some diseases are evident in infancy and others only in adults. Some have little effect and others are fatal. Some are slowly progressive and others remain constant for most of a lifetime. Many occur more often in certain racial and national groups.

Autosomal dominant

Autosomal inheritance means that the responsible gene is located on one of the 22 pairs of nonsex chromosomes. As we previously noted, a gene is *dominant* if the presence of the gene is always apparent in the features of the person. An autosomal dominant disease is one due to a single abnormal gene at one locus, the allele of this gene being normal. The individual with only one abnormal gene is *heterozygous* at that locus.

Autosomal dominant inheritance (Fig. 7.8) affects males and females with equal frequency. If the parent is affected, there is a 50 percent chance each child will be normal. It is important to remember that an abnormal gene must arise at some point in time. Therefore, an individual affected by a spontaneous mutation for an autosomal dominant gene will have normal parents and a 50 percent chance each of his or her children will be affected.

TYPE II HYPERLIPOPROTEINEMIA   This disease is probably the most common autosomal dominant disorder in the United States. It results from too much fat or lipids in the blood plasma. This excess fat is present in the blood of newborn infants, but its effects develop slowly over several years. The effects include deposits of the lipids in the skin, the tendons, and the lining of the arteries, especially the coronary arteries of the heart. As a result, affected individuals have a high incidence of heart attacks at an early age and a shortened lifespan. There is no effective treatment at this time.

NEUROFIBROMATOSIS   This disease has several different features including many brown "birth marks," numerous small lumps under the skin which are most common on the face and chest, deformities of bone, and many types of tumors. Only the brown marks are evident at birth; the other problems develop during childhood and adulthood. Fortunately the affected person may have only some of these problems. The only treatment is surgery to remove the tumors and some of the most bothersome lumps under the skin.

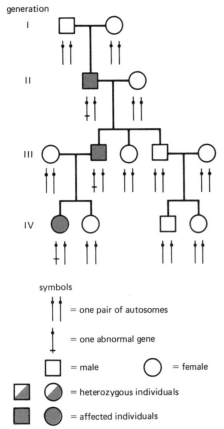

Figure 7.8. Autosomal dominant inheritance. The first affected family member represents a spontaneous mutation. The presence of male-to-male transmission confirms the fact that the mutant gene is located on an autosomal chromosome. The unaffected individuals do not have any affected children. The disease is present in each generation.

Figure 7.9. A polycystic kidney (left, cut surface, and center, external surface) from a 48-year-old woman undergoing a kidney transplant. The large size (900 grams in weight), numerous cysts, and lack of any visible areas of kidney tissue are evident. At right is a normal kidney weighing 140 grams which is normal in appearance except for a single and insignificant cyst (arrow). The centimeter rulers at the bottom show that the magnification is uniform.

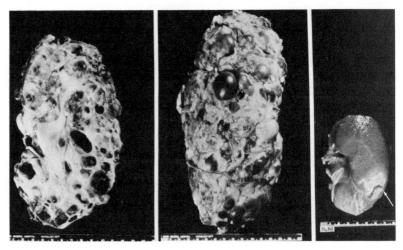

POLYCYSTIC KIDNEY DISEASE   The presence of this disease is not evident until the adult years. The kidney abnormality consists of structural defects that impair the proper functioning of the kidney, making it unable to clear the waste products from the blood and to excrete them in the urine. With time the defects develop into large cysts. The first sign in an affected person may be high blood pressure, which may be detected as early as the teenage years or as late as middle age. The cysts are present throughout the kidney (Fig. 7.9) and cannot be removed individually. Treatment can be given for the symptoms of high blood pressure, but the only hope for a cure is a kidney transplant. Unfortunately the affected individual may not be aware of this problem until after children have been born.

Autosomal recessive

In autosomal recessive inheritance an individual is affected when he or she has two abnormal genes: the same abnormal gene at the same locus on both chromosomes in a pair. A person with two abnormal genes at the same locus is said to be *homozygous* for the abnormal gene. If there

Figure 7.10. Autosomal recessive inheritance using symbols for a mutant gene on one pair of chromosomes. Note that the affected individual is only in one generation. All of his or her children must be heterozygous for this gene.

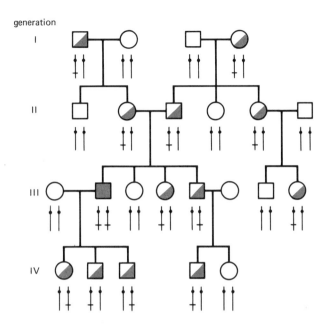

is only one abnormal recessive gene, the normal allele will dominate the abnormal allele.

The parents of the affected or homozygous person with two abnormal genes are heterozygous for the abnormal gene. As is shown in Figure 7.10, there are four ways in which the abnormal gene and the normal gene in each parent can combine in their children. This means they have a 25 percent chance any child will be normal, a 50 percent chance any child will be heterozygous, and a 25 percent chance the child will be homozygous and affected by the disease. Because of the low incidence of most autosomal recessive genes in the population, there is very little chance that a heterozygous child will marry another heterozygous individual and have affected children of their own. Therefore, typically autosomal recessive disorders occur in one or more brothers and sisters in only one generation of a family.

SICKLE CELL ANEMIA This disorder is the most prevalent recessively inherited disease in the United States today irrespective of race. As indicated in Table 7.2, it occurs almost exclusively in blacks. The term *sickle cell* is derived from the sickled shape of the red blood cells. The abnormality is present at birth, but the affected individual may not have symptoms until he or she is a few years old. During the usual childhood infections, these children may develop severe anemia from the sudden destruction of red blood cells. They also have frequent episodes of sudden pain in the abdomen and their arms and legs because of obstruction of blood vessels. The sickling of their red blood cells cannot be prevented, and they can only be helped to have fewer or less severe episodes of discomfort. Unfortunately the lifespan of an affected person is greatly shortened: half will die by age 20 and 90 percent by age 40.

CYSTIC FIBROSIS An infant may show signs of having cystic fibrosis in several different ways. For some infants the first sign is obstruction of the bowel at birth; for others the first sign may be repeated episodes of pneumonia in a young child (Fig. 7.11). The primary abnormality is not known. The most bothersome feature is thick, tenacious mucus in the lungs and intestinal tract. Treatment must be carried on twenty-four hours a day for some children: antibiotics to prevent infection, sleeping in a mist tent to combat breathing difficulty, and taking enzyme supplements with each meal so they can ingest food. Great progress has been made in the treatment of this disease: in the 1940s, 70 percent of the children died by age one and 95 percent by age five; in 1964 only 10 percent died in the first year, 25 percent by age five. In 1964, 25 percent of the affected individuals reached the adult years and at the present time the percent is larger. The affected adult females can have children, but most of the affected males are sterile.

Figure 7.11. Chest x-rays of an 8-year-old child with cystic fibrosis (left) and a normal 9½-year-old (right). The chest x-ray of the child with cystic fibrosis shows extensive scarring throughout both lungs and collapse of the upper lobe of the right lung. Because of the overinflation of the lungs, the heart appears smaller in comparison to that of the normal child.

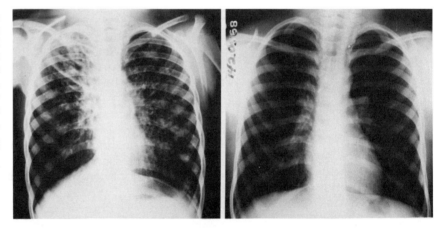

TAY-SACHS DISEASE This condition, which is untreatable and fatal, is named after two physicians who first described affected infants in the 1880s. Recently the disease has been shown to be due to the accumulation of a specific lipid called *ganglioside* in brain and nerve cells. The affected infant appears entirely normal at birth, but at around four to six months of age he or she begins to show signs of brain damage. The disease is steadily progressive with the infants gradually losing all awareness of and response to their surroundings. Death usually occurs between two and four years of age. The disease is not common, but for unknown reasons the gene is more common in Jews with Eastern European ancestors (Ashkenazi Jews) than any other ethnic or national group.

X-linked recessive disease

X-linked recessive diseases are due to one abnormal gene on one X chromosome of a male or two abnormal genes on both X chromosomes of a female. Since a female has two X chromosomes, each gene on one X chromosome has an allele on the other X chromosome. In contrast, a male has only one X chromosome (and one Y) and thus, the presence of the abnormal recessive gene on the male's X chromosome is always expressed (Fig. 7.12).

The expression of an X-linked gene in the female is more complicated. Unlike the male, the female inactivates one X chromosome in each of her cells. The choice as to which X is inactivated and does not express the effect of its genes is entirely random. This process, called the *Lyon hypothesis*, was first proposed by Dr. Mary Lyon. This is a very important phenomenon which explains why a female can express one abnormal X-linked gene in some of her cells and the normal allele of this gene in the remainder of her cells. Therefore, if a woman has an abnormal X-linked recessive gene, it will be inactivated in an average of half of her cells and expressed in the other half of her cells. Thus, the female carrier of the abnormal X-linked recessive gene is protected from its ill effects.

Each of the sons and daughters of a woman with an abnormal X-linked recessive gene has a 50 percent chance of inheriting her X-linked gene. There are no instances of a man having an affected son, and all the daughters of an affected male are carriers of the abnormal gene.

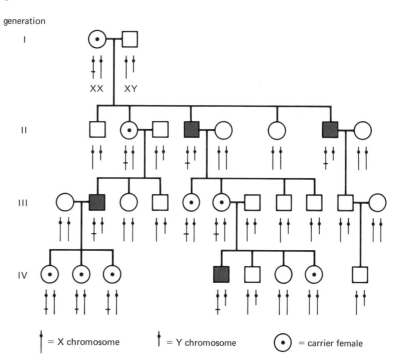

Figure 7.12. X-linked recessive inheritance in which only males are affected, and they are related to each other through maternal relatives. Note the absence of male-to-male transmission and that the daughters of affected males are always carriers of the abnormal gene.

A deficiency of a red blood cell enzyme (glucose-6-phosphate dehydrogenase) is the most frequent X-linked recessive disorder in the United States. There are at least 85 different alleles for this gene. Some of the resulting diseases are serious, such as chronic anemia and acute episodes of destruction of red blood cells in response to stress caused by medications such as antimalarial drugs and certain antibiotics. This was a problem during the Vietnam War when soldiers were routinely given medication to prevent them from developing malaria. Since the soldiers, blacks in particular, were not initially evaluated to see if they had a form of glucose-6-phosphate dehydrogenase deficiency, they only learned about the abnormal X-linked gene when they developed anemia following the use of this medication.

CLASSICAL HEMOPHILIA This disease (also called hemophilia A), accounts for about 25 percent of the blood used in the United States today. The primary abnormality is virtual absence of activity of plasma factor VIII which is essential for normal blood clotting. Most often the first signs are frequent and large bruises produced by insignificant falls as the male infant is learning to crawl and walk. The more serious subsequent problem is bleeding which occurs in the joints, such as the knee, hip, ankle, and elbow, following minor injuries to these areas. This bleeding causes serious damage to the joints. Treatment has improved in recent years with the development of better means of providing additional amounts of factor VIII by intravenous transfusion. Studies of the financial impact of this disease have shown that approximately 60 percent of the families spend an average of about $2,000 per year on medical care; to pay for the added expenses, 20 percent of the fathers obtain extra jobs and 30 percent of the mothers find employment.

X-linked dominant disease

In this mode of inheritance (Fig. 7.13) both the male and female show the effect of the gene because the gene is dominant. The disease results from one abnormal gene on one X chromosome. Because the affected male has only one X chromosome, all of his daughters will be affected but none of his sons will be. As previously noted few X-linked dominant genes have been identified in humans.

MULTIFACTORAL INHERITANCE Some of the most common diseases in man have been attributed to multifactorial inheritance (Table 7.3). The diseases include diabetes, schizophrenia and many of the most common birth defects like cleft lip and palate. In this type of inheritance, the condition is caused by the presence of several minor gene abnormalities and presumably by harmful environmental factors. While several genes are considered to be causes of the problem, they cannot be seen in chromosome analysis and the total number involved is not known. It is assumed that one minor gene abnormality does not cause any apparent effect. However, a number of gene abnormalities together results in a disease or abnormality.

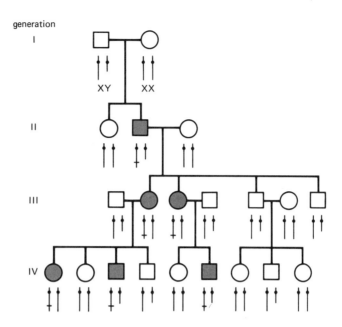

Figure 7.13. X-linked dominant inheritance with affected males and females in successive generations. Note that all daughters of affected men are affected.

Most multifactorial diseases are more common in certain national and racial groups.

The diseases attributed to multifactorial inheritance are quite varied in nature. The genetic aspects of multifactorial inheritance have been established from studies of large numbers of families. One can determine whether a disease is caused by multifactorial inheritance by identifying specific characteristics of the disorder. These characteristics are:

1. The chance that a parent, brother, or sister can have the same disorder is usually between 2 and 10 percent. A similar rate or recurrence is shown in the children of the affected individual. While the risk to these relatives is low, it is usually ten to fifty times the risk in the general population which is usually between 1 in 500 (0.2 percent) and 1 in 2,000 (0.05 percent).

2. The chance that other, more distant relatives, such as aunts, uncles, and first cousins, will have the same disorder is greater than the risk of the general population, but less than the risk for brothers, sisters, parents, and children.

3. Some multifactorial disorders occur more often in one sex. For example, *pyloric stenosis,* a muscular enlargement of the small intestine which causes vomiting in young infants, is five times more common in males. In multifactorial disorders, if a person of the less likely sex is affected, he or she is much more likely to have affected children. Therefore, a woman who had pyloric stenosis as an infant is four times more likely to have affected infants than a man who had this problem in infancy.

4. Different races are more prone to certain defects, even after migration. For example, the incidence of club foot deformity is low in Chinese and high among Polynesians, while the incidence among Hawaiians with mixed Chinese-Polynesian ancestry is intermediate between the two.

5. When one identical twin has a multifactorial disorder the other twin is often similarly affected. The rate of both being affected varies from 20 to 40 percent in different conditions. The reason why it is not 100 percent is thought to be the effect of variations in the rate of development and environmental factors of the twins. However, this rate is much higher than the rate for non-identical twins, which is 2 to 5 percent.

Table 7.3 Disorders due to multifactorial inheritance

Disease	Incidence in general population[a]	Rate of recurrence in brothers and sisters of affected persons	Rate of recurrence in children of affected person
Diabetes mellitus	1 in 2,500	6 to 9%	10%
Psoriasis	1 in 50	7.8	unknown
Schizophrenia	1 in 100	6 to 12	11 to 21
Cleft lip and palate	1 in 750 white Americans 1 in 2,500 black Americans 1 in 500 Navajo Indians	3.9	3.5
Cleft palate alone	1 in 2,000 white 1 in 2,500 black Americans 1 in 2,800 Navajo Indians	3	6.2
Congenital dislocation of hip	1 in 1,400	4.3	unknown
Congenital heart defects	3 to 7 in 1,000		
atrial septal defect		3	unknown
patent ductus arteriosus		2.3	2.8
Pyloric stenosis	1 in 500	4 (brothers)	16.2 (if mother affected)
		2.4 (sisters)	4.6 (if father affected)

[a] All data concerns white Americans unless otherwise designated.

Why marrying your first cousin might be risky

Many states have laws forbidding marriages of cousins, especially first cousins. The reason is that parents who are first cousins have a greater likelihood of having infants affected by (homozygous for) a rare autosomal recessive trait. These laws were passed mainly because of the fear that the affected children would be handicapped and mentally deficient. There is a basis for this fear, but the danger to society appears to have been exaggerated.

Many people do not realize that we all carry several rare autosomal recessive genes. The exact number is not known, but the estimates are about five to eight per person. (It is not possible to test people to identify the rare recessive genes they carry.) Being recessive, these genes do not cause problems to the carrier. However, if two persons who are carriers of the same recessive genes have children, they have a one in four chance any one of their children will be abnormal. Because these genes are rare, it is very unlikely

anyone will ever marry someone who carries the same rare genes.

First cousin marriages are of concern because each parent is more likely to have the same rare gene or genes. For example, as is shown in the pedigree, this couple has a 1/16 chance that each has inherited the same rare gene from their common grandfather. This is determined by calculating the probability the grandfather transmitted this gene to his son (1/2), the chance this gene was transmitted to his daughter (1/2), the chance his son transmitted the gene to his son (1/2), the probability his daughter transmitted the gene to her daughter (1/2), and then totaling these probabilities: $1/2 \times 1/2 \times 1/2 \times 1/2$ or 1/16. In turn, this couple has a 1/4 chance that any of their children will be affected by the rare gene of their common grandfather. The overall risk of this man's rare recessive gene being transmitted to his great granddaughter is $1/16 \times 1/4$ or 1/64. The same calculations can be used to determine the risk for

rare recessive genes in other ancestors of parents who are first cousins. Fortunately the total risk, although much greater than the risk for unrelated couples, is relatively low; the precise risk of first cousins having an abnormal child has not been determined, but it appears to be less than 10 percent.

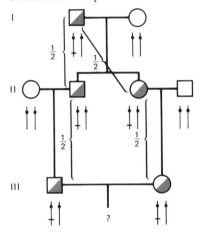

$\frac{1}{2} \cdot \frac{1}{2} \cdot \frac{1}{2} \cdot \frac{1}{2} = \frac{1}{16}$, probability both parents have inherited same autosomal recessive gene from their common grandfather.

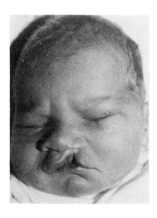

Figure 7.14. An infant with an isolated cleft lip deformity. Surgical closure of the cleft lip is usually carried out in the first few months of life.

It should be stressed that there are many unanswered questions concerning multifactorial inheritance. Studies of similar disorders in animals have clearly shown that many different environmental factors make the animal more likely to exhibit a particular multifactorial disorder. However, the factors that influence animals do not seem to affect humans in the same way. Unfortunately none of the environmental factors that contribute to people having multifactorial disorders has been identified.

Another major difficulty is that there is no way to pick out in advance couples who risk having a child with one of these disorders because their chromosomes show no abnormalities. All we can do is inform them of the possibility of having a second affected child. After the birth of the second affected child, we know the risk for a third increases. For example, it has been learned from experience with hundreds of families with one child with cleft lip and palate (Fig. 7.14) that the risk for a second child is about 4 percent. If a couple has two affected children, the risk of having a third child with cleft lip and palate is 9 percent. This means that some parents have a greater risk than others.

GENETIC COUNSELING   During the past ten to twenty years the greatest progress in medical genetics has been in recognizing the existence of hundreds of new genetic diseases. Only a few of these disorders can be prevented from having damaging effects by treating the affected individual. Because treatment is not often possible, the physician should help the family understand why the problem happened and inform them of the likelihood of its occurring in their future children. While some counselors consider it their function to tell the family members whether or not they should have more children, most do not. *Genetic counseling* is the art of communicating the facts about genetic diseases to those already affected or likely to be affected by them and helping each family to formulate plans that are most appropriate for its own situation.

Experience has shown that successful counseling is difficult. Some of the specific steps in the process of counseling are:

1. Having the individual or family available for counseling
2. Being certain the medical diagnosis is correct
3. Interpreting the genetic risk (Table 7.4) in terms that are meaningful to the family
4. Helping the family make plans that are appropriate and realistic
5. Seeing the counseled individuals subsequently to correct any misconceptions, to reinforce the correct information, and to add new facts.

Table 7.4 Genetic counseling—recurrence risks

Disease	Risk that any sister may be affected	Risk that any brother may be affected	Risk that any child of affected parent may be affected
Chromosomal abnormalities			
Trisomy 21 (Down's syndrome)	1%	1%	*
Multifactorial inheritance			
Diabetes mellitus	6 to 9	6 to 9	10
Cleft lip and palate	3.9	3.9	3.5
Single mutant gene diseases			
Autosomal recessive	25	25	0
Autosomal dominant (assuming one parent is affected)	50	50	50
X-linked recessive (assuming mother is a carrier)	0	50	0

* No males with Down's syndrome have had children. A few females have had children; of these children about half had Down's syndrome.

As one might expect, there are difficulties with many aspects of counseling. These are some of the problems that have been identified:

1. Individuals who have a genetic disease or who risk having affected children rarely seek genetic counseling. In some instances they are ignorant of their risk; often they are simply reluctant to ask about it.

2. Only in recent years have physicians received instruction in medical school about genetic counseling. As a result, many physicians are unaware of those diseases that are hereditary and do not feel qualified to provide genetic counseling.

3. Too few professional counselors and counseling facilities are available; when available, they are often located in urban areas associated with large medical centers and are difficult to find.

4. Many people have difficulty understanding the principles of inheritance.

5. A common reaction to counseling is to deny that the disease in question is hereditary in nature.

6. Many studies have shown that information provided verbally is not retained as long as visual or written reminders. Few genetic counselors provide reinforcement through letters or follow-up visits.

7. Many physicians use percentages to indicate the risk that a disease might occur, and often this terminology is not understood. Furthermore, the more important factor is the person's concept of the burden imposed by the disease and not the size of the risk.

8. Usually a follow-up visit for genetic counseling is not made. This prevents many dividends to the family: reinforcing information obtained, allowing the physician the opportunity to change the diagnosis in light of new findings or recent medical discoveries, and providing separate counseling to children who have become old enough to understand and benefit from the counseling.

Every aspect and step of genetic counseling has significant inherent difficulties, and only major and sustained efforts will improve the chances that more families will benefit from genetic counseling. Unfortunately at the present time the chances are slim that a significant amount of tax money will be spent on improving the situation.

One new dimension of genetic counseling that may eventually gain more support is prenatal diagnosis. During the past five years this has captured the imagination of the public and has given counseling a more exciting and innovative image in the medical community.

PRENATAL DIAGNOSIS The basic premise of diagnosing a genetic disease in an unborn child is that it allows the parents to selectively have only normal children. While this concept has been readily accepted by some of the public, it is vigorously opposed by others on ethical and religious grounds. Many people do not believe it is appropriate to carry out a therapeutic abortion on a fetus with an untreatable genetic disorder. Most genetic counselors feel that the decision to undertake prenatal diagnosis is an individual choice and that this option must be made available to everyone, but not imposed upon them.

There are several methods of prenatal diagnosis. The best known and most often used technique is *amniocentesis*. This process requires inserting a needle into the amniotic fluid which surrounds the fetus. It cannot be carried out until 14 to 16 weeks of gestation (the normal length of pregnancy is 40 weeks), because it is at this time that the mother's uterus is large enough to protrude above the front rim of the pelvis. The procedure does not necessitate hospitalization. Medication to decrease the pain caused by the needle is injected into the skin and the tissues just beneath. The insertion of the needle thereafter causes a sensation of pressure, but little else. Every effort is made to be certain the area is sterile so neither the fetus nor the mother will be infected by bacteria carried by this needle from the skin. After its insertion, a small amount of amniotic fluid is removed (Fig. 7.15). This fluid contains cells that have been shed by the fetus from his or her skin and intestinal and urinary tracts. At the present time the cells are of greatest interest because they can be grown in cell culture. Three to four weeks are required for a sufficient number of cells to grow from the original sample to permit chromosome analysis and biochemical studies. Because these cells have come from the fetus, the chromosomes and enzymes in these cells accurately reflect the fetus. One important aspect of amniocentesis is whether or not the procedure is hazardous. This is currently being carefully studied, and at this time the risk of serious complications appears to be less than one percent.

As has been discussed, the incidence of having a chromosomally abnormal child increases significantly in older women. Because of this,

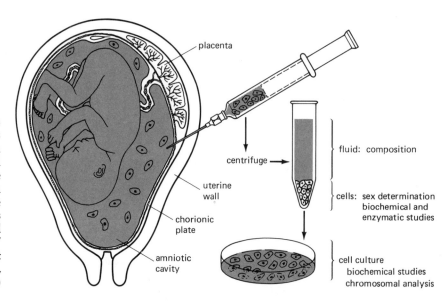

Figure 7.15. Amniocentesis. This schematic drawing shows a uterus and amniotic sac through which a needle has been inserted and fluid containing cells from the fetus is removed. The fluid is spun in the centrifuge to concentrate the cell culture. This drawing is not to scale. (From "Prenatal Diagnosis of Genetic Disease," by Theodore Friedman. Copyright © 1971 by *Scientific American*, Inc. All rights reserved.)

placenta

centrifuge

fluid: composition

uterine wall

cells: sex determination biochemical and enzymatic studies

chorionic plate

amniotic cavity

cell culture biochemical studies chromosomal analysis

amniocentesis is recommended by some geneticists for every woman over 35 years of age; there is little disagreement that it is appropriate for every pregnant woman 40 or older. While the woman's age is the most common indication, amniocentesis is most often used by couples who have had a child with Down's syndrome. Their risk that the subsequent child has Down's syndrome is only about 1 percent.

There are at least 40 inborn errors of metabolism that can be diagnosed by amniocentesis. These are autosomal or X-linked recessive disorders due to a marked decrease in the activity of a particular enzyme which can be determined in the cells of the fetus. While each of these diseases is rare, the affected couples have a 25 percent risk of having an affected child. In most situations the fact that the couple is at risk is only determined after the birth of an affected child. It would obviously be preferable to identify in advance couples liable to have a child with a serious and untreatable disease. This is only possible through systematic screening of individuals. Obviously the practicality of screening is related to the frequency of the abnormal gene and the ease with which susceptible individuals can be identified.

While screening programs are feasible for a disease such as Tay-Sachs, they are not for the two common hereditary conditions in the United States, sickle cell anemia and cystic fibrosis. In the case of sickle cell anemia, the carrier adult is detected by screening, but since it is not yet possible to test the unborn fetus to see if it has sickle cell anemia, parents cannot selectively have only unaffected children. In the case of cystic fibrosis, neither the carrier adult nor the affected fetus can be identified at this time.

Rh incompatibility

One of the most impressive stories of medical progress concerns the identification and development of successful treatment for Rh incompatibility. The problem was only recognized in the 1940s. It was learned that persons may have a particular characteristic in their red blood cells called the *Rh factor.* If red blood cells with this factor (Rh positive) were injected into a person who did not have this factor (Rh negative), the recipient developed antibodies to destroy the Rh positive red blood cells. Studies in the United States showed that 85 percent of the population were Rh positive and 15 percent were Rh negative.

The problem that led to these discoveries was *erythroblastosis fetalis.* In this disorder, the mother is Rh— and has developed antibodies to the Rh factor from a blood transfusion or a previous pregnancy. It was learned that most Rh— women had developed these antibodies from a pregnancy in which the child was Rh+. During delivery of the baby, some of the baby's Rh+ red blood cells went into the mother's blood stream. This brief exposure was sufficient for the mother to develop powerful antibodies. During the next pregnancy when carrying an Rh+ child, the previously formed antibody would cross from the mother into the child. The mother's antibody would destroy the child's Rh+ red blood cells. If this process was severe enough the unborn child would become severely anemic and die.

The first successful treatment of this process was giving the newborn child a blood transfusion (RH—) once or several times. Later the treatment was perfected to save more infants by giving them transfusions before they were born. This required passing a needle through the mother's abdomen and uterus and into the child's abdomen. While this process was often successful and many infants' lives were saved, it was not the final answer. In the mid-1960s complete prevention of Rh incompatibility between a mother and her baby became possible. By injecting the mother with serum containing antibodies to Rh+ red blood cells, the Rh+ cells which she received from her infant were destroyed and she never developed her own antibodies. The injection must be given within 72 hours of any birth, miscarriage, or abortion to be effective. With this treatment most instances of Rh incompatibility can be prevented.

Amniocentesis can also be used to determine the sex of the fetus. This is used to control the frequency of serious untreatable X-linked recessive disorders, such as Duchenne's muscular dystrophy. Unfortunately the disease itself is not detectable in the cells of the fetus. All the parents can learn is the sex of the fetus. They know that if the mother is a carrier, there is a 50 percent chance that each of her sons is affected; each of her daughters has a 50 percent chance of being a carrier, but no chance of being affected. Therefore, some parents have elected to abort all male fetuses to prevent having affected sons.

There are many problems associated with amniocentesis. One is the need to have a means of routinely localizing the placenta before the needle is inserted; at the present time the needle is inserted "blindly" and it is not known whether or how much of a risk this is to the fetus. Some obstetricians use ultrasound (sonar waves) to locate the placenta but this instrument is not widely available. Another problem is the need to know whether or not there are two fetuses present. Obviously the amniotic fluid and cells would reflect the status of only one fetus which in the case of nonidentical twins often does not reflect the status of the other twin. Again, the routine use of ultrasound would routinely identify the presence of twins. Another problem is the need for speed, care, and reliability in interpreting the results of biochemical studies in the cells of the fetus. Little time is available, after the three to four weeks required to grow a sufficient number of cells for studies, to inform the parents of the results, and, if the fetus is affected, to decide whether or not it will be aborted. Most obstetricians prefer to abort a fetus before it is 20 weeks old. An abortion at this time can be done by infusion of a salt water solution into the amniotic fluid itself. A later abortion often requires surgical removal of the fetus by making an incision in the mother's uterus and removing the fetus.

Several new methods of prenatal diagnosis are currently being developed. These include ultrasound, amniography, fetoscopy, and radiographs. With *ultrasound*, sonic waves are used to measure various parts of the body, such as determining whether the head is too small. *Amniography* requires the injection of dyes into the amniotic fluid to identify a physical abnormality by the outline of the dye on x-rays. *Fetoscopy* is the use of an elaborate optical device for examining the fetus directly. At the present time it is not known how hazardous it is to insert such an instrument into the uterus or how well one can examine the fetus. Prenatal *radiographs* could be used to detect the presence or absence of certain abnormalities of the fetus' skeleton known to be associated with certain hereditary malformations. With careful selection and control of the number of radiographs taken, the amount of radiation to which the fetus is exposed can be minimized. One technique for prenatal diagnosis that has not been developed is a means of taking blood samples from the fetus. This must be developed before couples at risk for serious, fatal, and untreatable blood diseases, such as sickle cell anemia, can benefit from prenatal diagnosis.

FUTURE DEVELOPMENTS   It is apparent from the pace of current research in the field of genetics that new discoveries will be made with amazing rapidity. The intricacies of how a specific defective gene alters the function of the genetic code will continue to be clarified. Hundreds of new genetic diseases will be identified. With this new ability come several controversial issues which the public and the medical profession must face. Three of these issues are the screening of newborns and adults for genetic disease, prenatal diagnosis of genetic abnormalities, and changing the methods for providing genetic counseling.

Screening for genetic disease

1. If a serious condition is detectable in a newborn infant, but no treatment is available, is detection justifiable? For example, 0.5 percent of newborns have significant chromosome abnormalities which can now be detected efficiently. Should this be done so that the parents will know the diagnosis as early as possible? If this is not done, how can treatments be developed?

In another case, between 0.5 and 1 percent of newborns has type II hyperlipoproteinemia,[6] discussed earlier. Often the detection of this lipid abnormality leads to the discovery that one of the parents has this problem and is thereby more prone to a heart attack at an early age. If a disease is untreatable, should the parents and their risk be identified? One can argue that by detecting the affected parent he or she is given the opportunity of limiting the number of children born who risk having a serious hereditary disorder.

2. If the individual subject to having any serious genetic disease can be detected, should everyone be tested? Should this be done for diseases like sickle cell anemia and cystic fibrosis which cannot be diagnosed in the unborn fetus and therefore the parents cannot control whether or not an affected child is born? Should detection be confined to those diseases for which prenatal diagnosis is possible, such as Tay-Sachs disease?

3. If screening is possible, should cooperation be mandatory or voluntary?

4. If screening is done, how can the identity of those who are found to have any serious recessive gene be protected?

Prenatal diagnosis

The expected developments in prenatal diagnosis are improvements in the ability to detect serious autosomal dominant traits such as neurofibromatosis and polycystic kidney disease. Also, it should be possible

[6] C. J. Glueck, F. Heckman, M. Schoenfeld, P. Steiner and W. Pearce, "Neonatal familial type II hyperlipoproteinemia: cord blood cholesterol in 1,800 births," *Metabolism*, Vol. 20 (1971), pp. 597–608.

to examine the fetus directly. Hopefully instruments will be developed for taking blood samples from the fetus to make it possible to diagnose serious blood diseases, such as sickle cell anemia. However, as the ability to make more prenatal diagnoses becomes available, greater centralization and quality control of the facilities will be necessary. Who should be in charge of these facilities? How can the perspective of and importance of the average individual be preserved in the face of these complex developments?

Genetic counseling

As has been stated previously, many persons with a genetic disease or at risk never seek genetic counseling. This raises several issues. Should a physician seek out family members at risk for a significant untreatable genetic disorder who do not wish to come to a hospital for counseling? Should there be a central registry in each large city, region, or state of each individual with a known genetic disorder? If there is such a registry, widely separated family members could be systematically contacted to be certain they understand their risk for a particular disease. Likewise should each woman be contacted at age 40 (or 35) to be told of her increased risk of a chromosomal abnormality in any subsequent child she may have? If these more aggressive approaches to counseling are undertaken, who should do it? How can the rights of the at risk individuals to remain uninvolved be protected? At the present time neither the state or federal public health programs are prepared to undertake such an aggressive role. Hopefully as more is learned about genetic diseases better means will be developed to make this information more useful to all concerned.

Questions

1. What is the difference between meiosis and mitosis?
2. Name one chromosome abnormality with an extra chromosome and explain how it could have been caused.
3. What are the major autosomal recessive and autosomal dominant diseases?
4. In genetic counseling there are many problems in communicating facts once the individual is available for a discussion. What are some of these?
5. Explain the most common basis for prenatal diagnosis by amniocentesis.

Key Concepts

Alleles – different and alternative forms of genes which occupy the same locus on both members of a pair of chromosomes

Autosome – a nonsex chromosome

Heterozygous – the state of having different alleles at a specific gene locus on a pair of chromosomes

Homozygous – the state of having identical alleles at a specific gene locus

Locus – the site of each gene on a chromosome

Mutation – a change in the genetic material involving a specific single gene and resulting in an abnormal gene

Translocation – the displacement of part or all of one chromosome to another chromosome

Selected Readings Bergsma, Daniel, M. D. (editor). *Birth Defects. Atlas and Compendium.* Published for The National Foundation—March of Dimes, The Williams and Wilkins Company (Baltimore), 1973.

Goldstein, J. L. et al. "Hyperlipidemia in Coronary Heart Disease." J. Clin. Inv. 52:1533–43, 1544–68, 1569–77, 1973.

Holmes, Lewis B., *et al. Mental Retardation: An Atlas of Diseases with Associated Physical Abnormalities.* New York: Macmillan, 1972.

Leonard, C. O., G. A. Chase, and B. Childs. "Genetic Counseling: A Consumer's View, *New England Journal of Medicine,* Vol. 287 (1972), 433–39.

McKusick, Victor A., M. D. *Mendelian Inheritance in Man. Catalogs of Autosomal Dominant, Autosomal Recessive, and X-Linked Phenotypes.*

Milunsky, Aubrey. *The Prenatal Diagnosis of Hereditary Disorders.* Springfield, Ill.: C. C. Thomas Publisher, 1973.

Olafson, Freya, and A. W. Parker. *Sickle Cell Anemia—The Neglected Disease.* Berkeley: University of California Press, 1973.

Smith, David W., M. D., and Wilson, Ann Asper. *The Child with Down's Syndrome (Mongolism). Causes, Characteristics and Acceptance.* W. B. Saunders Company (Philadelphia), 1973.

Stern, Curt. *Principles of Human Genetics,* 3d ed. San Francisco: W. H. Freeman and Co., 1973.

Warkany, Josef. *Congenital Malformations. Chicago:* Year Book Publishers, Inc., 1971.

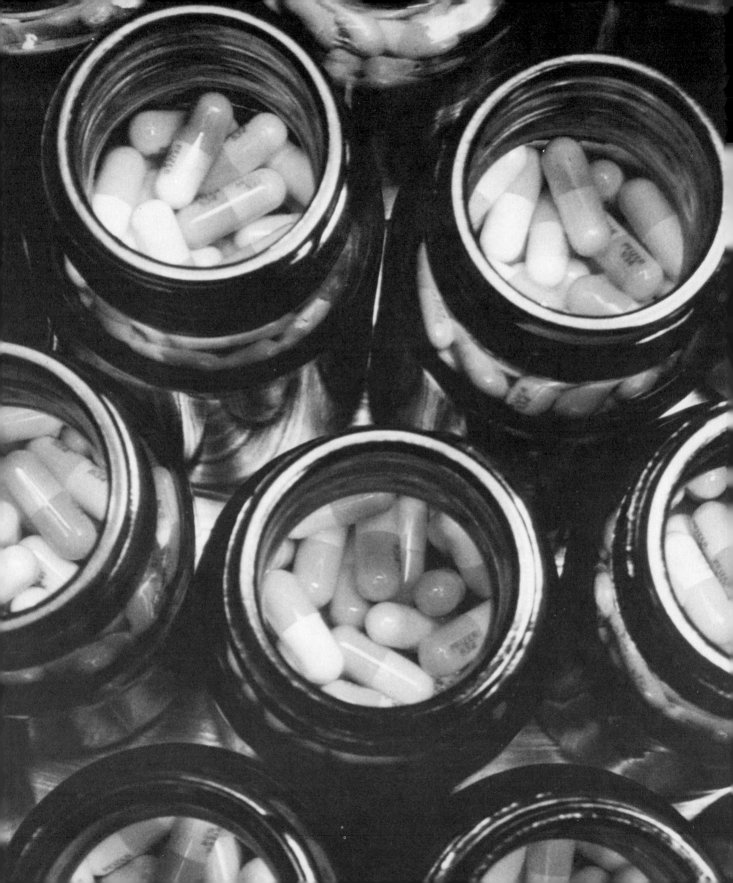

Part II

ILL HEALTH AND PREVENTIVE MEDICINE

Chapter 8

Epidemiology

"Each person in the world creates a Book of Life. This Book starts with birth and ends with death. Its pages are made up of the principal events in life. Record linkage is the name given to the process of assembling the pages of this Book into a volume."[1]

This view of life was written thirty years ago by the Chief of the National Office of Vital Statistics of the United States. A physician compiles such a Book for each of his patients. By referring to previous pages of the Book, the physician can review knowledge of a patient's history and prescribe the proper treatment of disease. The Book of Life for an individual, therefore, is of value in treating and curing disease.

The vital statistician uses the same process to create a different Book of Life. Rather than assembling the pages for an individual, the statis-

[1] H. L. Dunn, "Record Linkage," *American Journal of Public Health*, 36 (1946), pp. 1412–16.

This chapter was contributed by Richard R. Monson, M.D., Sc.D., Associate Professor of Epidemiology, Harvard School of Public Health.

tician gathers similar pages for many individuals. One volume is made up of the birth certificates of all newborn children, a second of marriage licenses, a third of death certificates. The Books of the statistician describe not the life of a man, but the life and death of a population.

In theory, these Books of Life can be used to study sickness and health. The lessons learned can be used to prevent or cure disease. Each of the Books has limitations, however. While a particular person's book may be complete, his pattern of sickness and health may not apply to others. The experiences of each man's life are unique. Conversely, while the statistician's Book may be complete for a population, no pattern of sickness and health can be deduced for a particular person. Knowing what diseases caused death in New York City is of no value unless each disease can be related to a prior experience in life.

The role of the epidemiologist is to link the pages of these two Books of Life. The patterns of sickness and health in a population must be studied and the causes of disease sought. If a cause can be identified, prevention is possible. Thus, while the physician attempts to cure illness, the epidemiologist's goal is to prevent illness.

THE HISTORY OF EPIDEMIOLOGY

Hippocrates and natural causes

Before Hippocrates, it was generally accepted that demons were responsible for disease. A person became ill when an imbalance of the four humors—earth, air, fire, and water—occurred. Since demons were the work of the devil, preventing disease or finding its cause was considered pointless. Instead, driving out the devil was held to be necessary to cure illness.

Hippocrates directed attention to the environment as a factor in the cause of disease. When the wind was hot, digestion suffered and the body became flabby. Pains in the chest resulted from cold wind. Malaria (bad air) occurred when water became stagnant. This latter observation predated by over 2300 years the recognition that malaria was transmitted by mosquitos growing in stagnant water.

Establishing a natural event as an important cause of disease was a major development in understanding the relationship between sickness and health. The realization that disease could be prevented by removing its natural cause was a necessary step in controlling illness. Hippocrates, however, merely *considered* the association between exposure and disease. While this consideration was a giant leap forward, the essential second step was not taken for over 2000 years. During this period the physician-epidemiologist, while continuing to be aware of the exposure-disease association, failed to *count* or quantitate its incidence.

John Graunt and the London Bills of Mortality

In 1532 an unknown person in London launched a revolution in epidemiology: the Bills of Mortality. For the first time, a tally was kept of the number of persons dying from different diseases. This tally permitted a quantitative study of the causes of illness. However, no scientific use was made of the Bills of Mortality for over one hundred years. Their primary purpose at the time seems to have been as a numbers game: bets were made to see who could best predict the number of deaths that would occur each week.

> Now having (I know not by what accident) engaged my thoughts upon the *Bills of Mortality,* and so far succeeded therein, as to have reduced several great confused *Volumes* into a few perspicuous *Tables,* and abridged such *Observations* as naturally flowed from them, into a few succinct *Paragraphs,* without any long Series of *multiloquious Deductions,* I have presumed to sacrifice these my small, but first publish'd *Labours* unto your lordship, . . .[2]

With these words John Graunt described the first effort to understand and quantitate the patterns of disease in a population. His analysis of the London Bills of Mortality is the foundation upon which present-day epidemiology is based. The realization that data on a population could be used to study the causes of disease had not previously occurred.

Graunt was the first to estimate the population of London, the first to count the number that died of specific causes, and the first to realize that more boys than girls are born. Between 1628 and 1662, 140,000 male infants were born in contrast to 131,000 female infants. All of the numbers that Graunt calculated are commonplace today, but in 1632 they were unique.

The pioneering work of Graunt was not continued. No effort was made to systematically collect data on health until the early nineteenth century. In 1837 the office of the Registrar-General was established to collect information on births and deaths in England. Comparable data were not collected in the United States until 1900, and not until 1933 was information on deaths in the entire country assembled.

John Snow and the sewage of London

> The most terrible outbreak of cholera which ever occurred in this kingdom, is probably that which took place in Broad Street, Golden Square, and the adjoining streets, a few weeks ago. Within two hundred and fifty yards of the spot where Cambridge Street joins Broad Street, there were upwards of five hundred fatal attacks of cholera in ten days. The mortality in this limited area probably equals any that was ever caused in this country, even by the plague; and it was much more sudden, as the greater number of cases terminated in a few hours. The mortality would undoubtedly have been much greater had it not been for the flight of the population. Persons in furnished lodgings left first, then other lodgers went away, leaving their furniture to be sent for when they could meet with a place to put it in. Many houses were closed altogether, owing to

Leading causes of death

London, 1632

Cause	Number
Diseases of early infancy	2,268
Consumption	1,797
Fever	1,108
Old age	628
Flocks and smallpox	531
Teeth	470

United States, 1969

Cause	Number
Diseases of heart	738,945
Cancer	323,092
Stroke	207,179
Accidents	116,385
Influenza and pneumonia	68,365
Diseases of early infancy	43,171

From John Graunt, p. 24, and "Ca—A Cancer Journal for Clinicians," American Cancer Society, Jan/Feb, 1973.

---

[2] John Graunt, *Natural and Political Observations made upon the Bills of Mortality* (Baltimore: Johns Hopkins Press, 1939), p. 3.

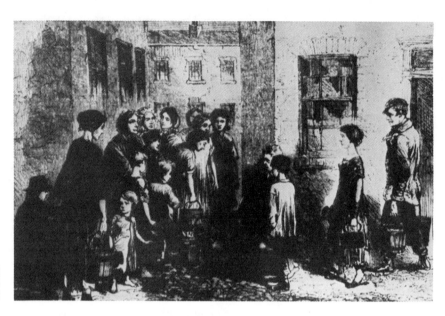

Figure 8.1. Water pump in London about 1850. (Courtesy of World Health Organization)

the death of the proprietors; and, in a great number of instances, the tradesmen who remained had sent away their families: so that in less than six days from the commencement of the outbreak, the most afflicted streets were deserted by more than three-quarters of their inhabitants.[3]

As this account indicates, widespread epidemics were not confined to the Middle Ages. London in the mid-nineteenth century was ravaged by infectious disease which killed many of its inhabitants in a matter of hours.

John Snow, a physician and anesthesiologist to Queen Victoria, was disturbed by the frequent epidemics of cholera. Through his clinical experience, he became convinced that cholera was transmitted by contaminated water. To prove his belief he not only collected data on the occurrence of cholera but also linked cholera death rates to the water supply used by the population. The associating of cause (water) and effect (cholera) was the first modern epidemiologic study.

Snow directed his attention to the water companies of London. In the mid-nineteenth century, there was no "city water." Under the free enterprise system, many companies had laid down pipes in direct competition and sought to outbid each other in selling water to individual households. In many districts, however, one water company was the predominant supplier. Each water company took its water from a specific point along the Thames.

Snow theorized that, as the Thames flowed to the sea, it became increasingly polluted. If cholera was caused by polluted water, persons

[3] John Snow, *Snow on Cholera* (New York: Hafner Publishing Co., 1965), p. 38.

Charles Babbage and the computer

The development of the computer over the past thirty years has caused a revolution in epidemiology. Studies involving more than a million people can now be performed with relative ease. Prior to the computer, epidemiological studies involved hand tabulation and calculation of data, making large-scale studies impossible.

Charles Babbage, a mid-nineteenth-century Englishman, was the first to attempt to construct what today is recognizable as a computer. Driven by a dream to calculate by machine, Babbage constructed a "Difference Engine" in 1822. This engine was used for many years, mainly in the calculation of logarithms.

Babbage next attempted to construct an "Analytic Engine," a prototype of today's digital computer. It used punch cards, had a memory, and was given instructions by a program.

Unfortunately, Babbage's efforts were doomed to failure because his engines were totally mechanical. The potential of Babbage's engines was never realized during his lifetime. Not until the mid-twentieth century with the development of electronics was adequate technology available to fulfill Babbage's dreams.

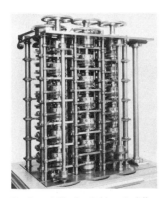

Portion of Charles Babbage's difference engine. (British Crown Copywrite. Science Museum, London, in the case of negative numbers 26592 and 508/54)

supplied by water coming from the lower Thames should have relatively high cholera death rates. Two companies were identified: one taking water from the high Thames and one from the low Thames. Each company was the predominant supplier of a defined part of London. As seen in Table 8.1, there was a major difference in the death rates according to water supplier. The persons supplied by the Southwark and Vauxhall Company had a strikingly high rate. That company took its water from the low Thames.

*Table 8.1 Cholera mortality in London according to water company**

District	Water company	Population	Deaths from cholera per 10,000 persons
A	Southwark and Vauxhall	167,654	114
B	Both companies	301,149	60
C	Lambeth	14,622	0

* From *Snow on Cholera*, p. 73.

This evidence was nevertheless not strong enough for Snow. There were differences other than in the water supply between these two areas that might account for the different cholera rates. Fortunately, there was one region in London that was supplied jointly by the two companies.

Although the facts shown in the above table afford very strong evidence of the powerful influence which the drinking of water containing the sewage of a town exerts over the spread of cholera, when that disease is present, yet the question does not end here; for the intermixing of the water supply of the Southwark and Vauxhall Company with that of the Lambeth Company, over an extensive part of London, admitted of the subject being sifted in such a way as to yield the most incontrovertible proof on one side or the other. In the sub-districts enumerated in the above table as being supplied by both Companies, the mixing of the supply is of the most intimate kind. The pipes of each Company go down all the streets, and into nearly all the courts and alleys. A few houses are supplied by one Company and a few by the other, according to the decision of the owner or occupier at that time when the Water Companies were in active competition. In many cases a single house has a supply different from that on either side. Each company supplies both rich and poor, both large houses and small; there is no difference either in the condition or occupation of the persons receiving the water of the different Companies. Now it must be evident that, if the diminution of cholera, in the districts partly supplied with the improved water, depended on this supply, the houses receiving it would be the houses enjoying the whole benefit of the diminution of the malady, whilst the houses supplied with the water from Battersea Fields would suffer the same mortality as they would if the improved supply did not exist at all. As there is no difference whatever, either in the houses or the people receiving the supply of the two Water Companies, or in any of the physical conditions with which they are surrounded, it is obvious that no experiment could have been devised which would more thoroughly test the effect of water supply on the progress of cholera than this, which circumstances placed ready made before the observer.

The experiment, too, was on the grandest scale. No fewer than three hundred thousand people of both sexes, of every age and occupation, and of every rank and station, from gentlefolks down to the very poor, were divided into two groups without their choice, and, in most, without their knowledge; one group being supplied with water containing the sewage of London, and, amongst it, whatever might have come from the cholera patients, the other group having water quite free from such impurity.

To turn this grand experiment to account, all that was required was to learn the supply of water to each individual house where a fatal attack of cholera might occur.[4]

Snow's survey produced strong evidence to support his theory that dirty water caused cholera (Table 8.2). As he states, "the experiment was on the grandest scale." The residents of the area were unaware of the source of their water. There was no difference in life styles or socioeconomic factors. The only difference was the water supply: one group received relatively pure water, while the other was drinking the "sewage of London."

[4] *Snow on Cholera*, pp. 74–75.

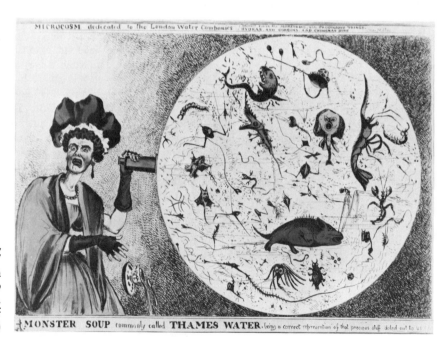

Figure 8.2. "Monster soup, commonly called Thames water" (1828). Caricature by William Heath on the contents of a drop of water from the Thames. (Courtesy of National Library of Medicine, Bethesda, Maryland)

Table 8.2 Cholera mortality in London within district B*

Water company	Number of houses supplied	Deaths from cholera per 10,000 persons
Southwark and Vauxhall	40,046	315
Lambeth	26,107	37
Rest of London	256,423	59

* From *Snow on Cholera*, p. 86.

The work of John Snow illustrates the methods of modern epidemiology. Based on clinical intuition, he formed the hypothesis that water caused cholera. He tested his hypothesis by relating water supply to cholera death rates. A cause-effect association was established. Note that he did not perform an experiment—he did not feed dirty water to a group to see if cholera was the result. He *observed* what nature had created. This is the basis for much of today's epidemiology: a study is made of the association between diseases and their causes. If an association is found and cannot be disproved, the credibility of the possible cause must be evaluated. At some point a decision must be made as to whether it is prudent to assume causality or to wait for further study. In the case of cholera and dirty water, it was clearly prudent to stop taking water from the lower Thames and to start taking it from farther upstream.

DESCRIPTIVE EPIDEMIOLOGY

Methods: measures of disease

The first step in studying the epidemiology of a disease is to *count:* the number of persons who die from suicide, the number of persons who develop syphilis, the number of persons who have diabetes, and so on. These counts, however, are not enough. The numbers must be related to a population. For example, if an epidemiologist found that 20 people in the city of Fargo developed lung cancer during 1973, he must relate that figure to the number of people living in the city (50,000).

The basic measure of disease in epidemiology is a *rate:* the number of persons with a disease divided by the number of people in the population. There are two basic types of rates: *incidence rate* and *prevalence rate.*

Incidence refers to the number of people in a population who *develop* a disease during a particular period of time and also predicts the chance of getting a disease. The incidence rate of lung cancer in Fargo during 1973 would be written as 20/50,000/year (20 cases per 50,000 persons per year). A *mortality rate* is a special type of incidence rate measuring the probability of *dying* from a disease.

Prevalence rate expresses the number of persons *having* a disease. If 500 people in Fargo have diabetes, the prevalence rate would be 500/50,000 or 10/1,000.

Measuring incidence or prevalence rates is essential to all epidemio-

Epidemiology and literature

Charles Babbage sent the following letter to Alfred, Lord Tennyson about a couplet in "The Vision of Sin":

"Every minute dies a man./ Every minute one is born:" I need hardly point out to you that this calculation would tend to keep the sum total of the world's population in a state of perpetual equipoise, whereas it is a well-known fact that the said sum total is constantly on the increase. I would therefore take the liberty of suggesting that in the next edition of your excellent poem the erroneous calculation to which I refer should be corrected as follows: "Every moment dies a man/And one and a sixteenth is born." I may add that the exact figures are 1.167 but something must, of course, be conceded to the laws of metre.

From P. Morrison and E. Morrison, eds., *Charles Babbage and his Calculating Engines* (New York: Dover Publications, 1961), p. xxiii.

logic studies. These measurements indicate the probability that a person gets or has a disease. These probabilities may be measured in different subgroups of a population, in the same group at different times, or in groups exposed to different causal agents. By comparing rates, information is assembled concerning the cause of disease.

How does one compare rates? There are two basic methods. Suppose that one wishes to see whether a disease occurs more frequently in women than in men and, if so, to quantitate the relationship. The first step is to measure the incidence rate of disease for each sex. Assume that the disease is infectious mononucleosis ("mono"), and that the yearly rate in men is 20/1,000 and in women is 15/1,000. If one rate is divided by the other, a *relative rate* is obtained: 20/1,000 ÷ 15/1,000 = 20/15 or 1.33. In epidemiologic jargon this is termed *relative risk* or *risk ratio*. The second method is to measure the difference between the two rates: 20/1,000 − 15/1,000 = 5/1,000. This is termed *attributable risk* or *risk difference*.

Risk ratios and risk differences are different measures of the risk of disease and are used in different ways. If one wishes to assess the role of a suspected agent in the causality of a disease, the risk ratio is most useful. For example, if a disease is ten times more frequent in men than in women, something about the male sex is a causal factor in the disease. In contrast, the risk difference is used to measure the cost to society of a disease. Even though there may be a small risk ratio (say 1.5) associated with a causal agent, the risk difference will be large if the disease is common. This will be illustrated below.

A problem: Cigarettes, lung cancer, and heart attacks

The relationship of tobacco and disease is presented in Chapter 16. It is the purpose of this section to illustrate how data studying these associations are collected and interpreted.

The possibility that cigarette smoking was a cause of lung cancer and heart attacks (coronary heart disease) first received serious consideration over forty years ago. As illustrated in Fig. 8.3, by 1945 a sharp increase in the death rate from cancer had been noted among white males aged 60 to 64. The increase has continued to the present day, even though the total death rate for men of the same age has fallen slightly. Evidence from descriptive epidemiology pointed up the fact that something of importance was adversely affecting the health of the population.

Because cigarette smoke comes into contact with the lungs, it was logical to postulate that cigarette smoke was responsible for the increase in lung cancer. It was first necessary, however, to determine whether smoking had also increased.

As seen in Fig. 8.4, the pattern of cigarette smoking paralleled that of lung cancer. Between 1910 and 1940, there was a twenty-five-fold increase in the annual per capita consumption of cigarettes. On the basis

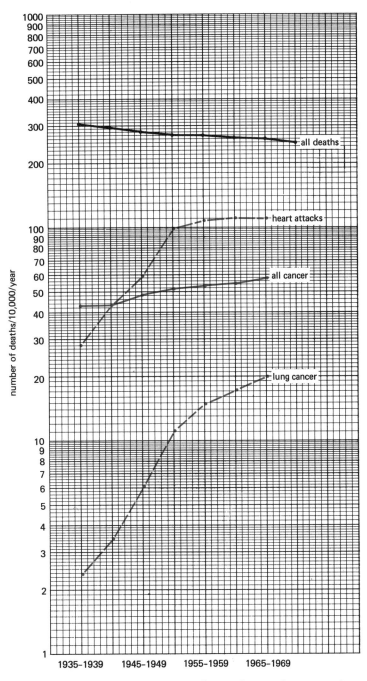

Figure 8.3. Death rates for white males aged 60–64 by year and age, 1925–1970

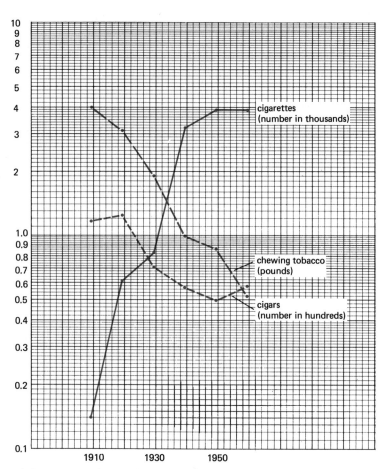

Figure 8.4. United States tobacco consumption per capita by year (*Smoking and Health*, Washington, D.C., Public Health Service Publication No. 1103, 1964, p. 45)

of descriptive data, a hypothesis could be formed that cigarette smoking caused lung cancer, but the evidence presented thus far is relatively weak. For example, if one plotted the curve of per capita refrigerator ownership over the same period, a similar increase could be noted. Such circumstantial evidence must be interpreted with caution.

To test the hypothesis, new studies must be devised. Fig. 8.5 gives an example of a descriptive study. A comparison was made between the rate of lung and larynx cancer in 44 states and the average per capita sale of cigarettes in 1960. States in which more cigarettes were sold were found to have the highest death rates for lung cancer. Thus, the hypothesis linking cigarettes and lung cancer is strengthenend. It is nevertheless important to further quantitate the magnitude of the increase in mortality from lung cancer, that is, how the risk of dying from lung cancer in 1965 compares with the risk in 1935. As shown in Fig. 8.3, the mortality rate in 1935–1939 was 2.4/10,000/year. In 1965–1969 the rate was 20/10,000/year. Expressed as risk ratio, the risk in 1965 was 20/2.4 or over eight times greater than in 1935. In other words, for every 10,000

Figure 8.5. Correlation between lung cancer death rates and per capita cigarette sales (1960) in 44 states. (Joseph F. Fraumeni, "Cigarette smoking and cancers of the urinary tract: geographic variation in the United States," *Journal National Cancer Institute,* Vol. 41, 1968, p. 1208)

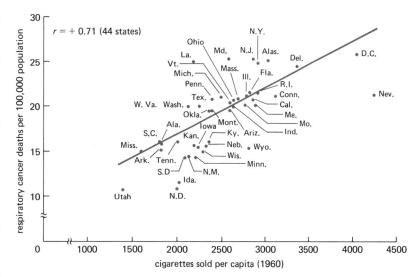

white males ages 60–64, 20 — 2.4 or 17.6 more died from lung cancer in 1965 than in 1935.

Figure 8.3 also contains time-specific mortality rates from heart attacks. During the period 1935–1965, about 10 times as many 60-year-old white males died from heart attacks as from lung cancer. Also, the death rate from heart attacks rose from 1935 to 1965. Expressed as risk ratio, the increase was 110/10,000/year ÷ 28/10,000/year—about four times greater in 1965. Thus, the increase in heart attacks was *relatively* smaller than that in lung cancer.

However, the risk *difference* between 1935 and 1965 was 110 — 28 or 72/10,000/year—four times greater than the risk difference for lung cancer. Which disease, then, showed the greater increase between 1935 and 1965?

This apparent paradox illustrates the importance of defining the units of measure when describing the occurrence of disease and in using common sense in interpreting the data. For example, if a Rolls-Royce cost $20,000, a Thunderbird $5,000, and a Honda $500, which is relatively more expensive? The Rolls cost $15,000 more than the Thunderbird or four times as much. The Thunderbird costs only $4,500 more than the Honda, yet costs ten times as much. Obviously, if one uses two different measures of comparison, the measures should not be compared themselves.

Similarly, risk ratios and risk differences should not be compared with each other. The first is a relative measure, the second an absolute measure. The concepts should be kept distinct. However, these are general concepts which do not belong exclusively to epidemiologists. Such comparisons form the basis for decisions in all of science, as well as in everyday life.

ANALYTIC EPIDEMIOLOGY

Methods: The study of exposure and disease in an individual

As noted earlier, descriptive data do not relate exposure and disease in an individual. Even though the lung cancer rate is highest in states where more cigarettes are purchased, there may well be other factors in those states causing lung cancer. It is necessary, therefore, to perform studies in which exposure and disease information are known for a particular group.

One way to approach this problem is to divide a population into two groups: the exposed and the nonexposed. For example, all members of the freshman class at a particular college could be divided into smokers and nonsmokers and the lung cancer rates determined for each.

In this study, termed *prospective cohort*, exposure information is collected before the disease occurs. Because the epidemiologist does not know the disease history of each individual, there is no chance for bias to be introduced. Such studies, however, frequently take a long time to complete. It would take 20 to 40 years to develop sufficient cases of lung cancer in the college group to relate cancer to smoking.

For this reason a second type of study—*case-control study*—may be done. Persons with and without disease are identified and their past history of exposure is determined. Persons with lung cancer and a similar group without lung cancer are questioned about their past smoking habits. The main advantage of a case-control study is that the time needed to complete the study is short. The obvious disadvantage is that people suffering from lung cancer may be more likely to report a high cigarette smoking history because they wish to blame their cancer on something.

Several modifications of these studies may be made to overcome some of their disadvantages. Cohort studies, in which exposed and nonexposed groups are assembled, may be based on past rather than current exposure information. For example, during the initial physical exam at Harvard in the 1920s and 1930s, freshmen were asked, "Do you smoke cigarettes?" The classes were then divided into two groups, smokers and nonsmokers. Twenty to forty years later when the decision to study lung cancer and smoking was made, sufficient time had passed for lung cancer to develop and the groups were traced to ascertain who had developed the disease. This type of study is called a *retrospective cohort study*.

The major problem in case-control studies is obtaining objective data on past exposure to a suspected cause of disease. Asking a person directly is unlikely to yield bias-free information. If possible, it is desirable to obtain records where exposure to the disease was recorded prior to its development.

Data obtained from a cohort or a case-control study are displayed in a "fourfold table," illustrated in Table 8.3. In this case-control study of smoking and lung cancer, men with lung cancer were asked: "Have you ever smoked cigarettes for at least a year?" The study took place in England 25 years ago, and it indicates that most of the men smoked cigarettes. Only 0.3 percent of lung cancer patients stated that they never had smoked, while over ten times as many noncancer patients were nonsmokers. The data from this analytic epidemiologic study are consistent with that from descriptive studies, that is, there appears to be an association between smoking and lung cancer.

Table 8.3 Smoking history of men with and without lung cancer*

	With lung cancer	Without lung cancer
Cigarette smokers	647	622
Nonsmokers	2	27
Total	649	649
Percent nonsmokers	0.3	4.2

* From Richard Doll and A. Bradford Hill, "Smoking and carcinoma of the lung," *British Medical Journal*, Vol. 2 (1950), p. 742.

Problem: X-rays and the unborn child

Early in this century medical X-rays were used in obstetrics. A picture could be made of the size of the mother's pelvis and the size of the baby's head. If the head appeared to be too big, a Caesarian section could be performed to prevent a dangerous labor. Because the dosage of X-rays used to take such pictures was very low, radiologists and obstetricians felt that the procedure was safe. However, during the middle 1950s evidence began to accumulate that all was not well. Several studies reported that children whose mothers were X-rayed while pregnant had an increased risk of dying from cancer.

Two types of studies, cohort and case-control, were performed to study this problem. In a cohort study, the rate of fatal childhood cancer was measured in exposed and nonexposed children. The rates were compared using risk ratio and risk difference.

In one study the children of approximately 10,000 women who were X-rayed during pregnancy and of approximately 20,000 women who were not X-rayed were followed for up to 10 years after birth. All fatal cases of cancer that occurred were identified. Among the 10,000 irradiated children, 11 cancers occurred; among the 20,000 nonexposed children, 17 cancers occurred. These data are shown in part A of Table 8.4.

It appears that the rate of cancer in the exposed children (11/10,000) is greater than that in the nonexposed (8.5/10,000). However, the rate 11/10,000 does not take into account the number of years each child lived. This is of importance because had the exposed children been followed longer than those not exposed, more cases of cancer would be expected.

Therefore, Table 8.4, part B, was constructed relating the risk of dying from cancer to *person-years*. The number of years lived is determined for each person, and all of the *person-years* are added together. The number of deaths divided by the number of person-years equals the mortality rate from cancer.

As seen in Table 8.4, the risk ratio is 1.3. In other words, the risk for cancer in children exposed to X-ray is 30 percent higher than that of nonexposed children. A risk difference of 2.8/100,000/year means that if the X-ray is causing the cancer, for every 100,000 children exposed to prenatal X-ray, 2.8 will develop cancer each year.

Table 8.4 Relationship between prenatal X-ray and childhood cancer from a cohort study*

	Cancer	No cancer	Total	
A. Using persons				
X-ray	11	9,989	10,000	
No X-ray	17	19,983	20,000	
Total	28	29,972	30,000	
B. Using person-years				
X-ray	11	—	87,740	12.6/100,000/year
No X-ray	17	—	175,608	9.7/100,000/year
Total	28	—	263,348	

Risk ratio = 12.5 ÷ 9.7 = 1.3
Risk difference = 12.5 − 9.7 = 2.8/100,000/year

* From E. L. Diamond, unpublished study, cited in Irving I. Kessler and Abraham M. Lilienfeld, eds., "Perspectives in the epidemiology of leukemia," *Advances in Cancer Research*, 12 (1969), pp. 225–301.

How is this problem approached using a case-control study? First, children with cancer are identified. Next, a control group of children without cancer is assembled for comparison. The control group children should closely resemble the children with cancer with respect to characteristics likely to be related to X-ray exposure. Finally, the X-ray exposure of the mothers of the two groups must be determined.

In this type of study, the method used to measure the X-ray exposure is important. For example, mothers of children with cancer might be more likely to recall the X-ray because they would be interested in identifying a cause of the cancer. Therefore, it is desirable to use a more objective method of estimating X-ray exposure. In one study, the mother's maternity records were reviewed and X-ray reports were noted. Of the mothers of children with cancer 15.8 percent had been X-rayed, while only 10.6 percent of the mothers of the control group had been X-rayed.[5] These data are consistent with those obtained in the cohort study.

[5] Brian MacMahon, "Prenatal X-ray exposure and childhood cancer," *Journal National Cancer Institute*, 28 (1962), pp. 1173–91.

A case-control study measures percentages of exposure rather than rates of disease. Dividing one percentage by the other to obtain the *exposure* ratio is analogous to obtaining the risk ratio. While these two ratios are not numerically equivalent, the interpretation of each is similar. If the risk ratio is 1.0, the exposure ratio is also 1.0. An increase in one ratio is accompanied by an increase in the other.

EXPERIMENTAL EPIDEMIOLOGY

Methods

An experiment in epidemiology is similar to those in biological fields. A biologist, for example, might assemble a population of rats, divide them into two groups, treat one group and withhold treatment or drugs from the other, and follow each group to see what happens. Several principles are basic to experiments:

1. Randomization. The two groups must be selected so that prior to the treatment they are similar. A common means of obtaining similarity is to select the members of each group from the total population at random.
2. Control treatment. A nontreated group is necessary because it must be established what the results would be if there were no treatment.
3. Blindness. It is desirable that the investigator not know which group is treated and which is not so that he will not—consciously or unconsciously—favor one group. If the experimental treatment is surgery, this is difficult. But if one group is being given a drug to assess its possible danger, the control group can be given a placebo—an inert substance such as sugar—known to have no effect.

Experiments in humans differ from experiments in animals in several ways:

1. Ethics (see Chap. 18). It usually is unethical to conduct an experiment on a human population when one believes that harm is possible. If a chemical is a suspected cause of skin cancer, it would be unethical to paint the skin of humans with the chemical to see what happens. While there has never been a study to see if surgery is a better treatment for appendicitis than drugs, antibiotics have been successfully used to treat appendicitis in sailors at sea. However, because surgery has become the accepted treatment for appendicitis, it would not be considered ethical by most physicians to use antibiotic therapy alone to see if it would produce similar or better results.
2. Informing the participants. It is important that each person in an experiment be informed of the reasons for and nature of the experiment. The person must be able to judge for himself and free to choose whether or not he wishes to participate.

   Randomization is done only after persons who do not wish to participate are removed from the study. By this procedure, comparability between treated and nontreated groups is maintained. However, the ability to generalize the results is reduced.

3. Ability to generalize. In any study the investigator desires to apply the results to a larger group. If the experiment is conducted upon a representative sample of the total population, generalizations can be made. If only a small sampling of persons participate, the results of the experiments will not be as widely applicable. The results will hold for the group, but applying the results to nonparticipants may not be warranted. For this reason, experiments in human beings frequently have only narrow applicability.

4. Double blindness. In a double-blind study, neither the investigator nor the subjects know who receives the study treatment and who receives the control treatment. Furthermore, the outcome is measured in such a way that the type of treatment is not known, and thus no bias is introduced by the investigator or the subject. Frequently, however, blindness becomes difficult. The treatment being studied may have some minor side-effect which indicates to the subject that he is in the treatment group. In the case of surgical treatment of a problem, it is not ethical to perform a placebo operation. Thus, while double-blindness is desirable in human experiments, it frequently is not feasible.

Experimental epidemiology, then, is an ideal against which observational or nonexperimental epidemiology must be judged. An experiment has advantages and disadvantages. An experiment is advantageous because random assignment and blind assessment of disease are possible. However, an experimenter is limited to doing prospective studies—he does not start with diseased and nondiseased groups and look back—and he must always conduct his studies in light of ethical considerations.

A problem: diabetes

Diabetes is a disease in which the level of sugar in the blood becomes abnormally high (see Chap. 11). As a result of long term diabetes, persons may develop blindness or gangrene of the feet and frequently die of heart attacks. The level of blood sugar is controlled by insulin, a hormone secreted by the pancreas. In diabetics, for some unknown reason, either the pancreas fails to secrete enough insulin or the tissues do not react properly to the insulin.

During the 1920s methods were developed to extract insulin from the pancreas of cows and pigs and to use this insulin in the treatment of diabetes. As a result, control of diabetes was a possibility and most patients were able to live relatively normal lives. Because the development of insulin meant a dramatic improvement in the treatment of diabetes, its value was generally accepted.

Insulin can be administered only by injection, and thus substitute drugs were developed. These "oral hypoglycemic agents," which lowered the level of the blood sugar, were felt to be of special value in persons who developed mild diabetes late in life.

One major problem, even in patients with treated diabetes, was the occurrence of disease in the blood vessels of the heart and legs. The extent to which the oral hypoglycemic agents were of value in preventing these vascular complications was unknown. Therefore, an experiment (clinical trial) was designed to compare the experience of diabetics treated with insulin, with oral hypoglycemic agents, and with a placebo.[6] The study proceeded as follows:

1. Persons with diabetes were told about the study and the reasons for it and that if they agreed to participate, they would be randomly assigned to one of four treatment groups: two types of insulin, an oral agent, or a placebo. If for any reason a patient did not accept this proposal, he or she was not included in the study.

2. Each person who agreed to the study was assigned one of the four treatments. When insulin was the assigned treatment, it was not possible for the patient or doctor to be blinded to the mode of therapy, because one or more shots per day were needed. However, neither the patient nor his doctor knew who was being treated with an oral agent and who was receiving a placebo. In addition to the treatment, each patient was placed on a specific diet that limited his sugar intake.

3. If a patient died, the circumstances of death were recorded and submitted to a panel of physicians who determined the reason for the death. Since the panel did not know the treatment group to which the deceased patient belonged, blind assessment of outcome was possible.

4. After about five years, it became apparent that patients treated with the oral agent (tolbutamide) were dying at a higher rate than patients treated otherwise. The major cause appeared to be cardiovascular disease. This difference continued to increase for eight years (Fig. 8.6), at which point it was decided to stop the study.

Interpretation of the data from this study has met with great controversy. Tolbutamide is a widely used drug and clinicians have become convinced of its value. However, the study suggests that people may be dying from it. The study further suggests that diet alone may be a sufficient treatment because there was no difference in the mortality rates of those treated with insulin and those treated with the placebo.

This study serves to illustrate the problems involved in experimental epidemiology. While on the surface the experiment seemed to be an

---

[6] University Group Diabetes Program, "A study of the effects of hypoglycemic agents on vascular complications in patients with adult onset diabetes," *Diabetes,* 19 (1970), Suppl. 2.

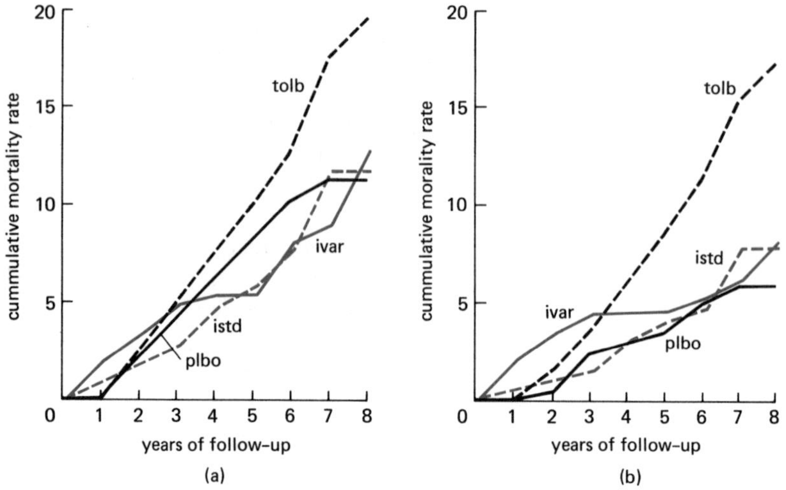

Figure 8.6. Cumulative mortality rates per 100 population by year of follow-up. TOLB—tolbutamide; IVAR—variable insulin; ISTD—standard insulin; PLBO—placebo. (University Group Diabetes Program)

appropriate way to answer a question, the realities are more complex. The design and execution of the study were well done. It is unlikely the results were biased because, if anything, the investigators expected to show that tolbutamide was of value in preventing cardiovascular complications of diabetes. The major argument against the study is that the circumstances of the study did not mimic clinical practice. Once a patient had been assigned to a treatment group, he remained there. In practice, a doctor has the option of switching therapies. Because the reasons for switching are frequently difficult to pinpoint, such a feature was not incorporated into the study design. An experiment is the model on which observational studies must be based; however, even well done experiments do not necessarily yield conclusive results.

PREVENTIVE EPIDEMIOLOGY

Methods

A doctor's primary goal is to cure disease, whereas the epidemiologist's prime concern is disease prevention. Most studies seek to identify factors associated with a disease in the hope that these factors can be removed or manipulated to reduce the risk of disease.

Most preventive studies involve research in which no direct service to the individual patient is provided. However, one type of study—a *screening program*—is geared to the direct prevention of disease. In a screening program an attempt is made to find persons in the early stage of disease. By so doing it is hoped that the disease can be treated in its early stage and be cured.

The main role of the epidemiologist in such a study is not to operate the program but rather to evaluate the results of screening. While it seems likely that finding a disease early in its course is of value, it is important to document that this is so. It is especially necessary if the screening procedure is of possible harm to the patient or if considerable

The contributions of epidemiology

In the short span of 30 years, epidemiologists have discovered the cause of the vast majority of cases of lung cancer; learned enough about the epidemiology of dental caries to be able to prevent a sizable portion of this disease; delineated the health effects of radiation exposures and stimulated adoption of control measures; discovered important risk factors in coronary heart disease and arrived at the point of testing the possibility of achieving effective preventive programs; enlarged considerably our knowledge of the various diseases caused by tobacco and alcohol; and begun to study a broad spectrum of diseases, including drug-induced and other iatrogenic disorders, in a serious way. Indeed, they have become bold enough to study medical care services from the epidemiologic standpoint, that is, with regard to impact on health status. Epidemiologists have moved beyond a preoccupation with disease to include violence—accidents, homicide, and suicide—among their concerns. And finally, they have begun to develop epidemiologic studies of healthy individuals, including major investigations of the relation of prenatal and infant nutrition to the mental and physical development of children.

From Milton Terris, "The epidemiologic revolution," *American Journal of Public Health* 62 (1972), 1439–41.

expense is involved. Also, if the screening test is positive in some people who do not have the disease, some persons may be treated unnecessarily.

A problem: X-rays and breast cancer

Cancer of the breast is the leading cause of cancer deaths among American women. Each year over 25,000 women die from breast cancer. Treatment involves removing the breast and frequently the muscles of the chest.

In recent years a new technique has been developed to identify breast cancer at an early stage. The procedure involves X-raying the breast, *mammography*, to detect cancer at an early stage. Because even low doses of X-ray may be harmful, as illustrated by prenatal X-ray, it is not advisable to expose women to additional X-ray unless there is evidence that there is some benefit.

To test whether or not early identification of breast cancer prevents death, the screening program must be evaluated. This is most easily done in an experiment. A group of women is screened for breast cancer using mammography and a comparison group is not screened. After a period of time the numbers of deaths caused by breast cancer are measured in each group. If the screened group of women has fewer deaths, the value of mammography would be shown.

Such a study was carried out starting in 1963.[7] Among 62,000 women who belonged to a prepaid group practice program, 31,000 were screened regularly for breast cancer by mammography and 31,000 were followed according to routine medical practice. After six years, 52 of the women in the control group had died from breast cancer in contrast to only 31 women in the mammography group. This is sound evidence that early detection of breast cancer using mammography is of value in curing the disease.

Evaluative programs such as this have only recently been done. Historically, whenever a new drug, surgical procedure, or diagnostic test comes along, its benefits are widely touted by the developer. Little thought has been given to establishing whether the procedure is indeed of value or, more importantly, whether there are any harmful side effects. Today, however, physicians and medical researchers are becoming convinced of the necessity for such programs, and it seems likely that the role of epidemiology in the evaluation of clinical practice will become increasingly important.

SUMMARY— INTERPRETATION OF DATA

This chapter has dealt primarily with the methods used to collect and analyze data involving sickness and health. Without such data it is difficult to make rational decisions concerning prevention and cure of

[7] S. Shapiro, P. Strax, and L. Venet, "Periodic breast cancer screening in reducing mortality from breast cancer," *Journal American Medical Association*, 215 (1971), 1777–85.

illness. Of equal importance is the interpretation of these data. Numbers may suggest an association between an exposure and an outcome, but this does not mean that action must be taken to eliminate the exposure. Careful thought is needed to decide whether the statistics reflect the true underlying situation being studied. In any study it is possible that the investigator has created an association through error or bias. In nonexperimental studies especially, the possibility exists that an unknown variable accounts for the results. Finally, even though a cause-effect relationship is established, there may be no easy way to correct the situation.

In spite of these caveats, decisions based on imperfect data must be made. At some point it becomes more prudent to assume that the data accurately reflect the true situation rather than some error or modifying factor. In the case of smoking and lung cancer, no experiment has or likely will be done on humans. Thus, this type of "proof of causality" will never be available. However, based on a large number of observational studies, it is accepted by most epidemiologists that cigarette smoking is a cause of cancer.

In spite of this strong evidence, the question still exists as to what is to be done about cigarettes. Clearly, everyone who smokes does not develop lung cancer. There are likely to be beneficial effects of smoking, but they are difficult to quantitate. How is a decision made on how to deal with this problem?

Currently, the decision is in the hands of the individual. Each person must judge whether the pleasure of smoking outweighs the risk of disease caused by smoking. Efforts are now being made to identify the components of cigarette smoke responsible for lung cancer.

The collection and analysis of data are essential if the processes of disease are to be understood. There are many pitfalls along the way and no one study is likely to be conclusive. Caution must always be exercised in interpreting and acting upon the results of studies. But without such studies, decisions would have little basis.

Questions
1. Compare and contrast the following: a. incidence and prevalence; b. risk ratio and risk difference.
2. Why is it necessary to compare rates rather than numbers in studying the occurrence of disease?
3. Discuss the advantages and disadvantages of case-control and cohort studies.
4. Discuss advantages and disadvantages of observational vs. experimental studies.
5. What criteria in a screening program should be used to evaluate the program?

Key Concepts

Case-control study – a study in which the percentages of exposure are measured in diseased and nondiseased persons

Cohort study – a study in which the rates of diseases are measured in exposed and nonexposed persons

Incidence rate – the number of persons who *develop* a disease per unit population per unit time

Prevalence rate – the number of persons *having* a disease per unit population

Rate – the number of persons with a disease divided by the number of persons in the population

Selected Readings

Fox, J. P., C. E. Hall, and L. R. Elveback. *Epidemiology—Man and Disease.* Toronto: Macmillan, 1970.

Hill, Sir Austin Bradford. *Principles of Medical Statistics*, 8th ed. New York: Oxford Univ. Press, 1966.

LeRiche, W. H. and J. Milner. *Epidemiology as Medical Ecology.* Baltimore: Williams and Wilkins Co., 1971.

Lilienfeld, A. M. and A. Gifford. *Chronic Diseases and Public Health.* Baltimore: Johns Hopkins Press, 1966.

MacMahon, B. and T. F. Pugh. *Epidemiology—Principles and Methods.* Boston: Little, Brown and Co., 1970.

Chapter 9

Infectious Diseases

We share this planet with a vast horde of tiny organisms which are invisible to the naked eye. Their existence was unknown until they were first seen by a Dutchman, Antony van Leeuwenhoek, in the microscope he had invented. He described the tiny creatures in a letter to the Royal Society in London on September 17, 1683. Many of their effects, however, have been known since man first emerged on earth. Certain of these microorganisms, as they are called, have made life more comfortable for mankind. Some kinds convert grape juice into wine, others wine into vinegar, grain into beer, milk into cheese or yogurt, while others cause bread dough to rise. Certain microorganisms living in the nodules in the roots of plants capture nitrogen from air and convert it into chemical compounds that enrich the earth for growing food crops. Other microorganisms break down the tissues of dead plants and animals and in the process release carbon dioxide, nitrogen, and water into the atmosphere to be recycled. Other microorganisms, notably the fungi, have

This chapter was contributed by J. William Vinson, D.S.Hyg., Associate Professor of Microbiology, Harvard School of Public Health.

been set to work manufacturing antibiotics, such as penicillin, and a variety of useful chemicals, such as citric acid.

We spend our lives among the vast population of microorganisms. A wide variety of them have found a home on man as well as other animals. They live and multiply on the skin and in the mouth and the intestinal tract. Most of them are harmless, living as guests at the expense of their host without doing any damage. They can even be beneficial. Some are potentially capable of injuring their host, but under normal conditions their numbers are kept too small by the population pressure from other harmless microorganisms to cause damage.

Other microorganisms, however, during the course of their multiplication in or on the body can cause damage to their host. When this happens they are called *pathogens*, and the damage to their host— together with the efforts of the body to block or repair the damage— is called *disease*. Each disease is caused by a specific microorganism and many of them are passed from one person to another, sometimes by circuitous routes. These diseases are called *infectious diseases*.

Disease is not the inevitable result of bringing together a human being and a microbe. Infectious diseases occur in a definite time and place and under certain sets of circumstances. These conditions can be sociologic, biologic, physical, or a combination of these, and together they compose the biosocial environment in which the diseases are transmitted to humans. A balance exists between the human host, the microbial agents of disease, and the biosocial environment. When this delicate balance is upset the individual can become ill. An epidemic can be ignited and sweep through whole countries, continents, or the world, leaving death and misery in its trail. This chapter is about the balance which exists between pathogenic microorganisms and human beings in a biosocial environment and about the sequence of events which ensue when this equilibrium is upset in favor of the pathogens.

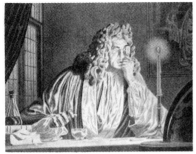

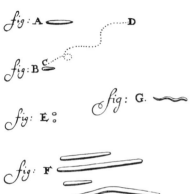

Figure 9.1. Using his microscope, Antony van Leeuwenhoek (1632–1723) was able to make the first drawings of bacteria.

AGENTS OF INFECTIOUS DISEASE

Microbial agents which under proper circumstances can cause disease in human beings come in a wide variety of shapes, sizes, degree of internal organization, and life processes. They vary widely in the relationships they can establish with their human hosts. All of them, with the exception of some of the worms, can be seen only in the light microscope or in the electron microscope.

Bacteria

Bacteria are divided into spherical forms called *cocci*, from the Latin word for berry, and into cylindrical forms called *bacilli*, from the Latin word for stick. Cocci are seen in characteristic groupings that result from the way in which they divide during reproduction (Fig. 9.2). Pairs of cocci are called *diplococci*, meaning double; pneumococci which cause pneumonia belong to this group. The cocci which cause scarlet fever or so-called strep sore throat are seen in chains and are called *streptococci*,

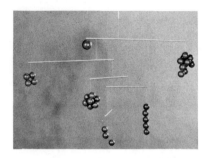

Figure 9.2. A mobile showing typical groupings of cocci in single cells, pairs, chains, tetrads, packets, and irregular clusters.

while the cocci which cause boils are found in clusters and are called *staphylococci,* from the Latin word for bunch of grapes. Bacilli come in several widths, lengths, and shapes. One kind which is curved into a commalike shape is the *vibrio* that causes cholera. Another, symmetrically twisted like a corkscrew, is called a *spirochete.* One kind of spirochete causes syphilis.

Some bacteria possess appendages called *flagella,* whiplike structures which function as organs of locomotion. Some bacteria are covered with tiny hairlike projections known as *pili.* These bacteria can reproduce with each other by means of the pili. A conduit is formed with the pili between bacterial cells. In this way, extrachromasomal genetic material can be passed from one bacterium to another. A mucous capsule surrounds some bacteria. In the pneumococcus, such a capsule defeats efforts of the human body to kill it.

All bacteria have an outer, rigid cell wall which helps protect them from environmental stress and an inner plasma membrane which regulates the passage of materials into and out of the bacterial cell. Inside the cell are ribosomes which are active in synthesizing protein and a naked chromosome which houses the genetic information of each species of bacterium.

Bacteria reproduce by dividing themselves into two daughter cells, a process known as *binary fission.* The time between cell divisions is called the *generation time* and varies among different kinds of bacteria. The coccus which causes gonorrhea has a generation time of about fifty minutes, while the generation time for the spirochete of syphilis is about thirty hours.

Sometimes, instead of dividing, certain bacteria form spores which are highly resistant to injurious conditions such as drying or heat. Under

Botulism

Many years ago in California Dr. K. F. Meyer investigated an outbreak of botulism which had afflicted most members of a family and caused the death of two. All the evidence indicated that canned string beans eaten by the family contained the poison. Almost to her last breath the mother protested. "It couldn't have been those beans," she whispered, "because *I canned them myself.*"

Primarily through the efforts of Dr. Meyer and other scientists the public became alerted to the dangers of botulism and laws were passed regulating the commercial processing of food to control this toxic disease.

The bacterium *Clostridium botulinum,* which causes the intoxication, lives in the soil and in the intestinal tract of animals and fish. The microorganism contaminates vegetables grown in the soil, meat, and fish processed for storage in various forms. It forms spores which are highly resistant to heat and other deleterious influences. They can survive canning temperatures usually achieved during home canning. In canned or processed food, the spores germinate into the vegetative bacterial form which starts producing the most potent toxin known to man. When swallowed in even minute amounts it kills within a few days.

The toxin, however, is easily destroyed by being boiled for ten minutes.

There are different antigenic types of toxin which are given alphabetical designations. Immune sera to the different types, which neutralize the toxins, are stockpiled around the country by the U.S. Public Health Service for emergency use in afflicted persons. While botulism is not a large public health problem, the potential for circumscribed epidemics remains whenever food processing is not maintained at a high level.

proper conditions the spores can germinate into the usual vegetative form and undergo division. Of particular importance to medicine is the fact that the bacteria causing lethal food poisoning (*botulism*) and lockjaw (*tetanus*), produce spores which remain alive for long periods of time in our environment.

Bacteria are classified according to the Latin binomial system invented by the Swedish scientist Karl von Linné to introduce order into the naming of all plants and animals. In this system each bacterium is assigned a capitalized *genus* name followed by an uncapitalized *species* name. Both are italicized. An example is *Shigella dysenteriae*, the bacterium causing bacillary dysentery. The genus was named in honor of Dr. Shiga, the Japanese scientist who discovered the causative microorganism, and the species name indicates the kind of disease this bacterium produces.

Rickettsiae

These microorganisms can be thought of as tiny bacteria which, with one exception, have lost their ability to live outside cells. They can live and multiply only within living cells. Members of this group produce some of the most severe infections of mankind, including louseborne typhus, which has caused devastating epidemics, and Rocky Mountain spotted fever (Fig. 9.3). This group of microorganisms is named after Howard Taylor Ricketts, who as a young man first elucidated the cause of Rocky Mountain spotted fever in Montana and shortly thereafter died of typhus fever while studying this disease in Mexico City. With the single exception of Q *fever*, the rickettsial agents are transmitted by body lice, rat fleas, mites, or ticks.

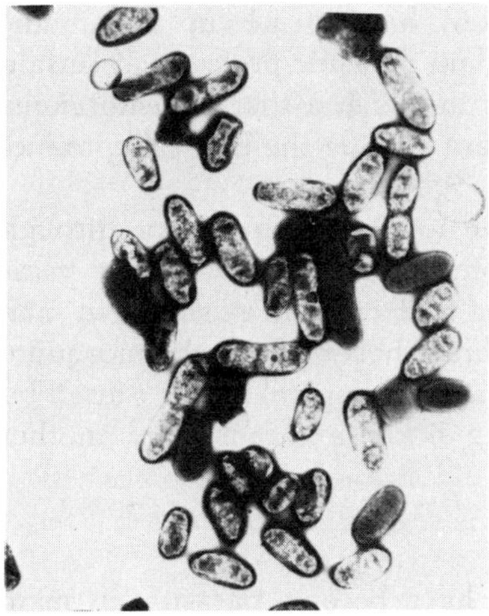

Fungi

Some members of this ubiquitous group of microorganisms, which includes mushrooms, produce a variety of human disease conditions. Officially classified as plants, they have a tough cell wall and a well-defined nucleus. There are two basic anatomical types of fungi. The filamentous form consists of hollow tubes which may or may not be interrupted at intervals by crosswalls called *septa*. Some organisms are simple but others produce a tangled mass of filaments. Individual filaments are termed *hyphae* and the mass of filaments a *mycelium*. The other type of fungus, or *yeast*, grows as spherical ovoid or elongated single cells which usually reproduce by budding.

Viruses

Viruses are composed of a core of genetic material wrapped up in a protective protein coat that serves as a vehicle for transmission from one person to another (Fig. 9.4). Each kind of virus contains only a single type of genetic material, either DNA or RNA (see Chap. 1). All viruses lack the necessary equipment for growth and multiplication; they can be

Figure 9.3. The rickettsia of Rocky Mountain spotted fever (*Rickettsia rickettsi*). (Courtesy of Dr. Erskine Palmer, Center for Disease Control, Atlanta, Georgia)

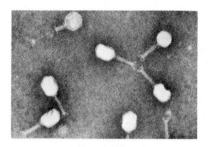

Figure 9.4. A bacterial virus. (Courtesy of Carl Zeiss)

replicated, that is, reproduced, only within a living cell. Some viruses can exchange genetic material with their host cells. Lacking any synthetic mechanism of their own, they depend entirely upon the cells for bio-synthetic machinery, diverting this for replication of themselves. Different parts of the virus are synthesized separately within the host cell, and these component parts are then assembled. Some viruses as they leave their host cell acquire an envelope that resembles the plasma membrane of their host cell. Viruses can infect every variety of plant and animal.

Protozoa

Protozoa are microscopic, single-celled animals which have a nucleus surrounded by a cytoplasm which contains various organelles. Movement is by cilia, flagella, undulating membranes, or by extension of the ectoplasm at the edge of the cell into pseudopodia (false feet). Most protozoa are free-living, but a few have struck up a parasitic existence in man and other animals. Certain parasitic protozoa at certain times enter into an inactive *cystic* state in which a tough membranous wall forms to protect them while they are outside the body. Reproduction may be either sexual or asexual.

Intestinal protozoa pass from person to person directly or through water or food that has left the body. Some protozoa have become parasitic in the blood and tissues. They pass part of their existence in man or other animals and part in an invertebrate host such as the mosquito. Malaria, one of the most important diseases of humankind, is caused by members of this group. African sleeping sickness is caused by another member.

Helminths

Helminths are worms, many of which have become parasitic in man. They exact a great toll in human misery. There are three major groups of helminths.

NEMATODES More than 80,000 species of roundworms are parasitic in vertebrates. The species which are parasitic in man range in size from 2 millimeters up to more than a meter. They have separate sexes and either a simple or a complex life cycle involving the human host and a free-living stage outside the host. Some species have an intermediate host, a second host besides their main, or definitive, host. Hookworms, pinworms, roundworms, and the worm causing trichinosis belong to this group. Another group, the filaria, live in the blood tissues and are transmitted by blood sucking insects.

CESTODES These ribbonlike flatworms have at their front end suckers and often hooks by which they attach themselves to the wall of their host's intestinal tract. The remainder of the adult body consists of segments, each containing both male and female reproductive organs. The worms absorb food from the intestinal tract into their bodies. In most parasitic cestodes, the adults inhabit the intestinal tract of man and other animals, while the larvae live in tissues of other vertebrates and invertebrate hosts. The tapeworms belong to this group of parasites.

TREMATODES The trematodes of interest to us include the intestinal, liver, lung, and blood flukes of man. They have an extraordinary life cycle which involves reproduction in man followed by asexual multiplication while they are in the larval stages nestled in the tissues of snails. The blood flukes cause schistosomiasis, a serious disease prevalent in areas of Asia, Africa, and South America where people come in contact with waters infested with snails that carry the parasites.

THE HUMAN BEING When a human being acquires an infectious agent, he becomes infected and may subsequently become ill. The time elapsed between acquiring the infectious agent and developing the symptoms of disease is called the *incubation period*. If the person can pass the disease to another person or animal he is said to be *infectious*, and the persons exposed to infection are called *contacts*. If, on the other hand, the person becomes infected but does not develop a recognizable disease his infection is *inapparent*, *subclinical*, or *silent* and can be identified only by laboratory tests. He may, however, still be infectious for other people. After a person recovers from an infection he is generally no longer infectious for other people. In some cases, however, an infection can persist in a person after symptoms of disease have vanished and the person can continue to infect other people. Such a person is referred to as a *carrier*. Perhaps the most famous carrier was Typhoid Mary, a cook who infected one household after another with typhoid fever.

When not infecting people, an infectious agent has to exist somewhere. The permanent home of the infectious agent, called the *reservoir*, may be human beings themselves, animals, insects or other arthropods, plants, soil, or inanimate matter.

If an agent of disease persists indefinitely in a geographic area the disease is said to be *endemic*. Thus Cape Cod, Massachusetts, is endemic for Rocky Mountain spotted fever. If a disease affects a number of people in a place where it has been absent, or appears in a greater number of people than usual for that time of year, it is said to be *epidemic*. World wide epidemics, such as those of Hong Kong and Asian influenza, are called *pandemics*.

Contamination refers to the presence of an infectious agent on or in something. Thus Typhoid Mary contaminated the food she prepared with her infectious feces by means of her unwashed fingers.

Interaction between host and agent
A *pathogenic* microorganism is one which can produce disease in a susceptible host. There are two basic mechanisms through which a pathogen can cause disease. It must first be able to invade the tissues

of the host. Some bacteria possess capsules which prevent them from being destroyed by the body's nonspecific defense methods. Others secrete enzymes which dissolve or destroy body substances or clot blood. Once the microorganism has successfully established itself in the body it may secrete toxic substances of two kinds. *Exotoxins* are proteins manufactured by living bacteria which act as cell poisons. In diphtheria, for example, the causative bacterium, *Corynebacterium diphtheriae,* grows in the throat and secretes a powerful poison which is absorbed into the body and produces disease. *Endotoxins,* on the other hand, are components of the cell wall of some bacteria which are released when the microorganism dies. Endotoxins cause a variety of pathologic effects, including shock, fever, and coagulation of blood.

The body has several mechanical and chemical barriers to invasion by microorganisms. The intact skin and mucous membranes prevent entry of many potential invaders. The normal flora of microorganisms which inhabit the skin, the intestinal tract, and the several orifices of the body secrete substances inimical to invading microorganisms. Secretions such as tears and saliva also contain antibacterial substances.

Should the microorganism invade the tissues, however, the body responds by producing an inflammation; boils and carbuncles are examples of this response. The features of inflammation—redness, swelling, heat, and pain—are familiar to everyone. Inflammation is the body's response to injury of any kind, including mechanical injury and burns, as well as to bacterial invasion. In the case of bacterial invaders, it is an effort to destroy them. Except against the most virulent microorganisms, this effort is successful.

The immune response

Our knowledge of the immune response began in the late eighteenth century in England when a young medical student named Edward Jenner observed that milkmaids who contracted cowpox were subsequently resistant to infection with smallpox. From this observation he went on to demonstrate that inoculation with cowpox crusts protected human beings from smallpox. Pasteur later named this procedure vaccination, from *vacca,* the Latin word for cow. This procedure is still in use today. Anyone who has been vaccinated against smallpox remembers the inflammed pox at the site of inoculation.

Inflammation initiates the complex sequence of events that results in the immune response of the host. The net result of these events is frequently that if ever the same pathogen tries to invade the body again, the body will recognize it and destroy it before it has a chance to cause disease. A person having this response is said to be *immune.* The drama resulting in immunity is enacted daily in our bodies. It is only now being understood in many of its ramifications, and it is the object of intensive research all over the world. A detailed description of the complex processes involved in the establishment of immunity cannot be presented here. In essence, however, immunity is based on the body's ability to discriminate between self and nonself.

Among the cells which migrate to the inflamed area are *macrophages*, large cells with a large, round nucleus. These cells have the ability to engulf small particles, including microorganisms, and to bring them into the cell in a little vacuole. The products of the digested microorganisms are released and taken up by smaller cells with eccentrically placed nuclei. These lymphoidal cells, as they are called, then undergo rapid, successive cell division. Some of the descendants manufacture proteins, called *antibodies*, in response to the digested fragments taken up by their forebears. The antibody is released into the blood stream and has the ability to recognize the microorganism from which the original fragment came. The antibody unites specifically with the microorganism to try to destroy it. The fragments of the microorganism, as well as the microorganism itself, are traditionally called *antigens*. The union of antigen with antibody, which removes or destroys the invading antigen, is one form of the immune response.

Figure 9.5. The immune response.

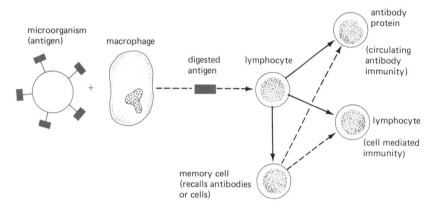

Other antigenic fragments processed by the macrophage are taken up by still other kinds of lymphoidal cells. Descendants of these activated *lymphocytes* recognize the antigen when it again appears on the microorganism. Any of several complex events will then occur in the attempt to destroy the microorganism or contain it. These events constitute *cell mediated immunity*. Circulating antibody immunity and cell mediated immunity together constitute specific defense against specific microorganisms. The events involved in the immune process are diagramed in Fig. 9.5. These motions have to be repeated for each different antigen as it invades the body.

Having the disease or being vaccinated with the disease agent generally results in *active immunity*, so-called because the body actively produces its own antibodies to fight the infection (Fig. 9.6). The agent can be dead, as in the killed bacteria of typhoid vaccine, or living but no

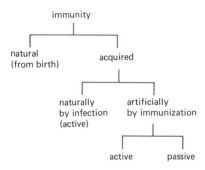

Figure 9.6. Natural and acquired immunity are differentiated according to the ways they are produced.

longer able to cause disease, as in the vaccines for poliomyelitis. In addition, products of the microorganisms, such as the exotoxin of diphtheria, can be detoxified and used as vaccines. Another form of immunity can be produced by inoculating antibodies from persons already immune into individuals threatened with disease. This is called *passive immunity* because the individual does not produce his or her own antibodies but rather uses other persons' antibodies temporarily. An example of passive immunity is the inoculation of gamma globulin, a substance containing antibodies derived from human blood, to prevent an individual from contracting infectious hepatitis.

BIOSOCIAL ENVIRONMENT

People's interrelationships, cultural backgrounds, socioeconomic condition, geographic location, associations with wild or domestic animals, and occupations all influence the pattern of infectious diseases. A few examples of the effects of biosocial environments on human disease are given below.

Poverty

The industrial revolution occurred during the nineteenth century in England and Europe. This development brought about major displacements in population as people left the country and crowded to get jobs in the mills, mines, and factories. There were soon fewer jobs than people, which meant a cheap labor market, low pay, and poverty. Chil-

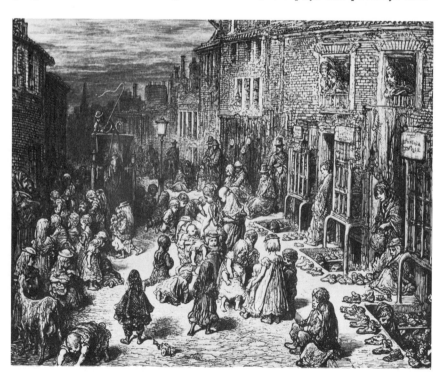

Figure 9.7. Tuberculosis—Disease of the Slums. Engraving by Gustave Doré showing the slums of London in 1875. At the time of the Industrial Revolution tuberculosis—as the disease was beginning to be called—raged everywhere in Europe. Toward the middle of the nineteenth century the death rate from the disease was as high as 500 per 100,000 in some places. (Courtesy of Radio Times Hulton Picture Library, London, and the World Health Organization)

dren, who were cheaper than adults, often were set to hauling coal carts in mines or were chained to looms to keep them working for fifteen hours a day. Malnourished hordes were huddled together in fetid tenements. The setting was ideal for the spread of tuberculosis, which is passed from one person to another in mucous droplets from the respiratory tract. It is no wonder that in the western world tuberculosis became the foremost disease of the nineteenth century. As economic conditions gradually improved, the rate of tuberculosis slowly began to decline, even without the intervention of public health control methods.

Culture

KURU In the highlands of New Guinea exist tribes whose cultural traditions have not yet been eroded by contact with outsiders. Some of the tribes are afflicted with a strange disease called *kuru*. It attacks children of both sexes, but after puberty the disease affects mainly women of the tribe. The disease begins insidiously with weakness and a sense of disequilibrium. As it slowly progresses, the body is set into tremors until finally the victims can neither walk, stand, nor sit up. Curiously, since they know death is inevitable, the countenance of the sufferers expresses contentment rather than terror, and they die with a beatific smile on their face.

After studying the disease for many years and living with the tribes, an American scientist, Carleton Gajdusek, worked out the epidemiology of the disease and finally succeeded in isolating the viral agent which causes this fatal affliction. It is classified as a *slow virus*, since the disease it produces has an exceptionally extended incubation period.

The tribespeople practice ritual cannibalism. Sacred tradition requires that any member of a family who dies, even members dead of kuru, must be eaten by the bereaved family. Considered the superior members of the family, men get the best cuts. Inferior portions, including the viscera and brain, are assigned to women and children. Although the diseased body is roasted, the heat does not penetrate sufficiently to kill the virus which is lodged in the brain, waiting to infect the children and women who eat it.

INFECTIOUS HEPATITIS The epidemiology of this disease has dramatically shifted during the last several years in the United States. Infectious hepatitis is generally transmitted from the intestinal tract of one person to others who are unfortunate enough to ingest the virus either in shellfish, in food and water contaminated with feces, or during gymnastic sexual activity with an infected person. The virus also circulates in the blood stream for fairly long periods.

During recent years, hepatitis has become a prominent disease of young adult urban males. This shift has paralleled the epidemic of drug abuse in large cities. When addicts are shooting drugs into their veins together, the virus of infectious hepatitis will contaminate the needle if one member of the group has the virus floating in his blood stream. His companions get inoculated with the virus and an epidemic of infectious hepatitis results. Syphilis can also be passed around in this fashion. Likewise, little epidemics of malaria have occurred when a member of the shooting party included a U.S. Army veteran who acquired both his habit and his malaria in South Vietnam.

Progress

Histoplasmosis is a respiratory disease caused by a fungus, *Histoplasma capsulatum*, which normally lives in the ground. The disease has frequently been confused with tuberculosis. For reasons not yet clear, the fungus grows particularly luxuriently in soil enriched with bird droppings. If the contaminated soil is disturbed by massive upheavals as by a bulldozer, the spores are borne aloft and carried through the air to the lungs of human beings. Epidemics can result.

Three recorded epidemics of histoplasmosis have involved school children. At one school the children engaged in a rigorous cleanup campaign to celebrate Earth Day. By accident they disturbed a *nidus* (nest) of *Histoplasma capsulatum* and many came down with the disease. In North Carolina, spores disturbed during construction of a new golf course blew through the open windows of a school and produced an epidemic of the disease among the children. In a northern state, a civic project to convert into a city park a dank, wooded area near a river, the abode of thousands of starlings, produced an epidemic of histoplasmosis in a nearby school. The project was halted.

Once a nidus (nest) of the fungus is discovered, the problem arises as to how to eliminate it without disturbing the soil and causing more disease. No perfect solution has yet been found. A windless day is chosen for the operation, surrounding people are evacuated, workers are equipped with spore-proof masks, and the soil is saturated with a potent germicide.

From these examples it is clear that patterns of human infection depend on the activities of human beings. *Histoplasma capsulatum* would exist harmlessly in the soil if human beings did not disturb the spores by constructing bridges, buildings, highways, and golf courses. The always fatal kuru would probably vanish within one generation if the tribespeople would stop eating their dead relatives. Young adult urban males would not take the chance of acquiring hepatitis if they did not feel the need to join their companions in a subculture of narcotic addiction. Improvement in general health and living conditions, which includes putting a certain amount of space between people, helps to slow the transmission of tuberculosis.

DISEASES TRANSMITTED BY THE FECAL-ORAL ROUTE

The intestinal tract begins at the mouth and extends through the body to the anus. It changes in character, function, and size as it passes through the body. Since it is open to the outside world at either end, it is, in effect, outside the body proper. Before a baby is born his or her intestinal tract is free from microorganisms. During birth and immediately thereafter, however, the intestinal tract begins to acquire microorganisms from food, water, fingers, nipples, skin, objects, and other people. Some of these microorganisms will find a comfortable home in the mouth and throat, many will be swallowed and survive the acidity of the gastric juices to establish colonies in the lower intestinal tract. The various populations of microorganisms are dynamic, shifting in kind as new strains are swallowed or internal environmental conditions change.

While most of the microorganisms that live in the intestinal tract are harmless, some can cause disease if the opportunity arises. Pathogenic microorganisms are excreted in the feces, and by means of vehicles such as water, food, and fingers they find their way into the mouths of other people. Wherever human beings live, the environment tends to be coated with a fecal veneer. In areas of the world where feces are not disposed of in a sanitary manner, the fecal veneer is thick. In highly sanitated areas like North America, northern Europe, and Australia, the veneer has become relatively thin. In some agricultural cultures, human excreta are highly prized because of their high content of nitrogenous compounds. Called "night soil," they are used for fertilizing crops. Pathogens in the night soil are carried on to the vegetables to be recycled through human beings who consume them.

A wide variety of organisms, including many viruses, bacteria, fungi, protozoa, and worms, infect human beings by the oral route. Some important causes of disease transmitted by the fecal-oral route are listed in Table 9.1. Control of many of these diseases consists essentially of preventing people from swallowing human feces. This is the reason for the treatment of sewage, the purification of drinking water supplies, sanitary measures controlling the production, processing, and serving of foods, and personal hygiene. Asiatic cholera is an example of a disease which is carried from the intestinal tract of an infected person to the mouths of other people by means of water and food.

Cholera

The present pandemic of cholera fanned outward from its traditional home in the East. When it reached Taiwan in 1962, the symbolic flaming red flag was raised to warn ships that an epidemic of cholera was rampant. The present cholera pandemic is the seventh in a series of pandemics which have spread from India and Bangladesh throughout much of the world. When the chief transportation between continents was by ship, ports were the site of entry of the disease into new countries. Ships carrying crews or passengers ill with cholera were not allowed to dock, and ports where cholera was present were required to warn ships not to land. These measures to prevent the spread of disease, called

Table 9.1 Some diseases transmitted by the fecal-oral route

Disease	Vaccine available	Specific therapy
Bacteria		
Typhoid Fever	Yes	Yes
Salmonelloses	No	No
Shigellosis (Bacillary dysentery)	No	Yes
Viruses		
Poliomyelitis	Yes	No
Infectious hepatitis	No[a]	No
Protozoa		
Amebiasis (Amebic dysentery)	No	Yes
Worms		
Enterobiasis (Pinworm disease)	No	Yes

[a] While no vaccine is available for infectious hepatitis, persons exposed to the infection or traveling to highly endemic areas such as North Africa, the Middle East, and Asia should be given a prophylactic inoculation of immune serum globulin, which aborts or prevents the disease.

quarantine, were first developed by the Venetians in the fourteenth century. Cholera is one of four internationally quarantinable diseases; the others are plague, smallpox, and yellow fever.

Cholera is caused by a comma-shaped bacterium which was named *Vibrio cholerae.* The cholera vibrios must reach the small intestine to cause disease. During an epidemic many people become infected without becoming ill, while others, especially children, may have only a mild disease. Other persons, however, experience a severe illness and, if not treated, more than half of them die. After an incubation period ranging from a few hours to several days, the illness begins abruptly with vomiting and intense diarrhea.

The cholera vibrios multiply rapidly in the small intestine and produce a toxin which acts locally on the wall of the small intestine to produce a massive outpouring of body water and salts. This process results in the copious diarrhea called "rice-water" stool because of its resemblance to the water in which rice has been washed or boiled. As water and salts are drained out of the tissues and blood, the dehydration causes the characteristic sunken appearance of the face. The patient rapidly goes into shock. Death may occur.

The mechanism by which the disease is produced has been understood only during the last decade. Treatment based on this knowledge results in rapid recovery from the disease. Simple replacement of the water and salts brings about recovery. In actual practice the patient is placed on a specially designed "cholera bed" which has a hole cut out for the buttocks. Below the hole a bucket catches the rice-water stools. At intervals the volume of liquid is measured and an equal volume of saline is administered to the patient. At first this must be given intravenously because the patient is usually in shock, but as he begins to recover the patient can drink the combination of water and salts with the addition of glucose, which helps to pull water from the intestine into the body. An appropriate antibiotic is given to reduce the number of cholera vibrios in the gut and consequently the concentration of toxin. The duration of diarrhea is thereby shortened. A laboratory diagnosis is made by growing the curved vibrios from the stool in special media.

Cholera control requires the interruption of the fecal-oral cycle of transmission. Interruption is effected by treatment of sewage combined with availability and purification of water supplies. Implementation of these procedures, in turn, is dependent on high socioeconomic development. So long as the high standards of hygiene remain intact in the United States and other economically advanced countries, it is unlikely that cholera can be again established in these areas. An occasional tourist catches the disease in a country where it is epidemic, but when he returns to his home, his disease will be treated and the infection will not spread. In impoverished countries, however, cholera remains a threat to life. Persons traveling to such areas should avoid drinking unpurified water and eating unpeeled fruits and vegetables. They should also be given a cholera vaccine which offers some, but not complete, protection against the disease.

DISEASES TRANSMITTED BY ARTHROPODS

Four international killer diseases are transmitted to man by insects: malaria, yellow fever, epidemic typhus, and bubonic plague. Many other diseases are also transmitted by insects as well as by their eight-legged relatives, the *acarines*. Both insects and acarines are classified together as *arthropods*. The organisms in this diverse group, which includes ants, spiders, butterflies, horseshoe crabs, and ticks, are among the most ancient of all living animals. During the course of their evolution, they have acquired microorganisms which live harmlessly in their tissues. When passed to man, some of these microorganisms, like the rickettsial agent of Rocky Mountain spotted fever, cause severe disease. Some members of almost all major groups of disease agents are transmitted by arthropods, including viruses, rickettsiae, bacteria, protozoans, and worms. In some instances the relationships among the human being, the agent of disease, and the arthropod vector (transmitter) of the disease have become exacting and elaborate. In malaria, for example, the infectious protozoa multiply asexually in man to produce sexual forms which then must be sucked up by a mosquito before sexual reproduction inside the mosquito results in a form of the parasite which is, in turn, infectious for man.

These disease-laden arthropods wing their way through the air to us, attach to our clothes as we pass through brush, crawl on us from an infested person, or leap on us as we go about our daily business. They are hungry, and in order to stay alive or to perpetuate themselves they must suck our blood. Some of the pathogens are injected directly into the puncture wound made by the arthropod's mouth parts, while others are excreted in the insect feces and get rubbed into the bite wounds. Some of these diseases are listed in Table 9.2, together with the arthropods which transmit them. One of these diseases, bubonic plague, is described in detail.

Table 9.2 Some diseases transmitted by arthropods

Disease	Vector	Vaccine	Specific treatment
Viruses			
Yellow fever	Mosquito	Yes	No
Encephalitis	Mosquito	No[a]	No
Dengue	Mosquito	No	No
Spirochetes (Relapsing fever)			
Epidemic form	Human body louse	No	Yes
Endemic form	Soft ticks	No	Yes
Richettsiae			
Epidemic typhus	Human body louse	Yes	Yes
Murine typhus	Oriental rat flea	No	Yes
Trench fever	Human body louse	No	Yes
Rocky Mountain spotted fever	Wood and dog ticks	Yes	Yes
Scrub typhus	Mites	No	Yes
Rickettsialpox	House mouse mites	No	Yes
Protozoa			
Malaria	Mosquito	No[b]	Yes
Leishmaniasis (Kala azar)	Sandfly	No	Yes
Trypanosomiasis (African sleeping sickness)	Tsetse fly	No	Yes

[a] Vaccines are available for horses which also can become infected.
[b] Prophylactic drugs which suppress infection during exposure are available.

Bubonic plague

The origin of plague is lost in antiquity. During the middle ages, the Black Death spread over Europe and much of the rest of the world. With our present knowledge of the cause of the disease and its manner of transmission, it is now difficult for us to understand the terror and panic created by the arrival of the Black Death in a town or country. Plague is supposed to have killed one-half to two-thirds of the population of Great Britain during the fourteenth and fifteenth centuries. As a major killer disease it has acted throughout the centuries as an effective means of population control.

The present pandemic of plague originated in the middle of the nineteenth century in Yunnan, near the Burma border, progressed slowly to the coast of China, and appeared in 1898 in Canton. From there it

The plague—1968

On June 11, 1968, a six-year-old girl living in the east central section of Denver, Colorado, was taken to the Children's Hospital with a high fever, painful swelling in her left armpit, pain in her left ear, and a sore throat. The next day she was worse and was given an antibiotic. Her blood was cultured on media in the laboratory and grew out bacteria which appeared to be plague bacilli. This diagnosis was subsequently confirmed when pus drawn from the swelling in her armpit was shown to contain an abundance of *Yersinia pestis*, the plague bacillus. She recovered after treatment with streptomycin and tetracycline and was discharged from the hospital on July 8.

An investigation revealed numerous dead fox squirrels in Denver, one found only three-quarters of a block from the girl's home. Laboratory tests showed that it had died of plague. It is known that a particular species of flea infests fox squirrels. Although the flea prefers to feed on fox squirrels, when hungry it will suck blood from other animals, including human beings. This flea becomes infected with plague and transmits the disease from one squirrel to another. It soon became apparent that an infected flea had abandoned its plague-killed squirrel host, and had fed on the little girl, infecting her with plague.

To stop the epidemic among fox squirrels, the health authorities placed baited DDT dust boxes in trees throughout the city. Before the squirrels could get to the bait, they first had to receive a dusting of DDT which killed the fleas. A possible outbreak of bubonic plague in Denver was averted.

was carried down the river to Hong Kong and fanned out to most of the port cities of the world as ships carried plague-infected rats and fleas along with commercial cargo. Bubonic plague arrived in San Francisco in 1900 and produced an epidemic that terrified the city. An intensive campaign of rat control stopped the epidemic. It is not clear whether the plague subsequently spread from the rats and their fleas to the wild rodents and squirrels in the western third of the United States, or whether, as seems more likely, the plague bacillus has existed there for centuries.

Every year there are a few cases of bubonic plague in the United States. The victims are hunters and trappers or Indians living close to nature on reservations in the southwest. Why is it that with a third of

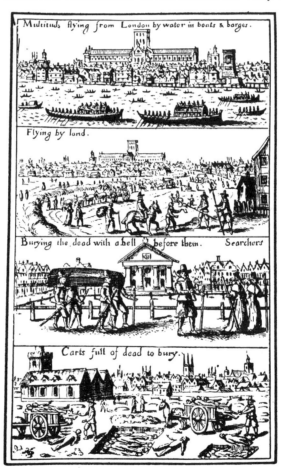

Figure 9.8. Scenes in London during the Great Plague of 1664. International quarantine measures were first instituted when a pandemic of bubonic plague—the Black Death—devastated Europe in the fourteenth century. (Courtesy of Clarendon Press, Oxford, and the World Health Organization)

the United States widely seeded with the plague bacillus we do not have the devastating epidemics of bubonic plague that have ravished mankind for as long as we can remember? The reasons for our present quiescent state of plague should emerge in the remainder of this section.

Cycles of plague infection

WILD PLAGUE Plague is a disease primarily of small wild mammals, especially rodents and their fleas. Over 200 species of rodents have been found infected with plague. During a plague *epizootic*, as an epidemic among animals is called, susceptible animals will die. Some animals, however, survive the infection. The progeny of survivors tend to become more and more resistant to fatal plague infection. Year after year they keep the disease going in its cyclical fashion from rodent to flea to rodent. If new susceptible animals enter this cycle they will contract the disease and there will result a die-off. Human beings entering such a natural cycle of infection can also contract bubonic plague.

URBAN PLAGUE Rats apparently evolved in Asia and, together with their cousins the mice, have become man's most prolific and tenacious companions. Rats have their own species of flea, *Xenopsylla cheopis*, frequently called the oriental rat flea. While preferring to feed on rats, it will suck blood meals from man and other animals as a second choice. It is a very efficient transmitter of plague.

If plague-infected wild rodents and fleas come in close contact with commensal rats, the plague bacilli can cross over to ignite an epizootic among the rats and their fleas. As rats begin to die of plague, fleas leave the chilling corpses to feed on human beings, infecting them in the process.

Like other mammals, human beings have their own special flea called *Pulex irritans*. Before effective insecticides were developed man's life was tortured by these voracious and omnipresent pests. During times when infestation with *P. irritans* was intense, the sequence of events which transported the plague bacillus from the wild rodent to the rat, to its flea, to man, could result in infection of *P. irritans* and so establish a human plague cycle.

From time to time a person with plague will develop plague-pneumonia. When the patient coughs, talks, or sneezes, plague bacilli are propelled from his respiratory tract in droplets of mucus. Persons close to the patient will breathe in the contaminated droplets and develop the almost certainly fatal *pneumonic plague*. Many physicians and nurses, as well as family members tending a pneumonic plague patient, have died from this form of the disease. Pneumonic plague is the most terrifying of all manifestations of plague. Under proper conditions of crowding and moisture it can spread rapidly from person to person to produce a giant, lethal epidemic such as occurred in Manchuria in 1910–1911.

Human plague

A person falls sick with plague three to five days after having been inoculated with the bacilli by an infected flea. Infection can also occur by handling infected tissues of an animal. Onset is sudden, with high fever, chills, and rapid pulse. A sore or carbuncle may occur at the site of the infected flea bite. The local lymph nodes draining the area of the bite—usually those in the groin or the armpit—enlarge, fester, and become extremely painful. These are the *buboes* which give the disease the name of bubonic plague. About one-fourth to one-half of people with untreated bubonic plague can be expected to die. Death, which may occur before the development of buboes, is the result of heart failure or collapse of the blood circulatory system. For reasons which are not understood, bubonic plague may change into the extremely contagious pneumonic plague which, if not promptly treated, is invariably fatal in one to four days.

As is true with most other diseases, mild cases of plague can occur, particularly towards the end of an epidemic. During the plague epidemic in Vietnam, apparently well human contacts of plague patients were discovered to be carrying fully virulent plague bacilli in their throats.

Diagnosis and treatment

Diagnosis of plague in this country may be delayed because physicians are not accustomed to think about the possibility of its presence. Physicians should remain alert to the possibility of plague, since a person in the incubation stage of plague can travel by jet in a few hours from an endemic zone to a place which has been free of plague for many years. For a laboratory diagnosis, pus is aspirated with a syringe and needle from the bubo. In the microscope, the stained plague bacilli in the pus have the characteristic look of a closed safety pin. Bacilli from the pus also grow into typical colonies on special media in the laboratory.

Plague patients, even those with pneumonic plague, can be saved if they are treated in time with an effective antibiotic such as streptomycin or tetracycline.

Control of plague

Methods for control of plague depend upon the plague cycle involved. Control of urban plague means, essentially, the control of the rat reservoir of the disease and the oriental rat flea. During a plague emergency, rat runs are first dusted with DDT or other insecticide to kill the fleas and then rats are trapped or killed with poisoned bait. It is mandatory that fleas be destroyed before the rats because fleas leave dead rats to feed on human beings. Other measures, which should be continued even

The infected flea

Fleas have a series of valves in the fore part of their intestinal tract which operate to prevent blood from flowing back into the puncture wound while they are feeding. Since plague bacilli are circulating in the blood stream of an infected mammal (as well as an infected human being), a feeding flea will suck them up in its blood meal. Some of the microorganisms colonize the spaces around the valves, and during their multiplication form gelatinous masses of plague bacilli which interrupt the function of the valves and prevent the flea from swallowing blood. When a blocked flea tries to feed, it sucks in blood, which sloshes against the mass of plague bacilli. Since the blood cannot be swallowed, it is regurgitated back into the puncture wound, carrying with it small clumps of plague bacilli broken off from the mass of organisms. A completely blocked flea will eventually die, but in the meantime hunger will drive it to try to feed many times. A partially blocked flea will continue to live and inoculate plague bacilli into animals or human beings as it feeds. Plague bacilli are also excreted with the flea feces and under proper environmental conditions the bacteria can remain alive for many months in rodent burrows. Some fleas can eventually overcome infection. A flea species is said to be an efficient vector of plague if it can be easily infected and can infect its host while sucking blood.

in the absence of plague, include rat-proofing of buildings and elimination of rat harborages, especially around docks and airports. Garbage should be disposed of rapidly in a sanitary manner.

PERSONAL PROTECTION Immunity to plague is only partial, since contracting the disease does not invariably result in protection from a second attack. Vaccines cannot be expected, therefore, to induce greater protection than the disease itself, but they offer some protection. When vaccinated persons do become infected, they apparently experience less severe disease than do nonvaccinated persons. Encouraging evidence that vaccines can afford protection have come from the experience of American servicemen in South Vietnam during the recent conflict. Even though bubonic plague was attacking the civilian population of South Vietnam, practically no cases of plague occurred among U.S. servicemen who had all received immunizing doses of vaccine.

A vaccine composed of killed plague bacilli was first made by Haffkine in India in 1896. Other vaccines have also been devised, including one composed of living plague bacilli which can no longer cause disease. For maximum effectiveness two or three doses of vaccine should be given at weekly intervals, and booster doses should be given every six months thereafter, since immunity conferred by vaccines is short-lived.

DISEASES AIRBORNE FROM PERSON TO PERSON

A wide variety of human infections including many so-called childhood diseases are passed from one person to another through the air. When people cough, sneeze, yawn, spit, sing, and talk they project droplets of mucus containing microorganisms which can land on the mucous membranes of neighboring mouths, noses, and eyes. This direct transmission of microorganisms from one person to another cannot extend beyond a distance of about three feet. The large droplets settle out fairly quickly. Microbial aerosols resulting from evaporation of droplets emitted by an infected host also contaminate the air. These aerosols are suspensions in air of particles consisting partially or wholly of microorganisms. Ranging in size from 1 to 5 microns, the particles are easily drawn into the lungs and retained there. They may remain suspended in the air for long periods of time, either retaining or losing infectiousness, depending on the microorganism. If the microorganisms are pathogenic, they will infect other susceptible people and possibly initiate an epidemic. Some of the diseases transmitted by this means are listed in Table 9.3. Influenza, a particularly interesting example of an airborne disease, will be discussed in greater detail.

Influenza

Influenza is not the common cold, it is not the usual less severe infections of the respiratory tract, and it is not what is loosely called "intestinal

Table 9.3 Some diseases airborne from person to person

Disease	Source	Treatment	Vaccine
Bacteria			
Tuberculosis	Respiratory secretions	Yes	Yes
Diphtheria	Nasopharyngeal secretions	Yes	Yes
Meningitis	Nasopharyngeal secretions	Yes	Yes (for one type only)
Pneumococcal pneumonia	Respiratory secretions	Yes	No
Whooping cough	Respiratory secretions	Yes	Yes
Streptococcal Diseases:		Yes	No
Scarlet fever	Discharge from nose, throat,		
Strep sore throat	or purulent lesions		
Viruses			
Smallpox	Respiratory dicharges and scabs of pox	No	Yes
Measles	Respiratory secretions	No	Yes
German measles (Rubella)	Nasopharyngeal secretions	No	Yes
Mumps	Saliva	No	Yes

Influenza A virus

Curiously, most new antigenic varients of influenza A virus have arisen in Asia. It is known that birds and domestic animals can become infected with human influenza virus. When this happens the viruses are apparently no longer infectious for human beings. A theory has been constructed to explain the antigenic shifts which enable the influenza A virus to be such a continuing scourge of mankind. The theory suggests that all the varied influenza strains now present in domestic animals were derived from human strains but that during their adaptation to animals they lost their ability to infect human beings. They can return to their primary, or human, host only after a fortuitous genetic recombination has produced a new subtype of influenza virus. The new subtype must be at once infective for humans and not destroyed by antibodies already present in the human host. A transfer of such a virus would most likely occur where humans are in close contact with domestic animals. In many parts of Asia, where the strains first appear, men share their houses with animals.

flu." Influenza is a brief but incapacitating disease with an incubation period of 24 to 72 hours. Its abrupt onset is signaled by chills, fever, headache, aching muscles, and intense fatigue. The patient then develops a running nose, sore throat, and cough. Influenza usually lasts from three to seven days but leaves the patient with a washed-out feeling after the disease has ended. Influenza is not usually fatal, except in persons already disadvantaged by chronic heart or pulmonary disease. Influenza weakens the patient, however, and sets the stage for secondary bacterial infections, many of which are severe and some lethal.

It is difficult to control this plague because of the versatile way in which the influenza virus changes its antigenic structure. As a strain of influenza virus shoots around the world—as fast as jet airplanes can carry infected human beings—a large percentage of the world's population becomes infected and thus immune. When this has happened, a new strain of the same virus appears against which the world's population is not protected or perhaps only partially protected. The new antigenic strain spreads through the population until it, like its predecessor, is halted by rising immunity in the population. A new cycle is then set in motion.

An influenza vaccine gives protection only against the strain of virus from which it was prepared. Made for the last strain that came around, it gives little, if any, protection against a newly arrived antigenic varient. Epidemics occur too rapidly for a vaccine made from the new strain to be useful. The new virus has to be isolated, compared with other known strains and types, produced on a massive scale, tested, and finally distributed. By the time the vaccine is in the physician's office the epidemic has already swept by.

DISEASES TRANSMITTED TO MAN FROM HIS ENVIRONMENT

Some microorganisms live tranquilly in the soil and produce disease only when circumstances bring human beings into contact with them (Table 9.4). Spores of the bacteria which cause gas gangrene live in the soil, for example. These can contaminate objects which make deep, penetrating wounds and cause infections like those which resulted in many deaths and amputations during World War I. Other microorganisms cause disease in wild, commensal, or domestic animals. If man enters one of these cycles of infection he may become infected. Rabies, one of the most terrifying diseases, belongs to this category.

Table 9.4 Some diseases transmitted to man from the environment

Disease	Usual source
Bacteria	
Tetanus	Spores in soil, derived from intestinal tract of man and other animals
Anthrax	Hides, hair, and wool of infected animals
Leptospirosis	Water and soil contaminated with urine of infected animals
Rickettsiae	
Q fever	Dust contaminated with placental tissues and birth fluids of infected cattle, sheep, and goats
Fungi	
Histoplasmosis	Soil
Coccidioidomycosis	Dust in arid and semiarid areas
Cryptococcosis	Soil and pigeon nests and feces

Rabies

Rabies in man is almost 100 percent fatal. The virus which causes the disease is widespread in a great variety of wild animals. The world is currently undergoing epidemics of rabies in animals, epidemics reaching from the arctic to the tropics in both old and new worlds. In 1972, 4,427 confirmed cases of rabies were reported in the United States, but there were many more cases in animals which escaped attention. The figure included 3,462 cases in wild animals, 963 in domestic animals, and 2 in human beings. Sixty percent of the wildlife cases were in skunks, 19 percent in foxes, 15 percent in bats, and 5 percent in raccoons. Infected domestic animals included cattle, dogs, cats, horses and mules, sheep, goats, and swine.

Rabies virus has a predilection for nervous tissue and for glandular tissue which secretes mucus, such as the salivary glands. The virus is shed in the saliva and when a rabid animal bites another animal or a human being the virus and saliva are deposited in the wound. The virus then begins its journey on or in the nerves which lead to the brain at a

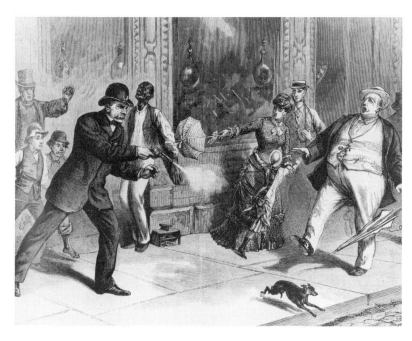

Figure 9.9. Shooting a mad dog. Wood engraving (1879) by I. Pranishnikoff, from a sketch by S. D. Ehrhart. (Courtesy of National Library of Medicine, Bethesda, Maryland)

Rabid animals

Rabies kills many species of animals, especially canines such as dogs, wolves, and coyotes. The disease in pet dogs is marked by personality changes, as it is in human cases; the dog becomes either abnormally quiet (dumb rabies) or violent, racing about and trying to bite all animals in his path. Even animals like bats which ordinarily eat fruit or insects can become violent and attack other animals, including human beings. Some bats do not die of rabies but continue to secrete the virus in their saliva and urine for the rest of their lives. In caves inhabited by enormous hordes of bats, the accumulation of virus can apparently be dangerous. Two men who entered the Frio cave near Uvalde, Texas, the abode of thousands of bats, later died from rabies apparently transmitted to them in the air.

In Latin America, vampire bats are infected with rabies. Contrary to popular belief, vampire bats do not suck blood. With their sharp fangs they make a razor-like slit in the skin of their victim and lap the blood as it pours out. This is done so deftly that the animal is usually unaware that it is happening. Vampire bats tend to return again and again to the same victim, reopening the wound and lapping the blood. Infected bats contaminate the wound with virus-laden saliva and the animal contracts the disease. Infection of cattle with rabies by this method results in death to the animal and great economic loss when whole herds are affected.

velocity of about 3 millimeters per hour. Symptoms of disease can begin from as early as ten days to as late as eight months after the infected bite, but the incubation period is usually from four to six weeks.

The human disease starts with fever, headache, fatigue, nausea, and sore throat. After several days of these symptoms an abnormal sensation around the site of infection occurs, followed by a phase of excitation with increasing nervousness, insomnia, anxiety, and apprehension. (At lease one individual in this phase of the disease has been admitted to a mental institution.) The patient may become stuporous, apathetic, and develop paralysis. The most famous symptom of the disease is *hydrophobia,* or fear of water. When fluid comes into contact with the patient's throat the muscles of swallowing go into violent, painful spasms. The reaction is so intense that even the subsequent sight, smell, or sound of liquid is sufficient to precipitate the spasms. The patient may die during a convulsion in the phase of acute excitation, or he may die from a progressive paralysis which ascends upward from the legs.

Formerly, most human rabies was contracted from rabid dogs. Current regulations requiring the vaccination and licensing of dogs, and the trapping and destruction of stray dogs, have greatly reduced the number of dogs infected with rabies.

If a person has been bitten by an animal suspected of being rabid, the animal should be detained by public health authorities to wait for symptoms of the disease to appear: excitability or paralysis followed by death. Heads of animals which have been killed should be iced until they can be examined for rabies in a public health laboratory. The wound of the person bitten should be thoroughly cleansed with water and soap or detergent. The decision made by the physician to treat for rabies is based on the findings in the animal and the circumstances surrounding the attack by the animal. Treatment is by vaccination using, in effect, the method developed by Pasteur almost 100 years ago. The generally long incubation period of rabies allows a person to be immunized against the disease *after* exposure. Vaccination consists of a series of fourteen or twenty-one daily injections of rabies vaccine. While immunity is developing the person can be further protected by being given antiserum against rabies. Vaccination is a painful and heroic procedure, not entirely without danger and not in every case successful. It is, however, together with immune serum, the only protection against a certain and terrible death.

A vaccine which provides protection against rabies before exposure has now been developed. Persons with high risk to exposure, such as veterinarians and Peace Corps volunteers entering an area where rabies is not well controlled, are given this vaccine.

Questions

1. Does contact between an infectious agent and a human being always result in disease? Why or why not?
2. Name three diseases which have profoundly influenced human history and describe how they have done so.
3. What are the relationships between control of infectious diseases and population growth?
4. How is the presence or absence of many infectious diseases in a country directly related to the socioeconomic condition of that country?
5. Do you think that any given disease can be completely eradicated from the earth? Why or why not?

Key Concepts   *Antibody* – protein manufactured during the immune response that can recognize the invading pathogen and is released into the blood stream to destroy it

Antigen – an invading pathogenic organism or one of its digested fragments that stimulates the production of antibodies

Immunity – the body's ability to resist infection from invading pathogenic organisms. The immune response to these organisms immediately recognized from a previous infection with them is to destroy them or to counteract the effects of their poisonous products (exotoxins and endotoxins) before they have a chance to cause disease. Immunity can be either active or passive

Pathogen (adj. *pathogenic*) – an organism capable of producing disease

Vaccination – generally, the inoculation of a person with the living or killed agent of a disease in order to induce an immunity to that disease through the production of antibodies; specifically, the inoculation of a person with cowpox virus in order to induce an immunity to smallpox virus

Selected Readings   Camus, Albert. *The Plague.* New York: Alfred A. Knopf, 1948.

Dauer, Carl C., *et al. Infectious Diseases.* Monograph. Washington, D.C.: American Public Health Association, 1968.

De Kruif, Paul. *Microbe Hunters.* New York: Pocket Books, 1959.

Garrison, Fielding H. *An Introduction to the History of Medicine.* 4th ed. Philadelphia: W. B. Saunders, 1960.

Jones, Kenneth L., *et al. Communicable and Noncommunicable Diseases.* San Francisco: Canfield Press, 1970.

Roueché, B. *Eleven Blue Men and Other Narratives of Medical Detection.* New York: Berkley Medallion Books, Berkley Publishing Corporation, 1947.

Walter, William G., *et al. Introduction to Microbiology.* New York: D. Van Nostrand Company, 1973.

Chapter 10

Sexually Transmitted Diseases

The germs of syphilis and gonorrhea have become so well adapted to their human hosts throughout the history of mankind that they seem to have evolved an almost sure-fire way of ensuring their own survival through continuous human protection. The microorganisms are so fragile that they cannot survive even a few moments' exposure to the drying and chilling effects of the air. They must be transferred from an infected person to a noninfected person during sexual contact, when the warm moist secretions of the genitals, mouth, or anus provide them with a protective environment. For this reason no one has ever caught syphilis, gonorrhea, or the other venereal diseases from a toilet seat, door handle, bathtub, drinking fountain, or any other place in popular mythology. There are a few minor exceptions to this rule, such as the accidental infection of physicians and dentists from direct contact with infectious

This chapter was contributed by J. William Vinson, D.S.Hyg., Associate Professor of Microbiology, Harvard School of Public Health.

sores in cases of syphilis or the transmission of the syphilis bacterium on needles and syringes among drug abusers who are shooting together. Syphilis can be transmitted from a mother to her unborn child, and a mother with gonorrhea can infect the eyes of her baby at the time of birth.

Sexually transmitted diseases are called venereal diseases, after Venus, the Roman goddess of love. Gonorrhea and syphilis are the two most important of these diseases. Three other venereal diseases occur infrequently in the United States. There are several disease conditions, however, which may be associated with sexual contact, but which can be transmitted by less intimate contact. This fact is important to know, because the diseases differ in symptoms, method of diagnosis, severity, and the kind of treatment required to cure them. It is also important to remember that a person can have more than one venereal disease at the same time. There are many look-alike disease conditions which can be differentiated from the venereal diseases only by a skilled physician. People should be acquainted with the existence and symptoms of these diseases so that if infection is suspected, prompt medical care can be sought.

About one in every twenty persons between fifteen and twenty-four years of age will catch a venereal disease this year. In the United States, somebody gets gonorrhea every fifteen seconds, right around the clock. Last year there were 718,000 reported cases of gonorrhea and 24,000 reported cases of infectious syphilis (Tables 10.1 and 10.2). The actual number of cases of the diseases is much higher, however, because physicians report only one out of every eight patients they treat. The epidemic of gonorrhea is now worldwide, and syphilis rates are increasing in many countries.

Table 10.1 Gonorrhea: reported cases and rates per 100,000 population in United States, fiscal years 1957, 1963–1972*

Year	Number of reported cases	Rate per 100,000 population	Percent change from previous year
1957	216,476	129.8	—
1963	270,076	145.7	+ 3.7
1964	290,603	154.5	+ 7.6
1965	310,155	163.8	+ 6.7
1966	334,949	173.6	+ 8.0
1967	375,606	193.0	+ 12.1
1968	431,380	219.2	+ 14.8
1969	494,227	245.9	+ 14.6
1970	573,200	285.2	+ 16.0
1971	624,371	307.5	+ 8.9
1972	718,401	349.7	+ 15.1

* From United States Public Health Service.

Table 10.2 Primary and secondary syphilis: reported cases and rates per 100,000 population in United States, fiscal years 1957, 1963–1972*

Year	Number of reported cases	Rate per 100,000 population	Percent change from previous year
1957	6,251	3.8	—
1963	22,045	11.9	+ 9.8
1964	22,733	12.1	+ 3.1
1965	23,250	12.3	+ 2.3
1966	22,473	11.6	− 3.3
1967	21,090	10.8	− 6.1
1968	20,182	10.3	− 4.3
1969	18,679	9.3	− 7.4
1970	20,186	10.0	+ 8.1
1971	23,336	11.5	+ 15.6
1972	24,000	11.7	+ 2.8

* From United States Public Health Service.

Many reasons have been given to account for the current epidemics, but none is definitive. Some contributing factors might be identified. There are more people in the world today than ever before, and many of them are in their most sexually active years. There have been large displacements of populations and greater mobility within population groups. Technological changes have encouraged urbanization of populations and introduced fast international travel.

Who gets venereal diseases? Anyone who has sexual contact can acquire one or more. It is not surprising that men and women in their most sexually active years have more venereal diseases than do those in younger or older age groups. Thus persons between twenty and twenty-four years of age have the highest incidence of sexually transmitted diseases, those between twenty-five and thirty years the second highest incidence, while those between fifteen and nineteen years run a close third (Figures 10.1 and 10.2). It is the increasing number of

Figure 10.1. Gonorrhea: age-specific case rates by sex, cases per 100,000 population in United States, calendar year 1971. (United States Public Health Service)

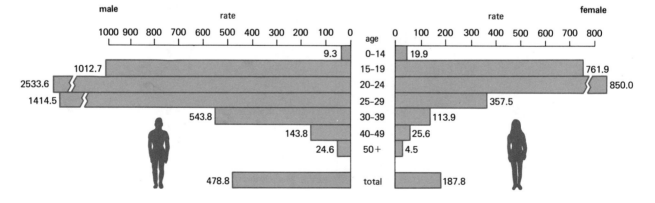

Figure 10.2. Primary and secondary syphilis: age-specific case rates by sex, cases per 100,000 population in United States, calendar year 1971. (United States Public Health Service)

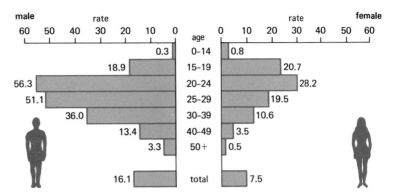

venereal infections in the last age group which generates the most concern.

Some of these diseases can have serious and tragic consequences if they go untreated. Fortunately they can all be completely and rapidly cured if promptly diagnosed and treated.

SYPHILIS   Syphilis begins with a sore. During the late fifteenth and early sixteenth centuries when a severe epidemic of syphilis first swept Europe, the sore was called a pox, and the disease became known as the Great Pox to distinguish it from the disease known as smallpox. One of the dire curses of the time was "A pox on you!" Why the disease suddenly appeared in Europe for apparently the first time at the close of the fifteenth century remains a mystery. Some medical historians think that it had been present for centuries but had not previously been differentiated from other diseases. Another school of thought, however, believes that the disease was present in the New World on the island of Hispaniola (now known as Haiti), and that Columbus's crew of sailors contracted the disease from the native Indians and brought it back to Europe with them. On the return voyage Columbus landed at Cape Palos, Spain, on March 15, 1493. Most of his crew remained there, but Columbus set off for Barcelona by way of Madrid with six of his sailors and six Indians whom he had persuaded to sail back with him. It is presumed that during the course of their journey across Spain these men, infected with syphilis, stopped at brothels and thus ignited the epidemic of the disease in Europe.

The disease had apparently already reached Naples when King Charles VIII of France laid siege to that city in 1494. His mercenary soldiers came from every part of Europe, including Spain. Syphilis broke out among his troops, and as these soldiers of fortune dispersed to their homelands, they took the disease with them. So rapid was the spread of the infection despite the slow methods of transportation then available that by 1497, only four years after Columbus had landed in Spain, it had reached as far as Scotland. Each country blamed the other for the

Figure 10.3. "Spaniard afflicted with the disease of Naples." During the Renaissance, each European country considered another country responsible for the spread of syphilis. Here syphilis is considered the disease of Naples by the French. (Bibliothèque Nationale, Paris, and the World Health Organization)

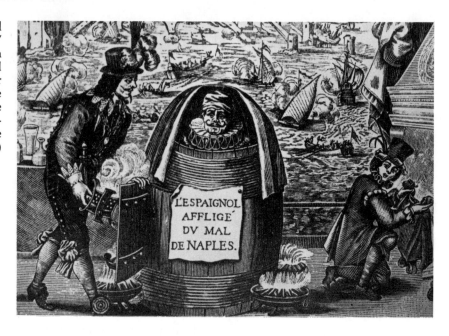

disease. The French called it the disease of Naples, while Italians called it the French disease, and the English called it the Spanish disease.

During the first decades after it swept Europe, syphilis was apparently an acute, painful affliction, and death was not infrequent during the early stages of infection. By the end of the sixteenth century, however, the disease had changed into the chronic form we know today in which the infection insidiously and frequently silently gnaws away at the body's tissues until the final stages of damage to vital tissues are reached. The destroyed tissues cannot be repaired or restored to function.

Although the microorganism which causes syphilis was not discovered until 1905, the physicians of the sixteenth century accurately described the disease itself and its transmission during sexual contact from an infected person to another individual. Much of the current knowledge was put into a poem written in 1530 by an Italian pathologist, Hieronymous Fracastorius. The poem is about a shepherd boy who tended a flock of cattle belonging to King Alcithous. During a severe drought the cattle died of thirst, and the shepherd lad became so angry that he cursed the sun-god for drying up the water and refused to worship the god again. Moreover, he successfully urged all the people to worship King Alcithous as a diety. Enraged at this impiety, the sun-god punished the people by afflicting them with a dread disease, and the shepherd lad, whose name was Syphilis, was the first victim. In 1563, an English surgeon, Thomas Gale, called the disease itself syphilis, after the unfortunate shepherd, and this became the name for the most severe of all sexually transmitted diseases.

This story is sadly prophetic because even today, almost 400 years after the disease first ravaged Europe, a stigma of retribution for sexual transgression is still attached to the disease. And the shame and guilt engendered by this attitude has made control of syphilis as well as gonorrhea difficult, if not almost impossible.

The causative microorganism

The microorganism which causes syphilis is called *Treponema pallidum* (Fig. 10.4). In Latin *treponema* means twisted string, which more or less describes the appearance of the bacterium. It belongs to a group of spiral, corkscrew-shaped microorganisms called spirochetes. Several of these live as normal inhabitants in or on the human body without causing any trouble, two in the mouth and one on the genitals. Three treponemes cause three diseases in human beings. Two of them are found only in the tropics and are not passed by sexual contact. The other one, *T. pallidum*, causes venereal syphilis and is found all over the world.

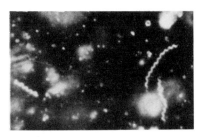

Figure 10.4. Darkfield photograph of *Treponema pallidum*, causative organism of syphilis. (Courtesy of Dr. T. Rosebury, A.S.M.)

T. pallidum will grow only in human beings, monkeys, and a few laboratory animals, notably rabbits. It has not yet been grown on artificial media in the laboratory. Failure to grow the spirochete outside an animal body has greatly retarded research on syphilis because it is difficult to obtain enough spirochetes to study in the laboratory.

T. pallidum multiplies by dividing itself into two every thirty hours. Like the gonococcus (the bacterium that causes gonorrhea), the treponeme of syphilis is so delicate that it cannot long survive outside the body and must be passed from one person to another by intimate body contact. Heat, drying, antiseptics, as well as soap and water kill it instantly.

Nonsexual transmission of syphilis can occur if the treponemes from an infected person are inoculated directly into the skin or blood stream of another person. This sometimes happens among drug abusers if one member of the group has syphilis and contaminates the equipment used for communal injection of the drug. The spirochetes can also be inoculated directly by tattoo needles if they are being used at the same time to decorate a syphilitic and a healthy person. The most tragic method of transmission is from an infected mother to her unborn child. This is called *congenital syphilis*. Syphilis caught from an infected person is called *acquired syphilis*.

Acquired syphilis

Untreated syphilis progresses in a leisurely fashion through an orderly sequence of events and symptoms which spans the life of the infected person. The stages of the disease are called primary syphilis, secondary syphilis, latent syphilis, and late syphilis. Primary and secondary syphilis may be so mild as to be missed or ignored by the infected person. Patients in the first two stages are highly infectious for other people.

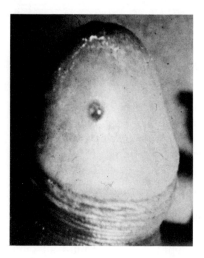

Figure 10.5. The painless chancre of primary syphilis, which appears at the site where the treponemes entered the body, as it appears on a penis. (Reproduced with permission of Technical Information Services, Bureau of State Services, Center for Disease Control, Public Health Services, Department of Health, Education, and Welfare)

PRIMARY SYPHILIS The treponeme causing syphilis can bore its way through the delicate mucous membranes or through microscopic breaks in the skin anywhere on the body. Some spirochetes remain beneath the skin where they entered, but others wiggle their way into the blood stream and within a few hours are carried to various parts of the body. No matter where they are, they begin multiplying at once. After an incubation period of about three to four weeks (but with a range of nine to ninety days), a sore develops at the site where the treponemes entered the body. At first there is a slight erosion of the skin. The rim of the eroded area then thickens and hardens and the center becomes scooped out like a tiny, shallow crater which may ooze fluid or crust over (Fig. 10.5). The round crater, from a few millimeters to one or two centimeters in diameter, contains millions of treponemes and thus is highly infectious. Oddly enough, this initial sore, or *chancre*, is completely painless unless it becomes secondarily infected with other common microorganisms. Chancres can occur in any orifice or on any part of the body. They generally occur on the genitals but they can also be found on the lips, tongue, tonsil, nipples, fingers, and anus. A chancre in the vagina or on the cervix would go unnoticed by the infected person, as would a chancre in the anal canal. About a week after the chancre develops, the local lymph node enlarges and becomes rubbery and hard but does not hurt. The chancre persists from one to five weeks and then spontaneously heals even without treatment. The disappearance of the untreated chancre is deceptive. A person may think he or she has recovered when in fact the spirochetes are continuing to multiply in every tissue of the body in preparation for the second stage of the disease.

SECONDARY SYPHILIS From a few days to several months after the chancre, but generally in six to eight weeks, the symptoms of secondary syphilis appear. They can vary widely and can involve any organ of the body as well as any skin or mucosal surface. The patient may have fever and headaches and experience some nausea. A rash evolves which can

The symptoms of syphilis

This anonymous verse was formerly used as an aid in teaching the symptoms of syphilis to medical students.

There was a young man from
    Back Bay
Who thought syphilis just went
    away.
    He believed that chancre
    Was only a canker
That healed in a week and a day.

But now he has "acne vulgaris"—
(Or whatever they call it in Paris);
    On his skin it has spread
    From his feet to his head,
And his friends want to know
    where his hair is.

There's more to his terrible plight:
His pupils won't close in the light
    His heart is cavorting,
    His wife is aborting,
And he squints through his gun-
    barrel sight.

Arthralgia cuts into his slumber;
His aorta's in need of a plumber;
    But now he has tabes,
    And saber-shinned babies,
While of gummas he has quite a
    number.

He's been treated in every known
    way,
But his spirochetes grow day by
    day;
    He's developed paresis,
    Has long talks with Jesus,
And thinks he's the Queen of
    the May.

From Theodore Roseberry, *Microbes and Morals* (New York: Viking Press, 1971).

be found on any skin surface, including the palms of the hands and the soles of the feet. The rash varies greatly in appearance and mimics almost every other skin condition known. Each spot of the rash is teeming with spirochetes. The rash can be present on mucous surfaces including the lips, mouth, throat, genitals, and anal canal. In such places moisture erodes the surface from the rash spots, leaving them highly infectious. Lymph nodes all over the body become swollen. Even without treatment the symptoms of secondary syphilis heal spontaneously within two to six weeks. The patient, appearing normal and without symptoms of disease, has emerged into the stage of latent syphilis.

LATENT SYPHILIS The patient in latent syphilis has no physical signs or symptoms of disease which could lead to a diagnosis of syphilis by a physician. The only telltale mark is a positive blood test. During the first year or two of latency, the patient may relapse and have the same symptoms as in the secondary stage. In addition, there may be a patchy loss of hair giving a "moth-eaten" appearance to the scalp, loss of eyelashes, and a partial loss of eyebrows. After two to four years the patient goes into late latent syphilis when he or she can no longer transmit the disease to another person. The only exception is that a woman with untreated latent syphilis can infect her unborn child. Latency can last the rest of a patient's life, or in from several years to more than twenty years, can be transformed into the late, disastrous injuries of late syphilis.

LATE SYPHILIS About one-third of untreated syphilitics are afflicted with the destructive lesions of late syphilis. The other two-thirds remain in the late latent period for the rest of their lives without showing further signs of syphilis. While they appear to have minimal physical inconvenience, their life span appears to be shortened. About one-fourth of all untreated syphilitics die of this disease. Unfortunately, there is no way of predicting which patients will die as a result of late syphilis.

The symptoms of late syphilis can mimic those of many other diseases. Almost any organ of the body can be affected. Massive destructive and disfiguring sores called *gummas* involve the skin, mucous membranes, and almost any organ of the body. Other lesions cause destruction of the heart and blood vessels, and others destroy the brain and nerves. Custodial care of the syphilitic insane in public institutions costs about $40 million a year, more than two to three times the amount spent to control the disease.

Congenital syphilis

After the eighteenth week of pregnancy, the treponemes of syphilis can pass from the mother to the fetus and infect the unborn child. The relationships among the mother, the fetus, and the treponemes are complex and depend somewhat on the stage of syphilis the mother is in during the pregnancy. Pregnancy can end in stillbirth or the birth of a congenitally infected baby with a wide spectrum of diseased and deformed tissues. Treatment of the mother before her eighteenth week of pregnancy prevents infection of the fetus. Treatment with penicillin after this time cures both the mother and unborn child.

Congenital syphilis is completely preventable if syphilis is diagnosed and treated during pregnancy. For this reason blood tests for syphilis should always be performed during pregnancy as a part of routine prenatal care.

Diagnosis of syphilis

Two laboratory tests are used to aid the physician in diagnosing syphilis. One is the direct observation of *T. pallidum* in the microscope by means of special illumination. The other is a blood test for telltale changes in the blood proteins.

DARKFIELD MICROSCOPY In the first test, a drop of fluid containing treponemes is scraped from the chancre of primary syphilis or the rash spots of secondary syphilis, placed on a slide, and examined. Because the treponemes are too narrow to be viewed through an ordinary, direct-light microscope, they are examined under a special light brought in at an angle. This procedure is called darkfield microscopy (Fig. 10.4). Darkfield examination cannot be used in latent syphilis because no sores are present or in late syphilis because too few treponemes live in the tissue to be easily found.

BLOOD TESTS Since 1906 when Wasserman developed the blood test which still bears his name, over 200 blood tests for syphilis have been described. Many are still in use today, and new procedures are still being devised. This array of tests suggests that none is completely satisfactory. The tests have been immensely useful in diagnosing cases of syphilis and in detecting the disease in large numbers of people unaware of their infection. About 40 million blood tests for syphilis are performed each year in the United States. Tests are done on people before marriage, on women at prenatal and family planning clinics, and on people being screened for jobs or inducted into the armed services.

Blood tests for syphilis are possible because the human body reacts to defend itself against the invading treponemes by producing a complex of antibodies which bind themselves to the treponemes. These antibodies react with two kinds of antigens administered for the test. The blood is first tested with a nontreponemal antigen. A positive reaction from this could indicate syphilis, but because it could also indicate other disease conditions, a second blood test using a treponemal antigen is usually performed if the first test is positive. This second test is not used as an initial screening test because it takes a skilled technician to interpret the results of each test, making it expensive and practical only for limited use.

When the chancre first appears, the blood test is usually negative, but it becomes positive a few weeks later. If syphilis is treated during the primary stage, the blood test eventually becomes negative again. Treatment for late latent syphilis and late syphilis usually has no effect on the blood test: it remains positive for life.

Treatment of syphilis

During its early stages, syphilis can be completely cured by penicillin. The physician follows one of several dosage schedules. One injection of a long-lasting preparation of penicillin is curative, but many physicians prefer to give an injection of penicillin every day for eight to ten days. Late syphilis requires more prolonged therapy with penicillin. The treatment will arrest the progress of the disease in late syphilis, but it cannot repair tissue which has been destroyed by the disease.

Treponemes are rapidly killed by penicillin and the treated person becomes noninfectious to other people. About half the patients with early syphilis will develop a fever during the first twelve hours after treatment with penicillin. Treponemes all over the body are killed, and their protein is released into the system to produce the temporary fever. This event, which is called the Jarisch-Herxheimer reaction, indicates that the treatment is working effectively.

As stated earlier, sexual contacts of persons with infectious syphilis are given penicillin to prevent their developing the disease. The dose of penicillin now being given to treat gonorrhea is so large that is it sufficient to cure syphilis in the incubation period.

Some people are sensitive to penicillin and cannot be given it without serious danger to their health or even life. For this reason, physicians always ask if the patient has ever had an adverse reaction to penicillin before prescribing it. Patients sensitive to penicillin can be treated with broadspectrum antibiotics.

GONORRHEA

Gonorrhea, a disease which goes back into the prehistory of the human race, is caused by the bacterium *Neisseria gonorrhoeae* named after Albert Neisser who discovered it in 1879. These bean-shaped bacteria, called gonococci, are generally found as a pair with their concave sides facing each other (Fig. 10.6). The delicate gonococci swiftly die on exposure to air and have to be transferred from one person to another on a moist, warm mucous membrane. This membrane, which consists of a single layer of column-shaped cells, lines the urethra, the cervix and some glands in the female, the rectal canal, the mouth and throat, and the eyes. Primary infection with the gonococcus occurs only at these sites. Once the infection is established, however, it can spread to other structures and enter the body proper to cause systemic disease. The gonococci rapidly reproduce by dividing into two every fifty minutes. Genital gonorrhea differs between male and female because of differences in sexual anatomy. During childbirth an infected mother can in-

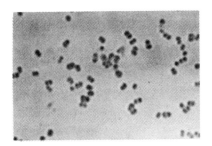

Figure 10.6. Neisseria gonorrhoeae, causative organism of gonorrhea. (Courtesy of S. S. Schneierson)

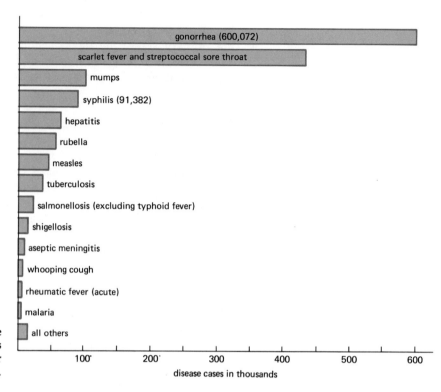

Figure 10.7. Communicable diseases: number of reported cases in United States, calendar year 1970.

fect the eyes of her baby. This form of gonorrhea, which rapidly destroys sight, was once the most common cause of blindness in infants.

Gonorrhea can be cured by antibiotics. Some strains of *N. gonorrhoeae* have become more resistant to penicillin than they were when this antibiotic was first introduced. It now takes about fifty times more penicillin to cure gonorrhea than it used to, but contrary to popular myth, no strain is completely resistant to antibiotics. The disease should be treated early because antibiotics obviously cannot repair tissues destroyed by the disease process.

One of the barriers to control of gonorrhea is people who do not have symptoms of disease and so remain unaware of their infection. About 90 percent of women with gonorrhea do not have symptoms, and it has recently been learned that about 10 percent of males with urethral infection have no symptoms. These persons can nevertheless transmit the disease to their sex contacts and together make up a vast reservoir of infection in our population.

Genital gonorrhea in the male

A wide range in degree of infection occurs in the male urethra. As mentioned above, the infection can produce no symptoms. Some men may develop a discharge from the penis which is so mild that they ignore it.

In both instances the man can and often does transmit the disease to his sex partners. On the other hand, a severe disease can develop two to five days after the infectious contact (although the incubation period can extend from one day to two weeks). There is scalding pain on urination, the head of the penis turns angry red, and heavy, thick pus drips from the urethra. These symptoms generally cause the patient to seek medical care as soon as possible. If treated with penicillin or other antibiotics at this stage, the infection rapidly subsides and no damage is done. If the disease is not treated, however, the gonococci can continue to invade the sex organs to cause prostatitis as well as sterility.

Genital gonorrhea in the female

The incubation period of gonorrhea in women is difficult to determine since most women develop no symptoms which would lead them to suspect an infection. Most women discover they have the disease either when their male sex partner(s) develops gonorrhea or during medical examination in prenatal, family planning, or other clinics. The urethra may become infected causing some pain on urination, and the glands in the genital area may also become involved. The vagina does not become infected because it is not lined with the single layer of column-shaped cells described above. The gonococci usually infect the cervix. Infectious pus leaks from the cervix into the vagina, where the male sex partner picks up the disease. Inflammation of the cervix—*cervicitis*—can become chronic. Backache is the chief and usually the only symptom.

Gonococci can spread from the cervix into the Fallopian tubes. These are the two tubes down which the ova travel from the ovaries to be fertilized by the male sperm cell. If inflammation of the tubes becomes chronic, they may become permanently closed and the patient then becomes unable to bear children.

Gonorrhea of the rectum and throat

Since the anal canal and rectum, as well as the mouth and throat, are lined by mucous membrane, these areas of the body can also become infected with the gonococcus. In women, anal infection occurs either by extension of an infection already present in the genitals or by direct inoculation of the microorganism during genital-anal contact. In men the infection follows direct implantation of the gonococci. In about half the cases of anorectal gonorrhea, there are no symptoms which would suggest to the person that he or she is infected. In other patients, the disease is mild, with moisture or irritation around the anus. In a few cases, the disease can be painful and severe, with blood and pus in the stool. Persons without symptoms join the growing infectious reservoir of gonorrhea. Men frequently learn of their anorectal infection only from a male sex contact to whom they have transmitted the disease.

In gonorrhea of the throat, the gonococci are implanted directly on the mucous membrane during fellatio. About half of infected persons do not have symptoms and thus are unaware of their disease. The remainder have sore throats in varying degrees of severity.

It is important to remember that several different sites of the body can be infected at the same time, depending upon modes of sexual behavior. In clinics which treat venereal diseases, it is now becoming almost routine to check for infection in the anal canal and throat as well as in the genital sites.

Systemic gonorrhea

For reasons which are not clear, the body sometimes cannot contain the gonococcal infection in the primary site—genitals, rectum, or throat. The microorganisms break away from the constraints on the local infection and escape into the blood stream. This can have several results. The gonococci can settle out in the skin to form pimples which turn into red sores that crust over as they heal. The gonococci can also cause a painful arthritis in the joints. This form of the disease generally begins with chills, high fever, swelling, and stiffness and pain in one or more joints, commonly those of the ankles, knees, hips, and wrists. If the arthritis is not treated, the condition can lead to permanent crippling.

Other rarer complications of gonorrhea include a life-threatening infection of the valves of the heart and a severe *meningitis*, an inflammation of the coverings of the brain and spinal chord. Before the discovery that sulfa drugs and penicillin could cure gonorrhea, about 400 people died each year in the United States from the severe complications of gonorrhea.

Gonococcal conjunctivitis

The eyes and eyelids are lined by mucous membrane and thus are vulnerable to infection by the gonococcus. The infection is extremely severe and if not treated promptly can lead to blindness. The infected eye or eyes become red and inflamed, a watery discharge begins, and the lids become stuck together. Soon the watery discharge gives way to thick, abundant pus. The head aches and the afflicted eye is painfully sensitive to light. Ulcers rapidly form on the cornea, the transparent covering which protects the eye. When the ulcers heal, scars are formed and vision is lost. The eyeball itself can also be penetrated, with resulting blindness.

Gonococcal conjunctivitis in adults occurs when gonococci in a genital discharge are carried to the eye, generally by the fingers of the infected person or his or her sex partner.

A woman with gonorrhea can infect the eyes of her baby during passage of the infant through the birth canal. For this reason all states have laws which require that at birth every baby's eyes must be treated to prevent gonococcal conjunctivitis. Such treatment is called *prophylactic* or preventive treatment. Immediately after delivery the baby's

Gonococcal vulvovaginitis in prepubital girls

Before puberty the vagina is lined with the single layer of column-shaped cells which are vulnerable to infection with the gonococcus. After puberty the lining changes into multiple layers of tightly adherent cells which cannot be penetrated by the gonococcus and so are not susceptible to infection. Girls before puberty can have a gonococcal vaginitis. Infection comes about by direct implantation of gonococci in the vagina during sexual contact or assault. Gonococci are also said to be spread in the discharge of infected parents to a daughter sharing their bed.

eyes are swabbed and a silver compound, such as silver nitrate, or an appropriate antibiotic is dropped into the eyes. This prophylactic procedure has saved many babies from blindness. Before it was instituted, almost 30 percent of blindness among children in schools for the blind was caused by gonorrhea. Since most women with gonorrhea do not have symptoms, pregnant women should be tested for infection towards the end of their pregnancy. If they are found infected, treatment will ensure that they will not transmit gonorrhea to the eyes of their babies.

Diagnosis of gonorrhea

When a male patient comes to the physician or clinic with pus dripping from his urethra, the physician must learn whether the symptoms are due to the gonococcus or to another microorganism before treatment can be started. A drop of the pus is smeared onto a glass microscope slide and allowed to dry. The slide is then rapidly passed through a flame to "fix" the pus on the slide, and then the smear is stained with several dyes and examined in the microscope. If it is gonorrhea, there will be many pink bean-shaped gonococci in pairs in the pus. There will also be many pus cells—large cells which the body has mobilized to help cope with the infection—and some of them will have gobbled up many of the gonococci. From this typical microscopic picture of the pus as well as from the clinical symptoms in the male, the physician can make a diagnosis of gonorrhea.

Diagnosis is more complicated if the infection is in the cervix, rectum, or throat. A great many other bacteria also inhabit these regions and some of them look like gonococci. In a chronic cervical infection, there may be too few gonococci to see in a smear of the cervical secretion. Consequently another method is used. The gonococci are grown in the laboratory on a special nutrient medium which suppresses the growth of all the other contaminating microorganisms and encourages the propagation of the fastidious gonococcus. This medium, solidified with agar and placed in a flat dish with a cover, is called Thayer-Martin medium after the two men who devised it. Their formulation represented a great advance over all the media which had previously been proposed because it increased the chances of making an accurate diagnosis of gonorrhea. A sterile cotton swab is inserted into the opening of the cervix during a pelvic examination or into the throat or anal canal and then rolled over the firm surface of the medium. A small, platinum, bacteriologic loop, sterilized in a flame, is then streaked back and forward across the medium to distribute the secretion which came off the cotton swab. The "inoculated" Thayer-Martin medium is then kept at 36° centigrade in an atmosphere of air containing 5 percent carbon dioxide. Steadily multiplying by dividing into two every fifty minutes, the gonococci by the end of eighteen to twenty-four hours have formed little colonies the size of a head of a pin which glisten like dew drops on the surface of the medium. For complete identification, they must be put through a few more tests to differentiate them from closely related bacteria. The report of positive or negative is then sent to the physician.

CONTROL OF SYPHILIS AND GONORRHEA

Sex and the law

Theoretically, the law regulates all sexual behavior. Throughout most of the United States, the only legal sex act is genital contact between a legally married husband and wife, and all other expressions of sexual activity, in or out of wedlock, are defined as crimes and are punishable by law. Despite the apparent relaxation of attitudes toward sex, people throughout this country are still being imprisoned for violations of the sex laws, many of which are cruel, vindictive, and archaic. These laws express the attitude of sex as sin which we have inherited as part of our Judeo-Christian culture. The feeling that sexual activity is somehow inherently sinful is unfortunately extended to those diseases which are transmitted by sexual contact.

A venereal disease is often taken as evidence that a person committed not only illegal but also immoral acts. Until recently, catching a venereal disease was considered a suitable punishment for such transgression, and it is still considered by some to represent a useful deterrent to sexual activity. Making people fearful of contracting a venereal disease has not been a notably successful method of controlling these infections, which, in view of the fact that sex is one of the most fundamental of all biological urges, is hardly surprising. The repressive legal and cultural attitudes toward sexual behavior create an atmosphere of fear, shame, and anxiety which severely hampers attempts to control sexually transmitted diseases (see Chap. 4).

Fiction and facts about VD

False: You can catch venereal diseases from contact with a toilet seat, doorknob, shaking hands, etc.

True: Fortunately not. Venereal diseases are transmitted through sexual intercourse.

False: You can't get a venereal disease again once you've had it.

True: There is no immunity to the venereal diseases—you can have a venereal disease any number of times.

False: Syphilis is hereditary.

True: Syphilis CANNOT be inherited. An expectant mother who has syphilis can transmit the disease to her unborn child, but this has nothing to do with the factors responsible for inheritance.

Methods of control

The aim of control is to reduce the chance of catching the disease. Every person who contracts a venereal disease received it from another person. Control of these diseases consists in treating the person with a venereal disease and in finding, examining, and treating the person from whom the patient acquired the disease and the person or persons to whom the patient may have transmitted the disease. Control begins when the physician diagnoses and treats a patient with a sexually transmitted disease.

Venereal diseases can be treated by a physician in his private office, in which case a fee is charged as for any other medical visit to the physician. Sexually transmitted diseases are also diagnosed and treated free of charge in public clinics strategically placed in centers throughout the United States (they are all listed in the local telephone books). The cost of diagnosis and treatment is paid by the federal government.

The physician, whether in private practice or in a public clinic, is

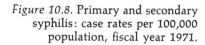

Figure 10.8. Primary and secondary syphilis: case rates per 100,000 population, fiscal year 1971.

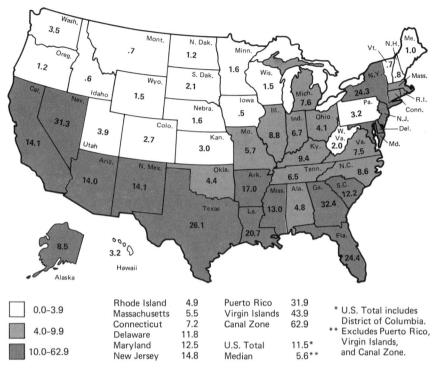

0.0–3.9	Rhode Island	4.9	Puerto Rico	31.9
4.0–9.9	Massachusetts	5.5	Virgin Islands	43.9
	Connecticut	7.2	Canal Zone	62.9
10.0–62.9	Delaware	11.8		
	Maryland	12.5	U.S. Total	11.5*
	New Jersey	14.8	Median	5.6**

* U.S. Total includes District of Columbia.
** Excludes Puerto Rico, Virgin Islands, and Canal Zone.

required by law to report all cases of sexually transmitted disease to the local Department of Health, just as he is legally required to report certain other specified diseases such as smallpox, plague, and poliomyelitis. Cases of venereal disease treated in a public clinic are automatically reported, while private physicians, at least in the past, have reported only some of the cases which they have treated.

What happens after a venereal disease is reported? In the clinic, the patient is interviewed by a specially trained nurse or social worker to learn the name of the person from whom the patient acquired the disease and the names of those with whom the patient has had sexual contact while he or she was infectious and could have transmitted the disease. This interview is confidential. The patient's name is never revealed to any of his or her sex contacts. An attempt is made to locate each sex contact in order to urge the person to visit the clinic for examination and, if necessary, treatment. Some of the contacts may be suffering from one or more venereal diseases without knowing it. If infected, each contact is asked to name his or her sex contacts who are then sought for examination and treatment where necessary. In this way the reservoir of infected persons in the population can be gradually reduced and the chances of acquiring a disease during sex contact decreased.

Figure 10.9. Gonorrhea: case rates per 100,000 population, fiscal year 1971.

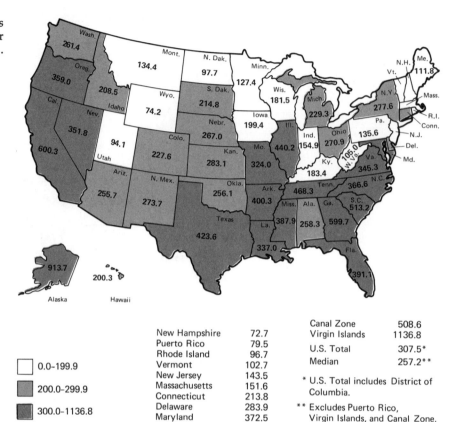

New Hampshire	72.7
Puerto Rico	79.5
Rhode Island	96.7
Vermont	102.7
New Jersey	143.5
Massachusetts	151.6
Connecticut	213.8
Delaware	283.9
Maryland	372.5

Canal Zone	508.6
Virgin Islands	1136.8
U.S. Total	307.5*
Median	257.2**

* U.S. Total includes District of Columbia.

** Excludes Puerto Rico, Virgin Islands, and Canal Zone.

0.0–199.9

200.0–299.9

300.0–1136.8

Persons who have been sexually exposed to an infectious case of syphilis are generally treated whether they show signs of syphilis or not, since they may be in the long incubation period of the disease. In some states women exposed to males with gonorrhea are also treated, since they frequently do not have symptoms of the disease and may transmit the disease before a laboratory diagnosis can be made.

If the patient is treated by a private physician and the case is reported to the health department, the authorities ask the physician's permission to interview the patient for sex contacts. If the physician agrees, as he should, the same procedures described for the clinic patient are applied to finding sex contacts of the private patient.

This method of control of sexually transmitted diseases requires tact and sympathy on the part of the health workers who interview the patient and the other workers who trace all named sex contacts and persuade them to come for examination and treatment. When successful, this method can reveal a chain of infection and stop transmission of the disease. An example is shown in Fig. 10.10, which traces the chain of syphilis through an American high school. Formerly, it was illegal to treat a minor without parental consent. In most states, however, this law has been changed, and minors can now be treated for venereal diseases without parental consent or knowledge. The remaining problem is that the legal age allowing such treatment varies widely from state to state.

The epidemiological method of control, as it is called, is time-consuming and expensive. The method has worked well for syphilis because of the long incubation period of this disease. It is almost useless in gonorrhea, however, because of its short incubation period. Several cycles of transmission of gonorrhea can occur before the machinery of

Figure 10.10. Syphilis epidemic in a U.S. high school. Syphilis was introduced into the school by an infected boy. During the flow of the disease through the school, 14 other persons became infected with syphilis. Another 26 exposed persons were treated preventively to keep them from developing the disease and transmitting it to other persons, while 25 were found not to be infected. ("Today's VD Control Problem—1971," American Social Health Association, 1740 Broadway, N.Y. 10019)

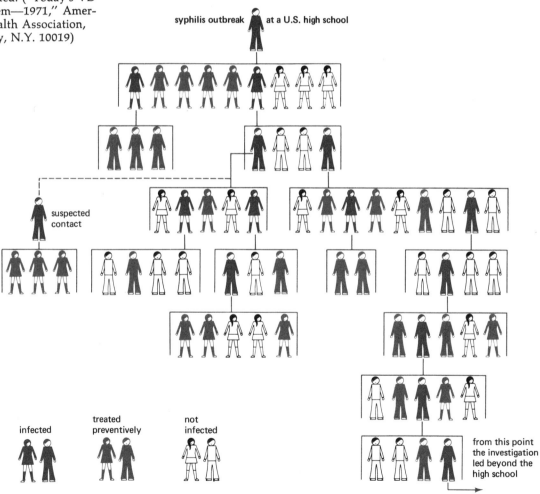

case-finding can be brought into action. The number of cases of gonorrhea now occurring would swamp present facilities and personnel.

Personal control

The only foolproof way not to catch a venereal disease is not to have sexual contact with a person who has one. The chief way to achieve this end is to avoid all sexual contact until married to a person who has done the same and thereafter to lead a completely monogamous life. Other solutions are theoretically possible. If all teenagers could manage to have sexual contact only within their peer groups and never with an older person, sexually transmitted diseases would vanish within a generation. These solutions are not likely to be applied on a universal scale since they do not allow for individual needs or behavior. The problem thus is one of minimizing the risk of contracting syphilis or gonorrhea and seeking rapid treatment should infection occur.

Given the present epidemic of gonorrhea throughout most of the world, it stands to reason that a person who has sex contact with a large number of partners will have a greater chance of catching the disease than will a person who limits contact to a single person.

When used properly, condoms can act as a barrier to the germs of syphilis and gonorrhea. They afford some but not complete protection, but the sale of condoms is illegal in many states. The vaginal jellies and foams sold as contraceptive agents contain chemicals which kill the gonococcus of gonorrhea and the spirochete of syphilis and thus can protect the female from infection (see Chap. 21). Certain antibiotics taken in proper doses just before or after sexual activity provide almost complete protection against infection, but their use is frowned on by the medical profession for two reasons. First, this method might increase resistance of the gonococcus to the antibiotic so that the antibiotic can no longer cure the disease. Second, a certain percentage of persons become sensitized to an antibiotic and can no longer be given that antibiotic without serious danger to their life.

Perhaps the most practical method for personal control is to recognize the possibility of catching a venereal disease, to seek prompt medical care if one has reason to believe one has been exposed to or contracted such a disease, and to persuade one's sex partner(s) to be examined and treated. It is a good idea for a person who has sexual contact with a variety of partners to have a blood test for syphilis performed at reasonable intervals. A person can be in the early stages of syphilis without knowing it, and the blood test is free at public clinics.

NON-GONOCOCCAL URETHRITIS IN MALES

The most prominent symptom of Non-Gonococcal Urethritis (NGU) is the dripping of pus from the lips of the urethra. The disease can be so mild that it is noticeable only as a small drop of whitish, sticky fluid on

Table 10.3 Other sexually transmitted diseases

Name	Causative agent	Incubation period	Early symptoms	Later developments	Treatment
Chancroid	Haemophilus ducreyi	1–7 days	Small, painful pimples where bacterium entered body become filled with pus and break down to form shallow ulcers.	Infection infiltrates lymph nodes in region causing abscess (bubo). Abscesses erupt, spreading ulcers over skin.	Sulfa drugs, broadspectrum antibiotics except penicillin
Lympho-granuloma Venereum	Chlamydia	1–6 weeks	Tiny pimple where bacterium entered body may be so insignificant as to be unrecognized or ignored.	Infection infiltrates nearest lymph nodes which may fester into abscesses. Abscesses erupt, leaking out blood-stained pus. If chronic, infection may cause gross swelling of penis and scrotum (*elephantiasis*) and may spread from vagina to rectum.	Sulfa drugs, broadspectrum antibiotics except penicillin
Granuloma Inguinale	Donovan body	unknown	Initial painless pimples where bacterium entered body break down into beefy-red, velvety raised masses which bleed and spread over body.	Scar tissue forms over wounds.	Broadspectrum antibiotics

the end of the penis. In other cases, the pus leaks out more or less continuously, without causing pain, and is considered a nuisance because it constantly stains the underpants. The disease can be severe enough to resemble gonorrhea, with discharge of thick pus from the urethra and painful urination.

A causative agent can be found in about 10 percent of cases of NGU. These include several kinds of bacteria as well as the protozoan *Trichomonas vaginalis* (see the section on Vaginitis). In the remaining 90 percent of the cases no specific microorganism has yet been identified as the cause of the disease. In order to make a diagnosis of NGU, the physician must first rule out all other known diseases. The pus must be examined as it would be for gonorrhea. If gonococci cannot be seen in the pus on examination in the microscope or cannot be grown on special medium in the laboratory, the physician can make a diagnosis of NGU. It is important to distinguish between gonorrhea and NGU because the treatment for each is usually different. Penicillin does not cure NGU. The infection is treated with a broadspectrum antibiotic, such as one of the tetracyclines. This treatment cures most cases. If a relapse occurs, the patient may have to go through another course of treatment.

As in gonorrhea, it is sometimes difficult to distinguish a relapse from a reinfection. It is a curious fact that while men appear to contract NGU from females, the woman herself (who in turn probably acquired the microorganisms from another man) shows no sign of having the infection. A man having repeated sexual contacts with the same infectious woman may become reinfected after successful treatment.

NGU generally comes on about eight days after the infectious contact, although the incubation period can extend up to a month or more. The infection is frequently acquired at the same time as gonorrhea. In such a case, the whitish, sticky discharge is first noticed after penicillin has cured the gonorrhea, or it appears after treatment has stopped. The physician must then differentiate between a relapse of the gonorrhea or infection with NGU.

Today NGU is the most common of all sexually transmitted diseases in the male. In England, where good records are kept on this disease, the incidence of NGU is greater than gonorrhea and is increasing every year. It is believed that the situation in the United States may be similar to that in the United Kingdom. Control of this condition, which seldom results in serious complication, is hampered by our ignorance of the cause or causes of the disease and by the fact that antibiotics do not cure all cases. The fact that antibiotics do cure most cases strongly suggests that in these cases the disease is caused by a microorganism (or microorganisms) other than a virus, since presently available antibiotics have no effect whatever on viral infections.

VAGINITIS

Vaginitis is an inflammation of the vagina which can be accompanied by a discharge of matter. It is an uncomfortable, bothersome, and sometimes painful condition. Vaginitis can result from a variety of causes including microorganisms and physical or chemical injury. Some of the microorganisms causing vaginitis are transmitted by sexual contact. A woman suffering from vaginitis can also be infected with one or more of the venereal diseases. The physician must determine the precise cause or causes of the disease before treatment can be started. The two most common causes of vaginitis are described below. One is a tiny animal and the other is a yeast.

TRICHOMONAS The one-celled organism first found in vaginal secretions in 1836 was somewhat misnamed *Trichomonas vaginalis*; the organism, however, is not limited to the vagina. This microorganism, probably the most common cause of abnormal vaginal discharge, is transmitted during sexual contact to the woman by her male partner. Curiously, most men who carry the protozoan are free of symptoms. They appear to carry the microorganism only temporarily. On the other hand, a small percentage of infected males may have a urethritis.

There is a wide range of disease in females. Some infested women may be without symptoms, others may have a slight discharge from the vagina, while still others may suffer a severe and painful infestation. In the latter case the disease begins from one to three weeks after the infectious sexual contact. A copious, greenish-yellow, frothy discharge leaks more or less continuously from the vagina. It has an offensive odor and is irritating to the tender membranes of the genitals and the skin of the thighs.

The diagnosis of trichomonas is made by examining a drop of the discharge in the microscope. The physician has several drugs in the form of tablets to be taken orally which effectively cure the disease. It makes sense to treat the male sex partner at the same time in order to prevent their ping-ponging the infestation back and forth between them.

VAGINAL THRUSH When a fungus called *Candida albicans*, normally found in the large intestine with other microorganisms, is allowed to multiply rapidly and become the dominant microorganism in the gut, vaginitis as well as other diseases can result. *Candidosis*, vaginal thrush, is not an infection ordinarily transmitted by sexual contact, but male partners of women with the infection can become infected and sometimes develop urethritis.

Underlying events which allow *C. albicans* to set up an infection in the vagina include pregnancy, diabetes, and the taking of certain contraceptive pills. The vaginal infection can be mild and induce slight or no symptoms or be severe and extremely painful. The discharge from the vagina may be scanty and watery or copious and flecked with white, curdlike material. Diagnosis is made by examining a drop of the discharge in the microscope. Treatment involves correcting the underlying condition and administering one of the few antibiotics effective against fungal infections.

DISEASES ASSOCIATED WITH SEXUAL CONTACT

The venereal diseases discussed in the preceding sections are, except in certain circumstances, transmitted only by sexual contact. In addition to these diseases, there are a variety of other disease conditions which can also be transferred from one person to another during sexual contact, although in some instances close bodily contact suffices. Four such conditions are described in this section. Two are caused by viruses, one by a louse, and another by a mite.

Herpes genitalis

Two closely related herpes viruses infect human beings. *Herpesvirus 1* causes cold sores and fever blisters on the lips and nostrils. In some people this infection remains silent for intervals and then flares again into action. The closely related *herpesvirus 2* is passed from person to person by sexual contact and causes sores on the genitals. About 90 percent of persons who become infected with herpesvirus 2 have no symptoms of disease. In the remaining 10 percent the disease ranges from a mild to a severe condition. In men the lesions are most frequently seen on the foreskin, head and shaft of the penis, and the scrotum, while in women they are generally found on the labia minora and majora and clitoris.

The disease appears four to five days after exposure as blisters which erode and leave small, shallow ulcers. The two major lymph nodes of the genital area may become painfully tender. If there are no further complications, the ulcers usually heal themselves in about ten days. In some cases, the infection goes "underground" and symptoms disappear, although the virus is still living in the cells of the skin. Periodically the virus may break out and produce a fresh crop of sores.

There is no drug to cure the virus infection. The sores should be kept clean and dry to prevent secondary infection with bacteria. Antibiotics can be used to control secondary infection, if it occurs, and painkillers lessen the discomfort of the raw ulcers.

Genital warts

Warts are caused by a virus. They can occur on the skin on any part of the body, but they tend to grow more luxuriantly on those parts of the body which are kept warm and moist. Favored places for genital warts are near the head of the penis, around the vagina, and around the anus. They can be found in the opening of the urethra and in the anal canal. The virus which produces genital warts is transmitted during sexual intercourse and the precise location of the warts reflects the type of contact which occurred. From one to six months after infectious contact, the wart begins as a tiny swelling which swiftly develops into a growth resembling a cauliflower. A group of such structures may fuse into one tumorlike growth which can grow to the size of a baseball. The physician has several methods for successful treatment of genital warts, including chemicals and electric cautery. A person with a developing genital wart should seek medical attention as early as possible.

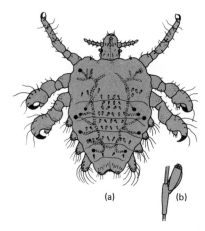

(a) (b)

Figure 10.11. The crab or pubic louse, *Phthirus pubis,* has claws which enable it to grasp the hairs of the body where it spends its entire life.

Crab lice

Crab lice, so-called because they roughly resemble miniature crabs (Fig. 10.11), are small insects which spend all of their lives on human beings and can pass from one person to another during sexual contact or less intimate physical contact. Unlike the bacteria of syphilis or gonorrhea, they are relatively hardy little beasts and can be acquired from a toilet seat if one or more happen to fall to the seat on a pubic hair of a prior user.

Because of humidity and warmth in the crotch, the crab louse prefers to live among the pubic hairs—those hairs which surround the genitals. This preference gives the insect its other common name, the pubic louse. Several times a day the lice crawl down these hairs to the skin, pierce it with their sharp mouth parts, and suck up blood from a small blood vessel by means of muscular pumps in their esophagus. If there are many lice, this intermittent stabbing of the skin with puncture wounds becomes irritating and causes itching and scratching. Under population pressure, the lice will migrate downward and upward from the crotch and can eventually be found nestling in the eyebrows, eyelashes, and hair in the armpits. For unknown reasons pubic lice do not appear to like the hair growing on the head; this area of the body is reserved for another kind of louse, the head louse.

Several chemical preparations are available for getting rid of the infestation. Some must be prescribed by a physician, while others can be bought over-the-counter in drug stores and pharmacies.

Scabies

Scabies is a disease caused by the female itch mite (Fig. 10.12) as she tunnels her tortuous way through the body just beneath the surface of the skin. The itching, especially at night, can be almost intolerable. Although the tiny insect frequently crawls from one human being to another during sexual encounter, sex contact is not absolutely essential for spread of the mite. Any close bodily contact suffices. Spread of the disease occurs in families and among children. Natural disasters of famine and earthquake or the man-made disaster of war furnish ideal conditions for epidemics of scabies. Normal community sanitation breaks down and people are huddled together with inadequate housing and facilities for washing either themselves or their clothes. Under these conditions the itch mite rapidly passes from one person to another. Scabies has been a traditional scourge of armies during wartime. The itch mite infests human beings all over the world. Small epidemics of the disease are currently reported in England and the disease appears to be on the increase in the United States.

A person does not generally realize that he or she has become infested until about a month after the first female has eaten her way into the skin. By that time, she has been able to lay her eggs in the burrows under the skin, and the larvae that survived have developed into adult mites and repeated the reproduction cycle. Once the infestation has

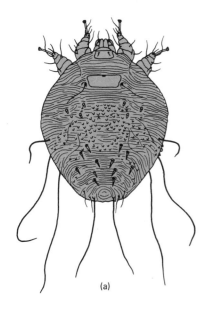

(a)

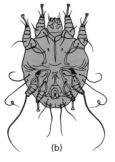

(b)

Figure 10.12. The female itch mite, *Sarcoptes scabiei*, burrows a tunnel just beneath the skin in which she lays her eggs. Note the backward-pointing spines which aid her progress through the flesh.

gotten underway, there are usually ten to fifteen adult mites burrowing their own tunnels through the skin, although there can be as many as one hundred.

Mites prefer thin, wrinkled skin. If transmission has been by familial spread, the burrows are found in the skin between the fingers, on the wrists, near the armpits, and on the buttocks. If transmission was by sexual contact, the tunnels are on the genitals. In men, the lesions are generally on the shaft of the penis, the foreskin, and the scrotum. The burrows appear as slightly raised lines on the skin. Sometimes, especially on the penis, the burrows will be scratched open because of itching, resulting in a long, shallow ulcer. The ulcer may become infected with bacteria.

The infestation can be eliminated by treatment with benzyl benzoate, several forms of organic sulfur compounds, and with preparations containing the insecticide lindane. All of these must be used under the direction of a physician. If the mite infestation is circulating in a family group or commune, all members as well as all sex contacts should be examined and treated.

Questions
1. Why should you know about sexually transmitted diseases?
2. How is it possible that a person can have syphilis or gonorrhea and not know it?
3. Both syphilis and gonorrhea can be cured with antibiotics. How do you account for the paradox that they are not, and probably cannot be, eradicated from our population?
4. How would you try to control venereal diseases?
5. What would you do if you thought you had been exposed to a venereal disease or that you had contracted one?

Key Concepts

Chancre – the initial, painless sore of primary syphilis which develops where the infectious spirochetes (*Treponema pallidum*) entered the body

Gonorrhea – an inflammation of the genital and other mucous membranes and the most widespread of all communicable diseases. The causative agent, *Neisseria gonorrhoeae*, is transmitted during sexual contact

Non-Gonococcal Urethritis (NGU) – a condition of urethritis for which the causative agent is unknown. Its symptoms, most notably a discharge of pus from the urethra, are often mistaken for those of gonorrhea. Women can be carriers for the infection, but they do not contract it

Syphilis – the most serious of all sexually transmitted diseases. Beginning with a chancre, the diseases progresses over a lifetime through four stages of increasing severity (primary, secondary, latent, and late). In the last stage it can cause insanity and even death

Vaginitis – an inflammation of the vagina which can be caused by various microorganisms and certain injuries. Men can be carriers of the causative agent, but they generally do not develop an infection from it

Selected Readings   King, A. and C. Nicol. *Venereal Diseases,* 2d ed. Philadelphia: F. A. Davis, 1970.

Morton, R. S. *Venereal Diseases.* Baltimore: Penguin Books, 1966.

Rosebury, T. *Microbes and Morals: The Strange Story of Venereal Disease.* New York: Viking Press, 1971.

"Today's VD Control Problem." American Social Health Association (yearly publication). This pamphlet can be obtained from the American Social Health Association, 1740 Broadway, New York, New York 10019.

"VD Fact Sheet." U.S. Public Health Service (yearly publication). This pamphlet can be obtained from the Venereal Disease Branch, Center for Disease Control, Atlanta, Georgia 30333.

Chapter 11

Noncommunicable Diseases

Although communicable diseases were the principal scourge of our ancestors, noncommunicable diseases are the major causes of death in the United States today: heart disease and cancer account for over half of all deaths in our society (Table 11.1). This shift to the noncommunicable diseases is due in large part to the successful control or elimination of many communicable diseases.

CARDIOVASCULAR DISEASE

The heart and blood vessels combined are referred to as the cardiovascular system. Like all organs and tissues of the body, they are subject to disease. The diseases may be inherited, but they may also develop during an individual's lifetime as a result of the way he lives. Whether genetically or environmentally determined, cardiovascular diseases are responsible for over a third of all deaths in the United States. However, evidence indicates that the number of these deaths can be greatly reduced through some simple, basic changes in many Americans' pattern

---

This chapter was contributed by Robert B. McGandy, M.D., M.P.H., Associate Professor of Physiology, Harvard School of Public Health.

of daily living, particularly in regard to eating, exercising, and cigarette smoking.

Table 11.1 Mortality for leading causes of death: United States, 1969

Rank	Cause of death	Number of deaths	Death rate per 100,000 population	Percent of total deaths
1	Diseases of Heart	738,945	359.9	38.4
2	Cancer	323,092	160.0	16.8
3	Stroke (Cerebrovascular Diseases)	207,179	102.6	10.8
4	Accidents	116,385	57.6	6.1
	Motor Vehicle Accidents	55,791	27.6	2.9
	All Other Accidents	60,594	30.0	3.2
5	Influenza and Pneumonia	68,365	33.9	3.6
6	Certain Diseases of Early Infancy	43,171	21.4	2.2
7	Diabetes Mellitus	38,541	19.1	2.0
8	Arteriosclerosis	33,063	16.4	1.7
9	Cirrhosis of Liver	29,866	14.8	1.6
10	Emphysema	22,939	11.4	1.2
11	Suicide	22,364	11.1	1.2
12	Congenital Anomalies	17,008	8.4	0.9
13	Homicide	15,477	7.7	0.8
14	Nephritis and Nephrosis	9,417	4.7	0.5
15	Infections of Kidney	8,750	4.3	0.5
	Other and Ill-Defined	227,428	61.0	11.8

SOURCE: Vital Statistics of the United States. Prepared by: American Cancer Society, Research Department, September, 1972.

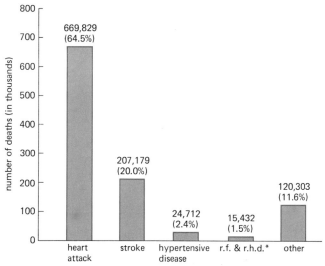

Figure 11.1. Deaths due to cardiovascular diseases by major type of disorder, United States, 1969. (National Center for Health Statistics, U.S. Public Health Service, DHEW)

*rheumatic fever and rheumatic heart disease

Figure 11.2. An eighteenth-century anatomical illustration of the heart. (Courtesy of the World Health Organization)

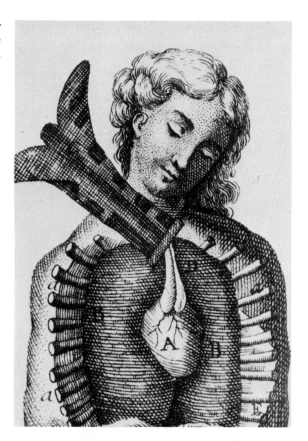

Congenital heart disease

Most congenital heart defects are caused by abnormal development of the human embryo. A disease, such as rubella (German measles), in the mother in the early stages of pregnancy may cause the abnormality. Generally, congenital heart defects are not inherited.

The blood in the fetus does not flow through the lungs because, being the mother's blood, it is already filled with oxygen. Normally when the infant is born, the blood begins to flow through the lungs. But for a variety of reasons, in certain infants some of the blood does not flow through the lungs and so the infant does not receive an adequate supply of oxygen. Without oxygen, the blood is blue and gives the infant a bluish appearance; thus we refer to a "blue baby." The condition can be corrected through open heart surgery.

There are thirty-five kinds of congenital heart defects. Some defects can be detected immediately after birth; others are detected only after many months or even years. There are an estimated 25,000 infants born each year in the United States with some form of congenital heart disease. Through medical advances in recent years, deaths from this disease have been reduced 65 percent.

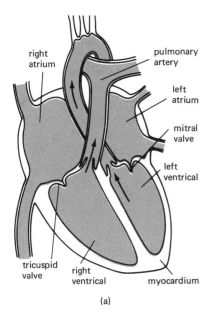

(a)

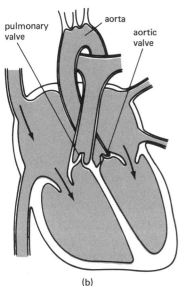

(b)

Figure 11.3. Direction of blood circulation through the heart. (a) Ventricle contraction. (b) Atrial contraction. The right atrium receives deoxygenated blood from the rest of the body; it contracts to let the blood pass through the tricuspid valve into the right ventricle. Upon contraction of the ventricle, the tricuspid valve is closed and prevents blood from seeping back into the atrium. Blood is transmitted into the pulmonary artery, then into the lungs for oxygenation, and finally into the left atrium. Upon contraction of the atrium, the oxygenated blood passes through the mitral valve into the left ventricle; upon contraction of the ventricle, the blood passes through the aortic valve and into the aorta (the body's largest artery). The blood is now ready for circulation throughout the body.

Rheumatic heart disease

Children between the ages of five and fifteen are the persons most apt to develop rheumatic fever. The disease usually begins one to four weeks after a streptococcal infection. (Fortunately, only a small percentage of "strep" infections develops into rheumatic fever.) The symptoms are pain and inflammation in the joints (rheumatism) and fever, but sometimes in the early stages of infection the symptoms are so slight they are overlooked.

If allowed to progress, the disease will infect the heart valves and permanently scar them. The valves as a result do not open and close properly, and blood that is being pumped out is often able to seep back into the heart. The sound from this backward seepage is called a heart murmur. To compensate for the decrease in the amount of blood being pumped out, the heart must pump harder and faster, causing a strain which can eventually lead to heart failure.

Rheumatic heart disease can be surgically corrected by removing the scar tissue or implanting artificial valves. But as with all diseases, rheumatic heart disease is more easily and effectively prevented than treated. The best method is the early treatment of all streptococcal infections.

Hypertension

Blood pressure, like atmospheric pressure, is measured in millimeters of mercury. Unlike atmospheric pressure, there are periodically two pressure levels in arteries. *Systolic* pressure is the pressure in the arteries when the heart is contracting and pumping blood into them. *Diastolic* pressure, which is lower than systolic pressure, is the pressure in the arteries between heart beats when the heart is relaxing. Blood pressure is read as systolic over diastolic pressure. A blood pressure of 120/80 is considered normal for a young man; the figure is somewhat lower for young women.

The level of arterial blood pressure represents a balance between the force of contraction of the heart and the amount of resistance (due to

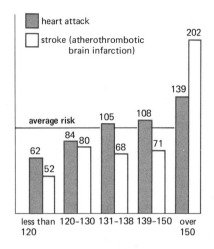

Figure 11.4. The relationship between blood pressure and risk of heart attack and stroke in men. (From The Framingham, Mass. Heart Study—16 Years' Experience)

the degree of narrowing) of the peripheral arterioles, the smallest arteries just before the capillaries arise. When these arteries are narrow, they hinder blood circulation. The heart must then pump harder to overcome their resistance, resulting in a condition known as hypertension. Hypertension means high blood pressure, which is defined as a systolic pressure of 140 or more millimeters of mercury and a diastolic pressure of 90 or more millimeters of mercury. This is a rather arbitrary definition, for the risk of heart disease or death is greater with every increase in blood pressure, not just with increases in pressure over 140/90 (Fig. 11.4). Except for a few instances in which greatly elevated blood pressure is a result of kidney disease or a tumor of the adrenal gland, the causes of elevated blood pressure levels are unknown; heredity may well be a factor, as may a habitual high level of salt intake.

High blood pressure greatly accelerates the rate of development of atherosclerosis (see below). Furthermore, it causes an enlargement of heart muscle mass which may result in a heart failure. Hypertension often may result in a stroke. It also may lead to sufficient impairment of kidney function to cause death from renal failure.

High blood pressure can be medically treated with relatively safe and effective drugs. Over the past few years, the decline in deaths due to hypertension has been ascribed to widespread use of these antihypertensive agents.

ATHEROSCLEROTIC CARDIOVASCULAR DISEASE

Arteriosclerosis means hardening of the arteries and refers to several degenerative diseases of the artery wall. The most important of these diseases is *atherosclerosis*, which is characterized by deposits of cholesterol (a large, complex, fat-related molecule) and other fats in the wall of arteries. These deposits cause the artery wall to thicken and thus cause the channel available for blood flow to narrow (Fig. 11.5). Accounting for over 850,000 deaths in the United States each year, atherosclerosis of the arteries supplying the heart muscles (coronary arteries) and of the arteries supplying the brain (cerebral arteries) is responsible for over 80 percent of all deaths due to cardiovascular diseases.

Coronary heart disease

Coronary thrombosis (commonly referred to as a "heart attack") results from a clot formation in a coronary artery. The clot, called a thrombus or occlusion, blocks the blood flow to the heart and kills the area of the heart muscle supplied with blood by the particular coronary artery. This area of dead muscle is called a *myocardial infarction*. Most individuals survive a first attack with myocardial infarction, but death can result either from a serious alteration in heart rhythm, caused by the interference with the heart's nervous system, or from "pump failure," caused by so great loss of heart muscle that the heart cannot maintain its usual work load.

The clot is much more apt to occur in a coronary artery narrowed by

Figure 11.5. (a) Cross section of a normal artery. (b) Atherosclerotic deposits formed in the inner lining. (c) The narrow channel blocked by a blood clot, depriving the heart muscle of blood and so causing a heart attack. (Courtesy of the American Heart Association)

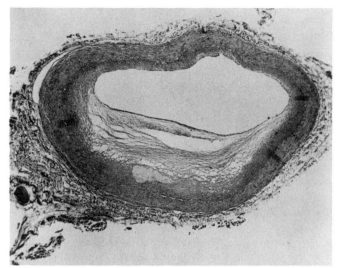

a

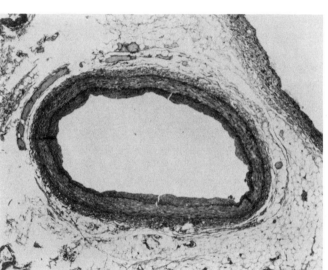

b

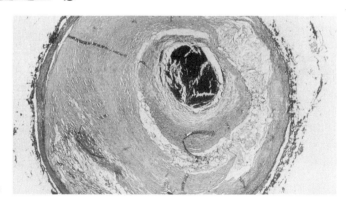

c

atherosclerosis than in a normal coronary artery. Though the attack is sudden, the underlying atherosclerotic condition is built up over many years. The most notable symptom of coronary thrombosis is *angina pectoris*, a severe pain resulting from the inadequate supply of blood (and therefore of oxygen) in the heart muscle tissue. The actual cause of coronary thrombosis has not yet been proved, but the mechanisms of the attack seem to be brought on by physical and emotional stress.

Cerebrovascular accidents

A cerebrovascular accident (commonly referred to as a "stroke" or "apoplexy") results from a clot formation or a hemorrhage in a cerebral artery usually weakened by atherosclerosis or hypertension. A stroke can also occur when a roving blood clot, called an embolus, lodges in a cerebral artery. The clot or rupture cuts off the normal flow of blood to the area supplied by the artery, causing the functioning of the nerves in that area rapidly to deteriorate. Death can occur. If the patient survives, the damage done to the brain may leave permanent neurologic impairments of which the most common are loss of muscle use, loss of sensation, loss of speech, hearing, or vision, and loss of higher intellectual function.

Incidence of atherosclerosis

The National Health Examination Survey conducted in 1960–1962 provided the basis for the estimate that 5.5 million adult Americans had definite or suspected atherosclerotic heart disease. This figure represented 5 percent of the population at that time. Twenty of every one hundred American males develop angina pectoris or a myocardial infarction by age sixty. Of these, one-third die within minutes to a few hours of the onset. Two-thirds of these deaths occur before hospitalization is possible. For those who survive an initial infarction, the risk of another is five times greater than for men of the same age who have not previously had an attack.

Atherosclerosis of some degree is universally present among postadolescents in affluent societies, particularly in the United States, Canada, and Northern Europe. The high incidence of atherosclerosis in these countries, and by contrast, the low incidence of it in developing nations, is related to certain environmental conditions that lead to the inception and progression of atherosclerosis. The disease tends to proceed more rapidly in the coronary arteries than in the cerebral circulation. This tendency is reflected by the fact that in the United States 25 percent of deaths resulting from coronary heart disease occur primarily in males under age sixty-five, whereas only about 15 percent of deaths from cerebrovascular disease occur in this "preretirement" age group. For this reason, the major emphasis of research and medical care has been on the study of coronary atherosclerosis.

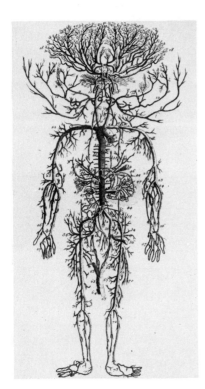

Figure 11.6. The arterial system. Illustration appearing in the *Medicinal Dictionary* by James Robert (1743–1745). (Courtesy of the World Health Organization)

Risk factors

Epidemiologic studies (cohort studies, described in Chap. 8), supported by clinical research and investigations using laboratory animals, indicate that certain hereditary and environmental factors increase the risk of atherosclerosis. A combination of these factors increases the risk still further.

SEX The severity of atherosclerosis and the frequency of atherosclerotic heart and brain disease is much less among premonopausal women than among men. However, by the time women reach age sixty or sixty-five, this early advantage is completely lost.

FAMILY HISTORY The risk of developing atherosclerotic heart disease is greater for persons with a maternal or paternal history of premature (before age sixty) heart attacks than for those without. But this increase in risk among certain families seems to be associated as much with environmental as with hereditary factors. In other words, both the genetic structure and the structure of home life, particularly as it concerns cigarette smoking, eating, and exercising, are shared in families.

BLOOD CHOLESTEROL AND TRIGLYCERIDES The principal blood fats are triglycerides, cholesterol, and phospholipids. These substances are not soluble in blood plasma; therefore whether ingested in the diet or synthesized in body tissues, they must be made soluble enough to be trans-

Dietary recommendations (American Heart Association)

With proper education, information and the availability of fat modified foods, it will be possible for most Americans to make desirable changes in their diets without major dislocation of personal eating habits.

Americans should be encouraged to modify habits with regard to all five major sources of fat in the U. S. diet—meats, dairy products, baked goods, eggs, table and cooking fats. Specifically a superior pattern of nutrient intake can be achieved by altering habits along the following lines:

Use lean cuts of beef, lamb, pork and veal, cooked to dispose of saturated fat and eaten in moderate portion sizes;

Use lean meat of poultry and fish;

Use fat-modified,* processed meat products (frankfurters, sausage, salami, etc.);

Use organ meats (e.g., liver) and shellfish in moderation since they are higher in cholesterol than muscle of red meat, chicken and fish;

Avoid fat cuts of meat, addition of saturated fat in cooking meat, large meat portions and processed meats high in saturated fat;

Use low fat and fat modified dairy products;

Avoid high saturated fat dairy products;

Use fat modified baked goods (pies, cookies, cakes, sweet rolls, doughnuts, crullers);

Avoid baked goods high in saturated fat and cholesterol;

Use salad and cooking oils, new soft margarines and shortenings low in saturated fat;

Avoid butter, margarine and shortenings high in saturated fat;

Avoid candies high in saturated fat;

Avoid egg yolk, bacon, lard, suet;

Use grains, fruits, vegetables, legumes.

* Throughout this set of guidelines *fat modified* refers to products made with reduced saturated fat and cholesterol content.

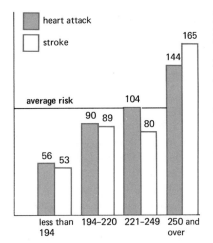

Figure 11.7. The relationship between the level of cholesterol in the blood and the risk of heart attack and stroke in men. Blood pressure is indicated by systolic pressure. (Courtesy of the American Heart Association)

ported through the blood stream. The body does this by wrapping large masses of triglyceride, cholesterol, and phospholipid in a protein coat. The resulting water soluble complexes are called *lipoproteins*. The accumulation of these liproproteins within an artery wall stimulates the atherosclerosis process. The concentration of lipoproteins circulating in the blood is determined by measuring the amount (in milligrams) of cholesterol or triglyceride in the lipoproteins per 100 milliliters of blood plasma. The result is called the serum cholesterol (or triglyceride) level. Though no specific level has been determined beyond which the risk of heart attack or stroke is certain, a man with a serum cholesterol level of 250 milligrams or higher is three times more apt to have a heart attack or stroke than is a man with a level of 194 milligrams or lower (Fig. 11.7).

In every segment of the American population, the higher the level of cholesterol or triglyceride, the greater the risk of developing angina pectoris, a heart attack, or a stroke. The blood levels of both fats also affect the development of atherosclerosis in laboratory animals. In both humans and animals, these levels are controlled by the kind and amount of dietary fat. Restricting the amount of cholesterol in the diet (mainly from egg yolks) and substituting polyunsaturated (vegetable) fats for saturated (animal) fats, can lower all blood fat levels (see Chap. 5). There is now good evidence that persons adhering to such a diet will lower their risk of heart attack.

BLOOD PRESSURE   The relationship of blood pressure to atherosclerotic vascular disease is similar to that of the blood fats—each elevation in level carries an increased risk of disease. Furthermore, the effects from the combination of a high serum cholesterol level with high blood pressure produce a higher risk of atherosclerotic disease than would be expected from a simple additive effect of either condition alone. Blood pressure is also influenced by dietary regulation. As mentioned earlier, a high sodium intake, mainly in the form of table salt, is associated with high blood pressure. A decrease in sodium intake will lower blood pressure. However, low sodium diets are difficult to maintain, and for persons with high blood pressure levels, modern, safe drugs can be effectively and more easily used.

CIGARETTE SMOKING   Repeated studies have shown cigarette smoking to be related to a higher risk of developing and dying from a myocardial infarction. The precise nature of the association between smoking and coronary heart disease has not been determined, but some evidence indicates that the nicotine absorbed by the body helps to constrict arteries already narrowed by atherosclerosis. Depending on the number of cigarettes smoked, the risk of developing coronary heart disease can be up to three times as high for smokers as for nonsmokers (Fig. 11.8). This subject is discussed in greater detail in Chapter 15.

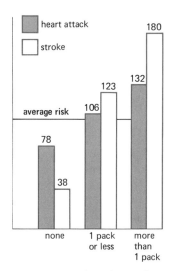

Figure 11.8. The relationship between cigarette smoking and the risk of heart attack and stroke in men. Note that compared to a nonsmoker, a man who smokes more than a pack of cigarettes a day has over five times the risk of stroke. (Courtesy of the American Heart Association)

OBESITY AND SEDENTARY LIVING When the number of calories consumed is greater than the number expended through physical activity, obesity results (Chap. 6). Obesity may enhance the progression of atherosclerosis through its association with elevated levels of blood fats and blood pressure. Weight reduction, either through eating less or exercising more (ideally both), leads to a lowering of blood cholesterol, triglycerides, and pressure. Furthermore, there is evidence that physical activity helps to increase the interconnections in the coronary blood supply and thus makes an occlusion at any point less likely to lead to a fatal outcome. The problems of obesity and sedentary living are hallmarks of affluent societies everywhere.

DIABETES This chronic disease, partly genetically and partly environmentally induced, causes widespread alterations in the body's metabolism. Although the inability to utilize sugar is the best known aspect of this disease, diabetes is also associated with elevations of blood fat levels. Even with careful management of dietary carbohydrates and insulin therapy, diabetics generally run a higher than average risk of developing atherosclerotic disease of the heart, brain, and large arteries supplying the legs. Currently, increasing attention is being paid to dietary regulation of blood fats in diabetics.

Diagnosis

A myocardial infarction is usually signaled by a pain in the chest (angina pectoris) which sometimes radiates to other areas of the body. An accumulation of fluid in the legs and lungs may indicate a heart failure, for as the heart pumps out less blood into the arteries, the pressure in the veins rises and water leaks out into the tissues. Changes in heart contractions are detected by a delicate machine called an electrocardiograph and recorded on a chart called an electrocardiogram. The recordings are used to diagnose an inadequate supply of oxygen to or the death of heart muscle. The death of heart muscle causes a release of enzymes into the general blood stream, and their measurement can lend support to the electrocardiographic findings. Advanced atherosclerosis of the coronary arteries can also be diagnosed from an exercise tolerance test, during and after which the physician looks for electrocardiographic changes resulting from an inadequate supply of oxygen to the heart muscle. Quite recently, techniques have been developed to inject an x-ray dense dye directly into the coronary arteries while simultaneously taking rapid x-ray pictures. This is called coronary angiography, and it allows a direct view of the points of narrowing and occlusion within the coronary circulation.

A diagnosis of a cerebrovascular accident depends on such symptoms as an alteration in the state of consciousness or a headache. If an artery becomes obstructed by a clot there is a rather sudden onset of localized nervous defects. If a hemorrhage occurs, there may be increased pressure of the spinal fluid and sometimes blood in this fluid.

Treatment and prevention

Over the past ten years, coronary care units (CCUs) have been established in many hospitals. The specialized, intensive care provided by these units has reduced "in hospital" death rates by 20 to 30 percent. Treatment is aimed at maintaining both the normal rhythmic beat of the heart and an adequate circulation. Under certain circumstances, electrical devices called pacemakers are used to overcome the interference with the normal sequence of nerve conduction to the heart which results from a coronary occlusion. Miniature electronic equipment and long-life batteries have made possible the implantation of devices that periodically stimulate the heart and maintain a normal, constant rhythm. Small, atomically powered devices are also currently being used.

In other cases, blocked or severely narrowed segments of the coronary arteries can be bypassed by grafting veins usually taken from the leg of the patient. This procedure can, for a while at least, reduce disability due to inadequately nourished heart muscle. Heart transplants and artificial hearts may hold some future benefit.

Most deaths from atherosclerotic cardiovascular disease occur before hospitalization is possible. Thus, the most significant approach to the tremendous problem of this form of heart disease is not in treatment but in prevention or retardation of the rate of development of the underlying atherosclerosis. This approach requires favorable alteration of those risk factors that are under environmental control. Already we know from small-scale studies that dietary changes to reduce the level of blood fats, the use of drugs to treat greatly elevated blood pressure, the cessation of cigarette smoking, and the permanent reduction of obesity will lower the rate of heart attacks. By inference, these same steps can also reduce the risk of atherosclerotic cerebrovascular disease. Considering the life-long course of atherosclerosis, attention should be paid to these factors in adolescence, perhaps even earlier.

CANCER   Though the chances of survival from cancer are greater today than they were forty years ago (one-in-three in the 1970s compared to one-in-six in the 1930s), the incidence of cancer, particularly in men, is also greater. Over half a million Americans will be diagnosed for the first time with cancer this year; over half of them (355,000) will die of the disease. Nearly one-third of those who will die (109,000) might have been saved by earlier diagnosis and treatment. To help prevent these unnecessary tragedies, the American Cancer Society has established extensive adult and youth programs throughout the United States to educate the public concerning the symptoms and early detection of cancer.

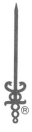

The Sword of Hope

The Sword of Hope is the symbol that to most Americans means "Help Fight Cancer." As the registered trademark of the American Cancer Society, it has for many years reflected the ACS image and identity. Today it remains the insignia of the national voluntary health organization that fights cancer on the broad fronts of research, education, service. It is the emblem that guides contributors who seek to make sure that their gifts go to the traditional ACS Cancer Crusade.

For this reason, the Sword of Hope is displayed in all Crusade materials, literature, posters, ads, films, etc., and is shown at meetings, lectures, exhibits, film showings.

The sword originated out of a nation-wide poster contest in 1928. The blade was meant to express the crusading spirit of the cancer control movement. The twin serpent caduceus forming the hilt emphasizes the medical and scientific aspects of the attack. The original insignia carried the slogan "Fight Cancer With Knowledge." Variations of this theme have been used by the ACS since then.

From *Cancer Facts and Figures, 1974,* a publication of the American Cancer Society.

Contributing factors

We still do not known the cause of cancer. Moreover, the types and courses of various cancers are sufficiently different so that we can assume there are probably multiple factors causing cancer which operate in a complex fashion and over a long period of time. It seems unlikely that identification of any single factor will yield complete information on all cancers. On the basis of epidemiologic evidence and experimental animal studies, we do know that there are several categories of factors that are strongly linked to cancer.

CARCINOGENS Carcinogens are chemical compounds capable of inducing cancer. Some of these substances have been identified in coal and tobacco tars. Cancer of the scrotum (commonly seen among chimney sweeps a generation ago) and lung cancer among cigarette smokers are examples of cancers in humans associated with carcinogens that are capable of inducing cancers in experimental animals.

RADIATION Ionizing radiation—whether from x-rays, radioactive atoms, or sunlight—has been associated with various types of cancer in man and with experimentally induced cancer in laboratory animals. That skin cancers frequently occur in sun-exposed areas of fair-skinned individuals is well known. Prolonged exposure to x-ray radiation is associated with both superficial cancers and leukemia. The occurrence of lung cancer among uranium miners is an example of the potential of radioactive compounds to cause cancer.

VIRUSES There is increasing evidence linking viruses to various cancers in experimental animals which suggests a link also to some types of cancer in humans. Intense research is currently being done on the relationship between viruses and cancer, especially because there is the possibility of using the immune mechanism to prevent or retard the cancer growth if the link exists.

HEREDITY In addition to the environmental factors already discussed, genetic factors may also contribute to cause cancer. There is good evidence in man that predisposition to certain types of cancer does run in families. In laboratory animals, inbreeding studies have produced strains very sensitive or very resistant to various induced cancers.

OTHER ENVIRONMENTAL INFLUENCES The epidemiology of cancer strongly suggests the presence of environmental factors of as yet unknown identity or mode of action. For example, among individuals working with asbestos there is a greater than average frequency of lung cancer as well as of a type of cancer arising in the layer of mesothelial cells lining the thoracic and abdominal cavities. This latter site is rarely a site of origin of cancer in persons never exposed to asbestos. How an inorganic fiber could cause cancer is still a mystery.

Geographic patterns of cancer as well as the way patterns of cancer change in migrating populations and in stable populations over a period of time provide further examples of the effects of the environment on cancer. Cancer of the liver is common in parts of Africa; cancer of the urinary bladder is common in persons in the Middle East who are infested with a particular parasite. The frequency of stomach cancer is high among Orientals living in their native lands, whereas among persons of oriental heritage living in the United States the frequency is comparable to that in Caucasians. Interestingly, cancer of the stomach has become steadily less common in the United States over the past fifty years. Conversely, the frequency of cancer of the large bowel is much higher in the United States and Europe than in any other areas of the world. This latter observation has been linked to dietary habits which affect the kind of bacterial population living in the bowel and possibly to dietary carcinogens.

The nature of cancer

A tumor or neoplasm is an abnormal growth of cellular tissue serving no physiological purpose. A tumor is said to be malignant if from its original location it can spread to other parts of the body. Cancer is a disease characterized by malignant tumors; a cancer refers to the malignant tumor itself.

Benign tumors rarely become malignant; their cellular characteristics remain similar to those of the surrounding normal cells from which they arose. They are usually well demarcated, grow slowly, and do not kill unless they occur in the brain or other location where they cause lethal pressure on a vessel or airway.

On the other hand, malignant cancers show cellular characteristics different from the cells from which they arose. The main difference is in the nucleus. The nucleus normally regulates the growth, development, and reproduction of the cell; but in a cancerous cell the nucleus becomes enlarged, loses its regulatory ability, and allows the cell to divide at random. Possibly this rapid, uncontrolled cell division is due to the large increase in the number of chromosomes (often twice the usual 46 and occasionally many times more) which also occurs in cancerous cells. Moreover, since the nucleus loses its ability to regulate not only the quantity but also the kind of cells that are reproduced, many people believe that the nucleic DNA and RNA (Chap. 1) which control cell differentiation are affected by cancer.

Normally, properly differentiated cells do not interfere with the functioning of cells that are not of their same kind. Liver cells do not associate with lung cells, for example. But, improperly differentiated, these cancerous cells ignore the kind of cells from which they originated and spread throughout the body, infecting other kinds of cells. Cancerous cells do not adhere as closely to each other as do normal cells, and so they are easily broken off from their original location and able to spread to other parts of the body. This spreading can occur in several ways:

1. Some cancerous cells may penetrate the blood or lymphatic vessels which distribute them throughout the body. The cells are then able to form new cancer masses elsewhere. This spreading of disease from its original location to distant parts of the body is called *metastasis*.

2. A tumor in a body cavity such as the thorax or abdomen may shed cells which implant themselves throughout the cavity or in nearby organs, multiply and produce new tumors, and so spread the cancer.

3. A tumor may so enlarge and expand in its original location that it is able to invade and infect surrounding tissue.

The rate of growth, the pattern of spread, and therefore the clinical course of cancers are generally characteristic of the tissue of origin. Early diagnosis and treatment can often arrest the growth of a tumor before widespread and irreparable metastasis, implantation, or invasion has taken place.

Ordinarily, the replacement of body cells lost by wear and tear and the new growth of cells to repair the injury are perfectly regulated events. The nature of cancer, in particular the process whereby cancer cells become independent of the body's control mechanisms that ordinarily regulate growth, is one of the leading challenges to contemporary biological research.

Types of cancer

There are two principal types of cancer. *Carcinomas* are cancers of the epithelial tissue (cancer of the skin, breast, lung, colon, rectum, prostate, uterus, and stomach) which metastasize primarily by means of the lymph vessels. *Sarcomas* are cancers of the connective tissue (bone, muscle, or cartilage cancer) which metastasize primarily by means of the blood vessels. The incidence rate of the different types of cancer varies according to age and sex (Fig. 11.9). Among adult males, the five most common sites of cancers causing death are the lung, large bowel, prostate, stomach, and pancreas. Among females the leading five are the breast, large bowel, uterus, lung, and ovary. Among children, leukemia (a third type of cancer which infects the blood-forming tissues) is the major cause of death from cancer; it is followed by cancer of the brain and nervous tissue.

Symptoms

With almost all cancers, the earlier a diagnosis is made, the better are the chances for successful treatment. For this reason, the American Cancer Society publishes yearly a series of pamphlets free to the American public outlining the seven warning signals of cancer as well as

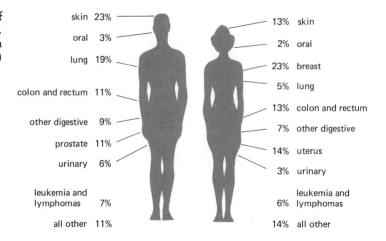

Figure 11.9. The percentages of cancer incidence by site and sex. (Courtesy of the American Cancer Society)

skin 23%	13% skin
oral 3%	2% oral
lung 19%	23% breast
	5% lung
colon and rectum 11%	13% colon and rectum
other digestive 9%	7% other digestive
prostate 11%	14% uterus
urinary 6%	3% urinary
leukemia and lymphomas 7%	6% leukemia and lymphomas
all other 11%	14% all other

providing general information on the nature of cancer. The alert individual is often the first to notice a warning symptom of cancer, and early personal recognition when followed by immediate medical care greatly increases the effectiveness of treatment. Many women have prevented widespread cancer of the breast by carefully checking each month for symptoms of breast cancer and seeking prompt attention if any unusual lump or thickening appeared. Though by knowing the seven warning signals an individual may detect a possible symptom of cancer, only a physician can make a sure diagnosis. The best precaution against cancer is a thorough, annual physical checkup by a physician.

Diagnosis

Blood tests can be used to diagnose leukemia (cancer of the blood cells themselves), but there are not yet any specific and reliable blood tests available for other types of cancer.

Table 11.2 Leading cancer sites, 1974

Site and estimated deaths, 1974	Warning signal	Safeguards	Comment
Breast (33,000)	Lump or thickening in the breast	Annual checkup; monthly breast self exam	The leading cause of cancer death in women
Colon and rectum (48,000)	Change in bowel habits; bleeding	Annual checkup including proctoscopy, especially for those over 40	Considered highly curable when digital and proctoscopic examinations are included in routine checkups
Lung (75,000)	Persistent cough, or lingering respiratory ailment	Prevention: heed facts about smoking, annual checkup, chest x-ray	The leading cause of cancer death among men, largely preventable

Table 11.2 Leading cancer sites, 1974 (Continued)

Oral (including pharynx) (8,000)	Sore that does not heal, difficulty in swallowing	Annual checkup	Many more lives should be saved because the mouth is easily accessible to visual examination by physicians and dentists
Skin (5,000)	Sore that does not heal, or change in wart or mole	Annual checkup, avoidance of overexposure to sun	Readily detected by observation, and diagnosed by simple biopsy
Uterus (11,000)	Unusual bleeding or discharge	Annual checkup, including pelvic examination with Pap test	Uterine cancer mortality has declined 65% during the last 35 years. With more application of the Pap test, many more lives can be saved, especially from cervical cancer
Kidney and bladder (16,000)	Urinary difficulty, bleeding—in which case consult doctor at once	Annual checkup with urinalysis	Protective measures for workers in high-risk industries are helping to eliminate one of the important causes of these cancers
Larynx (3,000)	Hoarseness—difficulty in swallowing	Annual checkup, including mirror laryngoscopy	Readily curable if caught early
Prostate (18,000)	Urinary difficulty	Annual checkup, including palpation	Occurs mainly in men over 60, can be detected by palpation and urinalysis at annual checkup
Stomach (14,000)	Indigestion	Annual checkup	A 40% decline in mortality in 20 years, for reasons yet unknown
Leukemia (15,000)	A cancer of blood-forming tissues characterized by the abnormal production of immature white blood cells. Acute leukemia strikes mainly children and is treated by drugs which have extended life from a few months to as much as ten years. Chronic leukemia strikes usually after age 25 and progresses less rapidly		
	If drugs or vaccines are found which can cure or prevent any cancers they probably will be successful first for leukemia and the lymphomas		
Lymphomas (20,000)	These diseases arise in the lymph system and include Hodgkin's and lymphosarcoma. Some patients with lymphatic cancers can lead normal lives for many years		

From *'74 Cancer Facts and Figures*, American Cancer Society.

Because cancer cells are shed so easily, an examination of cells lining certain organs, especially the lung and uterine cervix, has been useful in screening and therefore earlier diagnosis. The techniques of obtaining, preparing, and evaluating such preparations (a procedure called *exfoliative cytology*) were systematized by Dr. George Papanicolaou, after whom the "Pap test" was named. The Pap test is a simple, painless method of extracting and examining cells of the cervix for indications of

Cancer's 7 warning signals

1. Change in bowel or bladder habits
2. A sore that does not heal
3. Unusual bleeding or discharge
4. Thickening or lump in breast or elsewhere
5. Indigestion or difficulty in swallowing
6. Obvious change in wart or mole
7. Nagging cough or hoarseness
If you have a warning signal, see your doctor!

The 7 safeguards urged by ACS

Lung: Reduction and ultimate elimination of cigarette smoking
Colon-Rectum: Proctoscopic exam as routine in annual checkup for those over 40.
Breast: Self-examination as monthly female practice.
Uterus: Pap test for all adult and high-risk women.
Skin: Avoidance of excessive sun.
Oral: Wider practice of early detection measures.
Basic: Annual physical examination for all adults.

uterine cancer. Cells lining the cervix are shed normally and collect in the vagina as old cells die and new cells are produced to replace them. By inserting a cotton swab into the vagina and scraping the surface of the cervix, a physician can gather the cells for examination under a microscope. Not only can this method detect cancer before there are any symptoms, but also it can detect changes in the cells that may indicate a possibility of cancer developing. The Pap test thus can warn of cancer before the disease has a chance to begin. For this reason, an annual checkup is strongly recommended for all women. About 11,000 women die each year of uterine cancer; most of them could be saved by an early and simple examination with a Pap test.

Yet even with a suspicious or positive Pap test, a sure diagnosis depends on the microscopic examination of a part or all of the growth after surgical removal. This removal and examination of tissue is called *biopsy*. For the most part, the conditions that determine the appropriate therapy and the chance of successful treatment are the tissue of origin of cancer, the degree of spread, and the age and general condition of the patient.

Modes of death from cancer

Almost all cancers are associated with losses of appetite and weight. These can lead to generalized debility and poor resistance. Prolonged wasting away and undernourishment of a cancer patient eventually can cause his death.

Anemia is also common among cancer patients. It can result from malnutrition, cancer in blood-forming tissue, or cancerous erosion of a blood vessel. A cancer patient may experience intestinal bleeding which also causes anemia.

General debility or anemia can sufficiently lower the effectiveness of the body's normal defense mechanisms so that death may result from a bacterial or fungus infection.

Treatment

Once a new case of cancer has been diagnosed, the chance of a cure varies widely. A "cure" of cancer is defined as survival for five or ten years after diagnosis and treatment. Five-year survival is almost 90 percent for skin cancer and about 9 percent for lung cancer. This is the reason why the very common cancer of the skin is rarely responsible for death. The average five-year survival rates for the major types of cancer are shown in Figure 11.10.

The major modes of therapy have long been surgery and radiation. With a small, localized cancer, surgery can be completely successful; but with spread, the chances are less good, and often the extent of metastasis cannot be initially ascertained. Radiation treatment may utilize x-rays, radioactive elements such as cobalt, or laser beams. This approach is often effective because rapidly multiplying cancer cells are

Figure 11.10. Five-year cancer survival rates for selected sites (adjusted for normal life expectancy). (End Results Group, National Cancer Institute)

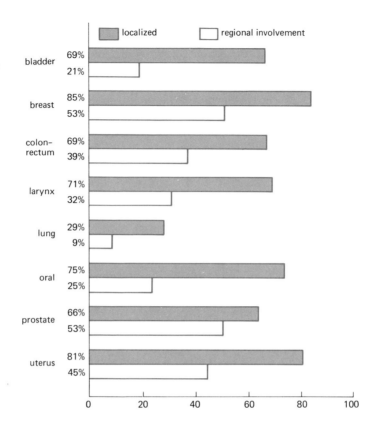

quite susceptible to lethal radiation damage. However, since other normally multiplying cells are also, though less, susceptible, there are often unfortunate side effects from radiation. The different types of cancers vary considerably in their response to radiation.

Some kinds of cancer are manageable by hormone therapy or by specific chemicals which, like radiation, affect cancer cells more than normal tissues. This latter approach—called *chemotherapy*—has been particularly useful in prolonging the survival of patients with cancers of the blood-forming and lymphatic system. In these cases, the disease has spread so extensively throughout the body that effective treatment through surgery or radiation is impossible.

Prevention

Though in many cases the initial cancer cannot be prevented, early diagnosis can greatly help to prevent death from cancer. There is much still to be done in applying present knowledge to population screening and early case-finding and in assuring an adequate periodic health examination for a larger proportion of our population. Widespread observance of the safeguards set forth by the American Cancer Society would lead to a tremendous reduction in cancer deaths.

Control of environmental factors associated with cancer may hold great future promise. At present, the most dramatic evidence that cancer is preventable through environmental alteration concerns lung cancer. There is strong epidemiologic evidence that cigarette smokers who have quit over a period of time have *less* risk of developing lung cancer than their counterparts who persist in smoking. Although the reduction in risk is greater as time passes from the moment a person stops smoking, he or she will never achieve the low risk of lung cancer enjoyed by those who have never smoked at all. Nonetheless, this evidence lends support to the theory that identifying and altering other environmental conditions that contribute to cancer will lower the incidence and death rates of cancer.

OTHER NONCOMMUNICABLE DISEASES

Diabetes

Diabetes mellitus originally referred to a condition associated with a larger than usual volume of urine that contained sugar. But this association accounts for only part of the condition. Diabetes is a systemic disease. It represents a defect in carbohydrate (sugar) metabolism resulting from a defect in or absence of the hormone insulin. Insulin regulates the level of blood sugar by allowing the sugar to enter the body cells where it can be metabolized. Not all diabetics have blood sugar levels high enough for sugar to spill over into the urine. Some diabetics exhibit higher than normal blood sugars only after a sugar-containing meal. These latter groups can be identified only through appropriate screening.

Much, but not all, of the tendency to develop diabetes is hereditary. Prolonged use of high-sugar diets, however, may induce the appearance of diabetes. Obesity also is associated with diabetes, and an important aspect of effective medical treatment for diabetes is weight reduction if the patient is obese.

Three types of defects have been noted in diabetic persons:
1. decrease or absence of production of insulin by the pancreas;
2. pancreatic production of an abnormal form of insulin that is less active in allowing dietary sugar to leave the blood stream and enter the cells;
3. circulation in the blood of substances that partly neutralize the effect of the body's insulin.

Insulin treatments, close attention to dietary sugar ingestion, and weight reduction have much improved the prospects of the diabetic patient. Antibiotics have reduced the hazards of infectious diseases to which diabetics are unusually susceptible. Nevertheless, even well-controlled diabetics have a significantly shortened life span. The major reason for this is that diabetes—even mild diabetes—predisposes to a more rapid progression of atherosclerosis, leading to the sort of premature death and disability discussed earlier in this chapter. More intense population screening and implementation of preventive measures against atherosclerosis could perhaps be the next great advance in aid for diabetics. It is estimated that some 8 percent of our population has some detectable degree of diabetes, thus making it a chronic disease of enormous significance.

Diseases of endocrine glands

There are other diseases of the endocrine glands which are less common than diabetes. Some of these result from the malfunctioning of the pituitary gland. The pituitary gland manufactures a variety of hormones responsible for normal growth and metabolic functions. A decrease or absence of the growth hormone leads to dwarfism; overproduction can lead to gigantism, which usually results from a tumor of the pituitary gland. In addition, there are many disorders related to either the under- or overfunctioning of the thyroid gland, the adrenal, the parathyroid, and the reproductive glands. Underproduction of a particular hormone can, for the most part, be presently managed by administration of that hormone (as with insulin for the diabetic). There is still no specific, effective therapy for the overproduction of these hormones.

Neurologic diseases

Multiple sclerosis is a disease involving the nerves of the base of the brain and spinal cord. The material that insulates the nerves, called myelin, is lost, causing the nerve fibers to degenerate. This in turn results in defects in sensory and motor nerves. The latter defect leads to impairment in walking, use of hands, vision, and speech. The clinical course of the disease is prolonged, progressive, and marked by cycles of remission and recurrence. The cause is still unknown, and there is as yet no treatment to arrest the process.

Parkinson's disease affects areas of the brain responsible for muscle control. Patients with Parkinson's disease show rigidity of muscles and a tremor most notable in the constant movement of the fingers. It is now known that the great worldwide epidemic of influenza following World War I led to a large proportion of the cases of Parkinsonism seen in the past few decades.

Degenerative diseases

The last category of noninfectious disorders of significant medical importance is arthritis. The term refers to inflammation of the tissues lining the joints between bones or to degeneration of the adjacent surfaces of the bones comprising a joint.

Rheumatoid arthritis is the leading example of the first type disorder. Affecting females about three times as frequently as males, this disease has both hereditary and still uncertain environmental causes. Perhaps the most widely accepted theory is that the immune response mechanisms (see Chap. 9) are involved. The disease takes a prolonged clinical course with remissions and relapses. The periodic inflammation of the joints leads to eventual destruction of the bone surfaces and eventually to permanent deformities which are most marked in the small joints of the wrist, fingers, and feet. Treatment with aspirin or with pituitary and adrenal hormones may give symptomatic relief as well as slow the progression of the disease, but these drugs do not cure whatever underlying process is responsible for it.

Osteoarthritis, on the other hand, occurs later in life and affects males and females with equal frequency. It also involves the large, weight-bearing joints. The disease is a result primarily of "wear and tear," and here again, the joint symptoms and deformities occur partly from atrophy of bone substance in older persons. So far, treatment is aimed only at symptomatic relief.

Key Concepts
Angina pectoris – a pain over the heart, often radiating to the left arm or abdomen, which results from inadequate oxygen supply to heart muscle; pain is produced by physical or emotional stress in individuals whose coronary blood supply is severely impaired by atherosclerosis

Atherosclerosis – a thickening of the artery wall which narrows the internal diameter of the artery and results from deposits of cholesterol and other fatty substances

Cancer – a malignant tumor or neoplasm whose growth is not regulated by normal body mechanisms and which often spreads either through the circulatory system to distant parts of the body or by direct invasion of local tissue. Cancers which arise from epithelial tissue are called *carcinomas;* those which are arise from connective tissue are called *sarcomas*

Cerebrovascular accident ("stroke") – the death of local brain tissue due to the sudden blocking of its blood supply, usually by a clot formation (thrombus) or by the lodging of a roving clot (embolus) in an area of severe atherosclerotic narrowing

Hypertension – the persistent elevation of blood pressure above a systolic pressure of 140 and a diastolic pressure of 90; the limit is an arbitrary but generally accepted definition of high blood pressure

Myocardial infarction ("heart attack") – the death of heart muscle due to the sudden blocking of its blood supply, usually by a clot formation in an area of atherosclerotic narrowing

Metastasis – the spread of cancer cells to distant body sites, often by blood or lymphatic vessels

Rheumatic fever – a disease affecting primarily children and characterized by inflammation of the joints and fever; if untreated, the infection can severely damage the valves of the heart, causing a heart murmur to develop and the heart thus to overwork

Questions
1. What environmental factors are associated with heart attacks? With certain types of cancer?
2. Discuss the problems of changing those factors in our present way of life which are associated with heart disease and cancer.

3. What are the merits of screening our population in order to identify persons with great risk of developing premature heart attack or stroke? Who should have responsibility? Who should pay the cost of screening?
4. How do malignant cancers spread throughout the body?

Selected Readings
American Cancer Society. *1974 Cancer Facts and Figures.*

American Heart Association. *1973 Heart Facts.*

Boyd, W. *An Introduction to the Study of Disease.* Philadelphia: Lea and Febiger, 1971.

Robbins, S. L., and M. Angell. *Basic Pathology.* Philadelphia: W. B. Saunders, 1971.

Selzer, Arthur. *The Heart: Its Function in Health and Disease.* Berkeley: University of California Press, 1969.

Chapter 12

Oral Health and Disease

THE HUMAN DENTITIONS

Although humans have two sets of teeth (primary and adult) to last throughout life, these appear to be far from adequate for most individuals due to the loss of teeth from *dental caries* (decay) or *periodontal disease*. The primary dentition, composed of ten teeth in the upper (maxillary) jaw and ten teeth in the lower (mandibular) jaw, should last from approximately six months to twelve years of age. At that time all of the primary teeth will have been replaced naturally by the growth, development, and eruption of the underlying permanent teeth (Fig. 12.1). The complete adult dentition which contains thirty-two teeth—sixteen in each jaw—starts to appear at age six with the eruption of the first permanent molar behind the last primary tooth. The third permanent molar or wisdom tooth should be in position during the late teens or early twenties, signaling the completion of eruption for the permanent dentition (Fig. 12.2).

Starting from the middle of the mouth and moving back, each half

This chapter was contributed by Paul Goldhaber, D.D.S., Dean and Professor of Periodontology, Harvard School of Dental Medicine.

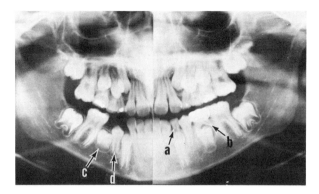

Figure 12.1. Panorex x-ray of ten-year-old child with both primary and adult teeth in position. Many adult teeth are still totally in the jawbone, where they are completing their formation and are in the process of erupting into the oral cavity. In some areas the roots of the primary teeth are being destroyed (a and b) so that the teeth will loosen and be shed and the permanent teeth can erupt into the vacated space; in other areas (c and d) the primary teeth have already been lost and the permanent teeth are about to erupt into the mouth.

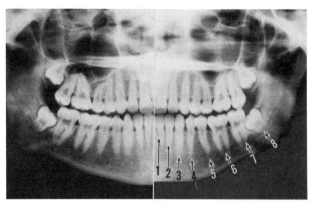

Figure 12.2. A healthy adult dentition of twenty-one-year-old individual. Each half of each jaw (quadrant) contains the following eight teeth: (1) central incisor, (2) lateral incisor, (3) cuspid (or canine), (4) first bicuspid or premolar, (5) second bicuspid, (6) first molar, (7) second molar, (8) third molar or wisdom tooth. Note that all four wisdom teeth are entirely embedded in the jawbone. Periodic examination will be needed to determine whether these teeth will erupt properly into the oral cavity or whether any of them will be trapped in the jawbone, possibly requiring extraction by the dentist.

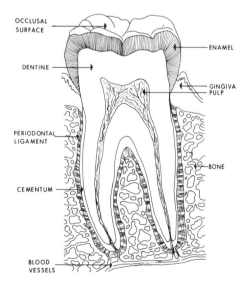

Figure 12.3. Diagram showing cross-section through a lower molar tooth and its surrounding tissues.

of each jaw (or quadrant) contains the following eight teeth: central incisor, lateral incisor, cuspid, first and second bicuspids, first and second molars, and third molar (or wisdom tooth). Each tooth is composed of a crown and root portion (Fig. 12.3). The crown has a relatively thin, extraordinarily hard, outer layer of *enamel*. The root has a very thin outer layer of *cementum* in which are embedded the fibers of the periodontal *ligament*. The periodontal ligament fibers are attached to the bony wall of the tooth socket in the jaw, forming a hammock or sling and enabling forces acting upon the teeth during chewing or clenching to be transmitted to the bone surrounding the roots of the teeth. The bulk of the tooth structure is *dentin*, which surrounds the central pulp chamber containing blood vessels, nerves, and other connective tissue elements. With age, the enamel on the chewing surfaces of the teeth wears down exposing the underlying dentin. New dentin is continuously laid down next to the pulp. This causes the pulp chamber to recede and become narrower, thereby accommodating for the wearing away of enamel and dentin on the biting surface.

STATISTICS ABOUT ORAL HEALTH PROBLEMS

By age two, when all twenty primary teeth have erupted into the oral cavity and are functioning, half of the children in the United States have at least one decayed tooth. On entering school, the average child has three decayed teeth, and by age fifteen the average child has eleven teeth that are either decayed, filled, or missing (primarily as a result of extraction due to dental caries). The statistics become more grim with increasing age. A total of 25 million people in the United States are completely without natural teeth: three of ten people past age 35, four of ten people past age 45, five of ten people past age 55 (Fig. 12.4). Dental caries accounts for about 36 percent of all tooth loss while periodontal disease is responsible for about 50 percent of tooth loss.

While the above statistics focus on the two most prevalent diseases of the oral cavity, dental caries and periodontal disease, it is important to note that there are several other more serious oral health problems. For example, cleft palate, with or without cleft lip, occurs about once in

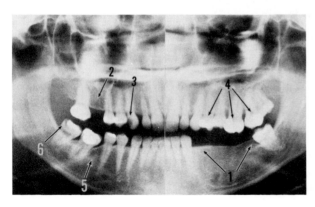

Figure 12.4. Twenty-five-year-old individual showing (1) extensive loss of teeth—4 teeth missing, (2) loss of upper first molar, (3) deep dental caries in upper cuspid, (4) extensive fillings in most of the remaining molars and premolars—white patches on crowns of teeth, (5) early loss of lower first molar with drifting of remaining molars forward and premolars backward to fill in space, (6) redecay under filling of lower third molar.

every 700 births and affects approximately 6,000 babies annually. Oral cancer occurs in approximately 14,000 new patients each year and accounts for over 7,000 deaths yearly, or one in every forty deaths from cancer throughout the body.

DENTAL CARIES

Causes

Dental caries is a localized and progressive destruction of the hard tissue of the tooth, usually starting on the biting surfaces of the rear teeth, the contact areas between adjacent teeth, or along the gum line. Demineralization of the tooth substance results from adherent bacteria. Destruction of the embedded tooth protein occurs as a result of continued bacterial action, leading to the formation of a cavity which will continue to expand if unchecked by a dentist.

During the past two decades, animal research has strongly supported the idea that dental caries is an infectious and transmissible disease. Attention has focused on a particular group of bacteria (*Streptococcus mutans*) that occurs indigenously in the mouth of humans in various parts of the world. This organism is the most common streptococcus found in dental plaque and has been shown to induce dental caries in rats and hamsters when the animals were fed a high-sugar diet. Future research in this area will be directed toward discovering measures for reducing colonization of bacteria causing decay on the teeth or for suppressing their effects through antibacterial agents, metabolic inhibitors, or immunological approaches.

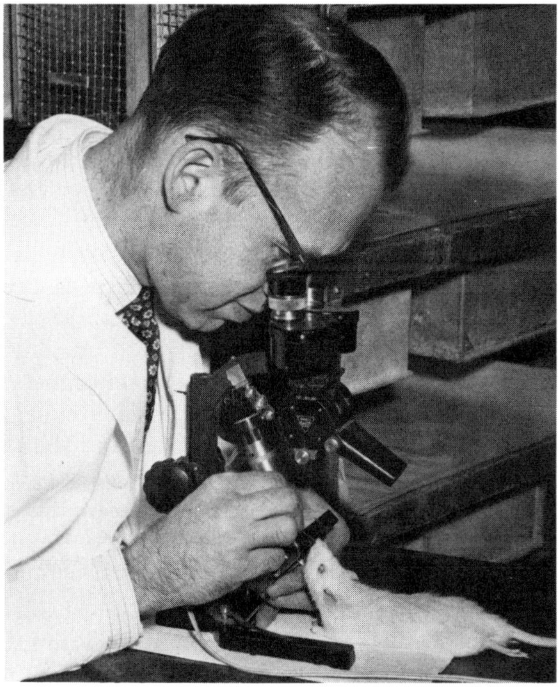

The discovery of general anesthesia Two dentists, Horace Wells and William Morton, are closely associated with the application of two well-known drugs to eliminate pain during surgery.

In 1844 Dr. Wells, one of the leading dentists of Hartford, Conn., was impressed by the pain-preventing potential of nitrous oxide gas during a demonstration of the effects of "laughing gas." He carried out several successful dental surgery procedures before making a demonstration at the Harvard Medical School. Unfortunately, the patient screamed out during the extraction and the experiment was deemed a failure—even though the patient later admitted feeling no pain and not knowing when the tooth had been extracted. Although this event resulted in the temporary abandonment of nitrous oxide as an anesthetic for general surgery, Wells must be credited with the concept of using anesthesia for such purposes.

Dr. Morton, a former partner and student of Wells, was more successful. On October 16, 1846, after a number of experiments with ether on animals, fish, and humans, Morton successfully anesthetized a patient for the removal of a jaw tumor at the Massachusetts General Hospital, thereby ushering in a new era in the control of pain and making possible the surgical advances of the past century.

Figure 12.5. A professor engaged in animal research to study the infectious and transmissible nature of dental decay and periodontal disease. Together these two forms of oral disease afflict 95 percent of the population.

Tooth implants

The transplantation of teeth from one person to another was carried out as early as the eighteenth century, but the process was abandoned because the teeth were usually rejected by the receiving patient. Reimplanting teeth—putting a tooth back into its original socket shortly following its loss as a result of a severe blow or accident, has been more successful. However, such teeth rarely last longer than five to six years.

In recent years, the polymer tooth implant procedure has been suggested as an alternate approach to the replacement of teeth. Briefly, this technique consists of fabricating an exact plastic replica of the extracted tooth and placing it in the socket within thirty minutes after extraction. Preliminary studies have shown that the plastic teeth become firm and can function as an integral part of the masticatory system. Should further controlled studies bear out these findings, it would provide a simple, relatively inexpensive approach to the replacement of missing teeth.

Treatment

The treatment of early or moderately advanced caries consists of cutting out the diseased portion of the tooth using a high-speed drill and rebuilding the missing portion of the tooth with an artificial substance such as amalgam (an alloy containing primarily silver as well as other metals), gold, silicates, or plastics.

As dental caries progresses and begins to advance closer to the pulp, pain will occur when cold objects such as ice cream or cold drinks contact the decayed tooth. At this stage, it may not be possible to see the cavity because of its small size or position between the teeth, and professional advice should be sought. A dentist will be able to determine whether a cavity exists by utilizing various diagnostic techniques, including X-rays. As the cavity progresses, pain may result from both heat and cold, and it may still be possible to treat the tooth by removing the decay and inserting a filling. However, when the symptoms change to pain from heat and relief from cold, the pulpal tissues are probably dead and the process of disease has become irreversible. The infection inevitably will engulf the entire pulp and affect the tissues around the end of the root resulting in abscess (*periapical granuloma*). An abscessed tooth is sensitive to pressure as slight as chewing or tapping and may cause excruciating pain due to the pressure exerted by the pus forming in the dead pulpal tissue. The pain may occur suddenly at night while asleep. If not treated, the abscess will penetrate the jaw bone and cause swelling in the surrounding soft tissues of the gum, the floor of the mouth, the palate, or cheek. If it is permitted to persist, the infection may spread through the tissue spaces and affect vital processes such as respiration, endangering the life of the individual. Once the pulpal tissue has died the only two possible methods of treatment are root canal therapy (a process where remaining pulpal tissue and infection are meticulously removed and replaced with an inert filling material to the apex of the root) or extraction.

Unfortunately, extraction of teeth, while solving the immediate problem of pain and infection, may create other long-term problems. For example, if a primary molar is prematurely lost, other teeth near the space created may shift position and prevent a permanent tooth from erupting in its proper position. This causes *malocclusion*, a condition in which the teeth fail to meet properly in closing the jaws. The loss of the lower first permanent molar frequently leads to the eruption of the upper first molar into the space and the shifting of the teeth on either side of the space. This not only leads to malocclusion but also encourages entrapment of food between the shifting teeth, subsequently causing dental caries and periodontal disease in those areas. For these reasons dentists prefer to avoid extractions. Where there is no alternative to extraction, a dentist will recommend inserting an artificial replacement, usually a *fixed bridge*, to fill the space of the missing tooth or teeth (Fig. 12.6).

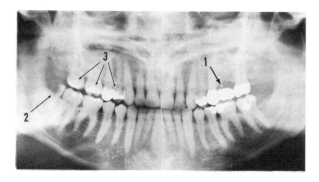

Figure 12.6. Panorex x-ray showing (1) three-unit fixed bridge in upper jaw replacing missing first molar, (2) badly decayed lower third molar with most of crown missing, (3) numerous fillings in the molar and premolar teeth.

PERIODONTAL DISEASE

Causes

There are several types of periodontal disease—diseases of the tissues surrounding the tooth, including the gingiva and supporting bone to which the tooth is attached. *Gingivitis,* the most common periodontal disease, is characterized by redness, swelling, and bleeding of the margins of the gums. About half of all school-age children in the United States have gingivitis, which, like dental caries, seems to be caused largely by the accumulation of oral bacteria and tartar (mineralized dental plaque) adjacent to the gum margin. *Dental plaque* is a soft, adherent deposit, composed primarily of bacteria, their extracellular products, and salivary proteins, that accumulates on the surfaces of teeth, especially near the margins of the gums. Apparently the presence of bacterial plaque is more important in initiating inflammation in the gum tissue than other factors such as tartar or overhanging margins of fillings or crowns. It is not clear how bacteria initiate the gum inflammation, but it is known that bacteria produce substances that have the potential to damage gum cells and cause an inflammatory response. The correlation of gingivitis with poor oral hygiene is striking. Experiments have shown that when oral hygiene procedures were not practiced by students with healthy gums, soft deposits of bacterial plaque accumulated around the gum margins and gingivitis developed within several weeks. These developments were completely reversed when supervised oral hygiene procedures were reintroduced. Clinical observations also show that gingivitis in children or adults is usually reversible in response to proper treatment and the institution of a rigid regimen of oral hygiene.

If ignored, the inflammation will eventually extend to the deeper periodontal tissues and will slowly destroy the underlying bones and periodontal ligament around the affected teeth, giving rise to *periodontitis* or *chronic destructive periodontal disease.* As the inflammation progresses, the gums become detached from the root surface and "pockets" form. Pus may form in the inflamed tissue, thereby accounting for the term "pyorrhea" (flow of pus). As a significant amount of the bony socket is destroyed and the periodontal ligament fibers lose their attachment to the bone, the affected teeth loosen (Fig. 12.7). If

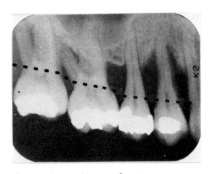

Figure 12.7. X-ray showing destruction of most of the alveolar bone around the two bicuspids and two molars. Only the tips of the roots are embedded in bone, leading to extreme looseness of the teeth. These teeth are beyond treatment at this stage and will be extracted. Dashed line shows where proper bone level should be.

this process is not intercepted by the dentist, the bone loss and tooth mobility will continue, accompanied by periodic episodes of periodontal abscess formation with pain and swelling, until the tooth must be extracted or is lost spontaneously.

Treatment

The treatment of periodontal disease consists of the careful removal of soft and hard deposits on the teeth. During the early stages, as in gingivitis, this is accomplished rather easily by periodic tooth cleaning (prophylaxis) by a dental hygienist and good home care. This treatment should bring the problem under control. In cases where the bone has been partially or more severely affected, periodontal surgery may have to be performed to remove tartar from the roots of the teeth and infected tissue adjacent to the destroyed bone and to eliminate the deep "pockets" created by the detachment of the gum tissue from the roots of the teeth. Pocket elimination is necessary to keep the area scrupulously clean and to avoid the accumulation of food debris and the growth of bacterial plaque. If the debris is left undisturbed under the protection of the gum flap, tissue breakdown will continue. Where tooth mobility has taken place it may be necessary to "adjust the bite" by grinding the biting surfaces of certain teeth to equalize the pressures of chewing or grinding. In cases where tooth mobility is great, the teeth may have to be temporarily splinted (tied together) using wires or other devices or permanently stabilized by an extensive fixed bridge. Treatment of advanced periodontal disease is complicated, time-consuming, and expensive, and not usually as effective as treatment administered in the earlier stages of disease.

PREVENTIVE DENTISTRY

In view of the national report that there are about one billion unfilled dental cavities in the United States, that periodontal disease accounts for about 50 percent of all teeth lost, and that the annual development of new dental disease is at least as great as the amount of disease treated annually, preventive dentistry becomes a prime factor in reducing the incidence of dental disease.

Dental caries

The evidence is striking that dental caries takes place when the following three conditions exist: a susceptible tooth, a cariogenic (cavity-causing) diet, and cariogenic bacteria. If any one of these conditions is not optimum, dental caries will be reduced. Let's examine each factor separately.

REDUCING TOOTH SUSCEPTIBILITY It has been definitely established by laboratory and clinical studies that incorporating fluoride into the mineral crystals making up the enamel of the tooth decreases the possibility of decay. A daily intake of approximately one milligram of fluoride lowers the caries rate by approximately 60 percent. This can be accomplished by fluoridating the public water supply or, if this is not possible, by dietary fluoride supplements. The application of fluorides in the dental office or the use of fluoridated toothpaste are also preventive measures, but they are less effective than fluoride obtained from the water supply. Other recent approaches to increasing the tooth's resistance to caries include the use of plastic sealants painted onto the surface of the enamel, with or without prior applications of fluoride. The sealants prevent food particles and bacteria from lodging in the pits and fissures of the biting surfaces of the teeth and keep freshly applied fluoride in contact with the enamel crystals for a longer period of time.

REDUCING THE CARIOGENICITY OF THE DIET Epidemiological and laboratory studies have shown that sucrose (table sugar) is the major dietary component that gives rise to dental caries (see Chap. 5). Both the form and frequency of sugar intake influence the caries attack rate. Between-meal eating of cakes, cookies, and candies, all of which stick to the teeth and are not readily cleared from the oral cavity, leads to high caries activity. The same amount of sugar in sweetened drinks is not as striking a decay producer because the sugar is not retained on the teeth as long. Heavily sugared breakfast cereals and sugared doughnuts are other examples of high decay producers. The cariogenicity of the diet can be reduced by substituting artificial sweeteners for the sugar, by cutting down on between-meal snacks, or by substituting potato chips, popcorn, and diet drinks for cakes, cookies, and candies. Practicing oral hygiene after meals and snacks should remove food particles and the bacterial plaque and contribute to the reduction of caries potential.

REDUCING CARIOGENIC BACTERIA Dental researchers are busily engaged in developing various antibacterial and antibiotic agents to reduce or eliminate cariogenic bacteria. A number of antibiotics have been tested in the form of mouthwashes or ointments, but no satisfactory long-term data have yet appeared to demonstrate their effectiveness and safety. The most effective means of reducing cariogenic bacteria to date are mechanical procedures: using the toothbrush and other oral hygiene aids such as dyes (to disclose bacterial deposits and food debris), dental floss, dental tape, water jets, and other devices for cleaning between the teeth and other hard to reach areas.

Periodontal disease

As pointed out earlier, bacteria in dental plaque appear to play a major role in the development of gum diseases. Prevention of gum inflammation and periodontitis consists primarily of the continuous removal of plaque, food debris, and tartar. Plaque formation can be prevented if a good, regularly applied oral hygiene program is followed, along with visits to the dentist for periodic check-ups and removal of dental tartar. The dentist or members of the staff should instruct each patient in the use of disclosing agents which make visible the areas of plaque missed during normal oral hygiene procedures. Several brushing techniques are effective. The easiest uses a soft nylon or natural bristle brush with a scrubbing motion that covers every surface of each tooth with specific emphasis on the border region between the tooth and gums. Electric toothbrushes are helpful for those who have poor manual dexterity. Because toothbrush bristles cannot adequately cleanse between the teeth, the use of dental floss, interdental cleansers, and water jets may be recommended. As with dental caries, eliminating or reducing sugar in the diet will lessen plaque formation. Including hard, fibrous foods such as apples in the diet may have some direct mechanical effect and may stimulate the flow of saliva which contributes to the washing away of food particles.

MALOCCLUSION (CROOKED TEETH)

The mouth is vital for taste, mastication (chewing), and speech, and, of course, is a part of the esthetic appearance of each individual. Malocclusion occurs in about 50 percent of the population, almost half of whom have serious problems. Malocclusion not only detracts from the individual's appearance but it may also interfere with chewing and speech. Correct tooth position is important because deviations lead to food impaction between the teeth, difficulty in removing bacterial plaque, and improper distribution of forces during chewing—conditions favorable to the development of dental caries and periodontal disease. It has been estimated that 25 percent of the malocclusions seen in some orthodontic practices are a direct result of premature loss of primary teeth from caries. The shifting and tipping of teeth already in the mouth following a premature loss frequently prevents the permanent tooth from erupting into proper position, thereby disrupting the exquisitely programmed eruption sequence and pattern.

An orthodontist, one who specializes in the proper positioning of the teeth, must be expert in the growth and development of the human skeleton as well as the teeth because skeletal growth influences treatment procedures and results. Orthodontic corrections can be accomplished more readily during puberty (eleven to thirteen and a half years of age in girls, thirteen to fifteen and a half in boys), usually the period of greatest head and facial growth. Ideally, the forehead, lips, and chin should be in a straight line when viewed in profile. A *convex profile* is caused by a relative prominence of the teeth and lips, while a *concave profile* is caused by a relative prominence of the chin (Fig. 12.8). Both conditions are abnormal, and the former condition is more prevalent. The orthodontist can reposition teeth in the jaws by putting on braces and exerting small, well-controlled forces over a period of one to two years. However, if there is a larger problem in the skeletal growth of the jaws, the results may not be favorable. This is particularly true in individuals with severe protrusion of the lower jaw. In such cases the orthodontist may collaborate with an oral surgeon to surgically remove

Figure 12.8. Three types of profiles: (a) *normal*, where forehead, lips and chin are approximately in a straight line, (b) *convex profile*, where there is a relative prominence of the teeth and lips, and (c) *concave profile*, where there is a relative prominence of the chin. (Reproduced and modified from "Diagnosis, Case Selection and Treatment Planning" by Anthony A. Gianelly, in *The Dental Clinics of North America*, W. B. Saunders Co., Philadelphia, Volume 16, Number 3 [July 1972], p. 415)

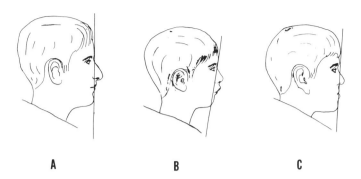

A   **B**   **C**

a segment of the lower jaw on both sides, moving the chin back to its proper position to produce a more esthetic profile.

CLEFT LIP AND CLEFT PALATE

Cleft lip and cleft palate occur once in every 700 births and are among the most common birth defects in the country. The defects occur in the early stages of development of the fetus in the uterus and represent a failure in the normal fusion of the tissues. An infant born with a cleft palate has a direct passageway between the oral cavity and the nasal cavity which makes breathing difficult and sucking impossible. Unless the cleft is surgically closed at an early age, eating will be difficult, speech will be nasal, and facial appearance, particularly when accompanied by a cleft lip (hare-lip), may be embarrassing.

The cause of clefting is unknown, but researchers have duplicated the condition in animals by injecting the pregnant mother with a variety of drugs at a specific stage in the development of the fetus. In 20 to 30 percent of the children born with a cleft there is a family history of this defect (see Chap. 7). While researchers are exploring the role of mechanical, infectious, and metabolic causes of this disease, surgeons, speech therapists, orthodontists, pediatricians, psychologists, and others are at work improving the management and treatment of affected patients.

ORAL CANCER

Oral cancer constitutes about 5 percent of all types of cancer and, like cancers elsewhere in the body, the outcome is more favorable when discovered and treated early (see Chap. 11). About half the tumors of the oral cavity and adjacent tissues occur on the lips, particularly the lower lip. In the mouth, about half the tumors involve the tongue, especially the back of the tongue. The major cause of lip cancer appears to be constant exposure to intense sunlight. Factors contributing to the development of oral cancer include tobacco (usually in the form of cigar and pipe-smoking) and excessive consumption of alcohol (see Chaps. 15 and 16). The most common precancerous lesion occurring in the mouth is *leukoplakia*, a whitish patch on the surface of the tissue lining the oral cavity. A small specimen of the patch can be surgically removed and examined under the microscope (a process known as biopsy) to detect cancer. All open sores which fail to heal in one to two weeks should be considered potentially malignant, and a biopsy should be performed to make a definitive diagnosis.

It is important to note that in the early stages the most common type of oral cancer is rarely as painful as other open sores in the mouth that result from trauma or infection. Treatment of patients with cancer of the lip is usually successful, but for patients with cancer of the tongue it is not as successful, especially if the cancer was not discovered early and has started to spread to other parts of the body.

INTERACTION BETWEEN ORAL AND SYSTEMIC PROBLEMS

Too often dentists and others forget that disease of the oral cavity may affect other systems of the body and that diseases elsewhere in the body may manifest themselves in the mouth. Perhaps the best example of the former situation involves *bacterial endocarditis,* a disease of the lining of the heart primarily caused by a strain of streptococci organisms commonly found in the mouth. These organisms usually enter the bloodstream in large numbers during tooth extraction. In patients having congenital or acquired heart disease such as rheumatic heart disease (see Chap. 11), this bacterial invasion could result in bacterial endocarditis, a disease which was 100 percent fatal prior to the discovery of antibiotics. To protect the patient with congenital or acquired heart disease, the dentist should obtain a complete medical history before starting treatment, cooperate closely with the patient's physician, eliminate all oral infection, and give adequate antibiotic therapy before any dental treatment that might release potentially damaging bacteria into the bloodstream.

An example of a bodily condition affecting the oral cavity is the treatment of epilepsy with sodium dilantin, a drug which cuts down the number and severity of seizures but which also gives rise to a marked

Choosing a dental profession

More than a decade ago, the major factors reported by dental students as having influenced their choice of dentistry as a career were:

1. desire to work for and with people
2. interest in content of the profession
3. desire to be own boss
4. desire to work with hands
5. prestige of the profession
6. monetary advantages of the profession

One-half of the 1958 freshman dental students came from families of middle or upper class status. Less than 13 percent of their fathers were dentists or physicians.

Some of these data may be changing in the near future. As students enter dental school with a greater concern for the lack of oral health care for a large segment of the population, a larger percentage will choose to work for neighborhood health centers or as public health dentists in city, state, and federal institutions. For some others, the advantages of private group practice may outweigh the advantages of being a solo practitioner and one's own boss. The "affirmative action" programs in dental schools have recently begun to change the composition of many student bodies by encouraging the enrollment of increased numbers of minority and female students. The changing attitudes and curricula of many dental schools have begun to afford dental students an opportunity to function in the community, to perform dental research, and to consider career goals and methods of practice quite different from the traditional.

overgrowth of the gum tissue around many teeth. This overgrowth may interfere with chewing and cause the patient embarrassment if it occurs in the front of the mouth. The treatment frequently involves the surgical removal of the excess gum tissue which, unfortunately, may regrow within several months.

PROBLEMS IN DELIVERING ORAL HEALTH CARE

The dental workforce

The grim statistics on the dental health status of the American people particularly reveal the wide gap between dental needs and services. It is difficult to escape the fact that any serious attempt to narrow this gap will require a significant increase in the dental workforce and the expenditure of enormous sums of money (Fig. 12.9).

The American Dental Association Task Force Committee on the Requirements for Dental and Dental Auxiliary Manpower has estimated the number of dentists available and the number needed for the period 1970–1990 (Table 12.1). The committee projects that there will be a deficit of more than 16,000 dentists by 1990 without the initiation of a national health program. The current dental workforce was considered adequate to meet the present *demand* for dental care. However, there is a great difference between the *demand* and the *need* for health services. It is a known fact that 50 percent of all children under the age of fifteen have never been to a dentist, a figure that is closer to 70 percent if one considers the children of poor families. The establishment of a national dental health program would *increase* the demand for care because one of the primary barriers to seeking care, the lack of financial resources, would be eliminated.

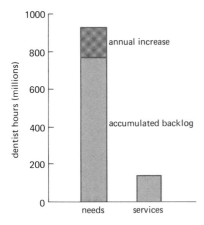

Figure 12.9. The backlog of accumulated dental disease—a backlog that includes 1 billion unfilled cavities—shows the disparity between dental needs and services. (Reproduced from "Dentistry in National Health Programs—Reports of the Special Committees," American Dental Association, Chicago, 1971, p. 8. Copyright by the American Dental Association. Reprinted by permission)

Table 12.1 Projected number of dentists available, number needed, and estimated deficits if no national health program is initiated, 1970–1990*

Year	Projected number dentists available	Projected number dentists needed	Projected deficits
1970	99,180	99,180	—
1975	107,325	113,311	5,986
1980	119,305	126,502	7,197
1985	132,740	142,620	9,880
1990	144,650	161,203	16,553

* Reproduced from "Dentistry in National Health Programs—Reports of the Special Committees," American Dental Association, Chicago, 1971, p. 31.

The problem of maldistribution of the dental workforce and the resulting shortage of dental workers in the inner cities and rural areas will probably not be solved merely by increasing the number of dental graduates and ancillary personnel, but will require new approaches such as that of the National Health Service Corps (Fig. 12.10). The increased use of auxiliary personnel to perform some of the simple, repetitive intraoral procedures previously reserved for the dentist, such as putting

Figure 12.10. Ratios of population per dentist, by state, 1968. (Reproduced from "Dentistry in National Health Programs—Reports of the Special Committees," American Dental Association, Chicago, 1971, p. 67. Copyright by the American Dental Association. Reprinted by permission)

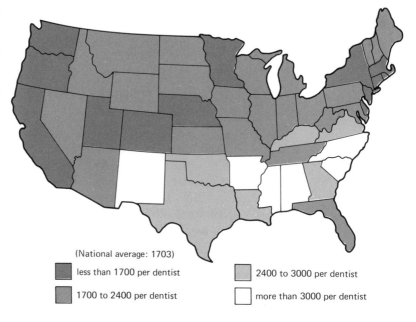

(National average: 1703)

less than 1700 per dentist

1700 to 2400 per dentist

2400 to 3000 per dentist

more than 3000 per dentist

National Health Service Corps

Physicians, dentists, and nurses serve in the Public Health Service in areas designated as critical health-manpower shortage areas. Their salaries are paid for a two year period. The community provides office space, equipment, and ancillary support. Usual and customary fees are collected from the patients. From the fees collected, an amount of money is returned to the federal government as reimbursement for its contribution to the program. The aim of the program is to retain these individuals in the community in private practice after they have completed their two year commitment. It should be noted that before going into any area, the federal government obtains the approval of the state and local professional societies, as well as that of the local government authorities.

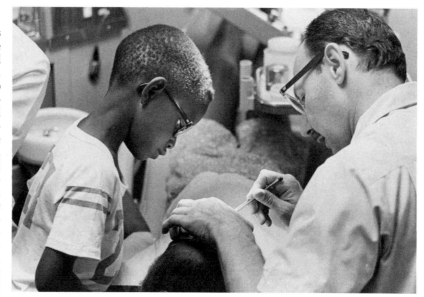

Figure 12.11. A dentist checks the completion of a dental procedure at a Neighborhood Health Center while an interested bystander looks on. (Photo by Bradford F. Herzog)

in fillings after the dentist has prepared the cavity for the filling material, could add significantly to the workforce and increase each dentist's productivity.

Cost of dental care

The cost of dental care in this country for 1970 has been estimated at $4.4 billion—approximately $50 for each person in the 42 percent of the population who saw a dentist at least once during the year (Table 12.2). On a per capita basis for the entire population, this would amount to about $22. It is of interest to note that in the three decades since 1940, while the per capita expenditure for dental care has risen seven-fold, the percentage of the "health dollar" going to dental costs has decreased from 10.9 percent in 1940 to 9.2 percent in 1970. Dental insurance programs, while still in their infancy as compared to medical insurance, offer a means of budgeting for dental care.

Table 12.2 Consumer expenditures for dental care*

Year	Total consumer expenditure for dentistry	Percentage of health dollar	Per capita expenditure
1970	$4,383,000,000	9.2	$21.74
1969	3,921,000,000	9.3	19.70
1968	3,461,000,000	9.3	17.57
1965	2,836,000,000	10.1	14.78
1960	2,007,000,000	10.5	11.27
1950	962,000,000	10.9	6.40
1940	419,000,000	10.9	3.18

* From "Survey of current business," U.S. Department of Commerce (various issues).

Prevention

One way to avoid sudden, large dental bills is to make regular, periodic visits to the dentist and to undergo corrective treatment at an early stage when it is relatively simple and inexpensive. In the final analysis, prevention of dental disease remains the best approach to better oral health and smaller dental bills. Effective approaches to prevention are now possible on both the public and private levels. As pointed out earlier, almost two-thirds of the dental caries problem could be prevented by fluoridation of the public drinking water. In spite of scientific proof of fluoride's effectiveness and safety, more than 12,000 city water systems remain unfluoridated, due in large measure to public apathy and a highly vocal antifluoridation minority. In addition to water fluoridation, if individuals carry out their prescribed oral hygiene programs and limit their sugar intake, there will be a pronounced, positive influence on maintaining oral health.

Questions   1. The adult dentition, in contrast to the primary dentition, is sometimes referred to as the "permanent teeth." Why is this a misnomer?
2. What is the role of bacteria in dental caries and periodontal disease?
3. What can you do to minimize the possibility that you and your children will be completely without teeth by age 65?
4. Why is it necessary for a dentist to be educated in the basic sciences and be knowledgeable about medical problems and human biology?
5. Discuss the factors involved in providing an adequate national oral health care program.

Key Concepts   *Dental caries* – a localized and progressive destruction of the hard tissue of the tooth usually starting on the biting surfaces of the rear teeth, the contact areas between adjacent teeth, or along the gum line
Dental plaque – a soft, adherent deposit, composed primarily of bacteria, their extracellular products, and salivary proteins, that accumulates on the surfaces of teeth, especially near the margins of the gums
Extrusion – the over-eruption of a tooth into a space created by the absence of an opposing tooth in the opposite jaw
Occlusal surface – the chewing surface of a rear tooth
Periodontal disease – disease of the tissues surrounding the tooth, including the gingiva and supporting bone to which the tooth is attached
Periodontitis – a chronic inflammation of the gingiva accompanied by the formation of periodontal pockets and the destruction of the supporting bone of the involved teeth

Selected Readings   "Dentistry in National Health Programs—Reports of the Special Committees," American Dental Association, Chicago, 1971.
Freedman, G. L. and J. R. Hooley, "Medical Contraindications to the Extraction of Teeth," *Dental Clinics of North America,* Vol. 13, No. 4 (October 1969), pp. 939–60.
Massler, M., "Teen-Age Cariology," *Dental Clinics of North America,* Vol. 13, No. 2 (April 1969), pp. 405–21.
Morris, A. L. and R. C. Greulich, "Dental Research: The Past Two Decades," *Science,* Vol. 160 (1968), pp. 1–7.
Scherp, H. W., "Dental Caries: Prospects for Prevention," *Science,* Vol. 173 (1971), pp. 1199–1205.
Shaw, J. H., "Diet Regulations for Caries Prevention," *Nutrition News,* Vol. 36 (Feb. 1973), pp. 1 and 4.

Chapter 13

Mental Illness

Throughout recorded history, people whose actions and speech were regarded as strange, peculiar, or unusual have been characterized as lunatic, crazy, insane, mad, or just plain "nutty." The extreme nature of their behavior and its unpredictability have always attracted an exceptional amount of attention from the rest of the population, chiefly because of society's fear of the crazy person. And because the lunatic seemed so threatening, society has been more concerned with the behavior itself than with the causes underlying it. Every culture has, indeed, sought reasons for insanity but from a viewpoint that was more often emotional than rational. As a result, society's explanations have sometimes been as bizarre as the insane behavior.

In its examination of unusual behavior, society has tended to study behavior as an entity. The "mystical" quality of man's mental processes and their unpredictable, complex nature have attracted the most attention in this examination. Human genetic and physiological attributes

This chapter was contributed by Ralph Minear, M.D., M.P.H., Director of Pediatrics, Roxbury Comprehensive Community Health Center, Instructor in Pediatrics, Boston University School of Medicine, and Assisting Physician for Pediatrics, Boston City Hospital.

have received relatively little consideration in relation to strange behavior.

Because of that bias, society's efforts to deal with strange behavior have generally followed a three-stage pattern. First is the attempt to isolate characteristics which can be labeled deviant as opposed to normal. That automatically creates problems because deviancy is not an absolute nor is it applicable in all cultures. Behavior that would be considered aberrant in western American civilization may seem perfectly normal on some Pacific island. The second general step has been to examine an individual's personal development or his relationships with others in order to locate causes for deviant behavior. Finally, treatment of the deviant individual has been approached primarily by assisting him to find ways to cope with his behavioral abnormalities.

The tendency to focus on behavior as a phenomenon exclusive of physiological determinants has been reinforced by the prevailing view of deviant behavior as an illness or disease of a mental nature. This labeling has prejudiced scientific observations with the result that the understanding of deviant behavior is far behind the knowledge that has been built up about purely physical infirmities. Only in recent years have discoveries in genetics, biochemistry, and psychology encouraged a view of mental illness that is broader than the purely behavioral one that has prevailed for so long.

One of the problems in dealing with mental illness has been that there are so many different ways of classifying and defining it. Aside from the general public, different professions view it from different perspectives and, even within the medical profession, there are a variety of definitions.

CLASSIFICATIONS OF MENTAL ILLNESS

Classification according to cause

In the ancient world—Egypt, Assyria, Babylonia, Biblical Israel, China— there existed a common belief that if a person acted crazy, his mind was possessed by a demon or evil spirit of some sort. The individual was seen as helpless to control his unusual behavior unless the offending demon was somehow removed or placated. To accomplish this priests and wizards invoked prayers, mystical incantations, herbal purgatives, and a variety of often elaborate counterspells. If those measures failed, the possessed person was whipped, beaten, even stoned to death. Demons had to be dealt with harshly lest they infect 'the rest of the populace.

Greek physicians, under the leadership of Hippocrates (c. 460–377 B.C.), were convinced that mental illness was the result of an imbalance of body fluids. Their methods—including baths, massage, diet changes, and exercise—were more humane and even made some sense in modern medical terms. But Hippocrates' theories did not spread very far, and during the Middle Ages in Europe superstition again guided the treatment of the mentally ill. In order to punish the demons and devils responsible for deviant behavior, the insane were beaten, generally abused, sometimes executed (as witches). This period also saw the birth of the asylum, and hundreds of "mad" individuals were chained in dark dungeons (where the demons could be held in check). Not only were they treated with the cruelty usually reserved for animals, they were, in some instances, exhibited to the "sane" members of the population as if the asylum were a zoo.

The demon theory began to wane late in the eighteenth century. Philippe Pinel, the administrator of a Paris asylum, demonstrated that patients humanely treated could improve and even return to society. Social reform movements in the nineteenth century generally improved the lot of insane persons even though the general public still regarded mental hospital inmates with fear and suspicion. If devils were discounted, there was still little knowledge of the actual causes of insanity.

New perspectives on mental health were opened up by Sigmund Freud late in the nineteenth century. Freud was able to identify episodes of behavior that might be called crazy at some point in everyone's life. He maintained that this aberrant behavior was produced by social and sexual conflicts that occurred during childhood development. According to Freud, such conflicts were repressed, buried in the subconscious, then emerged in later life in the form of deviant behavior. Freud's work generated a whole school of psychology that views personality composition as a major cause of strange behavior. Proponents of this theory believe that all individuals possess traits that can be classified as abnormal; but the mentally ill person is one who is dominated by the unresolved conflicts of early development. It is this theory, with numerous modifications, which underlies most psychiatric treatment today.

Modern medical research has brought forth additional causes underlying mental illness. In 1905 the syphillis spirochete (see Chap. 10) was identified as the reason for paresis, a steady mental deterioration marked by cloudiness of perceptions, disorientation, hallucinations, and other forms of aberrant behavior. Since then, peculiar behavior patterns have been linked with various bacterial or viral infections of the central nervous system, infectious mononucleosis, and infectious hepatitis. Similarly, mental and emotional changes have been associated with the ingestion of psychotropic drugs and alcohol in excessive amounts. These "outside influences" can produce behavioral changes that are both short-lived and permanent. Moreover, the changes produced are not uniform from one individual to another nor do they affect everyone. As such factors are identified and new vaccines and antibiotics are developed to counteract them, they have begun to diminish as causes of mental illness.

With the development of more sophisticated medical techniques, various physiological interactions inside the human body were identified as causative factors. For example, some of the frequently observed behavioral changes that accompany old age are due to arteriosclerosis. The reduction in blood flow caused by this condition damages tissue which, in turn, leads to mental deterioration. Some individuals may show only slight intellectual impairment while others with the same amount of damage exhibit psychotic behavioral disorders so severe they require hospital care.

Other behavioral oddities result from the compression of brain tissue that is secondary to brain tumor or trauma. Ironically, medical technology may sometimes be responsible for deviant behavior. Many babies who once would have died during birth now survive because of modern techniques; but, in the process of saving them, health personnel may unwittingly compromise the flow of blood and oxygen to the brain. Thus the babies survive but with an impairment that produces deviant behavior as they mature.

Most recently, physiological investigations have demonstrated that deviant behavior—particularly of a criminal nature—appears in individuals whose chromosomes are abnormal in both number and composition. Research with schizophrenic patients has led to a growing belief among investigators that this form of mental illness is caused by the inheritance of abnormal biochemical reactions. In general, the increased sophistication of biogenetic research seems likely to uncover additional causes of deviant behavior.

Classification according to degree of disability

A relatively small percentage of the people who regularly exhibit some form of deviant behavior are actually in mental institutions. Probably the majority "learn to live with it" in some way. It is not really known how many adapt to mental illness, but it has been estimated that as many as 60 percent of the people visiting physicians for medical care are actually seeking help for some mental condition. During World War II approximately 11 percent of the draftees were rejected for service on the basis of emotional problems. (However, authorities have challenged draft rejection as a reliable index of undetected mental illness.)

The degree of accommodation that an individual makes to his deviant behavior depends on how much of a social and financial burden it creates. Since it is impossible to determine how many people have made some sort of accommodation to their mental problems, it is equally impossible to assess their effects on others—the hazards to life and limb and the number of man hours lost to employers, for instance.

Among the people who do not try to "go it alone," a high proportion seeks assistance because modern pharmaceutical research has increased the likelihood of relief from their mental afflictions. New drugs may not resolve the causes, but they are often able to alleviate distressing symptoms. This is particularly true of physical manifestations of emotional upsets. Anti-inflammatory and antispasmodic medication provide effective treatment for spastic colon. Desensitization and antiallergic therapeutics are able to control allergic skin disorders and asthma. Even more

Facts about mental illness

On any one day, there are 753,000 persons under psychiatric care in hospitals alone. On that same day, there are about 173,000 who are on a "trial visit" or a similar form of supervised community care. In 1966 public and private mental hospitals, psychiatric services of general hospitals, and Veterans Administration psychiatric facilities admitted 867,000 persons. Of these, an estimated 300,000 have already been hospitalized one or more times. None of these figures accounts for the large number of people who are under treatment by private practitioners in an out-patient facility.

At least 7 out of 10 patients admitted to a mental hospital can leave partially or totally recovered with prompt and proper treatment. One large health insurance company reports that the average length of hospitalization for holders of its insurance is only 13 days, and about 80 percent leave the hospital within the first year. In 1947, a person with schizophrenia, the most prevalent mental crippler, faced a 50-50 chance of being hospitalized for more than a year. Today, provided he enters an adequately staffed institution, his chance for release within the year is increased to four out of five.

Mental illness occurs at all ages, including childhood. No one really knows how many mentally ill children there are. The estimates made by experts range from 500,000 to as many as 1,000,000.

About 473,000 children under 18 years of age received some service in a psychiatric facility in the United States in 1966. Of these children, 84 percent were seen on an out-patient basis and 14 percent were hospitalized.

The figures for 1966 show that 33,851 children and young adults were admitted to public mental hospitals—their first hospitalization for serious mental disorders. Of these 5,137 were under 15, and 28,714 were between 15 and 24.

From "Facts About Mental Illness," a leaflet prepared and distributed by The National Association for Mental Health, Inc., Arlington, Virginia.

common mental problems such as depression can now be effectively treated with mood elevation drugs and electroshock therapy. Depression causes as many as 8 million Americans to seek help from a physician each year, and approximately 250,000 individuals are hospitalized by this emotional condition.

There is also an alarming number of people who must be under constant care because of abnormal behavior. It may be a relatively small percentage of the total population, but United States mental hospitals hold about 750,000 patients. More people are hospitalized for mental illness than all other illnesses combined, and they occupy more than half of all hospital beds.

Classification according to law

The concern of law enforcement authorities with deviant personality is twofold: to protect society from danger and to guard the aberrant individual himself from exploitation and self-inflicted harm. The modern legal interpretation of mental illness had its origin in English law. A 1724 statute declared a man insane if he did not know what he was doing when he committed a crime. An 1843 ruling modified this view, allowing that a person could be acquitted of a crime if he did not know what he was doing at the time, or if, though aware of his action, he lacked the capacity to understand that it was wrong as perceived by society.

Individuals declared not guilty of crimes on the basis of their insanity are committed to mental institutions. Confinement for the treatment of their illness often lasts much longer than the prison term they would have received if convicted. The legal certification of insanity also prevents disturbed individuals from entering into a variety of activities—education, business contracts, estate management—that they could not comprehend because of their insanity.

Some authorities believe that the prevailing legal definition is too limited. Many individuals that any psychiatrist would classify as insane are able to make the moral distinction between right and wrong, but their compulsion is so great that they commit crimes anyway. Some efforts have been made to revise the legal definition, thus far with limited success.

Classification according to behavior

Mental illness is most often identified and classified in terms of observable behavior patterns. Such a definition is also subject to variations in meaning, even among professional psychologists, and has its limitations. It overlooks the fact that behavior may be a manifestation of the effects of environment on physiology, for example. Nevertheless, it is the frame of reference used by many investigators for most research done on mental illness, and it serves as a convenient means of identification.

The standards for classification are based upon the degree of deviation from what is considered normal behavior and upon the frequency and intensity with which deviation occurs. Basic to that consideration is the age-old question of what is and what is not normal. In part, normalcy depends on statistical frequency: how often a particular kind of behavior occurs within the population under scrutiny.

Closely connected to frequency is the context in which the behavior appears. Different societies have different standards. For some Central American Indian tribes, the total social isolation of children is a normal procedure. In the eyes of a North American city dweller, this practice seems abnormal. Even within societies, different cultural groups may hold widely divergent views of what, for example, constitutes normal and abnormal sexual behavior.

Within a somewhat smaller context, there is the question of how closely behavior patterns are related to the reality of a particular situation. For example, do the circumstances warrant crying or screaming or wearing shorts or carrying an umbrella? Given the same conditions, how would you react? If there is no apparent reason for the behavior, can a reasonable explanation be found? Sometimes, there are no answers. The more that behavior is removed from reality, the more likely that it will be called abnormal.

At one time or another, anyone is likely to exhibit abnormal behavior. What separates the person who is truly mentally disturbed from the majority is the frequency with which he repeats his behavioral peculiarities and the duration of his abnormal outbursts.

A final criterion for abnormality is the degree to which emotional problems prevent an individual from carrying out his routine responsibilities. If he is emotionally paralyzed or his actions threaten himself or others with harm, he is considered to be functioning abnormally. In general, all of the aforementioned criteria are involved in any judgment of behavioral abnormality.

TYPES OF BEHAVIORAL DEVIATIONS

Mental retardation

An estimated 1 to 5 percent of the population is mentally retarded and a high proportion of those individuals display behavioral abnormalities. The causes of this form of mental disability are found in: prenatal events (genetic factors, metabolic disease, infection, ingestion of foreign substances by the mother, plus many unknown causes); birth injuries; and postnatal events (infections, trauma, allergic reactions, and a variety of unknowns).

For administrative purposes, mental retardation is classified by four categories.

1. Profound. The I.Q. of these individuals is less than 20, and they are unable to take care of the routine matters of daily living for themselves. They may have some ability to make sounds or simple words, and frequently they suffer from physical handicaps.
2. Severe. Persons retarded to this degree have an I.Q. between 20 and 35. They are able to perform routine and repetitive activities, but they need some guidance in daily life.
3. Moderate. Persons in this group have an I.Q. between 36 and 50. They are able to care for themselves, and during childhood they can be trained to function with a reasonable degree of normality. As adults, they must live in a sheltered environment, and they are incapable of problem-solving.
4. Mild. The I.Q. level is between 51 and 70. Their educational limit is usually elementary school level. When they reach adulthood they are able to live independently, but they may require assistance if confronted with unusual social stresses. They have a general inability to succeed in school-related tasks.

Transitory deviancy

The stress of a crisis or an unfamiliar situation may generate striking changes in mood or behavior that is out of control. Usually these maladjustments are short-lived. Prolonged fatigue may trigger uncharacteristic hostility, for instance. During pregnancy, a woman experiences stresses that cause her to erupt in tears or anger that is quite unlike her usual personality. Periods of life such as adolescence are full of stressful situations. An adolescent who has not developed sexually, who has yet to menstruate, or who suffers from a severe case of acne may exhibit an overwhelming preoccupation with "normalcy."

These temporary conditions may also produce organic disturbances or physiological changes secondary to the emotional reactions. The "jitters," poor appetite, insomnia, or frequent trips to the toilet are but a few of the possible behavior patterns that might occur during the days preceding an important exam.

One of the most common behavioral deviations is depression which manifests itself as despair, loneliness, apathy, listlessness, and loss of weight (through loss of appetite). This mood alteration ordinarily involves the loss of something—a person, object, belief, sense of status, or value—which held a considerable attachment for the depressed individual. It may be anything from a failure to become a member of a prestigious fraternity to the break-up of a love affair.

Ordinarily the symptoms produced by stressful situations disappear once the crisis itself has disappeared or the individual is able to bring the conditions of stress under control. If they persist beyond that point, it is probably an indication of some form of mental illness.

The psychopathic personality

By the time most of us are two years old, we have learned that we cannot always have what we want when we want it. Unlike the newborn infant, we must defer our wants to the demands of our parents. Also at an early age we begin to develop a conscience and a moral code that guide us in our relations with others and prevent us from acting impulsively to gratify our own needs. Violations of personal morality can cause us considerable guilt and anxiety. In general we learn to relate to other individuals, to consider their wants, and to live more or less in harmony with society. The psychopath never learns any of these things.

Psychopathic individuals go through a lifetime of antisocial behavior. Concerned solely with their own needs, they almost never consider the needs of others. As a result it is virtually impossible for psychopaths to become involved in a close relationship with other persons. They may, however, develop a range of "unusual" sexual interests.

Psychopaths are not rebels. They simply never develop a conscience or code of ethics. Thus they are regularly in conflict with the laws and customs that govern the rest of society. In his eagerness to get what he wants instantly, the psychopath allows nothing to stand in his way. Should something frustrate him, it may unleash a burst of hostility. Such a person will lie, manipulate the feelings of others, steal, even kill to satisfy his needs—all without hesitation. Yet he does these things without intended malice. His antisocial acts are committed on impulse and his whole life pattern is a rather aimless, erratic one. Moreover, he commits even the most violent act without any evidence of guilt or anxiety. He knows the dictates of the law, but they are irrelevant to him. Because of this trait, he cannot be declared legally insane.

The underlying causes of the psychopathic personality are still largely a mystery. Some experts believe that they are products of loveless homes. Children who have no meaningful relationship with parents are unlikely to identify with their parents and absorb their parents' values. Thus such a child is not afraid of losing his parents' affection since they have given him none in the first place. Overall, he feels he has little to lose and behaves accordingly, without anxiety. The psychopathic personality requires considerably more research, particularly since it has proven difficult to treat effectively.

Neurosis

Anxiety plagues everyone at some time, but the neurotic individual is plagued by it most of the time. Neurosis appears as several types of deviant behavior, and while generally none of them is totally incapacitating, they do interfere with normal functioning. They are a barrier to building self-esteem, to working productively, and to forming close relationships with others, especially in the area of romantic love. Occasionally neuroses may produce physical reactions such as nausea, headaches, and loss of appetite. If neurotic disorders are severe enough, some form of therapy is required and sometimes hospitalization may be necessary.

To a large extent the deviant forms of behavior that characterize neurosis are exaggerated forms of the defense mechanisms employed by everyone to settle conflicts. The neurotic, whose life is dominated by unresolved conflicts, uses the defenses to avoid or overcome anxiety. Neurosis appears as a wide variety of behavioral reactions, but four types are most frequently observed. Most neurotics exhibit symptoms of more than one type.

ACUTE ANXIETY While anxiety is a common denominator of all neurotics, some are literally overwhelmed by it. They live in a chronic state of tension, fear overtakes them almost daily, and the ability to relax is all but unknown. Any sudden stress may precipitate an acute attack accompanied by such physiological responses as heart palpitations and nausea.

The typical anxiety neurotic creates a paradox for himself: he is burdened by a powerful sense of inferiority, yet he attempts to achieve unrealistic goals. As a result, he is never secure, even when he has achieved some measure of success. His anxiety may be set off by specific situations—a new boss, a first date—or it may be a sort of generalized condition, commonly called "free-floating anxiety." Among neurotics, acute anxiety is the most common type.

OBSESSIVE-COMPULSIVENESS Probably most of us have observed people who are compelled to check frequently whether doors and windows are locked, to repeatedly wash their hands, or to ritualistically arrange materials on top of their desks. Some compulsive actions may be a coverup for aggressive or sexual impulses that the individual cannot bear to consider (he may not be fully aware of them). The excessive hand-washer may be preoccupied with disease, or he may be washing away the guilt he feels over some of his activities.

The ritual of desk arranging is a way of keeping out of trouble. The neurotic avoids the possibility that he may act on the impulses that are unacceptable to him. Since he is also threatened by the confusing world around him, his activities are a way of establishing order.

Similarly, obsessive thoughts may frequently be connected to disturbing impulses of a sexual or hostile nature, sometimes both. Though the disturbed individual almost never acts on these impulses, he may repeatedly think about killing someone close to him or parading naked in public. While the thought is upsetting, it is usually an expression of an even greater hostility that the person has yet to admit to himself. The obsessed person feels out of control and is certain that he is losing his mind.

Obsessions and compulsions of this sort keep the neurotic so busy that he is unable to attend to his normal responsibilities. He realizes the futility of his behavior but has no control over it.

PHOBIAS   Some people see danger where there is none, or minimal danger at worst. Their fear of the imagined danger is so out of proportion to reality that their ability to function in even a routine way is stifled. They suffer from phobias. Some of the more frequently encountered are claustrophobia (fear of closed places), acrophobia (heights), ocholophobia (crowds), nyctophobia (dark places), hydrophobia (water), and zoophobia (animals, especially snakes).

Virtually any object, situation, place, or being can evoke excessive fear in the phobic individual. In some cases the fear stimulus may merely make the person tense and uncomfortable so that he cannot concentrate on the task at hand. More likely he attempts to ward off the misery of undue anxiety by avoiding situations where he is confronted by the source of his anxiety. Phobias can severely restrict his activities. The person who is uncomfortable with crowds, for instance, denies himself pleasure by staying away from concerts, basketball games, circuses, movies, and any number of potentially entertaining events. Most phobic individuals are well aware that their fear has no basis in fact, but that knowledge does not prevent anxiety.

Phobic reactions may be directly related to the stimulus itself—a bad scare while learning to swim may precipitate a lifelong fear of water—but not necessarily. Some phobias are similar to obsessive-compulsive behavior in that they are the means of shielding the individual from an undesirable impulse, primarily of a sexual or aggressive nature.

HYSTERIA   This type of neurosis manifests itself as physical symptoms, often very serious and disabling ones, even though there is nothing organically wrong with the person. Anxiety is the sole cause, and apparently these individuals convert their anxiety into illness, usually as a means of avoiding a frightening situation. These ailments often further benefit the individual by evoking sympathy from others.

The ills into which anxiety can be transformed cover a wide territory. It may impair motor coordination, paralyzing one or more limbs or a side of the body. The most familiar example is that of the soldier who becomes paralyzed in his legs, thereby becoming unfit for battle without having to admit that he is afraid of it. Anxiety also produces such motor problems as speech impairment, muscle spasms or tics, and "fits" like those of epilepsy. Other physical manifestations of anxiety include sensory difficulties as extreme as blindness or deafness, and a broad spectrum of visceral symptoms: spastic colon, coughing spells, fainting spells, unusual skin rashes, rapid breathing, and multiple aches and pains.

Though there are no organic causes behind hysteria, the physical symptoms are totally real to the patient. The paralyzed soldier is literally incapable of walking; he is not pretending.

Functional psychosis

Psychosis is the most disabling type of mental disorder and the most likely to require supervised care. It has been estimated that as many as 1 person out of every 20 will be so seriously affected by psychosis that hospital treatment will be necessary. "Functional," or psychogenic, means that the cause is purely psychological. It is distinct from organic causes, such as syphillis and arteriosclerosis, mentioned earlier. Those disorders are also referred to as psychoses since the behavioral symptoms are identical or very similar to the functional variety.

In its severest form the most notable characteristic of functional psychosis is a total withdrawal from reality. The psychotic may be untouched by his environment, living rather in a fantasy world. Even if he does respond to external stimuli, it is with emotions and resultant actions that are confused, impossible for others to comprehend, and way out of proportion to the situation at hand. In a sense they are psychological dropouts. By contrast, the neurotic individual may perform inefficiently, but he is struggling to deal with his environment and the anxiety it produces in him. He manages to cope to a limited extent, but the psychotic is too removed to even attempt to cope.

There are two types of functional psychosis that make up the bulk of cases: manic-depressive and schizophrenic. The division is somewhat artificial since each type of psychotic may exhibit traits of the other at some point during the illness. For convenience sake, however, they can be described separately.

MANIC-DEPRESSIVE This disorder can also be subdivided since most cases shift from a mood that can be considered normal to either the

Depression

Today depression is the most prevalent of all the psychic maladies in this country; it is so widespread it has been called the common cold of mental disturbances. Like the cold, it can lead to more serious consequences. A recent survey by the National Institute of Mental Health revealed that as many as eight million people a year may suffer depression severe enough to merit being treated by a doctor, and over 250,000 Americans were hospitalized for the ailment last year.

Yet despite the prevalence of depression and after a decade of the most intensive scientific research ever conducted into the nature of the disease, it has been relatively ignored by the public. Depression has always been a hidden disorder, its victims bewildered by their private hells and ashamed of their symptoms. "Depression accounts for a very large share of human suffering," says a special report put out this year by the N.I.M.H., and yet "it continues to be underestimated both by mental health professionals and by the general public."

Researchers disagree almost as much over a definition of depression as they do over its causes. Almost all stress the difference, however, between the everyday kind of mood drop commonly called depression and what doctors diagnose as "clinical depression." The brief fluctuations in mood that may trail a spell of dreary weather or the end of a vacation are not abnormal, and the person who occasionally feels down during the day or on his way home from work may be experiencing nothing more than the temporary effects of fatigue.

With a clinical depression, however, the blues become more and more intense until even the routine of dressing becomes impossible to perform. The depressed person can feel hopelessness, guilt, and self-loathing for periods of six months or more. He withdraws from the world and often loses interest in food, sex, and other people.... Insomnia is also common among depressed people. Their long nights are spent tossing and turning, and they are bedeviled by despairing thoughts.

Often, however, it is difficult for doctors to recognize depressed people because the disease can appear in the guise of other illnesses and pass purely as a physical problem. Most doctors are familiar with the famous "somatic mask of depression": The patient's true condition is often disguised by a host of physical symptoms such as fatigue, stomach cramps, and chest pains. Sometimes long and difficult investigations by doctors are necessary before the real difficulty is uncovered.

From R. Cherry and L. Cherry, "Depression: The Common Cold of Mental Ailments," *New York Times Magazine* (Nov. 25, 1973), p. 38.

manic or the depressive phase. Relatively few run the gamut, showing both manic and depressive tendencies.

Depression is the most frequently observed condition, and it goes far deeper than the type of "blues" that everyone experiences at one time or another. The depressive is so utterly lacking in self-esteem and enthusiasm, so guilt-ridden, and so hopeless and discouraged that suicide often seems the only answer. For such a person, life appears pointless. At its immobilizing worst, this degree of depression makes the patient withdraw completely, oblivious to anyone and everything around him, totally dependent on others for feeding and other aspects of survival.

On the other hand, the manic type (in milder cases) demonstrates such limitless energy and confidence that he seems to be "high" on alcohol or drugs like "uppers." Constant activity and incessant talking are his trademarks, though he actually accomplishes very little. More advanced manics are in such a state of frenzy that as they pace frantically, they shout, curse, scream, and babble. The hypermanic is a mass of confusion and is not oriented to time, place, or the person to whom he is speaking. He may have delusions (false beliefs) about his importance and abilities and may be further confused by hallucinations (a period during which he responds to nonexistent visual and aural stimuli). If such a person is not confined by custodial care, his lack of inhibitions and morality may result in sexual assaults or indiscriminate violence. Behaviorists who deal with such patients postulate that despite the fact that manics and depressives seem diametrically opposed, they are very closely related. The belief is that the wildness of the manic is an attempt to compensate for feelings of worthlessness that identify a depressive, and that this is why some patients swing from one phase to the other.

Unfortunately little is known about the reasons for this type of psychological disorder, but studies indicate two predominant factors. This type of psychotic feels compelled to achieve unrealistically high standards in everything he does and is plunged into guilt and feelings of inadequacy when he fails. Also, his conscience is so overpowering that any hostile feelings are blocked. Instead they are directed toward himself. In general, this type of psychosis seems to be triggered by a crisis situation such as the loss of a job or a loved one.

SCHIZOPHRENIA Contrary to popular belief, schizophrenia is not synonymous with split personality. It refers instead to a separation of the mental processes from the emotional so that the schizophrenic's emotional reactions seem to have no relationship to what he is thinking. The following are the most common symptoms (though a schizophrenic may not exhibit all of them).
1. Dullness, apathy, and emotions that are not appropriate to the situation. With the separation of thought and emotion, the schizophrenic may describe tragedy with an expression of glee on his face.
2. Lack of interest in everything and everyone in his environment. Patients may withdraw into silence and immobility (a catatonic state) for periods of several days.
3. Oblivion to surroundings, a life in a fantasy world. Since the schizophrenic is reacting to imaginary stimuli, his reactions are inappropriate to the "real" world. Time and place are obliterated by fantasy.
4. Delusions that someone or something is attempting to influence his thoughts and behavior or that various individuals or groups of people are persecuting him. The schizophrenic also hears voices, and they are usually saying "dirty things" about him. The extreme of the hallucination-delusion syndrome is paranoia: the psychotic believes that parents, other relatives, friends, doctors, etc. are spying on him, talking about him, trying to "get" him, possibly even to kill him. In reality, he is projecting his own hostile feelings onto other people.

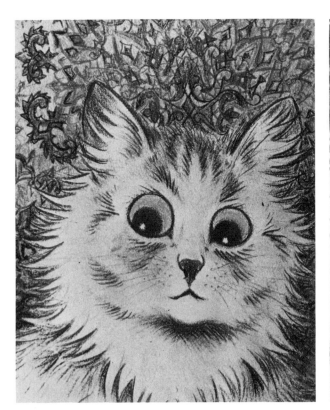 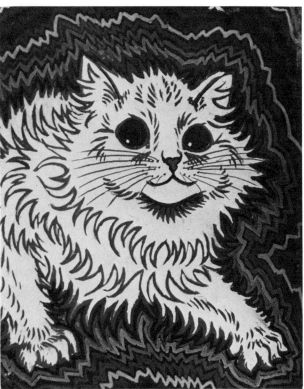

Figure 13.1. Schizophrenic cat paintings by Louis Wain, a British artist of the early twentieth century. Wain lived surrounded by cats, which he used as models for his popular drawings. In the early 1920s Wain had a schizophrenic breakdown with intermittent relapses until his death in 1936. These four paintings show the remarkable changes in his style during attacks. (© Guttmann Maclay Collection, Institute of Psychiatry, Univ. of London)

5. Behavior patterns, movements, and gestures that have no relationship to the schizophrenic's real environment but are instead responses to his own imaginary world.
6. Unintelligible speech. The schizophrenic may make up new words (that have meaning only in his fantasy world) and, even if he does not, his sentences are disjointed, incoherent, and peppered with undecipherable associations.

It may be an oversimplification but, for ease of discussion, it may be said that schizophrenics divide up into two types. Some have a long history of disturbed behavior and have steadily declined to their present schizoid state. These "process schizophrenics" almost always spend the rest of their lives in mental institutions. Others whose previous history was more or less normal seem to be jarred into a schizoid state by crisis events such as the death of a beloved relative. The recovery potential for these "reactive schizophrenics" is good.

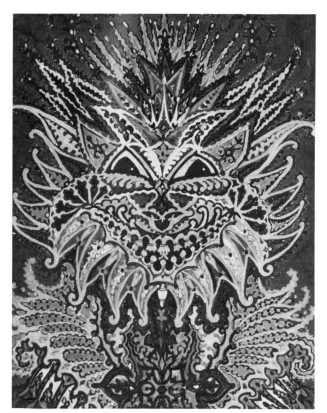 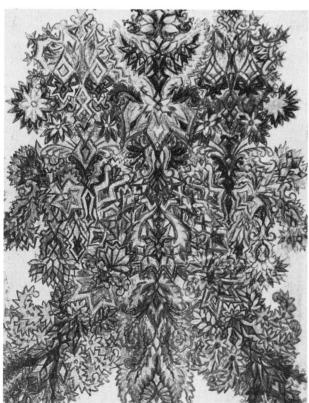

Establishing the source of either type of schizophrenia is another matter. An enormous amount of research needs to be done before a definitive answer can be supplied. There is a tendency currently among investigators to ascribe the cause of genetic factors (it may be organic, after all), but exactly how heredity plays a role is not known.

TREATMENT   The treatment of mental illness has traveled a long distance since the days when whips and branding irons were the primary therapeutic tools. Even though it is now a far more sophisticated (and humane) proposition, it still has a long way to go. Modern therapeutic methods can claim a considerable amount of success, yet the percentage of success is still relatively low, particularly in dealing with psychotics. Moreover, success can be measured more in terms of management than of cures for mental problems.

An extensive variety of techniques is used to treat mental disorders. Overall they can be divided into two categories: somatotherapy (treatment by physiological methods) and psychotherapy (treatment by psychological methods).

Somatotherapy

A growing number of physicians and psychologists are convinced that physiological factors are the major cause of psychological disorders, especially the psychoses. Consequently they concentrate on physiological methods, known collectively as somatotherapy. These techniques have been successful in some areas, such as the use of barbiturates to control epilepsy, but success in the treatment of psychosis does not approach the degree expected.

DRUGS OR CHEMOTHERAPY Drugs do not serve as a cure, but they can be very helpful as one aspect of a treatment program. The frenzied behavior of the hypermanic individual can be calmed with Paraldehyde, chloral hydrate, the barbiturates, and various major and minor tranquilizers. The amphetamines and such drugs as Elavil have succeeded in bringing depressives out of the depths of self-hate.

Perhaps the most dramatic results have been achieved with the major tranquilizers reserpine and chlorpromazine. Their ability to calm and relax patients has been notably successful with schizophrenics. They have, in some cases, not only eliminated hallucinations but even brought patients in touch with reality to the point where they can be reached by other treatment techniques such as psychotherapy.

Drug therapy is a mixed blessing, however. Chemical treatment can often produce dangerous side effects such as lowered blood pressure, jaundice, dermatitis, liver problems, anemia, and sometimes convulsions. Some therapists criticize their use in the belief that drugs merely mask the underlying causes of mental illness. Also, a patient who uses them regularly may become overly dependent on them.

SURGERY A once popular method for treating psychosis, the brain operation known as prefrontal lobotomy has generally fallen into disrepute. The procedure involved severing nerve fibers that connect the prefrontal lobes with the hypothalamus in order to reduce chronically agitated or violent behavior. Patients treated in this manner do lose their intense emotional reactions, but they also become apathetic. Other undesirable results include lowered intelligence and loss of self-control and judgment.

ELECTRIC SHOCK THERAPY This form of therapy is based on the idea that shock-induced convulsions seem to free a patient from some forms of his abnormal characteristics. An early type of shock therapy used an overdose of the hormone insulin, but this proved to be dangerous to patients. It was abandoned in favor of electric shock, a method developed in 1937 by a group of Italian physicians.

Standard shock treatment today involves a shock to the brain of 100 to 160 volts of alternating current. Usually within five seconds the individual has a seizure, and he spends the next one-half to one-and-a-half hours in a state of confusion and amnesia. Shock treatments have been used with some patients suffering from depression but exactly how this electric shock causes behavioral changes is not known. The method is not as successful with other types of mental disorders.

Psychotherapy

The emphasis in psychotherapy is on psychological factors with little or no consideration of possible physiological causes. It is the most popular form of treatment with both patients and therapists. Primarily its success lies in the treatment of neurosis, although a few therapists consider it applicable to psychosis (especially if used in conjunction with drug therapy). Many people have been helped by it, altering their behavior in ways that made life more rewarding and less anxiety-ridden. Others have merely developed a greater awareness and understanding of themselves without significantly altering behavior patterns.

Several different methods may be employed but all involve a relationship between patient and therapist in which the patient communicates his anxieties, fears, and experiences without fear of judgment. The therapist, while sympathetic, maintains an objective attitude.

PSYCHOANALYSIS An outgrowth of Freud's concepts, psychoanalysis is the most intensive, expensive, and often lengthiest form of psychotherapy. During several sessions each week, the patient begins by providing biographical information about himself. The analyst encourages him to "free associate" as he speaks—that is, to verbalize every thought and feeling that occurs to him no matter how absurd, outrageous, nonsensical, disturbing, or embarrassing it may seem. Since the natural tendency is to censor before speaking, it takes some time before the patient grows comfortable with his unedited thoughts. Often he becomes "blocked," his head empty of thoughts. It is the analyst's task to interpret by pointing out to the patient how he is resisting thoughts that may prove discomforting. He may also see behind the patient's statements and, by providing hints, set the associative process in motion again.

The next step is the process known as "transference." In the patient's eyes, the therapist acquires the characteristics of other individuals, such as his parents, and the patient reacts to his therapist accordingly. With continued therapy, the patient purges himself of long-buried emotions. He begins to gain insights into the sources of his problems. By repeatedly examining the conflicts that dominate his life, the patient eventually becomes able to confront them directly and realistically.

NONDIRECTIVE THERAPY Unlike psychoanalysis, the emphasis is on the patient's existing attitudes and behavior and does not require a detailed tracing of his emotional history. The topics under discussion are the patient's choice. The therapist does not direct them. It is the patient's job—with the aid of the therapist but without transference—to arrive at insights on his own. The therapist attempts to identify with his client, viewing things as the client does and clarifying feelings that person expresses without making judgements or interpretations. He is sympathetic and supportive yet objective. If therapy progresses properly, the patient is able to build a better self-image and the confidence that goes with it by using his own abilities to deal with his problems.

BEHAVIOR THERAPY A relatively new development, behavior therapy is not concerned with the kind of probing for insights that distinguishes psychoanalysis. Rather, it uses conditioning procedures to eliminate abnormal behavior patterns by replacing them with more desirable means of coping with conflicts. For example, in one popular method called counterconditioning, responses that are antagonistic to maladjusted behavior are strengthened until they take over. The therapist may train an anxiety-prone patient in relaxation techniques, then have him visualize situations which produce anxiety until relaxation (the antagonist) predominates.

GROUP THERAPY The therapy group provides an atmosphere somewhat closer to "real life" than the one-to-one relationship a patient has with his therapist. Members discuss their experiences and problems, react to one another's behavior and symptoms, test out different forms of behavior, try to assist one another in understanding and coping, and learn how others respond to their personalities and behavior. Once initial defensiveness is overcome, group members become more objective about themselves and, through this "laboratory situation," are able to develop behavior patterns that will foster better interpersonal relations outside the group.

ENCOUNTER OR SENSITIVITY GROUPS This fairly new and popular form of group therapy involves members in a more intensive relationship for a specified number of meetings or perhaps a single marathon weekend session. The goal is a completely uninhibited expression of emotion. Defenses are stripped away until the thoughts and feelings that are politely screened from everyday encounters come forth. Many leaders of this type of group employ a variety of "games" and role-playing techniques such as psychodrama in order to trigger the free expression of emotions. If the group functions properly, individual members should acquire a greater self-understanding through the reactions of other group members. Awareness will, hopefully, lead to a change in behavior and, from there, to better relationships with people outside the group.

THERAPEUTIC VARIETY No one method holds dominance or claims to greater success. Therapists tend to be selective, mixing techniques to find the most suitable combination for each patient. Individual personalities do not respond uniformly to different methods.

It is not possible for any given method to claim superiority. Success is a difficult thing to measure. It can not be quantified and subjected to biochemical examination. Behavioral changes may be vague and so are the subjective responses of patients. Success is often assumed on the patient's statement that he feels better. Whether he is "better" in an objective sense is an elusive proposition.

PREVENTION OF MENTAL ILLNESS

Defining mental illness is difficult. Partially because of that difficulty, preventing it is an even more formidable problem. One of the greatest barriers is the inflexible attitudes of society. The situation is not as bad as when demons prowled the earth, but mental disorders are still viewed with considerable apprehension. The admission that one is under treatment is still liable to produce raised eyebrows, and it has been known to be a barrier to professional progress.

A considerable amount of public education is required. It is necessary not only to stimulate a more positive, less prejudiced attitude toward mental disorders but to create a greater awareness of the symptoms of mental illness so that treatment may begin before the patient is beyond help.

The mental health movement, begun early in this century by a former inmate of a mental institution, has accomplished much along these lines. The group was the foundation of the National Association for Mental Health, formed in 1950. The organization has been instrumental in establishing child-guidance clinics and community mental-health clinics for the sake of treatment of existing mental disorders and the prevention of future cases.

One of the most important aspects of any prevention program is early detection of mental illness. In order to identify children with emotional problems at an early age, psychological services are becoming a feature of elementary school systems. However, they are not nearly widespread enough to be truly effective.

There are many reasons why more time, effort, and money must be expended in this cause. Though mental illness may not be directly responsible for death, it removes thousands of individuals from life as surely as cancer, heart disease, and other illnesses. The loss in talent and leadership is enormous. Aside from the disturbed individuals themselves, thousands of other lives are affected: grief-stricken families, parentless children, employers facing economic losses, law enforcement officials, and innocent victims of the more violent cases. The primary responsibility, however, is to the individual—to help him achieve his natural potential and share equally in the rewards offered by our society.

Questions

1. What are the major criteria that have been used to classify mental illness? What are the limitations of the various classifications?
2. How would you classify mental illness if management were the primary criterion?
3. What is the difference between psychosis and neurosis? Describe the major symptoms of neurotic and psychotic behavior.
4. Discuss the major types of psychotherapy. Why is there such a variety of therapeutic methods?
5. How would you develop a program to prevent mental illness? How would you measure the effects and success of such a program?

Key Concepts

Hysteria – a type of neurosis characterized by physical ailments that are caused by anxiety only and have no physiological basis

Manic-depressive – a type of psychosis characterized by behavior that is either manic (wild) or depressive (withdrawn) or both; both behaviors are believed to result from feelings of personal worthlessness

Neurosis – a behavioral disorder characterized by excessive and unreasonable anxiety

Paranoia – a type of psychosis characterized by a delusion of persecution and a general distrustfulness of other persons

Phobia – a type of neurosis characterized by an exaggerated fear of a particular object or situation

Psychopathic personality – a behavioral disorder characterized by an incapacity to cope with other individuals or society in general which results from a lack of a developed conscience or moral code and an uncompromising desire for immediate gratification

Psychosis – a behavioral disorder characterized by a total loss of contact with reality

Schizophrenia – a type of psychosis characterized by a separation of thoughts from emotions

Selected Readings

Eron, L. D., and R. Callahan, eds. *The Relation of Theory to Practice in Psychotherapy.* Chicago: Aldine Publishing Co., 1969.

Howells, John G., ed. *Modern Perspectives in World Psychiatry.* London: Oliver and Boyd, 1968.

Klein, D. F., and J. M. Davis. *Diagnosis and Drug Treatment of Psychiatric Disorders.* Baltimore: Johns Hopkins Press, 1969.

Martin, Lealon E. *Mental Health—Mental Illness: Revolution in Progress.* New York: McGraw-Hill Book Co., 1970.

Mendels, J. *Concepts of Depression.* New York: John Wiley and Sons, 1970.

Rachman, S. *Phobias: Their Nature and Control.* Springfield, Ill.: Charles C. Thomas, 1968.

Rycroft, Charles. *Anxiety Neurosis.* Baltimore: Penguin Books, 1970.

Chapter 14

Drugs

Knowledge and use of substances known primarily for their ability to alter the higher centers of man's central nervous system date to pre-Christian times. The substances, including stimulants, depressants, and hallucinogens, have been found in minerals, plants, and animals and have been synthetically prepared from chemical compounds. Culture, technology, and expediency have determined how the materials would be administered, i.e., smoked, chewed, ingested, sniffed, or injected by needle. Even though the existence and use of these materials dates to ancient times, their use has not always been condoned. It appears rather that their strong ability to alter man's sense impressions forced societies to control usage.

Mind-altering substances have been used by religious groups to intensify the religious feeling. In certain cultures these substances were used to enhance many social activities. It was acceptable, for example, for a peasant to smoke hashish while visiting with neighbors and for traders to smoke opium during business exchanges in village bazaars or during caravan rest periods. These uses, though not severely limited, were regulated by what was agreed upon as appropriate custom. Moreover, in these social activities the unwanted changes in behavior that resulted were largely ignored. As the structure of social activities

This chapter was contributed by Ralph Minear, M.D., M.P.H., Director of Pediatrics, Roxbury Comprehensive Community Health Center, Instructor in Pediatrics, Boston University School of Medicine, and Assisting Physician for Pediatrics, Boston City Hospital.

changed with economic development, however, so did society's willingness to accept the effects of these substances. Unwanted characteristics of drug use such as loss of control and unpredictability of behavior ceased to be ignored because they became detrimental to industrial and achievement-oriented cultures.

DRUG USE AND ABUSE Broadly defined, drugs are chemicals, natural or synthetic, that may alter the functioning of a person's body. The use of mind-altering drugs in America is legitimate if it comes as a result of a medical prescription. The medical uses of drugs include relief from pain (narcotics, cocaine), inducement of sleep (hypnotic-sedatives), and removal of anxiety and tension (tranquilizers). The stimulation of the amphetamines has been useful in preventing sleep and did have claims for decreasing appetite (supposedly causing weight loss). Also, hyperactive children have been successfully managed by the amphetamines. Legitimate users, however, are generally ignored in a discussion of drug use because of the preoccupation with the extreme result of illegal use—addiction. But legitimate and illicit users are not always different persons. Some legitimate drug users may give or sell their prescribed narcotics. In other cases, legitimate users who were not originally addicts may develop addiction and thereafter obtain illegally larger doses of their prescribed drug or other drugs.

Nonmedical use of drugs is for the purpose of achieving the mind-altering effects that make the drugs useful to medicine. The euphoria or sedation are sought in the absence of objective pain or tension in these circumstances. The fact that a drug may have a potential for illicit use is not known prior to its introduction to the general market. Only the market experience with a drug will demonstrate its vulnerability to illicit use.

Abuse of drugs

There is a potentiality for abuse whenever any drug is taken for any purpose other than its intended purpose and in any way that could damage the user's health or ability to function adequately. In the case of drugs lacking any legitimate "intended purpose" for the nonprofessional, such as hallucinogens, heroin, and cocaine, all use is abuse. Some substances, however, such as alcohol, caffeine, and nicotine were at one time deemed dangerous or unlawful by some cultures but were subsequently considered socially acceptable and not detrimental to health when used without excess. But what constitutes excess, and therefore abuse, for these substances is neither precisely defined nor universally accepted.

Administration of drugs

Drugs may be taken orally and then absorbed from the digestive tract into the bloodstream; they may be inhaled through the throat or sniffed

Figure 14.1. Injecting a drug into a vein produces the most rapid and potent effect. (Steve Rose, Nancy Palmer Photo Agency)

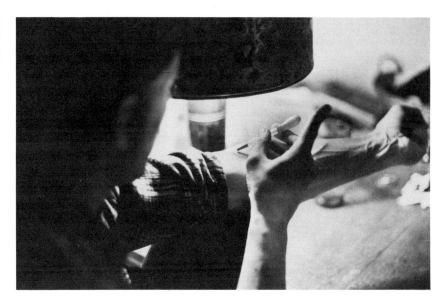

through the nose into the respiratory tract and lungs; or they may be injected into a muscle, under the skin, or into a vein. The last alternative, called *mainlining*, brings the drug most quickly into the bloodstream and tends to produce the most rapid and potent effect. In the case of drug abuse, this effect is usually the most harmful one.

Physiological effects of drug use

The effects of a particular drug depend upon the amount taken, the metabolism of the drug, and the response of the individual taking the drug. Because the conditions under which a drug is taken are not always the same, it is difficult to predict a normal response from any drug. But observations from a large group of individuals allow some generalizations (Table 14.1).

There is considerable evidence that addiction is more likely to occur if the mind-altering changes are spectacular and come quickly. If the drug is used frequently in large amounts and gains quick entry into the body, the chances of addiction are apparently increased.

Some observable effects of drug ingestion may be confusing. The polydrug habit (ingestion of more than one drug over a short time) decreases the ability to predict observable behavior. There are some drugs that increase the effect of another drug, and when two or more are combined, they may produce results that are far more harmful than those from the separate use of each of the drugs. Such an effect is called *potentiation*. For example, the combination of alcohol and hypnotics— a polydrug habit, incidentally most likely to be that of the legitimate drug user—may cause deep depression or even death.

Table 14.1 Drugs—source, classification, use, symptoms produced, and dependence potential*

Name	Slang Name	Chemical or trade name	Source	Classification
Heroin	H., Horse, Scat, Junk, Smack, Scag, Stuff, Harry	Diacetyl-morphine	Semi-Synthetic (from Morphine)	Narcotic
Morphine	White stuff, M.	Morphine sulphate	Natural (from Opium)	Narcotic
Codeine	Schoolboy	Methylmorphine	Natural (from Opium), Semi-Synthetic (from Morphine)	Narcotic
Methadone	Dolly	Dolophine Amidone	Synthetic	Narcotic
Cocaine	Corrine, Gold Dust, Coke, Bernice, Flake, Star Dust, Snow	Methylester of benzoylecgonine	Natural (from coca, not cacao)	Stimulant, Local Anesthesia
Marijuana	Pot, Grass, Hashish, Tea, Gage, Reefers	Cannabis sativa	Natural	Relaxant, Euphoriant, In high doses Hallucinogen
Barbiturates	Barbs, Blue Devils, Candy, Yellow Jackets, Phennies, Peanuts, Blue Heavens	Phenobarbital Nembutal, Seconal, Amytal	Synthetic	Sedative-hypnotic
Amphetamines	Bennies, Dexies, Speed, Wake-Ups, Lid-Proppers, Hearts, Pep Pills	Benzedrine, Dexedrine, Desoxyn, Methamphetamine, Methedrine	Synthetic	Sympathomimetic
LSD	Acid, Sugar, Big D, Cubes, Trips	d-lysergic acid diethylamide	Semi-Synthetic (from ergot alkaloids)	Hallucinogen
DMT	AMT, Businessman's High	Dimethyltriptamine	Synthetic	Hallucinogen
Mescaline	Mesc.	3,4,5-trimeth-oxyphenethylamine	Natural (from Peyote)	Hallucinogen
Psilocybin		3 (2-dimethylamino) ethylindol-4-oldihydrogen phosphate	Natural (from Psilocybe)	Hallucinogen

* Adapted from Resource Book for Drug Abuse Education, October 1969. Washington, D.C.: U.S. Department of Health, Education, and Welfare, Public Health Service, National Clearinghouse for Mental Health Information.

Medical use	How taken	Effects sought	Long-term symptoms	Physical dependence potential	Mental dependence potential
Pain relief	Injected or Sniffed	Euphoria, Prevent withdrawal discomfort	Addiction Constipation Loss of Appetite	Yes	Yes
Pain relief	Swallowed or Injected	Euphoria, Prevent withdrawal discomfort	Addiction Constipation Loss of Appetite	Yes	Yes
Ease Pain and coughing	Swallowed	Euphoria, Prevent withdrawal discomfort	Addiction Constipation Loss of Appetite	Yes	Yes
Pain relief	Swallowed or Injected	Prevent withdrawal discomfort	Addiction Constipation Loss of Appetite	Yes	Yes
Local Anesthesia	Sniffed, Injected or Swallowed	Excitation Talkativeness	Depression Convulsions	No	Yes
None in U.S.	Smoked, Swallowed, or Sniffed	Relaxation, increased euphoria, Perceptions, Sociability	Usually None	No	Yes?
Sedation, Relieve high blood pressure, epilepsy, hyperthyroidism	Swallowed or Injected	Anxiety reduction, Euphoria	Addiction with severe withdrawal symptoms, Possible convulsions, toxic psychosis	Yes	Yes
Relieve mild depression, control appetite and narcolepsy	Swallowed or Injected	Alertness Activeness	Loss of Appetite Delusions Hallucinations Toxic psychosis	No?	Yes
Experimental study of mental function, alcoholism	Swallowed	Insightful experiences, exhilaration, Distortion of senses	May intensify existing psychosis, panic reactions	No	No?
None	Injected	Insightful experiences, exhilaration, Distortion of senses	?†	No	No?
None	Swallowed	Insightful experiences, exhilaration, Distortion of senses	?	No	No?
None	Swallowed	Insightful experiences, exhilaration, Distortion of senses	?	No	No?

† Question marks indicate conflict of opinion.

Dosages of drugs

The dosage of a drug is the amount taken at one time or over a nearly continuous period. It is a significant factor in drug abuse since the effects of use may vary greatly according to the dosage. In the case of abusive use of a drug that has a proper intended purpose, the *abusive dose* is the amount needed to produce the special effects and actions desired by the user. This can become a *toxic dose*, severely damaging to the body, or even a *lethal dose*, producing death (especially with heroin and barbiturates) in many overdose cases. *Minimal dose* and *maximal dose* set the limits short of harmful special effects. It must be noted that in the case of drugs that may vary widely in potency because of differences in refinement or purity, the quantity of the drug by itself may not be the sole factor determining the kind of dosage. Other variable factors include different body chemistries between one user and another and in some cases the extent to which tolerance for the drug has been built up in the user's body cells.

Habituation and dependence

Habituation and *dependence* are terms often used interchangeably to describe a person's psychological dependence on a drug or other substance that is not physiologically addictive—a habit so deeply developed that he feels he cannot function at his best if totally deprived of it. The frequency and amount of use desired is not related to the strength of the drug. It can occur with the relatively mild drugs of caffeine, nicotine, and diluted ethyl alcohol (as in a cocktail) for which need is often felt daily. A habit involving marijuana, amphetamines, or cocaine is more likely to lead to a desire for use only at irregular intervals.

There is, however, clear evidence that the developing of habituation and dependency on certain drugs can lead to physiological addiction, notably with barbiturates, and possibly tranquilizers.

Addiction and withdrawal

The habitual user of certain drugs may develop both physical and psychological effects detrimental to his own health and to his nonuser associates. When the drug leads to actual physical dependence of his body cells, true addition is involved and the individual is not simply a drug user but a drug addict. The effect may develop soon after regular use starts, as in the case of heroin, or only through repeated excesses over a long period, as in the case of alcohol and barbiturates. Total withdrawal of the addict's drug produces a very real illness as the body cells, deprived of the substance for which they have developed an ever greater tolerance, try to return to normal. In the case of heroin, these withdrawal symptoms include insomnia, nausea, cramps in the abdomen, extreme nervousness, and symptoms resembling those of the flu victim. For barbiturate and alcohol addicts, symptoms include tremors, twitching, and even convulsions and hallucinations. Withdrawal symptoms, generally on a somewhat milder level, may also occur if the longtime addict, especially the heroin addict, fails to increase the dose for which tolerance has been established by his body cells.

CLASSIFICATION
OF DRUGS

The drug groups most associated with drug abuse are discussed in this section. The more potent members of each group have in common their ability to alter the higher centers of man's brain and central nervous system. The term *mind-altering* is most properly applicable only to the hallucinogenic group, but it is also frequently applied to the more potent members in the other groups.

Depressants are drugs which have the ability to decrease temporarily a body function or nerve ability—in particular, the central nervous system. The extreme of such action is to produce unconsciousness or coma, a beneficial function of anesthetics in major surgery. Narcotics produce marked insensibility to pain without loss of consciousness. Hypnotic-sedatives (primarily barbiturates) in their more potent form depress the central nervous system into a condition resembling normal sleep; in their less potent form they alleviate extreme nervousness. A similar function is performed by the recently developed milder drugs, the minor tranquilizers. (Major tranquilizers are properly used only in treating deep mental illness.) Antihistamines, as a side effect of their intended use, constitute the mildest of drowsiness-inducing drugs. Minor analgesics, notably aspirin, are the mildest of pain-killing drugs and constitute peripheral depressants. Ethyl alcohol decreases the functioning of the brain's master control center.

Stimulants are drugs which have the ability to increase temporarily a bodily function or nerve ability—in particular, the central nervous system. Unlike the depressants, their medical usefulness is limited. Caffeine and nicotine are among the milder stimulants widely used throughout the world. Cocaine and strychnine, a drug formerly widely used by physicians, are very potent stimulants. In between are the stimulant drugs most recently associated with drug abuse, the amphetamines.

Hallucinogens, also referred to as psychedelic drugs, produce vivid distortions of the senses and may also alter consciousness. Whether the distortions reach the level of hallucination and how greatly the consciousness is altered are among the variable effects of these controversial drugs. The drugs include marijuana, hashish, LSD-25, mescaline, peyote, and psilocybin. Normal medical use of hallucinogens is very limited and mostly experimental.

Tranquilizers

Tranquilizers were developed in the 1950s as a milder and safer alternative to the milder barbiturates as sedatives. Minor tranquilizers include Miltown, Librium, Equanil, and Valium. Major tranquilizers, whose much greater potency makes them as dangerous as barbiturates, are properly used only in the treatment of mental illness. There is evidence of addiction in cases of extreme overuse of tranquilizers, but tranquilizers have not been significant in illicit drug abuse.

Barbiturates

Barbiturates are the most versatile of all the drugs whose effect is to depress the central nervous system. Their action ranges from the sedation of emotional disturbance or even epileptic fits to inducing sleep to deep anesthesia—or even to death in overdose by accident or intent. By the beginning of this century, when German scientists had developed heroin as a supposed cure for morphine addiction, they had also derived, from substances in apples and animal urine, barbituric acid as a safer substitute for bromides. Over 2500 compounds have been developed from barbituric acid, and as with morphine and heroin, the safety record of the alternative drug has been far from clear.

The best known of the long-acting barbiturates, Veronal and Luminal, are generally used as hypnotics or sleeping-pills to relieve insomnia. Seconal and Nembutal are the most familiar of slower-acting barbiturates, used more for sedation than for sleep-inducing.

The effect of barbiturate abuse is somewhat similar to that of alcoholic intoxication. In depressing the part of the brain controlling inhibitions, it gives the user of small abusive doses temporary feelings of excitement along with relief from anxiety before he becomes sleepy. But for the chronic user of large dosages, the result is grogginess, moodiness, lack of coordination, and slurred speech—when the user is not collapsed into a deep sleep. A dose of about ten times the medically recommended dose for sleep will generally lead to death if medical aid is not administered. Unlike heroin, barbiturates produce a tolerance that is relatively fixed and does not necessitate increased doses that may eventually prove lethal. Each year there are over 3000 suicides in the United States from an overdose of barbiturates. Death may also result from a smaller overdose if the user has also had a high alcoholic intake.

Chronic abuse of barbiturates does lead to addiction, with withdrawal symptoms which are similar to those of an alcoholic and nearly as dangerous as abuse of the drug itself. These symptoms include violent tremors, convulsions, and hallucinations. Like the alcoholic, the barbiturate addict may neglect his appearance and his job and in his moodiness alienate his family and friends. Barbiturate addiction has sometimes been the result of excessive use to counteract excessive use of amphetamines.

Medical authorities consider that the chronic overuse of barbiturates, even where there is no abuse in terms of overdosage and no physiological addiction, nevertheless represents psychological dependence which is unhealthy and should be properly diagnosed and treated, if necessary by hospitalization and/or psychotherapy.

Narcotics

Narcotics, the drug family consisting of opium and its derivatives (opiates), originate as the dried juice of the Asian poppy, *Papaver somniferum*, grown throughout southern Asia from Turkey to southern China. For more than a thousand years, it has been smoked in a pipe to provide feelings of euphoria, or pounded into a powder for processing into a drug for relief of bodily ailments. In modern times opium derivatives were developed. The earliest of such opiates was laudanum, in wide use since the 1500s in many prescriptions and patent medicines. In the 1800s paregoric, a mild compound of opium and camphor, came into use. In the same period, pharmaceutical advances led to the development of a potent and highly concentrated derivative of opium: morphine. It was widely used for pain relief during the Civil War, but it made addicts of the wounded who had benefited from its use.

Intended to cure the addiction caused by morphine, heroin, a drug derived from morphine and about three times as potent, was developed by the Germans around 1900. (Another morphine-derived opiate, codeine, is used in some cough syrups and is too mild to be a significant drug abuse problem.) When heroin was found to be also addictive and offering medical science little advantage over morphine, heroin became exclusively a drug of use only to addicts. Recently there have also been developed synthetic opiate derivatives. They include Demerol, Dolophine (methadone), and Nalline. All but the last are as addictive as natural opiates.

The essential medical use of narcotics, especially morphine, is to decrease greatly the perception of pain without producing loss of consciousness or muscular weakness. This results from the drug's action in depressing the central nervous system. When a mild dosage is taken, there is also a sedative effect whereby the emotions are calmed and the mind freed from anxiety. In a more potent dosage, this sedative effect becomes euphoria, the exaggerated sense of well-being and contentment, the "high" that precedes drowsiness. Morphine is more frequently administered orally for a longer lasting effect than by injection. Heroin has its maximum effect when injected into a vein, although it is sometimes ingested orally or sniffed. There is very strong evidence that the severity of the addiction is related to the method by which the drug is taken as well as to dosage and tolerance factors.

Heroin is banned for medical use in the United States. It has been established for many years as the classic drug of drug abuse and drug addiction. In the early 1970s there were estimated to be about 300,000 heroin addicts, with perhaps as many as half in New York City.

In the United States, heroin is generally "cut" or adulterated with lactose (milk sugar) and sold as white crystalline powder. The uncertainty about the amount of adulteration presents extra hazards for the heroin addict. An amount of intake based on previous experience with highly adulterated heroin may prove fatal if the addict happens to get a supply of much purer heroin and he does not note that it is more grayish-brown and know that this indicates purer heroin. On the other hand, for the short-term addict, such adulteration may prove a blessing:

if he seeks to break his addiction, his withdrawal symptoms may be milder and briefer. It has also been observed that withdrawal symptoms are milder for users who have taken it by sniffing or smoking, as was the case with many servicemen who used heroin in Vietnam.

The immediate effect of the heroin injection is a great sense of well-being and relief from all anxieties. The user becomes relaxed and feels detachment from the world. As time passes, he may become drowsy. With continued injections, the heroin addict eventually loses interest in sex and food, becomes constipated, perspires greatly, and suffers feelings of restlessness and anxiety. He loses weight and finds his mental aptitude and physical coordination impaired. After the effects of an injection have worn off, the addict may suffer withdrawal symptoms.

Other opiates such as morphine have been relatively rare on the illegal market; they tend to be a drug abuse problem of doctors and other medical world personnel with access to supplies. However, such supplies are sometimes stolen for sale to addicts unable to obtain heroin. The same applies to the new narcotics, the synthetic opiates, especially methadone.

Methadone, most widely known for its use in the treatment of heroin addicts, is a synthetic opiate similar in appearance and effect to heroin and causing an addiction with withdrawal symptoms said by some users to be worse than those associated with heroin. It is usually ingested orally, like morphine, but can also be injected. Its greatest advantages are that it produces less euphoria than heroin, has a much longer-lasting effect, and enables the user to function adequately in some sort of productive work.

Nalline, a synthetic opiate that differs in being neither addictive nor a true depressant, is used to treat heroin overdose victims or to identify addicts by the reaction it causes.

Cocaine

Cocaine is usually classed by itself for a number of reasons. It is a powerful stimulant of the central nervous system, but also something of a hallucinogen. In various legal codes it has been classed as a major narcotic, though its effect is the opposite of that of narcotics. Because of its high cost (coca leaves from which it is derived grow in Peru, Bolivia, and Indonesia and effects of each use are brief) which is increased by vigorous law enforcement crackdowns against it, cocaine is a major item in underworld drugs. Among its variable effects is a sharpening of the mind, which has appealed not only to professional criminals but to some artists and intellectuals of the past and present. At one time cocaine was used as a local anesthetic because a side effect experienced by its Indian users was a numbing of certain parts of the body.

Cocaine is usually sniffed. The immediate effect is a euphoric excitement and feeling of great mental and physical energy with an impulse to be talkative and active. However, the effect may last as little as 10 to

Chapter 14 / Drugs 323

30 minutes. If repeated with frequency, such sniffing is likely to produce a deterioration of the nose's lining.

When cocaine is injected, the effect is more violent. The chronic user of cocaine is likely to be subject to fits of depression, convulsions, sudden hallucinations, and loss of appetite and weight with attendant malnutrition and possibly anemia. Cocaine is not addictive, however.

Amphetamines

Amphetamines (popularly called "pep pills" and "uppers") are a large group of synthetic drugs that were first developed in the 1930s as stimulants of the central nervous system. In this connection, they have been used to relieve symptoms of alcoholism, fatigue, depression, and prolonged grogginess after anesthesia. Since they have the side effect of reducing the appetite, they were long prescribed in weight-reducing programs, though there has been a phasing-out of this use recently. The longtime best known of the amphetamines were Benzedrine ("bennies") and Dexedrine ("dexies"). They were often sold "under the counter" to students wanting to stay awake to study for exams or to truck drivers anxious to avoid falling asleep at the wheel.

During World War II, German scientists perfected a more potent amphetamine, Methedrine, for use by troops engaged in prolonged missions with little time for sleep. Two decades later, Methedrine ("speed") became the favored amphetamine, frequently taken by intravenous injection. This drug, taken in this manner in repeated doses, has proved to be one of the most hazardous of abused drugs. Recognition of this danger by the young amphetamine users came when in 1967 they coined the slogan "Speed kills."

Taken as pills, and even more so when injected, amphetamines in abusive doses produce feelings of euphoria, exhilaration, talkativeness, and a sense of having better perceptions of and self-confidence to deal with any persons, things, or issues. While taking the drug in abusive doses can be lethal for someone with high blood pressure or certain heart disorders, the hazards derive primarily from what the user may do while his brain is under the influence of the drug. Prolonged use with increasing doses, as tolerance builds up, will keep the user awake for days. Acts of bad judgement, such as "defying death" at the wheels of an automobile, obviously may prove fatal. After the stimulant effects wear off, the user is often exhausted and may go for days into an on-and-off coma. The user may take barbiturates alternately with amphetamines as "downers" to give him periodic deep sleep after prolonged use of "uppers."

There is every indication that peer education has resulted in a sharp drop in extreme abuse of amphetamines by young people. Most problems now center on ethical and good-health aspects of use in individual cases, especially among athletes who may take amphetamines to get an extra edge towards the most successful performance possible. Even though there is no clear evidence of physiological addiction, the quick build-up of tolerance for amphetamines by the body makes the dividing line vague between occasional moderate use with somewhat increased doses and chronic use of abusive and hazardous dosages.

Hallucinogens

Hallucinogenic drugs have two types of sources. The first is *Cannabis sativa*, the Indian hemp plant, with a long history of use in the civilized world, containing the chemical tetrahydrocannabinol (cannabinol or THC), the active factor in a number of preparations from hashish to marijuana. The second is a group of alkaloids derived from an assortment of beans, seeds, shrubs, mushrooms and other funguses, and even a cactus. They have been used by some primitive and rural societies for an unknown number of centuries, often in connection with religious practices. Laboratory processing has derived from these alkaloids new potent preparations, such as LSD-25 of which the tiniest quantity is many times more potent than the purest and most concentrated cannabinols.

CANNABIS SATIVA Although variations of the plant are found all over the world, sometimes growing profusely like weeds, the most potent variant of this Indian hemp plant is grown in India and North Africa. Unfertilized female plants are specially cultivated to yield a heavy resin coating on their fruiting tops. From this concentrated resin, hashish is made. The top stems and leaves are dried and shredded to make a substance that when smoked is called marijuana.

Hashish, the most potent of the cannabinols, provided the origin of the words *assassin* and *assassinate*. At about the time of the Crusades, the head of a secret society of Moslem terrorists in the Far East built up his power through assassinations of his enemies carried out without fail by followers under the influence of the drug, thereby earning them the name *hashshashin* (assassins). In the nineteenth century there was some use of hashish in prescriptions in Europe and the United States as well as in the Orient. Hashish has no present-day use in this country other than as an illegal import taken for its hallucinogenic or mind-altering effects.

The effects of smoking hashish—which is estimated to be about ten times as potent as American marijuana—are typical of all hallucinogenic drugs: distortions of time and space, delusions, perceptions of sounds as colors and of the user having an additional body or parts and of others having grotesque faces. With some users, feelings of anxiety and dread follow. If the drug is ingested orally rather than inhaled as moke, the effects are often increased to approximate those of LSD.

While hashish is not addictive, individuals with previous emotional problems may accentuate and aggravate them by using this, or any, drug.

Under other names marijuana was already familiar in the United

Marijuana and health

The second annual Report on Marijuana and Health by the Department of Health, Education and Welfare, concludes that there are probably no unhealthy effects from moderate use of the drug by normal adults. Prepared by the National Institute of Mental Health and based on more than 100 scientific studies, the report does not find sufficient evidence to support theories of genetic damage or birth defects. Marijuana use was found to be as high as 90 percent among some young adult groups. This high use is clearly associated with the use of other drugs but "there is no evidence that the drug itself causes such use," and "marijuana does not appear to have a causal role in committing crimes." Further research into possible therapeutic uses of the drug was recommended by the NIMH. Favorable results have been reported from limited studies on depression, alcoholism and epilepsy and other research indicates that preparations from the drug have an antibacterial action in the treatment of certain skin diseases, inflammation of the ear and sinusitis, might be used in developing an anti-hypertension agent and in treating glaucoma.

From "No Unhealthy Effects from Marijuana: HEW Report," *Science News*, Vol. 101 (February 19, 1972).

States in the last century. In the Old West it was known as "loco weed" which caused grazing cattle that strayed on a patch to behave in unusual ways. In the latter half of the century marijuana was touted as "Indian cigarettes" by an enterprising pharmaceutical firm, appealing to those with respiratory problems.

In the twentieth century marijuana was introduced into the Southwest by Mexican laborers. In the 1920s it spread from Latin Americans and Jamaicans to New Orleans-based black musicians and then to many young jazz-oriented groups. In the 1930s reports of a crime wave in New Orleans by school children using marijuana produced widespread concern over the substance. In 1937 marijuana was banned for the first time under federal law with sale classed as a felony, though a few state laws had previously made it illegal.

Marijuana is usually smoked in a pipe or as a cigarette. The typical user, after inhaling, feels some distortion of perception and his sense of touch and of time and space. In a congenial environment among friends, he may feel relaxed, released from inhibitions, intensely sensuous, happy, and talkative—and eventually, after a number of marijuana cigarettes, he may simply go to sleep. However, if he is in an unpleasant mood to begin with, or in an uncongenial environment, he may remain quiet, absorbed in introspection, or become irritable, confused, anxious, and disoriented. The hallucinogenic effect of marijuana, generally the mildest of hallucinogens, is likely to be strongest after a very large dosage. In some cases, the user feels dizziness, ringing in the ears or a buzzing sound, loss of coordination, and blurry vision. There are some persons who claim to feel no effects at all from marijuana, especially when first using it.

The total effect of the marijuana experience, whether a good one or a bad one, generally lasts three to five hours. Except for the small percentage of users who do suffer immediate bad effects from smoking marijuana, there is no clear and obvious harmful result for the occasional user. Unlike alcoholic intoxication to which the experience is often compared, there is no hangover afterwards. Feelings of being drowsy and hungry are a frequent aftermath. There is no tendency to physiological addiction or the build-up of any significant increases in tolerance. Nor is there any tendency for most users, as has been charged, to go on to hard drugs.

LSD Among the most potent of the alkaloids associated with abusive use in the drug culture is LSD-25, derived from the lysergic acid produced from the ergot alkaloid in the fungus or rust of a rye plant. Records of outbreaks during the Middle Ages of mass hallucinations in certain communities are now attributed to the effects of this substance in rye flour. However, it was identified as a hallucinogen only in 1943 when the Swiss Dr. Jekyll who had developed LSD (in 1938) inhaled fumes from the colorless and odorless liquid. LSD is so potent that it is

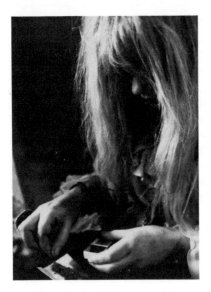

Figure 14.2. Rolling a marijuana cigarette. (Courtesy of E. Mandelmann and the World Health Organization)

usually taken only as a drop impregnated in a sugar cube, slice of fruit, candy, or chewing gum. It is about 5000 times as potent as mescaline, with 1 ounce sufficient for 300,000 doses.

The effects of LSD start in about 1 hour and normally last six to fourteen hours. With a "good trip," all sensory perceptions are vastly intensified, sounds appear as colors or even smells, all objects emanate bright colors, time seems to stand still, and the user often has full confidence that he can do anything—even fly.

The effects of a "bad trip" include overwhelming anxiety, depression, panic, delirium, convulsions, and efforts to commit suicide. Committing suicide can also be a result of a user having a "good trip" and stepping out of a high window to prove his conviction that he can fly. The familiar shakes of the alcoholic may also appear during the period of delirium. The "bad trip" is sometimes attributed to an impurity in the dose, to an overdose to which this superpotent drug is especially susceptible, or to the user having been previously in imperfect mental health. A result of LSD use by some people is the "flashback," when part of the experience under LSD may suddenly recur days or months after the last dose was taken. The charge that LSD produces chromosomal damage has not been proved.

PEYOTE, MESCALINE, AND STP Peyote, a carrot-shaped, spineless cactus found in the southwestern part of North America, was known for its hallucinogenic properties by the Aztecs, who used it in religious ceremonies to facilitate communication with spirits. In traditional use by the Indians, the button of the cactus (part of the above-ground portion) is sliced up, dried, and either chewed or brewed as a broth. Peyote has a bitter taste, and nausea with vomiting often precedes the heightened sensory perceptions that are similar to but less intense than those already noted in connection with LSD.

LSD and psychotherapy

The use of LSD has been investigated in the treatment of a wide variety of mental illnesses. This includes schizophrenia and other psychoses, various types of neuroses, and personality disorders such as sexual deviation. It has also been used to treat certain mental disorders in children.

Some investigators doubt the usefulness of LSD in psychotherapy. In one study of ten patients with sexual deviation, for example, only two improved. Others were reported to have improved, although subsequent behavior did not confirm this.

The use of LSD as an aid in psychotherapy lies in its ability, under the proper therapeutic setting, to release unconscious material from the mind, thus exposing it to the patient's full view so that he becomes aware of its implications. Long buried thoughts, deepseated wishes, and dreams are brought to the conscious level. Thus exposed it becomes possible for the patient to recognize and understand the real nature of his problem.

When used in psychotherapy, LSD is given to the patient once or twice weekly for several weeks or months, rather than in one intensive treatement. This is called the "psychotic" use of the drug. Used in this way, LSD has reportedly been beneficial to some patients with mental disorders.

From Louise G. Richards; Milton H. Joffe; and George R. Spratto, *LSD-25: A Factual Account* (Washington, D.C.: Bureau of Narcotics and Dangerous Drugs, 1969), pp. 15–16.

The active agent in peyote is mescaline, a derivative processed in the form of a soluble crystalline powder. Taken in fairly large doses, it produces a stronger effect than peyote, with less tendency to nausea, and similar to LSD for the same period. Chemically, mescaline has affinities to the amphetamines and produces some of their stimulant effects also.

"STP," an experimental mescaline derivative even more potent than LSD, got into the illegal drug market in the late 1960s. For those who have a "good trip" (estimated at fewer than 50 percent), the effects of benign hallucinations and energy without disorientation may last for several days, being present even after a period of sleep. For the less fortunate, hospitalization has been a result, with mental breakdown and even death in some cases.

OTHER ALKALOID HALLUCINOGENS Psilocybin is derived from a Central American mushroom and, like peyote, has had some religious ritual usage by American Indians. Its active agent was isolated in 1958 by the same Swiss researcher who had developed LSD twenty years earlier; later he synthesized it. The effects of psilocybin are similar to those of mescaline.

DMT is a laboratory-processed derivative of the cahobe, a sacred bean of Indians of the Caribbean area. DMT produces its hallucinogenic effects in about two minutes; they usually end in thirty minutes. Whether its hazards are substantially less than those of kindred drugs remains undetermined.

Among other substances used to produce alkaloid hallucinogens are the seeds of the morning glory plant. Various methods of preparation have been used, but sometimes the user merely swallows 300 seeds to produce an effect equivalent to one dosage of LSD-25, to which they are chemically related. Variations in effect match those of LSD.

DRUG USERS There are no proven reasons for why individuals use drugs, only speculations as to the causes for use. Because drug use is currently identified with youth, most explanations for its use are tied to the adolescent's emotional development. For example, models for developing appropriate adult roles come from belonging to groups and sharing their behavior patterns. In order to be an active participant in these groups, quite frequently it may be necessary to use drugs—in the same way that liquor consumption was required when it was in vogue. To some degree this might account for youth's acceptance of marijuana as a recreational drug for promoting a good time and an expansion of consciousness.

Some type of youth identification and youthful protest is also a part of an adolescent's personal development. During the 1960s this process took an unusual course. For many youth marijuana was used as a symbol of identification as part of a new generation refusing to accept old taboos.

There are others, however, who may use drugs—particularly "hard

Figure 14.3. (Steve Rose, Nancy
Palmer Photo Agency)

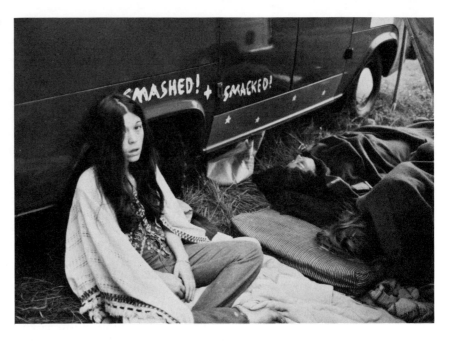

drugs"—out of desperation or because of an inability to cope with the
stresses associated with passing through adolescence or into a place
in adult society. These individuals are the ones who may have underlying difficulties in acquiring normal emotional development, and consequently they may be the most severely damaged by drugs. Yet anyone
may have an experience with drugs, no matter what his occupation,
socioeconomic status, or educational affiliation. If there is no common
type of drug user, there is also no common age for drug abuse.

The user's life style depends upon the drug used, the frequency of
use, his physical and emotional status, and whether he loses control to
the drug. Accordingly, some users of drugs may rely upon the euphoria
or well-being that follows the drug's use to carry them through subsequent psychological stresses and pressures. Other users are unable to
return to those intervals where they are not euphoric.

The economic stability of a drug user depends upon the extent of
his use and the type of drugs used. It also depends upon the degree of
support available to him. If his existing economic resources are insufficient, it has been believed, this lack leads him to resort to theft or even
violent crimes. Indeed, one study indicates that as many as 67 percent
steal in order to pay for drug use. However, when we consider that
another study indicates an equal percentage with criminal records before
drug use, it becomes unclear whether criminal activity of drug users was
developed to support their habit or whether it predated their use of
drugs.

There is a strong belief that anyone's experimentation with drugs, particularly heroin, has irrevocable results implying that any experimenter will become an addict and will have a degenerate life filled with criminal acts in order to support the habit. This belief is being challenged by our experience with Vietnam veterans. Of the heroin users in Vietnam, only slightly over 1 percent remained habitual users once they returned to the United States. However, the method of use apparently can be a determining factor in what happens to the drug user—only 8 percent of the users injected heroin while in Vietnam; the remainder sniffed or smoked it. Another popular theory—the inevitable escalation or progression from one type of drug ("soft drugs," such as marijuana) to more serious drugs ("hard drugs," such as heroin)—does not seem to be supported by significant evidence.

Yet certain generalizations can be made about the results of heavy drug abuse on the drug user apart from the varying physiological effects of each specific drug. Though the user may not have committed a crime to obtain his drug, jail or the court costs of seeking to avoid it is a prospect hanging over the head of the user, especially if he has in his possession a quantity large enough to justify a charge of intending to traffic with it. (The specific quantity varies according to different drugs and different laws.) Health deterioration in general is also a likely result of heavy use of many drugs, including inadequate sound sleep, overstimulation, loss of appetite and malnutrition, and in some cases damage to such organs as the liver, kidneys, or brain. An additional hazard, hepatitis (and in some cases syphilis), is a threat to those whose habit involves group injections with the same unsterile needle. The health consequences of drug abuse can even be passed to the unborn. One out of every forty babies (approximately 1,300 each year) in the hospitals of New York City is addicted to drugs. Many of these babies are premature and suffer undiagnosed withdrawal symptoms.

LEGAL CONTROLS

As early as 1912, the Hague Convention developed an international treaty to govern the use of narcotics. This treaty, which was intended to protect individuals from drug hazards, did not provide means for enforcement. In the United States, the Harrison Act of 1914 placed the control of narcotics in the hands of the federal government, even though some individual states had narcotic control laws already. The aim was to restrict narcotics to legitimate professional use in a uniform manner throughout the United States. This was done by establishing a unit for enforcement and requiring professionals to register and maintain a log of narcotics prescribed. Legal controls have been escalated since then in order to prevent the unknown dangers of nonmedical or unsupervised narcotic use. In 1946 the number of drugs subject to international control was approximately 20, but this number had increased to 90 by 1966.

In 1965–1966 a comprehensive surveillance of drug dangers was placed in the hands of two United States government agencies—the Food and Drug Administration and the Department of Health, Educa-

Reducing diet pills

Last year the Food and Drug Administration reviewed the use of amphetamines for diet control and concluded that they are of little value. Accordingly, production quotas for the drug were cut back by 83 percent . . . Now the FDA is requesting another 50 to 60 percent reduction in amphetamine production. Recommendations sent to the Justice Department's Bureau of Narcotics and Dangerous Drugs call for a 20 percent cut in production of orally taken amphetamines and the complete elimination of all amphetamines prepared to be taken by injection or in combination with other drugs.

Not only are the amphetamine diet pills of little value, says the FDA, they are unsafe in the injectable form and have a great potential for abuse. Reds and uppers, however, will still be available on the black market and abuse of these drugs will probably continue.

From "Reducing Diet Pills," *Science News*, Vol. 103 (February 3, 1973), p. 73.

tion and Welfare. After investigation the Secretary of HEW could specify any volume of a substance as having a potential for hazard because of its depressant, stimulant, or hallucinogenic effect on the central nervous system. The FDA was to enforce the recommendations.

Another method of controlling the use of narcotics is to restrict the production of narcotics. As early as 1949, opium production was restricted by the Economic and Social Council of the United Nations. At present there are ten international treaties regulating the production and use of narcotics. Just this year production of amphetamines has been curtailed, and amphetamines already on the market are to be recalled by the Food and Drug Administration and the Justice Department's Bureau of Narcotics and Dangerous Drugs.

Because the use of narcotics was a complex and seemingly unsolvable problem the President established two study groups—in 1962, the White House Conference on Narcotic and Drug Abuse, and in 1963, the President's Commission on Narcotic and Drug Abuse. These groups recognized the failures in enforcement when they recommended a more effective framework for regulation and a stronger unit to combat the large volume of illicit drug traffic. Further, the Presidential Commission suggested that the National Institute of Mental Health become involved in sorting out the problems of narcotic use. This recommendation cited narcotic use as a health as well as a crime-related problem.

These recommendations and others contributed to the decision for a large reorganization in the management of narcotics use by the federal government. It provided for a new Drug Enforcement Administration within the Justice Department. This unit would include four federal agencies (the Bureau of Narcotics and Dangerous Drugs, the Office for Drug Abuse Law Enforcement, the Office of National Narcotics Intelligence, and the Investigative Unit of the Bureau of Customs) all working with the problem of illicit drug traffic, but under separate supervisions.

Penalties for drug violations

Under the *Narcotics Control Act* of 1956, a second offense of illegal sale or a third offense of possession of heroin, cocaine, or marijuana brought a minimum of 10 years and up to 40 years, with no probation or parole permitted. Imprisonment for life, on the recommendation of a jury, was stipulated for repeated offenses of possession and sale. Heroin was separated for the most stringent provision: for acts of any sort leading to heroin being taken by someone under 18, a jury might recommend a sentence of death.

The Comprehensive Drug Abuse Prevention and Control Act of 1970 made the penalties less inflexible and severe than the 1956 law (especially in eliminating the mandatory minimum sentence) and provided sounder reclassifications concerning more dangerous and less dangerous drugs. Marijuana involvement was reduced to a misdemeanor except for trafficking, with no mandatory minimum sentence and a maximum of one year for the first offense. However, trafficking penalties remain heavy in a scale rising to 20 years to life and a $200,000 fine for repeated and regular trafficking. Almost as heavy is the penalty for second and subsequent sale to one under age—which is 21 in this law, as opposed to the previous 18. This can bring up to 15 years and a $45,000 fine.

In the case of heroin, penalties for possession are similar to those covering marijuana. But unlawful distribution, sale, or give-away brings up to 15 years for the first offense, up to 30 years for the second, and up to life for a repeating enterprise. Distribution to someone under 21 brings up to 30 years for the first offense and up to 45 years for subsequent offenses. Trafficking in LSD is penalized heavier than marijuana though somewhat lighter than heroin, but still with a double penalty if the drug goes to someone under 21, and up to life for a continuing criminal enterprise.

In order to cope with the continued illicit use of narcotics, each individual state has continued to enact legislation that either supplements or augments the federal narcotics laws. Enforcement of these laws is by local police as well as state agencies. An especially stringent law was enacted in New York State in 1973. Like the superseded 1956 federal law, it provided mandatory minimum sentences, with a complex scale based on the type of drug, the amount involved, possession or sale, and the previous record of the offender, ranging up to life imprisonment for the maximum sentence. However, marijuana was excepted for a first offense where probation is authorized. On the other hand, a judge is authorized to sentence up to 15 years for sale of any amount of marijuana or for possession of as little as one ounce at his discretion—in practice applicable to the offender with a previous drug-law violation record.

Drugs and Americans abroad

Almost 950 young Americans are presently languishing in foreign prisons around the world on drug charges. There are about 200 imprisoned in Europe and the Middle East. Some . . . have received draconian sentences—30 years in a Turkish prison—and others . . . are confined to windowless cells in what are described as unsanitary, disease-ridden jails in Spain. In many countries, there is no differentiation between hard and soft drugs and possession might carry much greater penalties than at home.

The U. S. embassies say there is virtually nothing they can do about the plight of these people; when an American is in another country he is subject to the laws of that country, with no exceptions—unless, that is, he has diplomatic immunity. The most they can do, the U. S. consulates say, is to make occasional visits of charity to the imprisoned.

Although Spain, Turkey, and Britain are three of the most publicized places where frequent drug arrests of Americans occur, in fact they are relatively far down on the list of countries which have imprisoned the most U. S. citizens.

Mexico tops the list, followed by Canada, and then Germany, with 110 civilian Americans, including four young women, serving time on narcotics convictions.

A U. S. State Department spokesman sums up the drug sentencing situation like this:

"Young travelers better know what they are up against when they travel. What happens to you in court depends on where you are and how the officials of that country feel on a particular day.

"If a judge feels particularly hostile to hippies, or drugs, or even Americans, then you might find yourself in the position of the mouse being hit with a sledgehammer."

From Lucinda L. Franks, "U. S. Family Goes Broke Trying to Free Drug Offender in Europe," *The Boston Globe* (October 27, 1973).

Changing attitudes about drug use since the sixties

The traumatic experience for the United States caused by the epidemic of narcotic use during the 1960s led to an all-out war on drugs. The confrontation demonstrated 1. that the use of drugs involved something more than simply a crime; 2. that the law enforcement approach alone was not totally effective; and 3. that all of the mind-altering substances were not of equal severity in their effects. Thus, solid public support for the existing approaches to controling the use of narcotics was undermined.

In response to new ideas about controlling drug use, the states began to require compulsory treatment for those individuals found to be using narcotics. The burden of care was transferred from law enforcement to medicine, but always with the threat that legal action would intervene if medical care failed. The premise was that the threat of confinement would reduce drug use. Because of the variable results with this restricted medical management, other ideas were introduced. For example, the Federal Drug Education Act of 1970 furnished large sums of money to be used in schools for the purpose of teaching students about the dangers of drug use.

The failure of law enforcement to control drug use has by no means been universally accepted. But those who strongly support reliance on the law-enforcement approach welcomed a new sharp distinction between two types of persons involved with drugs: the pusher (seller) and the users, especially youth, who experiment with or occasionally use narcotics. To enforce the credibility of this dichotomy in the definition of narcotic use, many politicians are demanding extremely severe sentences for individuals who sell drugs or participate in major drug trafficking. The most difficulty in the application of this approach occurs when the user is found in possession of an amount of drugs that qualifies under the law for trafficking intent, even if he claims it was only for his own use.

Previous legal controls of narcotic use were based on the premise that any use leads to the most severe of dangers, drug addiction. Also, all substances that had a potential for being dangerous were thought to be equally hazardous. These concepts were changed by a large-scale, "spontaneous" experience with drugs, the polydrug culture of the 1960s. Consequently, there is a trend to remove marijuana from the list of drugs that are considered severely dangerous. The trend results in a confusing status for marijuana; laws which consider its possession and use a crime are being reduced but its use as a product similar to alcohol and tobacco has not been legally condoned.

PREVENTION
AND TREATMENT

The prevention of drug use in the United States has been subject to federal law since 1914. Because most of the public felt that illicit use of drugs was a moral crime, the legal system long continued to be virtually the sole preventive tool for many decades. However, our experience with drug use over the last ten years has led to many preventive measures being explored aside from the legal ones which demand abstinence.

Under state laws, treatment was oriented toward graduated withdrawal, under medication, with success measured by the patient's professed lack of any further interest in narcotics or need for them. However, in many cases where freedom was a probable consequence of such a "cure," the patient often became an addict again after leaving his treatment institution. In recent years, there have been two new types of programs to tackle this problem. The first is the maintenance program, which grew out of the search for a cure for narcotics addiction by means of a drug—chemotherapy. It is designed for the addict who cannot permanently break his habit but wants to function as a useful member of society. The second is the psychological therapy center designed for the addict who has gotten rid of his addiction but needs months or years of assistance to avoid returning to it.

Chemotherapy

The prevention of unwanted drug effects is based on the principle of antagonism or of substitution by another substance. This material may be taken before or subsequent to the use of an illicit drug.

An antagonist is a chemical agent designed to counteract the effects of a drug. Most work with antagonists is directed against narcotics, especially opiates. A narcotic antagonist, such as Nalline or cyclazocine, occupies the same place in the central nervous system as would a narcotic normally, but it has almost none of the narcotic effects. There is also no threat of addiction from these antagonists. Administration of a narcotic antagonist to a narcotic addict who has decided to stop abusing the drugs can help him through his withdrawal and rehabilitation periods.

Heroin was developed as a substitute drug to cure morphine addiction, but boomeranged in presenting an even worse addiction problem. Several drugs were developed from synthetic opiates that did indeed eliminate the withdraw symptoms when the addict took them, but once again the most effective drugs proved addictive also. The best known application of the substitution principle in the United States and Great Britain is the use of one of these synthetics, methadone, as a substitute for opiates, especially heroin. Though it is addictive, methadone does offer advantages: the effect of an adequate dosage lasts several times as long as heroin, it does not involve the high of heroin addiction, and the addict who takes it can function effectively at a job while he continues to take his prescribed doses.

Methadone, however, cannot be considered a cure-all for every heroin user. For example, it appears more effective for older than for younger users. The substitution works best for those who participate in a drug treatment program but are unable to detoxify themselves by discontinuing their use of heroin. Before being admitted to a methadone program, the drug user must undergo careful screening in terms of age, background, sincerity about cooperation, and potential for social rehabilitation which depends in large part on appropriate support from a family and an employer. Many suitable candidates have had to be denied admission because of limited capacity throughout the major urban centers of heroin addiction.

Psychological rehabilitation

Efforts directed toward treatment of addiction, especially heroin addiction, cannot be based upon a premise that absolute abstinence means success. The failure to achieve this in many treatment programs serves to challenge such a premise. Instead, success has been found in the rehabilitation of the addict to some life style better than the one he had when he was addicted to drugs. The rehabilitation programs are directed at developing vocational skills, learning to have some experience at living in a viable group, and learning to cope with personal weaknesses.

The treatment programs most often begin under the jurisdiction of some sort of institution. While in these institutions, addicts are detoxified and a program of psychotherapy is begun. From here the individual may move to residential centers or "half-way houses." Synanon, founded in California in 1958, is the original model for these programs involving residential centers for reformed addicts. One of the largest is Phoenix House, begun in 1967 with funding from the municipal government of New York City. Odyssey House also serves New York. Among others of the better known ones are Gateway Houses in Illinois, Renewal House in Atlanta, Habilitat in Hawaii, and Renaissance in Washington, D.C. Most of the programs will not allow any use of an addictive drug, even methadone, under a maintenance program.

Though no one is required to join or to stay after being admitted, once in the program, the former addict must submit to the regulations of the program and to the discipline of being led through stages of ever-increasing responsibility within the community. Group therapy through encounter sessions is a major feature, and all residents are required to attend and participate in the sessions. Ex-addicts are used to participate in the small groups that seek to maintain a rigid and supporting community. In many programs, if a "graduate" does not have the needed outside family and job, he may be encouraged to stay on as a permanent resident to help others as he has been helped—or to work in a similar program elsewhere.

Questions   1. Name the major groups of drugs most associated with drug abuse and the primary physiological effects each produces. Which drugs are depressants? Which are stimulants? Which are hallucinogens?
2. What is meant by abuse of drugs? What are the various dosage levels of drugs and what are the physiological effects at each level?

3. What is meant by addiction? Which drugs are addictive?
4. Many people, hopeful that heroin addicts eventually will come voluntarily to treatment centers for rehabilitation, advocate free distribution of heroin to addicts in the meantime to keep them from stealing to support their habit. In light of what you know about heroin and heroin addiction, what is your opinion of this proposal?
5. What are various methods of controlling the use of narcotics in the United States today? How could more attention and funds be directed toward prevention rather than control of drug abuse?

Key Concepts

Addiction – a physiological dependence on a drug which if taken away causes severe physical discomfort and illness in the user

Depressant – a substance which has the ability to decrease body functioning temporarily

Hallucinogen – a substance which has the ability to cause distortions of the senses and perception

Potentiation – the combination of two or more drugs which produces more severe physiological effects when administered than are produced by each drug individually

Stimulant – a substance which has the ability to increase body functioning temporarily

Tolerance – the condition of body cells so accustomed to a drug that they no longer respond to the original dosage of the drug and an increased dosage is required to produce the intended effect

Withdrawal symptoms – the severe physiological discomfort and illness resulting from total or partial abstinence from an addictive drug, including nausea, stomach cramps, and extreme nervousness

Selected Readings

Blakeslee, Alton. *What You Can Do About Dangerous Drugs.* New York: Associated Press, 1971.

Drug Abuse: Escape to Nowhere, 3rd ed. Philadelphia: Smith Kline, and French Laboratories, 1968.

Endore, Guy. *Synanon.* New York: Doubleday, 1968.

Grinspoon, Lester. *Marijuana Reconsidered.* Cambridge, Mass.: Harvard University Press, 1971.

Jurgensen, Warren P. *Problems of In-Patient Treatment of Addiction.* New York: New York State Narcotic Addiction Control Commission, 1968.

President's Commission on Law Enforcement and Administration of Justice. *Task Force Report: Narcotics and Drug Abuse.* Washington, D.C.: U.S. Government Printing Office, 1967.

Chapter 15

Tobacco and Alcohol

Since man first discovered tobacco and alcohol centuries ago, he has been fascinated by their uses. Society's view of what constituted proper uses for these substances has varied considerably at different times and has included a wide range of possibilities, many of them based on ignorance or very skimpy knowledge at best. Alcohol, for example, has been accepted as everything from a universal solvent to a mystical ingredient in religious ceremonies. Even within societies, different segments of the population may take opposing views about what is and what is not a proper use. Adults and adolescents often conflict over the virtues and vices of social drinking versus marijuana smoking.

Degree of use raises other questions. Drinking cocktails and smoking cigarettes are generally regarded as normal aspects of the contemporary scene, but excessive use—chain-smoking or alcoholism—is considered abnormal. The problem lies in defining excessive. One man's excess is another man's mild indulgence. As a result, public policy governing usage of these substances tends to be contradictory, simplistic, unenforceable, or obscured in rhetoric.

This chapter was contributed by Ralph Minear, M.D., M.P.H., Director of Pediatrics, Roxbury Comprehensive Community Health Center, Instructor in Pediatrics, Boston University School of Medicine, and Assisting Physician for Pediatrics, Boston City Hospital.

TOBACCO

Learning to use tobacco

The plant from which tobacco products are made—a species from the nightshade family (Solanaceae)—was prescribed for medicinal purposes by physicians in ancient Greece. The same plant, now called Nicotiana, was introduced to western Europe as something to be smoked after the expeditions of Columbus. Its botanical name came from Jean Nicot, a French nobleman who popularized tobacco derivatives as both medical cures and pleasure products. The more common name, tobacco, originated with a Y-shaped pipe used by American Indians to inhale smoke through their nostrils.

Depending on the intended use, people learned to prepare tobacco in a variety of ways over the centuries: as rolled, dried leaves for smoking; as shredded leaves for chewing or smoking; or as pulverized leaves for sniffing or retaining in the mouth or on the body. In spite of the alleged values of tobacco as a therapeutic aid for everything from skin ulcers to plague, smoking became its most popular use wherever it was introduced.

Initially, smoking was associated with cultural ceremony—a means of demonstrating good faith and peaceful intentions among a group of individuals, for example. Changing life styles and periods of stress—such as wartime—led to new ritualistic and social uses as well as increased consumption. Ultimately, the act of smoking came to be regarded exclusively as a pleasurable self-indulgence.

Tobacco as industry

Smoking as a mass pleasure (or evil, depending on one's point of view) was an outgrowth of two developments: the increased mechanization of our society in the nineteenth century and, more recently, the growth of mass communications. The invention of the cigarette manufacturing machine during the 1870s made large-scale production possible and lowered the price of cigarettes. Annual production in the United States averaged 4.2 billion cigarettes in the first decade of the twentieth century. In 1973, the United States Department of Agriculture estimated that domestic consumption of cigarettes would hit an all-time high of 583 billion.

With the introduction of mass production, tobacco became a significant American farm product and a major contributor to the economic well-being of such states as North Carolina, Virginia, Kentucky, Georgia, Tennessee, and South Carolina. When tobacco prices fell during the Depression, the U.S. government began to subsidize tobacco farmers. This assistance program began as payments for diverting acreage from tobacco to other crops and later changed to price supports. By the mid-1960s tobacco ranked fourth among agricultural products as a recipient of U.S. government loans, and there was more tobacco on inventory than any other U.S. farm commodity.

Concurrent with the growth of the tobacco industry, the mass media

Table 15.1 Per capita consumption of cigarettes, 1925–1971*

Year	Cigarettes
1925–29 [a]	1,285
1930–34 [a]	1,389
1935–39 [a]	1,779
1940–44 [a]	2,558
1945–49 [a]	3,459
1950	3,522
1951	3,744
1952	3,886
1953	3,778
1954	3,546
1955	3,597
1956	3,650
1957	3,755
1958	3,953
1959	4,073
1960	4,171
1961	4,266
1962	4,265
1963	4,345
1964	4,195
1965	4,259
1966	4,287
1967	4,280
1968	4,186
1969	3,993
1970	3,985
1971	4,040 [b]

[a] Annual Average.
[b] Subject to revision.
* U.S. Department of Agriculture. Population 18 years of age and over.

expanded enormously in size and influence, and advertising agencies developed sophisticated techniques of selling. The cigarette companies took full advantage of both, projecting an image of smoking as a stimulus to friendship, a cure for shyness, an entree to joining the "in" group, a tension-breaker, and even as an aid to digestion and health in general. Advertising can take the greatest share of credit for pushing cigarette sales into the billions. In 1963 approximately 3.5 percent of the money spent by smokers went into advertising, and cigarettes ranked fourth among all products in terms of advertising expenditures.

Opposition to smoking

Despite widespread use and the general acceptance of smoking, its pleasures have not received universal approval. Beginning decades ago, large segments of public opinion, including many religious groups, branded smoking as immoral, unproductive, unhealthy, and unfit as an activity for well-bred individuals. Smokers have been punished by social ostracism, heavy fines, and expulsion from home or school. Protective laws were passed to prohibit the sale of tobacco products to minors and, at one time, to women. Taxation has also been used to curb smoking, but today it is largely a means of exploitation (for the sake of revenue).

During the 1930s the medical profession began to grow suspicious of the effect of cigarette smoking on health, mostly because of a rapidly rising number of cases of lung cancer. By the 1950s the general public began to worry about the effects of tobacco on health and, even though cigarette consumption continued to increase, it did so at a slower rate.

The evidence that these fears were correct arrived in 1964 when the "Surgeon General's Report" was released to the public. Research by a select group of scientists (approved by the tobacco industry, incidentally) showed that "cigarette smoking is a health hazard of sufficient importance in the United States to warrant appropriate remedial action." Follow-up studies by the U.S. Public Health Service and thousands of private agencies have confirmed those findings. The results were enough to make millions of people swear off cigarettes. Nevertheless, a decade later, 42.2 percent of the men over 21 and 30.5 percent of the women over 21 in America were still smoking.

Smokers

The habit of smoking—cigarettes for the most part—is usually acquired during the teenage years. The first experimentation comes around the age of twelve. Each year, approximately one million teenagers become smokers, according to estimates from the U.S. Department of Health, Education, and Welfare. Statistics reveal that 75 percent of the male and 46 percent of the female population of the United States have smoked regularly at one time or another, although 26 percent of those men and 11 percent of the women have quit.

Men smoke more than women. Twenty-six percent of American

males smoke more than a pack of cigarettes a day while only 18 percent of the women puff away at that rate. Rural areas have a lower percentage of smokers than cities—a comment, perhaps, on the tensions of urban living. People who are low on the socioeconomic scale and have less formal education are the most likely to smoke. That is true of both adults and teenagers. However, in terms of the amount of cigarettes smoked, there are more heavy smokers—both men and women—among people who have high incomes and high educational achievements.

Studies demonstrate that adolescents are more likely to smoke if their parents do. Older brothers and sisters, aunts, uncles, other family members, and admired adults such as teachers and athletic coaches can also influence the decision to smoke or not to smoke. All those people serve as models of adult behavior, and over the years smoking has come to be regarded as an adult prerogative. Teenagers, therefore, see smoking as a symbol of maturity and a way of experimenting with adult roles. By the same token, adolescents also use smoking as a device for expressing anger and rebellion against adult authority.

Regardless of where parents and other adults stand on the issue, young people frequently take their first puffs because friends urge them to try it. Social acceptance is a matter of crucial importance to most adolescents, and smoking often seems like the key to belonging. Adver-

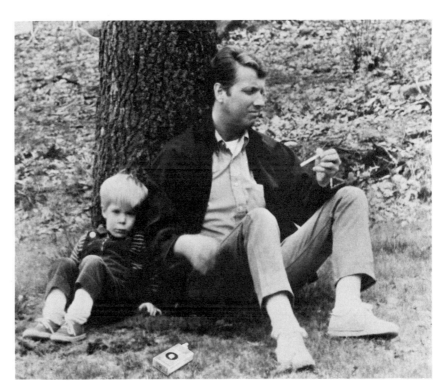

Figure 15.1. A scene from the American Heart Association's television spot film, "Like Father, Like Son," which makes the point that youngsters will follow the example of their elders in developing good habits, and bad ones, like smoking cigarettes. (Courtesy of the American Heart Association)

tising, the most inescapable influence of all, makes it a point to reinforce the aspect of social acceptability in smoking.

Reasons for smoking

As far back as the seventeenth century, long before cigarettes as we know them appeared, tobacco was recognized as a stimulant. The development of cigarettes enhanced this effect, most because the smoke was inhaled. Smoking does boost the pulse rate, probably because of the nicotine in the smoke.

Something in cigarettes—again, nicotine is the most likely candidate —is mildly addictive. Once an individual is initiated into the rites of smoking, he continues simply because it becomes a habit like any other habit. But it is a habit that soon becomes closely linked with psychological dependence, a need satisfied by the oral and manual gratification that comes from handling a cigarette, lighting it, placing it between his lips, inhaling, exhaling, and so on. It becomes connected with social drives: a link to one's peers, a source of security at parties. Smoking seems to relieve tension (at least people are convinced that it does) and, as the habitual smoker gets used to the effects of his habit, the absence of a cigarette creates tension which can be calmed, in turn, only by another cigarette.

It is a self-perpetuating phenomenon, and the longer it continues, the more the psychological dependence is strengthened and the more difficult it is to break. It becomes an addiction but not in the sense of physiological dependency. A smoker trying to quit will probably experience some uncomfortable moments, but his discomfort is not like the agony of a heroin addict trying to free himself from his habit.

Composition of cigarettes and smoke

As agriculture grew more sophisticated, the tobacco plant was developed in a variety of strains, each with its own properties and uses. Every cigarette manufacturing concern has its own highly classified recipes that blend tobacco types to give each brand a unique flavor. In a typical year the industry as a whole made its cigarettes from 53 percent flue-cured tobacco leaves (cured over heated metal pipes), 36 per cent burley (air-cured tobacco leaves), 1 percent Maryland, and 10 percent Oriental tobacco leaves. To make cigarettes, the leaves are shredded and flavored with any number of ingredients: fruit juices, honey, maple sugar, vanilla, tonka beans, wines, cocoa, tongue, and menthol. The mixture is given a moisture treatment before it is formed into cigarettes.

If a lot goes into cigarettes, more comes out. More than 270 distinct chemical compounds have been identified in cigarette smoke. At least 15 of these are known carcinogens—that is, cancer-producing agents. About 8 percent of the smoke is formed by particulate matter, better known as tar. (Nicotine is one of the elements in tar.) Tar contains most of the carcinogens, the most dangerous of which are the polycyclic aromatic hydrocarbons.

The smoke also contains chemical substances known as co-carcinogens which interact, like catalysts, with the cancer-causing agents to stimulate cancer growth. Phenol is one of these, and when very small amounts of a carcinogen (polycyclic aromatic hydrocarbons comprise only 0.03 percent of the tar) are exposed regularly to phenol, they will cause cancer. The remainder of the smoke is made up of gases such as nitrogen, carbon dioxide, oxygen, and carbon monoxide.

EFFECTS OF SMOKING
ON HEALTH

Many cigarette smokers rationalize their habit with the belief that city smog is such a health hazard that they might as well smoke—it cannot make things any worse. While it is true that air pollution is harmful, it plays a lesser role in illness than cigarette smoking.

In general, death rates are much higher among smokers. Young men who smoke over two packs a day will have their life expectancy reduced by eight years on the average. Cigarette smoking affects primarily the respiratory and circulatory systems, and 80 percent of the excess deaths caused by smoking are associated with three diseases: lung cancer, coronary heart disease, and respiratory diseases (chronic bronchitis and pulmonary emphysema).

LUNG CANCER Approximately 90 percent of all cases of lung cancer originate in people who smoke cigarettes. It is the primary cause of cancer death among American men and a rapidly growing one among women. In 1959, it was predicted that one million American school-children would die of lung cancer before they reached the age of 70. Yet lung cancer was a relatively rare disease as recently as 50 years ago.

The bronchial tubes, which carry air into the lungs, are protected by millions of tiny, hairlike structures called cilia which move constantly (as often as 1,000 times a minute). The cilia guard the delicate tissue of the tubes and lungs by sweeping out foreign particles such as dust, pollen, soot and propelling them back to the throat where they are easily expelled in mucous. However, when cigarette smoke enters the bronchial tubes, it causes conditions which eventually paralyze the cilia. Their failure to function slows down the macrophages, cells which help to keep the lungs clean. As a result, tar accumulates along the lining of the bronchial tubes, allowing cancer-causing and cancer-promoting substances to remain in contact with the sensitive cells over long periods of time. Most cases of human lung cancer begin this way in the bronchial tubes and spread into the lungs as more and more cells are attacked.

The smoking of cigarettes, cigars, and pipes is also a major cause of cancer of the larynx, esophagus, and oral area (mouth, pharynx, and cheek). Pipe smokers are particularly vulnerable to cancer of the lip. Research studies have also linked smoking with cancer of the urinary bladder, the pancreas, and the kidney.

HEART AND CIRCULATORY SYSTEM DISEASES Male smokers have a 70 percent higher rate of death from coronary heart disease than nonsmokers. For men between the ages of 45 and 54, death rates from coronary heart disease are 3 times as high among heavy smokers as nonsmokers. Women in the same age group who are heavy smokers have death rates twice as high.

Research is currently probing the exact nature of the relationship between smoking and coronary heart disease. Nicotine and carbon monoxide, both present in cigarette smoke, are believed to be the major

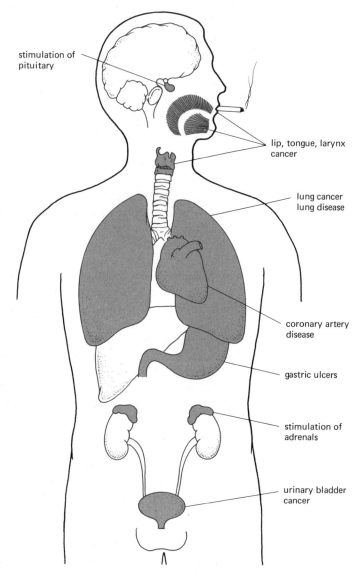

stimulation of
pituitary

lip, tongue, larynx
cancer

lung cancer
lung disease

coronary artery
disease

gastric ulcers

stimulation of
adrenals

urinary bladder
cancer

Figure 15.2. The effects of smoking.

causative factors. Nicotine increases the requirement of the heart for oxygen while carbon monoxide inhibits the ability of the blood to supply the oxygen that is needed. These two factors working in opposition exert tremendous strain on the heart, ultimately causing coronary heart disease. This is especially true when the heart is also under strain from high blood pressure, overweight, an excess of high serum cholesterol, and lack of exercise. Moreover, smoking can accelerate an already existing coronary condition and contribute to sudden death.

Smoking also strongly increases the risk of death from cerebrovascular disease (usually known as "stroke"), aortic aneurism (an enlargement of the wall of the aorta which blocks the flow of blood), and peripheral vascular disease (which affects the circulation of blood through the arms, hands, feet, and legs).

RESPIRATORY DISEASES   Cigarette smoking is the major cause of pulmonary emphysema and chronic bronchitis in the United States. It increases the risk of death from both. Even if death is not immediate, many thousands are so crippled by these diseases that they must retire at an early age.

Smoking promotes both diseases in much the same way that it promotes lung cancer: it renders the cilia powerless to perform their natural cleaning function. Foreign matter is allowed to penetrate deep into the lungs, irritating them and increasing the production of mucous which clogs the small bronchial tubes. Emphysema occurs when the walls of the air cells of the lungs are destroyed and large air sacs are formed by collections of damaged cells. The lungs lose their elasticity, and exhaling becomes extremely difficult.

Chronic bronchitis is caused when the mucous membranes of the bronchial tubes become inflamed. Bronchitis, which usually begins as a cold, can develop into emphysema when the nutrition of the lungs is blocked.

Other health problems which are associated with smoking include:

PEPTIC ULCERS   There seems to be a strong link between smoking and peptic ulcers, particularly gastric ulcers, both in terms of higher death rates and aggravation of the condition. Whether smoking directly causes ulcers—and if so, how—is not known. But the correlation exists. Among male smokers, the number of peptic ulcer cases is 100 percent higher for smokers than for nonsmokers. For women it is over 50 percent higher.

NONCANCEROUS ORAL DISEASE   Smokers seem to be afflicted with poor oral hygiene. Evidence suggests a causative relationship between smoking and edentulism (tooth loss), jawbone deterioration and loss, gingivitis (inflamed gums), slow healing after tooth extractions, and sores on the palate. It may also lead to pyorrhea, an infection of the gums which weakens the support of the teeth. Pipe smokers frequently suffer from stomatitis nicotina, an inflammation of the palate.

SMOKING AND PREGNANCY Research has shown that low birthweight babies (less than the normal average at birth) are more common among mothers who smoke during pregnancy. Smoking mothers also have more premature babies, and the cigarette habit has been implicated as a cause of stillbirth, spontaneous abortion (miscarriage), and neonatal death.

As a rule, people who do not smoke are healthier than those who do. The National Health Survey showed that men between the ages of 45 and 64 are disabled by illness at a rate 28 percent higher than men in the same age group who do not smoke. It may be that smokers are more vulnerable to infectious diseases such as pneumonia and influenza even though smoking is not the cause of those illnesses. Smokers are almost always in poorer physical condition than those who abstain—less "wind" leads to less exercise. Certainly they cough more, an effort by the body to clear the lungs of foreign matter when the cilia have ceased to function. Smokers frequently complain of headaches or "hangovers" after overindulging in cigarettes. The likelihood is that the headaches are a by-product of the tension which caused excessive smoking in the first place.

Whether or not anyone develops a smoking-related disease depends on several variables. The average number of cigarettes consumed daily is a major factor (Table 15.2). The length of time people have the habit also plays a vital role. The more years a person smokes, the greater the probability of disease. Those who inhale deeply are also more prone to disease.

*Table 15.2 Life expectancy (years) at various ages estimate for United States males**

Age	Never Smoked Regularly	Cigarette Smokers By Daily Amount			
		1–9	*10–19*	*20–39*	*40+*
25	48.6	44.0	43.1	42.4	40.3
30	43.9	39.3	38.4	37.8	35.8
35	39.2	34.7	33.8	33.2	31.3
40	34.5	30.2	29.3	28.7	26.9
45	30.0	25.9	25.0	24.4	23.0
50	25.6	21.8	21.0	20.5	19.3
55	21.4	17.9	17.4	17.0	16.0
60	17.6	14.5	14.1	13.7	13.2
65	14.1	11.3	11.2	11.0	10.7

* From Hammond study. Reprinted from World Conference on Smoking and Health, A Summary of the Proceedings. September 11, 12, 13, 1967.

Despite all the damage that can be done to health by smoking, the body also has remarkable restorative powers. If an individual manages to stop smoking before serious harm is done, the effects are largely reversible. The sensitive lining of the bronchial tubes becomes healthy again. The cilia are revived and once again able to sweep foreign matter out. of the lungs. The progression of conditions toward lung cancer or some form of respiratory disease is halted. The individual finds that he breathes easier and is no longer troubled by "smoker's hack." While all the effects of smoking on the cardiovascular system may not disappear, the heart is under less strain because circulation is better, and the flow of oxygen to nourish the heart is freer. Overall, an ex-smoker can look forward to better health and longer life.

BREAKING THE HABIT

Clearly there are many good reasons not to smoke. The problem lies in stopping. The first step is somewhat similar to that of the alcoholic who wants to reform: He must recognize that he has a problem—a potential one at least. He must become aware that, by continuing to smoke, he is virtually guaranteeing himself ill health and, very likely, an early death.

Even faced with those consequences, some people find it impossible to stop (that is, they are psychologically unable or unwilling). But they may attempt various alternatives that stop considerably short of outright quitting. They switch to pipe or cigar smoking and don't inhale (at least not at first); they "cut down" and smoke intermittently; or they use all sorts of gimmicks to decrease their cigarette consumption (smoke half the cigarette, hide their cigarettes from themselves, hold a cigarette in the mouth without lighting it, etc.). The probability is strong that, within a relatively short time, they will be right back where they started.

They may switch to a different type of cigarette. When evidence against cigarette smoking began to build up, the manufacturers inundated consumers wtih new types of cigarettes which presumably offered fewer health hazards. Filtered cigarettes, for example, reduce the amount of tar and nicotine that is inhaled in smoke. Similarly, extra-long cigarettes were introduced on the theory that people would not smoke them down to the very end where there is a high concentration of hazardous compounds. (The last half of a cigarette contains about 60 percent of the tars and nicotine.) Whether or not either filters or extra length reduce the intake of harmful substances sufficiently to lessen the probability of lung cancer or respiratory disease is open to considerable debate. These measures to reduce the harmful effects of tobacco have changed smoking habits, but they have not provided documented security to the smoker.

The ability to give up cigarettes is influenced by several factors: how much the smoker smokes; how long he has smoked; the reasons why he smokes in the first place; the degree of his psychological dependence; and whether or not he is surrounded by other smokers at home and at work. Some people find it far more difficult than others to give up cigarettes.

People determined to quit often find it helpful to consult first with their doctors, for psychological support if no other reason. Quitters generally employ a variety of substitutes to satisfy oral cravings: chewing gum, candy mints, snack foods, cloves, and bits of fresh ginger root. Some use pacifiers—noncombustible plastic cigarettes—to keep the mouth and the fingers busy. Many people claim that nonprescription lobeline sulphate tablets (sold under various brand names) make it easier to stop smoking because they serve as a nicotine replacement. Authorities disagree on whether or not these pills actually satisfy this craving and, in any case, a physician should be consulted before they are used because they can aggravate stomach ulcers. Other drugs, including alcohol, have also been used as substitutes, a questionable practice since it may create a whole new health problem.

Several more elaborate techniques have been developed to help people stop smoking, and their proponents claim varying degrees of success. Behavioralists have used mild electroshock to the hands in an attempt to create a negative association with smoking. Many doctors are encouraged by the use of hypnosis to create an aversion to cigarettes, particularly with addictive smokers. Antismoking clinics supply a form of group therapy which is similar to the programs of Weight Watchers and Alcoholics Anonymous. Smokers meet regularly to compare withdrawal problems and encourage one another in their mutual efforts to quit. Though many smokers have found these clinics helpful, they offer no guarantee of success—a fact that is true of any of the methods mentioned above. None of them will work unless they are backed up by personal ability and willingness.

Preventing the use of tobacco

Ideally the best way to stop smoking is never to start. If smoking is to be eliminated as a health hazard, the public must somehow be persuaded, preferably at an early age, not to light that first cigarette. Experience with a total ban on the sale of liquor during Prohibition in the United States indicates that the smoking habit cannot be legislated out of existence. Such laws often create more problems than they cure. Furthermore, a substantial body of law already exists to prohibit the sale of tobacco products to minors. Enforcement of those statutes is virtually nonexistent.

There are some formidable barriers to any program aimed at preventing the use of tobacco. The United States government displays an ambivalent attitude toward the subject. On the one hand, it supports research to study the harmful effects of smoking, but, on the other, it has a vested interest in the tobacco industry because of its subsidy programs. The government is also heavily dependent on tobacco as a major source of revenue (approximately 2 billion dollars annually).

Congressmen from tobacco-growing states, aided by industry lobbyists, do everything in their power to block legislation that might be harmful to the livelihood of their constituents. The production of tobacco products generates thousands of farm and factory jobs. The growers and

Nonsmokers' rights

Politely, and sometimes not so politely, the nonsmokers of America are taking on the puffers and hackers with a new zeal. Nonsmokers, once timid closet characters content to simply leave a smoke-filled room, are now demanding, and getting, equal but unpolluted indoor air.

So-called "nonsmokers' rights" legislation has been passed or is pending in several cities and states. On July 10, the Civil Aeronautics Board made a nonsmoking section mandatory on commercial airlines.

Some entertainers, such as Vicki Carr, the singer, tell nightclubbers to stop smoking during their acts. And growing numbers of cocktail party hosts simply prohibit smoking in their homes.

Perhaps more significantly, proprietors, previously afraid of offending smoking customers, are experimenting with nonsmoking sections in hotels, restaurants, beauty parlors and other establishments. And they say they are finding it profitable.

From James P. Sterra, "Nonsmoker is Winning Right to Clean Indoor Air," *The New York Times* (September 30, 1973), p. 1.

manufacturers certainly will not ignore any serious threat to their enormous investments. Moreover, they have the financial wherewithal to create massive, multimillion dollar advertising campaigns that render the educational efforts of health organizations and consumer groups ineffectual.

Nevertheless, a few steps have been been taken. Free distribution of cigarettes to Public Health Service hospitals and Indian hospitals was discontinued in 1964. Not long after, commercial airlines, colleges, and military installations began to eliminate long-standing policies of free-cigarette distribution. As public concern over smoking grew more intense, a law was passed that required cigarette packaging and advertising to display the statement: "Warning: The Surgeon General has determined that Cigarette Smoking is Dangerous to Your Health." Though that was a major victory for antismoking forces, its impact was not nearly so great as the 1969 ban on television advertising of cigarettes. The industry was forced to do without the advertising medium that reached the greatest number of potential customers. However, the ban does not extend to other communications media, and there is still plenty of cigarette advertising. Most recently agitation by consumer organizations has forced higher taxes on cigarette brands that contain a relatively high proportion of tar and nicotine. Antismoking advertising, particularly television commercials, that stresses the inherent dangers of cigarettes has expanded in recent years. But such campaigns are largely dependent on donations of public service air-time, and they cannot begin to compete with the promotional efforts of the big cigarette companies.

Though all these measures have helped to make the public aware of the problem, an enormous number of people are still smoking, and each year another million take up the habit. It would seem that, if this situa-

Figure 15.3. From "Johnny Smoke," an animated anticigarette television spot prepared by the American Heart Association using Western themes to discourage smoking. "Out of the land of the tobacco plant comes a tall, fast-drawing, long, lean bloke, feared by his friends and enemies alike," says the Song of Johnny Smoke. It also asks: "How many saddles will be empty tonight? How many men will lie still beneath the sky? How many tears will be shed because of you? How many more will die?" (Courtesy of the American Heart Association)

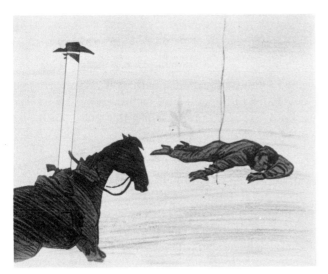
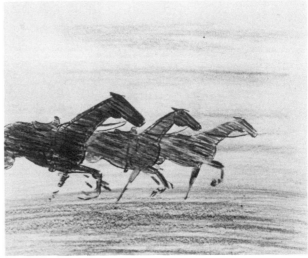

Figure 15.4. (Photo by Ingeborg Tallarek. Nancy Palmer Agency)

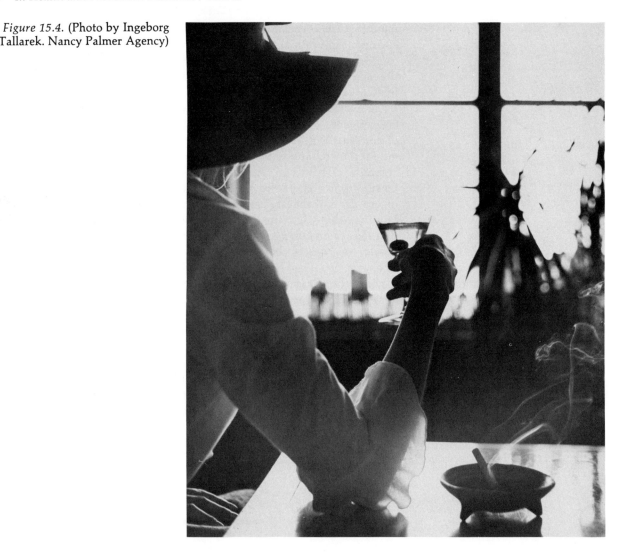

tion is ever to be reversed, public education must begin at an early age. Programs need to be developed to foster a long-lasting, negative association with cigarettes and other tobacco products. At this point, such programs on any significant scale seem a long way off.

ALCOHOL The origins of alcohol are lost in unrecorded history, but the discovery appears to have been an accidental one. The first prehistoric batch probably emerged from the natural fermentation of a supply of fruit in storage. Once people consumed this "new" substance, they realized that it had some strange effects on their behavior. It made them feel elated, even giddy, relaxed them, deadened pain, put them to sleep, and, if they weren't careful, made them ill. In some cultures these effects of fermented fruit juices were attributed to ghosts or evil spirits in the substance.

The use of alcohol spread throughout the ancient world where it was incorporated into social customs and religious ceremonies. To a great extent these ritual uses came from alcohol's ability to change behavior. In ancient Greek civilization wine was an integral part of a social and intellectual gathering known as a symposium. Under prescribed conditions, the mind-altering qualities of alcohol were used to encourage a freer, more uninhibited exchange of ideas.

As an aspect of religion, alcohol served as a symbol of homage to the gods who controlled man's destiny. Wine was an important feature of harvest festivals celebrating the bounty of the particular deity that was worshipped locally. The pagan cultures that flourished in the eastern world employed alcohol in the orgiastic fertility rites that were central to their religions. Monotheistic Judaism also used wine in its ceremonies, but with an emphasis on solemnity and sobriety. Overindulgence was sharply condemned. Later, wine figured prominently in the Christian faith as an element in the celebration of the Eucharist.

Eventually, other properties of alcohol became evident and important to mankind. During the Middle Ages, alchemists were fascinated by its ability to mix with water to dissolve many substances not normally soluble in water. They called alcohol "aqua vitae" (water of life).

Almost from their beginning alcoholic products were a major item of trade between nations. Over the centuries, the use of alcohol in beverage form came to be less ritualistic and more informal, as a prelude or accompaniment to meals and as an essential element at social gatherings. As use grew more widespread, alcohol evolved into a major industry and a vital factor in the economies of many countries. The United States alone produces 24 billion dollars worth of alcoholic beverages a year. In addition, it became an important source of revenue. Alcohol taxes accounted for 3 percent of the total U.S. federal tax receipts for the fiscal year 1966. Despite its contributions to the economy and the fact that it has added to many people's enjoyment of life, alcohol has not been an unmixed blessing to civilization.

Composition of alcohol

Alcohol is an organic compound created naturally through the process of fermentation: the action of yeast spores growing in a solution of sugar and water, such as fruit juice. There are many kinds of alcohol, and the use of any given type is determined by the concentration of alcohol by volume. Higher concentrations (60 to 90 percent) generally have a medical or pharmaceutical use, such as rubbing or surgical alcohol. Alcohol at this strength dries or hardens tissues by removing water and precipitating proteins out of the tissue. This type kills nonsporing bacteria, hence its use as a disinfectant. It is not very good for drinking, however, because it can irritate the mucous membranes rather severely.

The alcohol we drink is ethyl alcohol, a clear, inflammable liquid with an aromatic odor and a burning taste. By contrast with medical types, it does not exceed 50 to 53 percent by volume. Alcoholic beverages come in two basic types: those which are strictly the product of natural fermentation (wines, beers, ales) and those which are carried a step further through distillation (whiskey of all kinds, gin, rum, brandy, vodka, cordials, and liqueurs).

Distilled liquors have a much higher concentration of alcohol, about 45 percent on the average, than wine or beer. *Proof* indicates the alcoholic content of a liquor with a figure that is double the amount of alcohol. That is, a 100 proof whiskey is 50 percent alcohol by volume.

Figure 15.5. Alcoholic percentage (by volume) of principal alcoholic beverages.

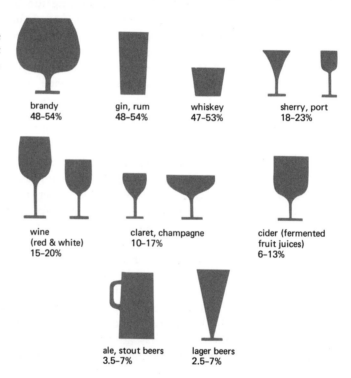

brandy
48–54%

gin, rum
48–54%

whiskey
47–53%

sherry, port
18–23%

wine
(red & white)
15–20%

claret, champagne
10–17%

cider (fermented
fruit juices)
6–13%

ale, stout beers
3.5–7%

lager beers
2.5–7%

Alcohol in all its forms is technically a food because it contains calories (7.1 per gram). Wines and beers do contain some nutritional elements used by body cells, but the amount is very meager and is certainly not enough to rely on for significant energy support. Distilled spirits have no nutritional value.

Since alcohol also affects the central nervous system and causes other physiological changes, it is also considered a drug. It can serve as a sedative by inducing sleep, an analgesic by lowering the perception of pain, or a tranquilizer by reducing emotional tension. Alcoholic drinks are frequently prescribed for elderly patients suffering from artherosclerosis (hardening of the arteries), digestive ailments, and arthritis.

EFFECTS OF ALCOHOL

Alcohol moves fast. As you sip beer or a cocktail, 20 percent of the alcohol in it is absorbed instantly into the bloodstream through the walls of the stomach or small intestine. It does not have to waste time being digested like other foods. The gastrointestinal tract processes the remaining 80 percent at a rate that is only slightly slower, moving it into the circulatory system. The bloodstream carries the alcohol directly to the brain. There it acts on the central control area and depresses the functioning of the brain.

Outwardly the first reaction may seem like stimulation. This is because alcohol strikes first at the part of the brain that controls inhibitions. In the course of human evolution, the brain has developed in layers of tissue, and learned behavior patterns are "stored" in the outer or "newer" layers. Despite the stimulating feeling, alcohol is actually a central nervous system depressant. Thus, a pace of about a drink an hour maintains a low level of alcohol in the blood and produces a mild tranquilizing effect. As the concentration of alcohol in the bloodstream increases, it depresses the cerebral cortex which controls memory, reasoning, and muscular coordination. Normal control of speech and movement disappears until the alcohol level goes down. This is the step into *intoxication:* temporary loss of physical and mental powers due to overconsumption. If more alcohol is consumed relatively quickly, the deeper, more primitive parts of the brain are depressed. Sensory perceptions are

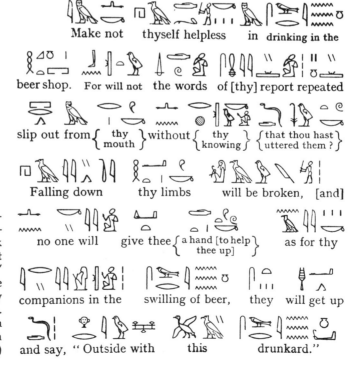

Figure 15.6. Beer was more common in ancient Egypt than wine— and usually more potent. A book of etiquette dating from about 1500 B.C., "The Precepts of Ani," included a warning about the effects of overdrinking. (Courtesy of Lutterworth Press, Sir E. A. Wallis Budge, "The Dwellers on the Nile," and the World Health Organization)

dulled and judgment is impaired. After continued heavy drinking at a steady pace, alcohol will penetrate the inner parts of the brain and anesthetize them. The drinker loses consciousness. The anesthesia of the deepest levels of the brain can also cause death if the drinker has ingested enough before he passes out. It should be noted that a recent theory contends that alcohol does not progress through this series of brain levels but rather that its affect is concentrated directly on the reticular formation, a sort of "master control" section of the brain.

In moderate quantities, alcohol produces a feeling of warmth because it causes an increase in blood flow which relaxes and dilates the blood vessels in the arms, legs, and skin. That reaction can lower body temperature, which is why hot alcoholic drinks are sometimes used to relieve a fever. The effect on blood vessels also increases the pulse rate and lowers blood pressure slightly.

Alcohol acts as a diuretic: it increases production and elimination of urine. This reaction is presumed to be a result of alcohol's effect on the pituitary gland which regulates urine production in the kidneys. Since the liver is the organ that does the major work of metabolizing alcohol, it can become swollen and tender if it has to handle excessive amounts. In the stomach, large amounts of alcohol over an extended period can cause gastritis, a chronic irritation of the stomach lining.

Rate of absorption

Only seconds after alcohol is ingested, it appears in all the organs, tissues, and secretions of the body. How quickly it goes to work on the brain depends on the interaction of several factors:

1. Rate of consumption. It takes most people about an hour to burn less than an ounce of alcohol. Drinking at a faster rate will produce some degree of intoxication.
2. Quantity of food in the stomach. Food slows the rate of absorption of alcohol into the bloodstream. Drinking on an empty stomach causes the alcohol to reach the brain faster and so causes a faster response.
3. Kind of alcohol. Distilled spirits are absorbed into the bloodstream faster than wine or beer. The latter are less concentrated and have small amounts of nonalcoholic substances which are removed during distillation that slow down the absorption rate.
4. Additional mixers. Water dilutes the alcohol and slows the rate of absorption. Carbonated mixers speed it up.
5. Body weight. Alcohol is distributed rapidly and uniformly throughout the circulatory system. A small person who is drinking the same liquor at the same rate as a large person will have higher concentrations of alcohol at every point in his bloodstream because he does not have as much blood or tissue to dilute the alcohol.
6. Emotional condition. During periods of anxiety, stress, or fatigue,

The sober side and the morning after

Though alcohol hurries its way into the bloodstream, it takes its time getting out. The general rule of thumb is that it takes a number of hours equal to the number of drinks consumed to reach sobriety again. A lot depends on how big a drink you pour. The average person can metabolize between one-half ounce and one ounce an hour. The liver handles most of the metabolism of alcohol, and 2 to 5 percent is eliminated through perspiration, urine, and breath.

None of the popular home remedies can speed up the process. The caffein in black coffee may make an intoxicated person feel more aware, but it has absolutely no effect on the amount of alcohol in his bloodstream. Cold showers and breathing pure oxygen are just as ineffective. The only way to sober up is to wait.

A hangover—extreme fatigue, nausea, headache, and general misery—is the body's reaction to overconsumption of alcohol. The likelihood of a hangover is large if the drinker is tired, under stress, or engaging in an unusual amount of physical activity at the party. Quiet drinking is less liable to produce a hangover. Like sobering up, the only cure is to wait, while alleviating the suffering as much as possible with aspirin, rest, and bland solid food. There is no scientific evidence to support the curative powers claimed for coffee, raw eggs, vitamins, oysters, and a variety of spicy foods.

the chances are alcohol will go to work faster than under comfortable and relaxed circumstances.

7. Body chemistry. There are apparently some differences in individual body chemistry that affect the rate of absorption. Even when all other conditions are the same, alcohol can have a stronger impact on one person than another.

When the percentage of alcohol in the blood stream reaches 0.02 or 0.03 percent, the average person will begin to feel the effects. Depending on the individual, a blood-alcohol level of 0.05 percent can affect reflexes enough to cause an auto accident. Between levels of 0.05 and 0.15 percent, most everyone will begin to lose control of speech and motor coordination. Intoxication is beginning, and by 0.20 percent it is obvious. If the level reaches 0.40 percent, the drinker loses consciousness.

Alcohol drinkers

According to surveys, about 68 percent of the adults in the United States drink alcohol at least some of the time. The roughly 85 to 100 million Americans who enjoy alcohol spend more on it (about 10 billion dollars annually) than they do on public education at all levels. A recent study which traced drinking trends from 1946 to 1963 showed a bigger increase in male drinkers than in female drinkers. This report indicated that, unlike the smoking habit, people with more formal education are more likely to drink alcohol. Roman Catholics consume more than Protestants, and there is more drinking among city dwellers than those living outside urban areas. Geographically, the highest incidence of alcohol use is in the northeastern United States (65 percent of the population), and the lowest is in the south (37 percent).

Other research indicates that the average age for taking the first drink is 13 to 14 years. The first exposure to alcoholic beverage is likely to occur at home in the presence of parents. The number of users increases with age so that virtually every young person has had at least one alcoholic drink by the time he or she graduates from high school. This varies by community but is most prevalent in metropolitan areas. Most teenagers who use alcohol do so with their parents' permission whether they are at home or away. Problems caused by alcohol (breaking laws, drunken driving, uncontrolled and undesirable behavior) involve approximately 2 to 6 percent of the young drinkers.

Reasons for drinking

For millions of people it is impossible to think about a social event without some sort of alcohol. Much of the time, most of those millions drink in conjunction with some other activity: at family gatherings; during card games; while watching television; at parties with friends; as part of religious feasts. Celebrations of any sort are reason for a drink, and often so are meals. People drink cocktails before dining to sharpen appetites (alcohol stimulates the flow of digestive juices) and wine or beer during a meal to enhance other flavors. Social drinking is based primarily on alcohol's ability to tranquilize. The individual's decision to drink is heavily influenced by his own personality and by his environment; ethnic group, family, neighborhood, friends, religion, and job all affect drinking behavior.

Adolescents are drawn to drinking for much the same reasons they take up smoking. Alcohol is viewed as an adult prerogative, and teenagers drink as a means of testing adult behavior and challenging adult authority. Thus, an adult who is concerned about teenage drinking will accomplish more if he attempts to establish responsible adult patterns for drinking in a young person than if he attempts to prevent drinking altogether.

The alcoholic

Most drinkers enjoy a lifetime of frequent but moderate drinking accompanied by occasional hangovers. They derive pleasure from drinking, and they do no harm to themselves or anyone else. The alcoholic is a compulsive drinker who repeatedly and deliberately drinks to the point of intoxication. He drinks not for pleasure but to get drunk. Alcohol is his means of coping with life, his only way of facing even the most minor conflict or distress. In a sense it is his nourishment, for without it he cannot function. Perhaps the most notable characteristic of the disease is the total loss of control. The alcoholic's compulsion is such that he cannot stop overdrinking no matter how destructive it is to himself or others, even though he is well aware of the destructiveness. But not every heavy drinker is an alcoholic. There are people who go through life consuming large quantities of liquor without the alcoholic's compulsion and without becoming addicted. There is no clearcut line that separates the alcoholic from the nonalcoholic.

Probably most of us tend to think of lonely Skid Row derelicts as typical alcoholics. Yet they represent only about 3 to 5 percent of the alcoholic population. The majority of alcoholics holds jobs, at least marginally. Many professionals, people in top executive positions, home owners, and heads of families are alcoholics. Though there may be a tendency to think of alcoholism as largely a male problem, women, too, are victims of the disease. The number of female alcoholics has increased in recent years. But knowledge of women alcoholics is skimpy; there probably are more than statistics reveal, but they have hidden the problem more successfully than have men.

There are an estimated 6 to 9 million alcoholics in America, and according to the most recent report of the President's Commission on Drug Abuse, alcohol is the number one drug problem in the country today. It can also be classified as the leading mental health problem. A 1964 study showed that one out of every seven patients entering state mental hospitals was an alcoholic. In terms of all health problems, it ranks fourth.

Alcoholism

For a disease that is so widespread, there is an amazingly small amount of research on alcoholism relative to other psychological disorders. The indications are that alcoholism cannot be attributed to any single cause.

Therapists, physicians, and psychiatrists who specialize in treating alcoholics claim that their patients reveal lives characterized by a great deal of deprivation and an exceptional amount of stress. They have yet to isolate what might be called an alcoholic personality that would distinguish alcoholics from other mentally ill people.

Investigators are studying a variety of possible physiological causes for alcoholism including poor nutrition and chemical and genetic abnormalities in the body. Some theorists believe that alcoholism is produced by allergic reactions to alcohol or other chemicals in alcoholic beverages or by addiction to nonalcoholic elements in these drinks. Thus far, those theories remain unproved. Vitamin deficiencies and hormone imbalances have also been considered, but evidence indicates that they are a product of alcoholism rather than a cause.

A hereditary link to alcohol problems has been investigated frequently, because the children of alcoholics also show a fairly high rate of alcoholism. Some researchers believe the hereditary association is a liver condition called hyperlipidism (see Chap. 7). This is an abnormality in fat metabolism which leads to the development of an abnormal (fatty) liver after alcohol is ingested. Approximately 15 out of every 100 people have hyperlipidism. If such a genetic link could be clearly established, it would provide at least one means of identifying potential alcoholics.

Research studies have also delved into influences of a more external nature such as childhood deprivations and environmental factors such as overexposure to drinking. Nothing conclusive has been established yet.

Alcoholism and health

Alcoholics are particularly vulnerable to a variety of physical and neurological disorders. One of the most common, cirrhosis of the liver, occurs eight times more frequently among alcoholics than nonalcoholics. Exactly what causes cirrhosis (a hardening and contraction of the liver) is not known. It may be a result of excess alcohol or some allied factor, but the association with alcoholic addiction is clear. Delirium tremors (DTs) also are a widespread ailment of alcoholics.

Alcoholics eat badly if at all. Vitamins and other nutrients are virtually nonexistent in their diets, and malnutrition is one of their commonest afflictions. Polyneuropathy, caused by lack of vitamin B_1, affects the nerves producing pain and burning sensations. Pellagra, which appears as skin rash and upsets in the digestive system, results from a

Alcoholism and ethnic groups

There is one direction in research that holds promise of a better understanding of the causes of alcoholism. Sociologists have traced alcoholism rates among various nationalities and ethnic groups. The French, for example, are well known as the world's largest producers and consumers of wine. French workingmen consume several quarts a day on the average, and the northern French have a high rate of alcoholism. (France also has the world's highest incidence of liver ailments.) Yet the Italians, who are the second largest wine consumers, have a relatively low rate of addiction. There is little alcoholism among Orthodox Jews but a high incidence among Roman Catholics. In fact, the National Clergy Council on Alcoholism admits that about 12 percent of America's 58,000 Catholic priests are problem drinkers. The Irish have a reputation for being heavy drinkers, but it is Irish-Americans who demonstrate a high rate of alcoholism. It remains for further research to determine whether these relationships are based on genetic or cultural factors.

deficiency in B-complex vitamins. "Beer heart," an enlargement and weakening of the heart, is another result of the alcoholic's vitamin-poor diet. In general, nutritional deficiencies among alcoholics lead to greater susceptibility to such infectious diseases as pneumonia, influenza, and tuberculosis.

Treatment of the alcoholic

Authorities disagree on how thoroughly alcoholics can be cured. Some insist that not more than one out of three recovers while others state that the rate is as low as one in ten. Yet even alcoholics who were severely addicted for several years have been rescued and returned to a more or less normal life.

Successful treatment usually involves a combination of methods:

HOSPITAL CARE For the chronic alcoholic, round-the-clock medical supervision is necessary to help him "dry out," to restore his physical health, and to prevent death. Tranquilizers and sedatives can be administered to alleviate hallucinations, tremors, delirium, and other agonizing withdrawal symptoms. A proper diet with plenty of fluids and vitamin "cocktails" will counteract nutritional deficiencies he has developed. Overall, he will be brought back to the point where he can undergo other forms of treatment that will rid him of his addiction.

DRUGS Aversion therapy is a conditioning procedure in which the patient is given certain drugs simultaneously with an alcoholic drink. The drugs induce nausea, creating a negative association with alcohol. Since drinking equals illness, many alcoholics will avoid future drinks, at least until other forms of therapy have taken hold. Aversion therapy has potential side effects and must, therefore, be administered by a doctor.

PSYCHOTHERAPY The therapist's aim is to help the patient understand his problems and, most importantly, to assist him in finding ways of either eliminating those sources of anxiety or of coping with them by some less destructive means than alcohol. This may involve individual therapy, group therapy, or both. In some instances, the alcoholic's family may be included in the counseling.

ALCOHOLICS ANONYMOUS Easily the most publicized form of therapy, the organization has chapters in communities all across the country as well as in prisons and hospitals. The program is designed to promote personal recovery without the use of drugs and, to be successful, it demands a compulsive preoccupation with sobriety. Thus the first step toward participation is for the alcoholic to admit that he allowed alcohol to overpower him, that it made his life chaotic and self-destructive, and that he now needs and wants help.

Breath analyser test

The Alcoholic Safety Action Program, sponsored by the U.S. Department of Transportation, has allotted funds to 34 American cities to establish programs aimed at reducing dangers produced by intoxication. A major aim of the program is to get drunken drivers off the streets by arresting any individuals whose conduct at the wheel looks suspicious. Those arrested are required to submit to a breath analyzer test. If the driver refuses the test, his license may be suspended. The test simply involves blowing breath into a balloonlike device attached to a meter which registers the blood-alcohol level (air in the lungs is in equilibrium with alcohol in the blood). If the driver's breath reveals a "dangerous" amount of alcohol, that is sufficient evidence for a drunken driving conviction. His license will be taken away temporarily and he may be required to undergo rehabilitative care. The danger level of blood-alcohol, according to law, varies from state to state, ranging from 0.10 to 0.15 percent.

Using a somewhat informal version of group therapy, addicts and reformed alcoholics meet to share their problems and support one another in their efforts to remain sober. There is no attempt to dig out the root causes of the addict's alcoholism and find solutions for them. Since AA believes that to be an impossible task, the society's sole aim is to help its members abstain from alcohol for the rest of their lives.

This does not mean that there is no backsliding among members. Records show that less than 20 percent have maintained total abstinence from alcohol for longer than five years. Should one succumb to the impulse to drink, he is still welcomed back so long as he has a sincere desire to end his dependence on alcohol. It may take many such attempts before a life pattern without alcohol is established and an alcoholic can be considered "saved." Moreover, he will probably have to continue participating long after he has had his final drink in order to reinforce his resolve.

PREVENTING THE PROBLEM

Since alcohol was discovered there have been people who drank too much too often. Societies have tried to deal with them in various ways. The Israelite prophets, Christ, and Muhammed were all concerned about drunkards in their communities, yet moral strictures have had little impact on personal intemperance.

A reform movement swept the United States early in this century with a goal of forced abstinence rather than temperance. The "Drys" gathered enough political support to pass the eighteenth amendment to the Constitution (better known as "Prohibition") in 1919. The sale, manufacture, and import of all beverages with a content of more than one percent alcohol was banned. Enforcement proved complicated and impracticable. Drinking not only continued, it seemed to increase and badly made "bathtub hootch" frequently caused serious illness or death. Black market activities proliferated and organized crime reaped a bonanza in profits. Pressure mounted until the amendment was repealed in 1933.

Even though this government attempt to regulate social behavior was a disaster, laws still exist to control the use of alcohol. For example, state and local statutes prohibit the sale of intoxicating beverages to a minor (which used to be defined as 21 years of age in most localities but has been lowered to 18 generally). Yet evasions are numerous.

Laws are limited in their effect. Alcoholics are arrested, convicted, punished, and released with their problems unsolved. Even the development of better methods of treatment is no solution. That helps only those who are already victims of the disease. The prevention of alcoholism demands a vastly expanded research effort to determine the character and causes of the disease as well as more effective cures. Coincident with that, a massive dose of public education is necessary to increase awareness of the threat posed by alcohol.

The most comprehensive program underway is administered by the National Institute on Alcohol Abuse and Alcoholism, a subdivision of the National Institute of Mental Health. One of the Institute's chief thrusts at the problem is through grants to universities, medical schools, and other research institutions for the study of alcoholism from biological, behavioral, and sociocultural points of view.

The Institute sponsors programs to develop new techniques of prevention, treatment, and rehabilitation and to train professionals in their use. NIAAA also subsidizes community rehabilitation and treatment services and collaborates with other federal agencies in programs aimed at controlling and reducing alcoholism among several categories of citizens where addiction is high. Several other agencies of the federal government and numerous local agencies have developed programs of public education in order to prevent alcohol abuse, alcohol problems, and alcoholism. It is a problem that will require many years and millions of dollars to solve. But there is only one truly effective solution: alcoholism must be stopped before it starts.

Questions

1. Do you believe that the reasons for the use of tobacco and alcohol are appropriate and reasonable today? Explain.
2. What physiological effects are produced in the body by smoking? What are the health consequences of continued smoking?
3. What physiological effects are produced in the body by the consumption of alcohol? What are various factors which influence the rate at which alcohol creates these effects?
4. How may the public management of the use of tobacco be compared with that of alcohol?
5. Do you think that increased public awareness of the dangers of cigarettes and alcohol will decrease the consumption of these products or that the increasing tensions and stresses of contemporary urban society that cause so many people to take up the habits will outweigh the health considerations? Explain. How does your opinion affect the program you would design for management of these products and prevention of the dangers associated with them?

Key Concepts

Alcoholic – a compulsive drinker who repeatedly drinks to the point of intoxication

Intoxication – temporary loss of physical and mental powers due to overconsumption of alcohol

Proof – indicates the alcoholic content of a liquor with a figure that is double the amount of alcohol

Selected Readings

Block, M. A. *Alcohol and Alcoholism: Drinking and Dependence*. Belmont, Calif.: Wadsworth Publishing, 1970.

Borgatta, Edgar F., and R. R. Evans, eds. *Smoking, Health, and Behavior*. Chicago: Aldine Publishing, 1969.

Chafetz, Morris E., and H. W. Demone, Jr. *Alcoholism and Society.* New York: Oxford University Press, 1962.

Diehl, Harold S. *Tobacco and Your Health—The Smoking Controversy.* New York: McGraw-Hill Book Co., 1969.

Jellinek, E. M. *The Disease Concept of Alcoholism.* Highland Park, N.J.: Hillhouse Press, 1959.

U.S. Department of Health, Education, and Welfare. *The Health Consequences of Smoking: A Report of the Surgeon General.* Washington, D. C.: Government Printing Office, 1971.

Wilkinson, Rupert. *The Prevention of Drinking Problems: Alcohol Control and Cultural Influences.* New York: Oxford University Press, 1970.

Chapter 16

Accidents and Health Risks

Everyone faces substantial risk from living and working. This chapter focuses on three important risks—occupational risks, risks of ionizing radiation, and risks of accidents.

OCCUPATIONAL RISKS

Every occupation has inherent risks whether it be the coal miner who faces cave-ins and black lung or the physician or nurse who has frequent exposures to infectious diseases such as tuberculosis or hepatitis. This section considers the magnitude of the problem and some of the conditions, the strategy and rationale for control, and the administrative and legal problems in effective control.

Magnitude of the problem

In a society where productivity .is as highly valued as in the United States, it should not be surprising to learn that occupational health is a

This chapter was contributed by John B. Little, M.D., Associate Professor of Radiobiology, Harvard School of Public Health, Lecturer on Radiology, Harvard Medical School, and director of the research and training program in Radiation Biology; and John M. Peters, M.D., Associate Professor of Occupational Medicine, Harvard School of Public Health.

problem of no small magnitude. At least 24,000 Americans are killed each year because of their jobs. Some 14,000 die as a result of accidents, while another 10,000 deaths are directly traceable to occupational disease. This latter figure represents a conservative estimate based on known effects of known hazardous exposures, mostly physical or chemical in nature. It is very likely that the number of deaths would be substantially higher if more were known about the subtle effects of other exposures not yet identified or thought to be hazardous. Figures on disease or injury are even more difficult to obtain but are nonetheless impressive: for example, seven million American workers are regularly exposed to hazardous noise levels sufficient to produce some degree of deafness. While we are beginning to compile estimates of the morbidity and mortality wrought by some physical and chemical agents, other surfaces have not even been scratched. Attention is just beginning to focus on such factors as the psychological effects of working. Few investigators have examined the dangers of high noise levels, psychological stress, and boredom, and even less has been done to explore the potential relationships between psychological factors and various physical or chemical stresses.

The 24,000 occupational deaths might seem low when compared to the morbidity and mortality produced by cigarette smoking and automobile accidents. However, from the standpoint of prevention, the situations are very different. The prevention of occupational disease depends largely on nonpersonal factors; it is almost always possible to create a work environment that is safe and healthy without relying on the be-

Facts and figures

Three and a half million American workers are exposed to asbestos and subject to asbestosis, a severe lung scarring, and to lung cancer. Recent studies of insulation workers in two states showed that 1 in 5 deaths was from lung cancer, 7 times the expected rate; half of those with twenty years or more in the trade had X-ray evidence of asbestosis; 1 in 10 deaths was caused by *mesothelioma*, a rare malignancy of the lung or pleura which strikes only 1 in 10,000 in the general working population—an increase in risk of 1000.

Of 6,000 men who have been uranium miners, 600 to 1,100 will die during the next 20 years from lung cancer.

"Black lungs," "grinder's rot," "potter's asthma," "stone mason's phthisis" are ancient terms for the progressive crippling lung damage which has afflicted thousands of workers exposed to various dusts over the years. The state of Pennsylvania in 1968 paid more than 16,000 persons $55 million in compensation claims for these occupational lung diseases.

Among soft coal miners, the death rate from respiratory disease is five times that of the general working population.

Fifty percent of the machines in industry generate noise levels potentially harmful to hearing. Seven and a half million workers are exposed to hazardous noise levels.

Hundreds of thousands of workers each year suffer skin disease from contact with materials in their work. Cases of dermatitis are the most common of all occupational illnesses.

The list of known or potential health hazards in industrial use is long, and it is growing longer—solvents, plastics, resins, lasers, masers, microwave, ultrasound, ultraviolet. Every 20 minutes, it is estimated, a new and potentially toxic chemical is introduced into industry.

havior of the worker. On the other hand, reducing the devastation from automobile accidents or cigarette smoking requires major changes in the life styles of many people, and thus far this has not been possible. However, once problems are found in the area of occupational health, preventive measures can be introduced and practiced. Since most of the diseases produced by the working environment are chronic and untreatable, it is especially important and logical to prevent them.

The relatively simple problem of assessing the effect of a specific chemical or physical agent on the human body is often not adequately understood, especially with regard to the relationship between acute (intense or short-term) and chronic (continuing) exposure to chronic disease. The mobility of the work force complicates this further. If a specific exposure does not produce a chronic disease until twenty to thirty years have elapsed, the discovery of such a relationship is delayed by the rapid turnover of labor. This turnover phenomenon may retard the understanding of the connection between exposure and disease, but it may also inadvertently serve to protect the worker. On the other hand, multiple exposures could be theoretically worse than a sustained dose if they produce additive or synergistic effects. The number of variables to be considered in various combinations becomes overwhelming.

Identifying occupational health problems

When a problem or potential problem arises, the investigator usually follows three basic steps: (1) he identifies and quantifies the stress, be it chemical, physical, or psychological, (2) determines the health effect, and (3) establishes proper control or preventive measures.

Step 1 involves establishing the parameters of the exposure or stress. Let us assume that a group of workers is exposed to some dust. Since this constitutes an airborne exposure with the lung as the route of entry, it would be important to know how much dust the worker breathed and where in the respiratory system the dust would be deposited. The general approach would be to quantify the dust concentration in the air in the worker's breathing area and to determine the size distribution of the particles so that the pattern of deposition in the lung could be estimated. The industrial hygienist, usually an engineer or a chemist with additional training in biology and toxicology, is responsible for compiling this information. However, if the occupational health problem involves radiation, a health physicist would provide the exposure information.

The second step, identifying the health effect of the exposure or stress, usually is the job of a physician. It may be necessary to employ toxicology, physiology, psychology, or other disciplines, depending on the nature of the problem. Dust exposure might involve physiology (lung capacity tests) if the dust had a primary effect on the lung, or it could involve toxicology if it had a primary effect elsewhere. Once health effects are identified, it must be determined at what levels of exposure health effects are produced.

Figure 16.1. A granite cutter at work. Granite contains silica, a mineral that can cause severe scarring of the lung. Notice the exhaust ventilation which sucks away the dust as it is generated to protect the worker.

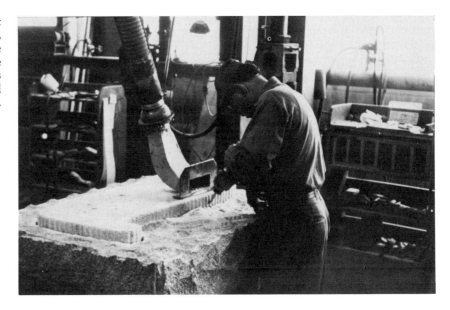

With these two pieces of information the third step can be undertaken; this involves control of the problem. In the case of dust exposure, the industrial hygienist is called upon again to engineer the control. Controls vary depending on the nature of the problem. In the dust example, local exhaust ventilation is the most likely mode of control.

Safe exposure limits

There are presently about 5,000 chemical substances in common use in American industry, and each year about 500 new ones are introduced. Unfortunately, we know very little about the effects of many of these compounds. The American Conference of Governmental Industrial Hygienists (ACGIH) has set safe exposure limits, called "threshold limit values" (TLV's), for about 500 substances. TLV's, which refer to time-weighted, airborne concentrations of substances, are set to protect "nearly all workers" who may be exposed and are described by the ACGIH as "guides in the control of health hazards."

Consideration of the basis for the TLV's illustrates the paucity of knowledge concerning chronic exposures to many materials, even to substances that have been around for many years such as silica and lead. Approximately 38 percent of the TLV's are based on human experience and give consideration to the chronic (long-term) effects of exposure. However, many of the data on which the TLV's are based lack sound epidemiologic studies. Eleven percent of the TLV's are based on experiments involving human volunteers. However, because volunteers cannot be exposed to a chemical substance for forty years, TLV's for the most

Table 16.1 Some chemical agents producing occupational disease

Agent	System(s) affected	Principal manifestation(s)	Representative occupations in which exposure occurs
Metals			
Lead	Gastrointestinal	Abdominal pain (colic)	Battery makers
	Neuromuscular	Palsy (wrist drop)	Enamelers
	Blood forming	Anemia	Painters
	Central nervous system	Encephalopathy	Welders
Mercury	Central nervous system	Tremor	Dentists
	Oral mucous membranes	Inflammation of mouth	Fluorescent lamp makers
	Renal	and gums	Thermometer makers
		Erethism	
Cadmium	Pulmonary	Pulmonary edema (acute)	Cadmium smelters
	Renal	Emphysema (chronic)	Engravers
		Nephritis	Solderers
Chromium	Respiratory	Dermatitis	Dye makers
	Cutaneous	Skin ulcers	Leather tanners
		Nasal septal perforation	Printers
		Lung cancer	
Beryllium	Pulmonary	Pulmonary inflammation and scarring	Ceramic makers
			Neon tube workers
			Nuclear physicists
Solvents			
Benzene (benzol)	Hematopoietic	Aplastic anemia	Organic chemists
	Central nervous system	Leukemia	Furniture strippers
		Narcosis	Rubber makers
Carbon tetrachloride	Hepatic	Toxic hepatitis	Dry cleaners
	Renal	Kidney shutdown	Ink makers
			Wax makers
Carbon disulfide	Central nervous system	Mania	Glassmakers
	Renal	Acceleration of atherogenesis	Rayon makers
		Chronic renal disease	Rubber makers
		Parkinsonian syndrome	
Methyl alcohol	Ocular	Blindness	Rubber workers
Gases			
1. Irritants			
Ammonia	Upper respiratory	Irritation	Refrigerator makers
Sulfur dioxide	Middle respiratory	Bronchospasm	Smelter workers
Ozone	Lower respiratory	Delayed pulmonary edema	Welders
2. Asphyxiants			
Carbon monoxide	Blood-oxygen transport	Headache	Auto mechanics
		Dizziness	Policemen
Hydrogen sulfide	Respiratory center paralysis	Decreased ventilation	Miners
		Irritation of respiratory tract	Sewer workers
Cyanide	Cellular enzymes	Deficient oxygen in tissues	Nylon makers
			Plastic workers

Table 16.1 *Some chemical agents producing occupational disease (Continued)*

Agent	System(s) affected	Principal manifestation(s)	Representative occupations in which exposure occurs
Dusts			
1. Inorganic			
Silica	Pulmonary	Nodular fibrosis or scarring (silicosis)	
		Chronic obstructive lung disease	
Asbestos	Pulmonary	Diffuse fibrosis or scarring (asbestosis)	Pipe insulators
			Textile workers
	Peritoneum	Lung cancer	Floor tile sanders
		Mesothelioma (rare malignant tumor)	Brake liners
Talc	Pulmonary	Fibrosis or scarring	Talc miners
		Pleural thickening	Rubber workers
Coal	Pulmonary	Chronic obstructive lung disease	Coal miners
		Coal worker's pneumoconiosis (black lung)	
2. Organic			
Cotton	Pulmonary	Chronic obstructive lung disease (byssinosis—brown lung)	Textile workers
			Weavers
Detergent enzymes	Pulmonary	Bronchitis	Housewives
		Pneumonitis	Detergent packers
		Asthma	
Hay	Pulmonary	Granulomatous reaction (farmer's lung)	Farmers
Sugar Cane	Pulmonary	Granulomatous reaction (bagassosis)	Bagasse processors

part exclude the possibility of effects due to chronic exposure. Even more upsetting is the fact that 51 percent of the TLV's are based only on animal experiments (27 percent) or chemical analogy (24 percent). Given the assumption that animal data apply to humans, which is a large assumption, most animal experiments do not adequately examine the question of the effects of chronic exposure. It is obvious that if we do not have a clear understanding of the effects of one substance, we have little chance of predicting what the interactions of two or more might be, and it is common in industry to see workers exposed to several substances.

Another problem for setting limits is the difficulty of measuring suspected health effects. It is easy to understand how an occupational exposure which doubled or tripled the risk of a certain type of cancer could go unrecognized. The discovery of excess bladder cancer in the leather industry required highly sophisticated techniques, even when the risk to leather workers was twenty times that of another working group. It is thus now known how many less overt risks are being overlooked.

It becomes obvious that our knowledge of hazards which confront workers is severely limited and that we rely more on the inherent toughness and resiliency of humans than on knowledge of occupational exposures and their effects.

Some problems in effective control

Would a corporation knowingly allow a working environment to produce a chronic occupational disease in a worker? Would a worker knowingly take a job that could affect his health? Would the federal government permit these things to happen? Are the universities failing to provide the training and research information necessary to make meaningful decisions? The answer to all these questions is an unfortunate yes. And in the answer lies a large part of why occupational disease still occurs with appalling regularity in the United States.

Until very recently, there were more federal game wardens in the United States than federal industrial safety and health inspectors; the abuse of birds and game received more attention than workers. The situation in most of the states is not much different. Should an industry that provides jobs be allowed to continue if its workers suffer disease because of their job? Who will make that determination?

While significant strides have been made, and while some large industries are admirable, there is still an inexcusable amount of abuse of the worker's health perpetuated by private industry. This happens for many complex reasons, a number of which are discussed below.

SIZE AND NUMBER There are 3.5 million employers of 80 million workers in the United States. Only 26,000 of these employers have more than 250 workers. There is an inverse relationship between the size of the industry and the rate of occupational disease; the larger an industry, the better it can afford to secure the expert service it needs to provide safe and healthful working conditions.

COMPETITION Because safe working conditions require investment, the industry that de-emphasizes safety and health could theoretically undersell a more conscientious competitor. This translates into money and profits—the hallmark of American industry. Moreover, there are major economic drawbacks which may discourage a corporation from even acknowledging that an illness may be work-related, such as the fear of incurring severe penalties through workmen's compensation. The coal mine owners of West Virginia refused to recognize the relationship between black lung (pneumoconiosis) and working in the coal mines.

Figure 16.2. A typical work site in a tire building plant. In this area, where various materials are mixed together, there is always a large amount of dust.

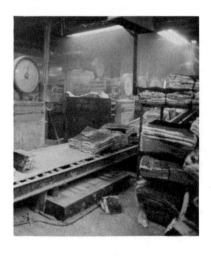

The companies operating uranium mines have refuted all efforts to link higher rates of lung cancer to the radioactivity in the air of the mines.

Once a causal link is established between occupational exposure and illness, the company becomes liable for the costs of maintaining the employee affected as well as the costs of his care. The threat of such a liability should serve as an impetus to seek more effective preventive measures, but too often it only stimulates more intense defensive litigation.

WORKERS   Traditionally workers and trade unions have not been very interested in health. The general reaction of the worker when confronted with a hazardous job has been to request and receive "hazard pay." This is changing—perhaps as a result of the general "environmental awakening." The worker, like all other human beings, is beginning to question the effects of his job on his life and future. The achievement of occupational health in America rests more with the worker than with any other sector. If the worker stays concerned and interested, he will get the working conditions he deserves.

TRAINED PERSONNEL   Even if an industry wants to supply the best and safest working conditions for its employees, it is sometimes difficult to find the necessary experts. Occupational medicine is not a popular medical specialty; in 1972 there were fewer than 300 physicians with specific training in this field. This deficiency may be due in part to the expectations of industry in regard to industrial physicians. Too often they are placed in a position of divided loyalties to their patients and their employers. Too often this field seems to attract the less competent physicians. Unfortunately many of the same deterrents appear to apply to the field of industrial hygiene as well.

Universities likewise have been negligent. Most medical schools teach little or no occupational medicine and have little or no competence in occupational medicine in their faculties. While many medical schools are developing programs in community medicine, many of these exclude occupational health problems. Schools of public health have done only slightly better. The number of full-time academic persons interested primarily in occupational medicine is small indeed. This may be due in part to lack of federal support for research in this area, lack of access to industrial problems, and a general lack of interest on the part of academicians.

INSUFFICIENT GOVERNMENTAL SURVEILLANCE   Until the passage of the Occupational Safety and Health Act of 1970 (see below), the federal government had minimal involvement in occupational disease surveillance. The most remarkable thing about state surveillance has been its complete lack of uniformity. Some industrialized northern and eastern states have good state programs; most southern states do not. This variation has resulted in some appalling adventures to the detriment of the worker. One example will illustrate this. A large eastern state outlawed the production of the chemical dye beta naphthylamine because it produced bladder cancer in many workers. The eastern factory closed and reopened in a southern state where no such ban, much less an occupational health surveillance system, existed. As a result, southern workers have been developing bladder cancer at an unconscionable rate. Lack of uniformity in workmen's compensation laws has also been a paramount feature of our patchwork state pattern. The OSH Act of 1970 yields the promise of wholesale change in both areas.

The Occupational Safety and Health Act of 1970

This federal law supplies the machinery to eradicate many of the problems described above. Successful enforcement will require many years and much money and manpower. The act sets mandatory occupational safety and health standards for businesses and provides for the necessary enforcement program and reporting procedures. It also provides for research in the field of occupational health and for training programs necessary to increase the number of competent workers.

The act established the National Institute of Occupational Safety and Health (NIOSH), which is responsible for health research, including studies of psychological factors and methods for dealing with occupational health. NIOSH is also responsible for determining safe exposure levels and for annual reports on chronic and low-level exposure to industrial substances. NIOSH prescribes regulations requiring employers to

Occupational Safety and Health Act, 1970

The Act provides for the preservation of human resources:

1. by authorizing the Secretary of Labor to set mandatory occupational safety and health standards applicable to businesses affecting interstate commerce, and by creating an Occupational Safety and Health Review Commission for carrying out adjudicatory functions under the Act;

2. by providing for research in the field of occupational safety and health, including the psychological factors involved, and by developing innovative methods, techniques, and approaches for dealing with occupational safety and health problems;

3. by providing medical criteria which will assure insofar as practicable that no employee will suffer diminished health, functional capacity, or life expectancy as a result of his work experience;

4. by providing for training programs to increase the number and competence of personnel engaged in the field of occupational safety and health;

5. by providing for the development and promulgation of occupational safety and health standards;

6. by providing an effective enforcement program which shall include a prohibition against giving advance notice of any inspection and sanctions for any individual violating this prohibition;

7. by encouraging the States to assume the fullest responsibility for the administration and enforcement of their occupational safety and health laws by providing grants to the States to assist in identifying their needs and responsibilities in the area of occupational safety and health, to develop plans in accordance with the provisions of this Act, to improve the administration and enforcement of State occupational safety and health laws, and to conduct experimental and demonstration projects in connection therewith;

8. by providing for appropriate reporting procedures with respect to occupational safety and health which procedures will help achieve the objectives of this Act and accurately describe the nature of the occupational safety and health problem.

submit reports on the exposure of employees to potentially harmful substances.

If adequately carried out, the OSH Act of 1970 could circumvent most of the problems attributed to private industry, governmental agencies, universities, and workers. This important and significant piece of health legislation will require much effort to implement, but it represents the beginning of what someday might be adequate surveillance.

RISKS OF IONIZING RADIATION

Ionizing radiation can be neither seen, felt, nor heard. Its unusual characteristic is its ability to penetrate tissue and deposit its energy at random within cells by producing ionization of cellular molecules. The usual body defenses against attack by chemical agents (such as barriers to absorption, detoxification, and immunological mechanisms) are ineffective against radiation. Moreover, a small amount of energy is required to damage cells by radiation.

The fundamental unit of radiation dose is the *rad*. Five hundred rads of X-rays to the human body will kill approximately one-half of people so exposed. Yet 500 rads will ionize only about one molecule per 40,000,000 in each cell.

Worldwide interest in ionizing radiation developed rapidly after the discoveries of X-rays by Wilhelm Roentgen in 1895, and of radioactivity from uranium by Becquerel less than a year later. In sufficient doses radiation may produce acute effects which can lead to death. More ominous, however, are its long-term effects—particularly its ability to induce cancer. These "late effects" occur many years after irradiation, may be lethal, and can result from doses far below those necessary to cause any symptoms at the time of exposure. Compared to other environmental and industrial hazards, however, there is extensive information about the effects of ionizing radiation on human health. In addition, the presence of radiation can be readily detected and exposure levels precisely measured. For these reasons precise and consistent international safety and protection standards exist for radiation exposure.

In a broad sense, the term *radiation* means any emission of energy from a point of origin. Heat from the sun, light from a lamp, and radio waves from a transmitter are all forms of radiation. If the radiation is of a type that is capable of penetrating matter and causing ionization along its path, then it is called *ionizing radiation*. One type of ionizing radiation is that emitted from an X-ray tube; another is that which is released from the nucleus of an atom. Such radiation represents a release of energy accompanying the transformation of atoms from unstable to stable states. Unstable atoms are called *radioactive elements* or *radioisotopes*, and the energy they release may be in the form of electromagnetic waves or particles. The rate of transformation or decay of an unstable element is measured in terms of its *half-life*, the time it takes for 50 percent of a radioisotope to decay.

Radiation dosage is properly expressed in *rads*, a unit related to the amount of energy absorbed by the tissue. Some radiations are more efficient at destroying human cells than others, however, and produce more biologic damage per rad dose. The *rem* is a unit of biologic dose used in the field of radiation protection that takes into consideration the differing efficiencies of the different radiations.

Natural sources of radiation exposure

The entire world population is continuously being exposed to background radiation from natural sources. Background radiation arises from three general sources: cosmic rays, external radiation from radioactive materials in the environment, and internal radiation exposure from naturally occurring radioisotopes deposited in the body by ingestion or inhalation.

Primary cosmic radiation from outer space interacts with nuclei of the upper atmosphere to yield secondary radiations. These consist of gamma rays, neutrons, protons, and electrons and they constitute the cosmic radiation received at the earth's surface. Owing to absorption of this radiation by the atmosphere, the dose rate from cosmic radiation varies considerably with altitude. A person living in Denver, for example, will receive nearly three times the radiation dose from this source as one living at sea level. Likewise, it has been calculated that a commercial jet pilot receives about six to eight times the sea-level dose.

External exposure from radioactivity in the environment results from naturally occurring radioactive elements present in soil, rocks, and the atmosphere. These radioisotopes are primarily uranium, thorium, radium, and ^{40}Potassium.

Naturally occurring radioactive materials are inhaled or ingested in food and water and incorporated into body tissues. Variations in internal exposure therefore depend on eating and drinking habits as well as the mineral content of water and foodstuffs. An extremely wide range of naturally occurring radioactive isotopes exists in water supplies, and variations may be large among water supplies in neighboring communities. The primary source of radiation from this source is ^{40}Potassium.

In the past, small groups of individuals have been occupationally exposed to high levels of the naturally occurring heavy istopes. A well-known example is that of the radium dial painters. Owing to the habit of licking the paint brush to make a fine tip, more luminous paint containing radioactive thorium and radium was apparently ingested by the workers than was actually painted on the dials. A continuing problem involves underground workers in mines with high concentrations of radon gas and its radioactive daughter products in the air. Radon gas is liberated into the mines from naturally occurring heavy isotopes in the mine walls or in stored uranium ore or radium-enriched residues. Owing to poor ventilation, it cannot escape into the atmosphere. There is thus an accumulation of radioactivity in the air of the mines, and the miners develop lung cancers at much greater rates than expected.

Medical X-rays

Medical X-rays constitute by far the largest man-made source of radiation exposure to the general population. About 40 percent of the genetically significant dose from medical X-rays arises from films of the lower back (lumbar spine). About 60 percent of the entire population dose arises from the irradiation of males between the ages of 15 and 29. Although usually of little diagnostic value, lumbar spine films have become a routine part of many preemployment physical exams because of the fear of law suits arising from the development of lower back pain later on. One lateral lumbar spine film yields a radiation dose to the patient equivalent to 50–100 regular chest X-rays, and a dose to the gonads in the male about 500 times that received from a chest X-ray.

Man-made sources of radiation exposure

Medical X-rays, both diagnostic and therapeutic, represent by far the largest man-made source of radiation exposure to the general population at the present time. The total skin dose to the exposed areas during X-ray examinations requiring fluoroscopy and several X-ray films can reach very high. For the patient, therefore, diagnostic X-ray examinations may yield radiation exposures many times above the normal background radiation that he will receive throughout his lifetime.

Of equal concern, however, is the average gonadal dose received by the population as a whole since it will determine the rate at which genetic mutations are introduced into the population pool. From this standpoint, it is the total population dose that is important; the effects are similar if 1 person receives 20 rems, or 20 persons each receive 1 rem to the gonads. Estimates of the average annual genetically significant dose to the general population from various sources are presented in Table 16.2.

Table 16.2 *Average annual genetically significant dose to each person in the general population from various sources*

Source	Dose (millirem)[a]/yr
Natural background	
Cosmic radiation	40
Radioactive elements in environment (external exposure)	40
Radioactive elements in body (internal exposure)	20
Medical sources	
Diagnostic X-rays	20–50[b]
Therapeutic X-rays	3–5[b]
Radioisotopes	0.2
Other sources	
Occupational (medical, industrial, and nuclear energy workers)	0.2
Fallout (from 1954–1962 period of testing)	1.5
All other man-made sources	2.0

[a] Rems measure the biological effect of ionizing radiation.
[b] Approximate range of estimates from several different countries.

Sources other than medical X-rays currently add little to background radiation exposure. Miscellaneous sources include television sets, increased cosmic radiation to passengers in aircraft, and luminous markings on clocks and watches. However, there is considerable uncertainty over the pattern of future radiation exposure from other man-made sources. Detectable increases in background radiation to man have been measured in many parts of the world because of radioactive fallout after atomic-bomb detonations. In general, however, radiation exposure due to fallout that has occurred up to the present time represents only a small fraction of background radiation to most of the world population.

The major potential new source of man-made radiation arises from the various uses of nuclear energy. The hazard to the general population is mainly from internal exposure to inhaled or ingested radioactive products. These products are derived from the normal disposal of radioactive wastes or the accidental release of radioisotopes into the environment from reactors or nuclear-power plants. Radioactive wastes are usually discharged into rivers or oceans or into the atmosphere, or stored until sufficient radioactive decay has occurred. To the present time, these sources have not added significantly to background radiation exposure. It has been calculated, for example, that conventional fossil-fuel power plants discharge relatively greater quantities of radioactive materials into the atmosphere than nuclear-power plants of comparable size. Experience with contamination of the environment both accidentally and through disposal of radioactive wastes is still very limited, however, compared with the potential magnitude of the problem.

Factors governing internal radiation exposure

With continued bomb testing and the increased use of nuclear energy, the problems involved in the control of radiation exposure due to internally deposited radioisotopes may become of major importance. Unlike X-ray machines, such radioisotopes cannot be "turned off." They are either inhaled from the atmosphere or ingested in food or water. The problems of radiation protection against internal emitters are entirely different from those for external radiation exposure, and have led to detailed studies of the way the body handles specific radioactive elements and to the emergence of the field of *radiation ecology.*

The first concern is the way in which isotopes derived from reactor wastes, nuclear-power plants, fallout, or natural sources reach the individual. For inhaled isotopes, this may depend on atmospheric mixing, the physical and chemical state of the isotope, and the living and working habits of the individual. For ingested isotopes, two general processes are involved: the introduction of the isotope into a "food chain" and its subsequent passage to the final food product.

FOOD CHAINS   The importance of food chains is perhaps best illustrated by examples. During the Windscale nuclear-reactor accident in England in 1957 large quantities of an isotope (^{131}I) were released into atmosphere. Because of the short physical half-life of this isotope (eight days), one might assume that most of the activity would have decayed before significant exposure to the population occurred. Due to a combination of circumstances, however, the isotope was rapidly brought to earth from the atmosphere and absorbed by plants and grass. The grass was eaten by cows, and the isotope appeared in significant quantities in their milk, which was rapidly processed and sent to the consumer. The hazard would not have arisen if a delay had occurred before consumption—for example, if the milk had been canned or converted into butter or cheese.

A different situation exists with the Eskimos near the Arctic Circle, where the main plant life is lichens, which, unlike seasonal plants, live for many decades. During their long lifetime, their leaves accumulate fallout products from atomic bomb tests as well as high concentrations of naturally occurring isotopes from the atmosphere. Lichens constitute the principal dietary constituent of caribou and reindeer, the main food of the Eskimos. Through this food chain, the Eskimos have accumulated high concentrations of radioisotopes.

ISOTOPES IN THE BODY The second area of importance in determining internal exposure is the fate of the isotope once it reaches the body. The physical, chemical, and biologic properties of an isotope determine its effect on the body. Physical factors include the half-life or rate of decay of the isotope, and its energy and type of emission. Isotopes with very short half-lives (less than one or two hours) offer little internal hazard since physical decay occurs before significant incorporation in the body. Chemical factors include the chemical form and solubility of the isotope as they affect absorption, transport, and excretion by the body. Biologic factors, usually the most important, include the regulatory mechanisms determining the absorption and excretion of the particular isotope and thus its biologic half-life, and the degree of concentration of the isotope in one or more body tissues. For example, ^{131}I selectively concentrates in the thyroid gland and ^{90}Sr concentrates in bone, whereas radioactive water distributes itself throughout the body and is relatively rapidly excreted. When concentration in specific tissues does not occur, local radiation doses are much lower and the eventual hazard generally less.

Biological effects of environmental radiation exposure

The biologic effects of radiation may be divided into two major categories: acute and delayed effects and late effects. The first are related to the killing of cells and occur after exposure to high radiation doses. Late effects may result from much lower doses and dose-rates. The important late effects of radiation are cancer induction (carcinogenesis) and genetic abnormalities in offspring. These are thought to result from irreparable damage to the genetic material of cells that survive radiation and remain capable of reproducing. When the germ cells in the ovaries or testicles are irradiated, the damage is passed on to the offspring.

A number of studies have related radiation exposure to the development of cancer in man, and the results of these studies allow us to estimate the risk of cancer from a given radiation exposure. These exposures have arisen from occupational, medical, and accidental sources.

There are several examples of cancers arising in human beings after localized exposure to high doses of radiation from environmental sources. Notable among these are the radium dial painters with a high incidence of bone cancer and underground mine workers with a high incidence of lung cancer.

The most important sources of data for carcinogenic effects have come from therapeutic medical exposures and from survivors of the atom bomb explosions in Hiroshima and Nagasaki. From these studies, it is estimated that doubling the level of background radiation would lead to 2000 additional cases of cancer among the United States population. This figure compares with 600,000 new cancer cases and 350,000 deaths yearly in the United States.

The genetic effects of radiation may not be seen for many generations, and as yet no definite radiation-induced abnormalities have been observed. This is not unexpected, as such mutations are difficult to detect, particularly in early generations. Experiments suggest that rather high doses are required to double the spontaneous (natural) mutation rate, and there is no general agreement as to the seriousness to the human population of even doubling the spontaneous mutation rate. It has been calculated, however, that tripling the natural background rate would eventually lead to an increase of between 0.5 percent and 5.0 percent in all illness.

Radiation protection and safety standards

Radiation protection standards are set by agreement between the International Commission on Radiological Protection (ICRP) and the National Council on Radiation Protection and Measurements (NCRP) in the United States. Those used by the federal government are based on recommendations of the Federal Radiation Council (FRC) which generally endorses the recommendations of the ICRP and NCRP. Originally, the setting of maximum permissible doses for radiation workers was based on the belief that radiation in doses below a certain level produced no biologic damage of consequence in man. Recent studies suggest that there is no threshold for the important long-term effects of radiation, and any additional radiation exposure above background is potentially harmful and protective measures should be as strong as possible.

Maximum permissible doses (MPD) for occupational exposure and to the general population are set at the minimum levels that are practically and economically feasible. The philosophy becomes one of an "acceptable risk"—that is, doses below the MPD are estimated to incur risks that are small compared with the other hazards of everyday living. The current maximum permissible doses are compared with radiation exposures for various environmental and medical sources in Table 16.3.

For medical patients, the question is one of weighing the possible risks from radiation exposure against the benefits of the diagnostic examination. In most cases, the radiation risk should be small in relation to that incurred if an indicated examination is not performed. However, many simple measures can markedly reduce radiation exposure from external sources. For medical X-rays, the use of properly designed equipment and optimum radiographic and processing techniques may greatly reduce both patient exposure and scattered radiation without affecting the quality of the examination. Exposure to personnel can be reduced by proper use of lead shields and lead rubber aprons. As medical X-rays constitute a large fraction of the overall population exposure, it is of particular interest to reduce this source of radiation as much as possible.

Table 16.3 Comparison of radiation exposures from various sources with permissible levels

Source	Dose (rems)
Annual whole-body dose from background radiation	0.10
Maximum permissible average annual exposure to any group in the general population[a]	0.17
Maximum permissible annual dose to any individual in the general population[a]	0.50
Mean annual doses currently received by occupationally exposed persons including medical, industrial, and nuclear energy workers	0.2–1.0
Maximum permissible annual dose for occupationally exposed persons to gonads and blood-forming organs (whole body)[a]	5.0
Diagnostic X-ray examinations (typical skin doses to exposed areas utilizing modern radiographic equipment)[b]	
Single X-ray film	0.02–3.0
Fluoroscopy (*dose per minute*)	1.0–7.0
Complete gastrointestinal examination (films and fluoroscopy)	6.0–30.0
Maximum permissible annual dose for occupationally exposed persons localized to hands	75.0
Approximate whole-body dose to produce acute radiation sickness	above 150
Approximate whole-body dose which may cause death	above 500

[a] These maximum permissible annual doses exclude the exposure received from natural background and medical X-rays (deliberate exposure of patients by physicians).
[b] The dose to tissues beneath the skin will be less. At a depth of 15 cm, for example, the dose will be about 10% of the skin dose.

Since the physical, chemical, and biologic properties of each isotope must be considered, safety standards for internal radiation exposure are more difficult to set than for external exposure. Protection against internal exposure primarily involves ingestion or inhalation of the isotope. This is aided by knowledge of the sources and the food chains involved. For now, little can be done to prevent radiation exposure once the element is deposited in the body.

RISKS OF ACCIDENTS

Accidents are the biggest public health problem in the United States today for those through age thirty-eight. In addition to the loss of life, accidents cost the United States $29.5 billion per year. This is spread out over wage losses ($7.8 billion), medical and hospital fees ($3.1 billion), insurance and claim settlement ($7.3 billion), property damage ($5.0 billion), fire damage ($2.2 billion), and other costs ($4.1 billion).

Table 16.4 Principal categories of accidents (1971)

Category	Deaths	Disabling injuries
Motor vehicle	54,700	2,000,000
Work (occupational)	14,200	2,300,000
Home	27,200	4,200,000
Public	22,500	2,800,000
Total	115,000	11,300,000

Facts and figures

For youths aged fifteen to twenty-four, accidents claim more lives than all other causes combined, and nearly seven times more than the next leading cause. Four out of five accident victims in this age group are males.

Accidents are the leading cause of death among all persons aged 1 to 38. For persons of all ages, accidents are the fourth leading cause of death.

In 1971 it was estimated that our nation lost 29.5 billion dollars from accidents. More than half of this total is accounted for by motor vehicle accidents. Deaths from accidents numbered 115,000; about one-half of these deaths were caused by motor vehicle accidents.

Every 10 minutes two persons will be killed and more than 200 injured. This results in a cost of $560,000 per 10 minutes or $3,360,000 per hour.

Lap-type safety belts if used by everyone would save between 10,000 and 20,000 lives per year. Drinking of alcohol is an important factor in at least one-half of the fatal motor vehicle accidents.

Between 1961 and 1971 bicycle deaths rose 70 percent. Urban fatalities increased 88 percent while in rural areas the rise was 54 percent. During this period bicycle sales more than doubled.

By analyzing the accident facts that exist, some clear-cut possibilities for reducing this devastation emerge. Since accidents are caused both by behavioral and environmental factors, it is possible to effect change by modifying either of these factors. The major categories of accidents will be discussed to point out their relative importance and to suggest ways in which frequency and severity of accidents can be reduced. It is important to keep in mind both the behavioral and environmental elements, as strategies depend on the ability to modify these two major factors.

Motor vehicle accidents

There were about 54,700 deaths from automobile accidents in 1971 (Table 16.5). If ways could be devised to reduce this devastation, there would be a huge impact on public health in the United States.

Table 16.5 How people died in motor vehicle accidents (1971)

Category	Deaths
Collisions of 2 or more vehicles	23,300
Noncollision	13,700
Pedestrian	10,600
Collisions with fixed objects	4,650
Collisions with trains	1,500
Collisions with bicycles	850
Other	100
Total	54,700

PHYSICAL ASPECTS Physical considerations are clearly responsible for the injuries produced from automobile accidents. When a collision occurs, there is rapid deceleration. The automobile stops, but the passengers and driver tend to remain in motion. If severe enough, the driver and passengers may be propelled into some fixed object—usually the steering wheel, windshield, or dashboard. This is the *two-collision concept*—a driver of an automobile that crashes into a cement wall is not injured or killed by the car hitting the wall; he is hurt by his body making a second collision with whatever is in front of him. There are thus two methods for reducing collision injuries. First, deceleration in the event of a collision may be reduced through highway design. For example, a guard rail in front of a cement wall may cause a car merely to glance off, instead of coming to a full stop. Second, the two-collision concept leads to several important safety devices among which are seat belts, shoulder harnesses, padded dashboards, and the experimental inflatable air bag. Eliminating projecting objects in the interior of the car also reduces the second-collision impact.

HUMAN ENGINEERING In human engineering the machine is regarded as an extension of man, whether that machine be an automobile, an industrial lathe, or a motor boat. Human engineering works to fit man to his machines so that errors are reduced and efficiencies enhanced. This applies to automobile safety in several ways. For example, the steering wheel, driver's seat, and brake, clutch, and gas pedals should be designed to minimize fatigue, a frequent cause of accidents. Seat belts and shoulder harnesses can be designed to be both comfortable and efficient. Unfortunately, style considerations receive more attention than safety. Most drivers of American cars have experienced ill-fitting shoulder harnesses and hard-to-reach controls. Attention to these matters could have a significant impact on accident frequency and severity.

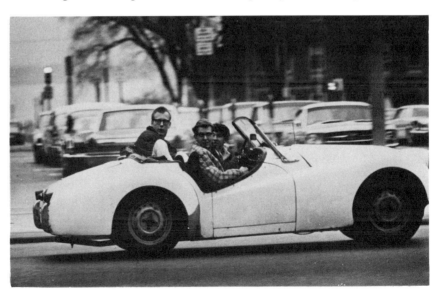

Figure 16.3. Automobile accidents— the leading cause of accidental deaths in the United States. (Courtesy of World Health Organization, photo by Jean Mohr)

EMERGENCY CARE While primary emphasis should be on accident prevention, the need for prompt, competent medical care when accidents occur is obvious. This implies both trained personnel and good equipment, but emergency care after accidents has received very little attention. It may be surprising that many members of the medical profession are not trained in first aid. Ambulances often are not suitable for transporting the injured properly, and even hospital emergency facilities are often inadequate. In addition, hospitals are often poorly located to receive accident victims. It would make good sense to consider training a large segment of the population in first aid. It goes without saving that medical and paramedical professionals should likewise be trained.

It is obvious that a full-scale attack needs to be made on both accident prevention and on rapid and appropriate treatment of the accident victim. This will require much planning, coordination of existing agencies and facilities, and the practical application of research studies.

Motor vehicle accidents: behavioral factors

The previous discussion has considered some aspects of the automobile accident problem that can be modified by altering the environment. Thus they are outside of the direct control of the individual. However, there are a number of the behavioral factors in the individual's control that influence automobile accidents.

SEAT BELTS The topic of seat belts deserves special mention. Of those preventive devices which are available and have proved to be of worth, the seat belt shows the greatest potential to reduce injuries. The behavioral problem is to get people to use them. Although it is estimated that seat belts could save 10,000 to 20,000 lives per year, only 20 to 30 percent of drivers consistently wear them. If anyone could think of a way to induce all drivers and passengers to use such devices, a fantastic impact on the public health of Americans would occur. But, even though 1974 American cars will not start unless the seat belts are fastened, it is expected that many drivers will devise means to avoid their use.

ALCOHOL DRINKING Alcohol drinking is an important factor in at least half of all motor vehicle accidents and fatalities. Of those involved in accidents, the highest rates of alcohol use occurred in the group aged twenty to thirty-four years. In the United States people do drink and drive. Most state laws governing drinking drivers are permissive. Definitions of drunkenness vary from state to state, but most are set considerably above levels at which significant performance impairment occurs.

It is clear that drinking of alcohol is associated with greater accident frequency. Just what are the risks? Data recorded in Table 16.6 shed light on the relationship between blood-alcohol levels and automobile accident risk. While most states (twenty-eight) use 0.15 gm alcohol/ 100 cc blood to define drunkenness, it can be seen that this level repre-

Table 16.6 *Accident risk in relation to blood alcohol*

Alcohol in blood mg/100 cc	Percent of 432 drivers in accidents[a]	Percent of 2015 drivers not in accidents[b]	Ratio accident/ nonaccident	Ratio hazard
0.00–0.05	77.5	91.3	0.85	1.0
0.05–0.10	7.1	5.4	1.31	1.5
0.10–0.15	4.0	1.9	2.1	2.5
0.15+	11.3	1.4	8.1	9.7

[a] 432 accident victims had blood alcohol measured.
[b] 2015 random drivers not involved in accidents had blood alcohol measured.

sents a hazard of almost ten times the sober state. Even at alcohol levels below 0.10 percent (a level used by fifteen states) there is a significantly increased accident ratio. Other experimental data substantiates this finding. For example, the scores of drivers taking driving skill and performance tests averaged 25 to 35 percent poorer at blood alcohol levels of as low as 0.04–0.06 percent. Some drivers even scored significant negative effects at 0.032 percent. What is equally important to the loss of performance is the loss of insight by the drinker that this impairment has occurred. In fact, many drivers under the influence of alcohol believe themselves capable of even greater driving skills while their judgment is severely impaired.

Although there are many reasons why alcohol affects people differently, it is reasonable to consider some general rules about the levels of drinking that produce "legal drunkenness." The two major factors that determine the blood level of alcohol from a given amount consumed are weight and whether the stomach is full or empty. However, the same blood alcohol level in the old (over seventy-five) or young (less than twenty-five) produces greater effects.

OTHER DRUGS A recent study of fatal single vehicle accidents revealed that 13 percent of the victims had been using identifiable drugs, usually tranquilizers and barbiturates. Of these victims over 60 percent had substantial blood alcohol levels in addition. While we have recently collected good information on alcohol and some sparse information on a few other drugs, there is incomplete or a total lack of information on most. For example, the effect of marijuana—a widely used substance—on automobile accident rates is not fully known. The effect of other mood-changing or mind-expanding drugs is equally unknown. Even the use of common medications such as tranquilizers or antihistamine could influence behavior and alertness. These problems have been inadequately studied.

Work accidents

At least 14,500 workers are killed and 9,000,000 injured at work each year. When considering work accidents, it is important to consider both frequency and severity. For example, in a coal mine an accident is likely to be very severe in terms of lost time, while in some industries injuries are frequent but minor.

If one examines statistics on accident frequency, depending on the source of data there can be wide variation in the industrial accident problem reported nationally. This relates to the way accidents are defined. It is relatively easy to count deaths, but when it comes to nonfatal injury, definition is highly important. For example, is a foreign body in the eye an accident? Is a splinter in the leg an accident? It is important to remember that definitions vary according to agency and source when assessing risks for any occupational groups. The National Health Survey (NHS), for example, defines a "bed-disabling" injury as requiring confinement of the injured to bed for more than half of the daylight hours on the day of the accident or some subsequent day. The National Safety Council (NSC) defines a disabling injury as an injury which prevents a person from performing any of his usual activities for a full day beyond the day of the accident. Difference in NHS and NSC definitions would thus yield different injury rates.

Another important point about industrial accidents is that the accident frequency and severity vary widely among types of industry and even within the same industry. This strongly suggests that programs for accident prevention can and do work. Those companies belonging to the NSC have lower accident frequency and severity (Table 16.7). For manufacturing, frequency rates of NSC members are about 70 percent lower, while for mining the frequency is about 40 percent lower.

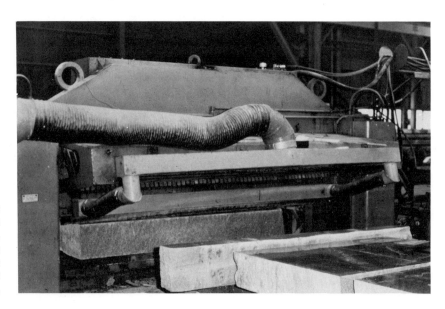

Figure 16.4. A large granite guillotine. Each time the blade strikes the granite to split it, hazardous dust is released; the exhaust vent prevents the release of the disease-producing dust into the workroom.

Table 16.7 Comparative injury frequency rates of
National Safety Council (NSC) members vs. nonmembers

Year	NSC	Non-NSC	Percent NSC rates are lower
Manufacturing			
1968	5.3	17.9	−70
1969	5.7	18.9	−70
1970	6.0	19.1	−69
Mining			
1968	22.2	36.7	−40
1969	21.8	37.6	−42
1970	22.2	39.2	−43

As with automobile safety, good engineering can contribute to a reduction in accidents—it is possible to design safer machines and safer methods of operating them. For example, if a guillotine is used to cut some substance such as rubber, it can be adjusted so that to lower the cutting blade, two switches must be actuated simultaneously by both hands. If the switches are placed well away from the dangerous part of the machine, there would be no chance for accidental amputation. There are many other common-sense prevention devices that have been developed to make the work setting safer.

Questions
1. What are some of the difficulties involved in determining whether a given substance is harmful? Why have save exposure limits been determined for so few substances?
2. Name the two types of effects that ionizing radiation may have. What is the most important controllable source of ionizing radiation?
3. What are the two factors responsible for accidents? Which one is easier to control?
4. From the point of view of prevention, how do occupational deaths and diseases differ from deaths due to cigarette smoking or failure to use seat belts?

Key Concepts
Human engineering – the science that deals with the design of machines for efficient use by humans

Isotope – atomic species differing in atomic weight, but having the same atomic number

Synergism – cooperative action such that the total effect is greater than the sum of the parts

Toxicology – the science which deals with poisons and their effects and with the problems involved (as clinical, industrial, or legal)

Selected Readings
Hunter, Donald. *Diseases of Occupations*, 4th ed. Boston: Little, Brown, 1969.
International Labour Organization, *Encyclopedia of Occupational Health and Safety*, 2 vols. New York: McGraw-Hill, 1972.
The Effects on Populations of Exposure to Low Levels of Ionizing Radiation. Report of the Advisory Committee on the Biological Effects of Ionizing Radiations. Washington, D.C.: Division of Medical Sciences, National Academy of Sciences, National Research Council, 1972.

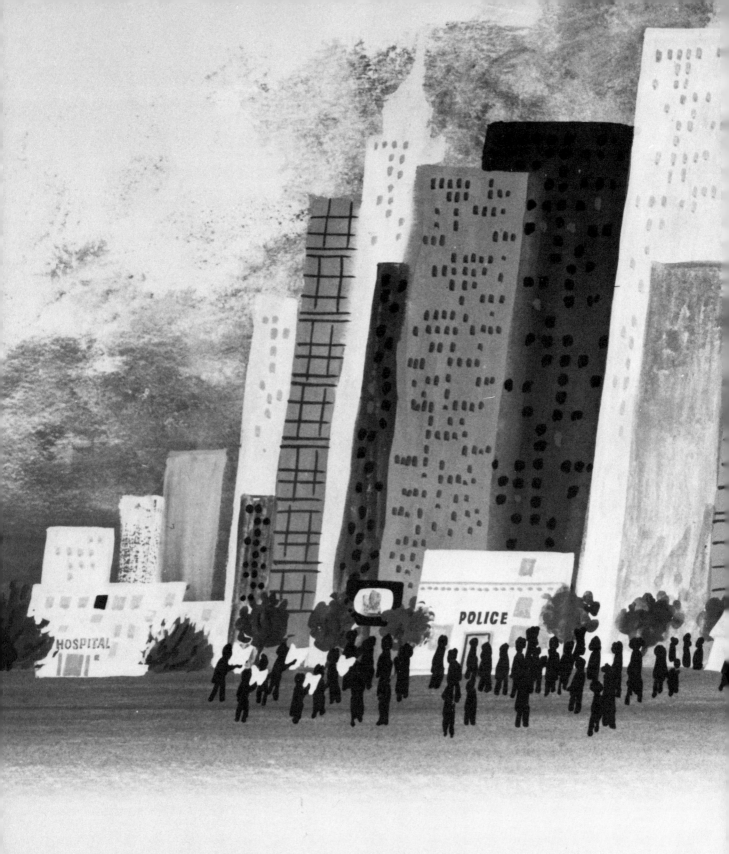

Part III

HEALTH AND THE COMMUNITY

Chapter 17

Ethics and the Law

MEDICAL ETHICS, OLD AND NEW

The historical ethical foundation of medical practice is the Oath of Hippocrates, the ancient doctrine of the Greek physicians who practiced their art from about the sixth century B.C. to around the first century A.D. Hippocrates himself is said to have lived from 460–379 B.C.

The genius of the Hippocratic Oath is not so much in its particular principles as in its overall philosophy: the devotion of the physician to his patient and to the healing process.

Prior to Hippocrates, the physician was hardly distinguishable from other tradesmen or, more commonly, from the unscrupulous magicians who preyed upon the troubles and superstitions of the sick. Indeed, the Hippocratic group was a minority in medicine even in its own time. It took great pride in its own high standards and looked upon other medical practitioners as little more than charlatans.

This chapter was contributed by William J. Curran, J.D., LL.M., S.M.Hyg., Frances Glessner Lee Professor of Legal Medicine, Harvard Medical School and Harvard School of Public Health, and Director of Interfaculty Program in Medical Ethics, Harvard University.

The doctor's oath

I swear by Apollo the Physician, by Aesculapius, by Hygeia and Panacea and by all the Gods and Goddesses that, to the best of my power and judgment, I will faithfully observe this oath and obligation.

My teacher in the art I will esteem as my parents, and share my resources with him, if he is short of the necessities of life. His children I will regard as my own brothers; and if they desire to learn I will instruct them in the same art without any reward or obligation. The precepts, the explanations and whatever else belongs to the art, I will communicate to my own children, to the children of my master, to such other pupils as have subscribed the Physician's Oath, and to no others.

I will treat my patients to the best of my power and judgment, in the most salutary manner without any injury or violence; neither will I be prevailed upon by another to administer pernicious physic, nor be the author of such advice myself; nor will I recommend to women a pessary to procure abortion.

I will live and practice chastely and religiously.

I will not cut a person suffering from the stone, but will leave this to such as are skilled in the task.

Whatever house I enter, I will always make the patient's good my principal aim, avoiding all mischief and corruption, and any irregular relations with females or males, bond or free.

And whatever I see or hear in the course of a cure, or otherwise, relating to the affairs of life, no one shall ever know it, if it ought to remain a secret.

May I be prosperous in life and business, and for ever honoured and esteemed by all men if I observe, and not confound, this solemn oath; and may the reverse of all this be my portion, if I violate it.

Hippocratic medicine was based on direct observation of the patient rather than on predetermined rules for diagnosis, on interest in the patient as a whole person rather than on the particular complaint, and on conservative, unharmful treatment taking advantage of the natural healing processes of the body. The principle of the relationship between doctor and patient was mutual respect. The patient was fully informed of what the physician was doing, what methods he was using, and what he expected from the treatment. Plato, ever the political philosopher, compared this sharing of information with the patient to the preamble of a statute, a statement of purpose intended to encourage the people to obey the law. In like manner, telling the patient the purposes of the treatment and what it was expected to achieve was intended to motivate him to take the medicine voluntarily, or to follow the regimen, as in diet, that the physician recommended.

During the Middle Ages, the Greek ideals went into some decline. Whereas pre-Christian physicians had concentrated all of their attention on the patients' human problems, medieval doctors were expected also to be concerned with their immortal souls. A Spanish law of Ferdinand and Isabella imposed a fine of ten thousand marevedis against any physician who attended a seriously ill person twice without encouraging him to call a priest and make his confession and receive Holy Communion. This act by the physician was considered not only a religious duty but also good medicine: the troubled sinner could not be expected to concentrate on getting well until he had made his peace with God.

With the Renaissance, the Hippocratic principles again gained ascendency and were accepted throughout the Western world as the ideal of all physicians. In fact, the Hippocratic Oath became the basis of the professional status and prestige of the medical doctor. With the prestige went an honored place in society, an established educational prerequisite, and a self-regulating guild controlling who could practice.

In the nineteenth century, medical ethics took on the character of professional etiquette and became more concerned with relations among physicians than between the doctor and his patient. Physicians were admonished not to advertise, to split fees, or to criticize the methods of fellow doctors. In the United States, enforcement of medical ethics in the interest of a close-knit medical profession was one of the major purposes in the organization of the American Medical Association (AMA) in 1846. There was clearly a need for such an organization at that time because of the poor condition of medical practice in this country, the lack of standards for medical schools, and the prevalence of medical cults. In 1873, the concern for ethical and legal regulation of medical practice was centralized in the Judicial Council of the American Medical Association.

In the meantime, the Hippocratic Oath had become more ritual than regulation, more pomp and circumstance than moral persuasion. The tradition of having medical students at commencement exercises solemnly swear to observe its ancient principles eventually began to break down in the face of the more informal styles of present-day graduates. The World Medical Association made a gallant attempt to revive the Oath by modernizing its language and updating its principles, but with only limited effect. In the 1970s, the growing acceptance of abortion and euthanasia as ethically and morally justifiable in medical practice has made universal adherence to the Hippocratic ideal even more embarrassing to the profession. Ironically, the Hippocratic condemnation of both of these practices was a minority philosophical position in Hippocrates' time as well.

THE OBLIGATIONS OF THE PHYSICIAN

In the United States today, the obligations of the physician to his patients are largely determined by law. All physicians must be licensed by the state or states in which they practice. The licensing laws spell out the areas of practice and conditions of practice. Essentially, the relationship between physician and patient is contractual. The patient pays the doctor for a service to be rendered within the expected range of medical competence. Furthermore, the relationship is one of trust and confidence. The patient often gives information to the doctor which is private and confidential, to be used by the physician only as necessary to the treatment. The physician is bound ethically and legally not to reveal these confidences.

The licensing of a physician to practice medicine does not require that he or she accept every person who comes for treatment. The physician is still free to refuse to enter into a treatment relationship. Once that relationship is entered, however, the physician is bound to continue treatment until the patient's problem is alleviated or until the patient is referred, with adequate notice, to another physician. This principle presents difficulties in emergency situations. The AMA Code admits that the physician has no obligation to aid in emergencies, but strongly recommends voluntarily rendering aid. In recent years, fear of malpractice suits has led to the refusal of many doctors to stop at roadside accidents or to answer a call in a crowded theater.

To encourage doctors to help in these situations, state legislatures have passed what are called "Good Samaritan Laws" which give an immunity from a malpractice suit to any physician who gives medical treatment in good faith in emergencies. Investigations by the American Medical Association and a National Malpractice Commission have indicated that doctors' fears of law suits arising from emergency aid are totally unfounded. There has not been a single recorded case of a suit against a doctor in such a situation. In 1973, the medical magazine *Emergency Medicine* offered a reward of $100 to any of its 160,000 readers who could document a case. In over five months there were no takers.

THE LAW OF MEDICAL MALPRACTICE

Americans are becoming increasingly conscious of their legal rights. One of the consequences of this awareness is a rise in law suits for personal injury damages. Physicians and hospitals have not been left out. There has been a significant increase in the number of medical malpractice suits and in the size of the settlements and court awards in such litigation in many parts of the United States over the past twenty years. One index of the increase is the cost of liability insurance to doctors and hospitals. In the 1960s, the insurance rates for surgeons rose 949.2 percent nationally; for physicians other than surgeons the rate rose 540.8 percent, while for hospitals they rose 262.7 percent.

The basic purpose of a malpractice suit is to recover money damages for an injury received by a patient because of the intentional wrong or the negligence of a physician or a hospital in caring for that patient. If such a wrong is committed, it is proper that the patient sue.

In the early decades of our country, the American courts established legal doctrines which favored the growth of industry and the professions in the interest of a growing continental nation. Medicine was among the favored areas. The courts granted immunity from personal injury suits to all charitable and governmental hospitals. For physicians, the courts created the "locality rule" under which all doctors could be judged only on the basis of the quality of care rendered in their own locality, be it a small village or a large city. Not only did this rule limit the standard of care applied, but it made it virtually impossible to prove a doctor guilty of malpractice. This was because in practice the suing patient could rarely find any other local doctor willing to testify against a local colleague. Slowly, the courts expanded the rule to allow proof of the standard of care in similar communities to that of the defendant-doctor, thus expanding somewhat the opportunity of the plaintiff-patient to find another doctor willing to testify.

There were other technical rules which also favored the practitioners. For example, the courts held that a physician could not be sued for any injury due to a mistaken professional judgment. The suit had to involve an affirmative action resulting in injury.

This protective attitude in the courts towards the professions did not begin to change until the Roosevelt years beginning in 1933, the rise of trade unionism, and the civil rights movement after World War II. The pendulum has now clearly swung in the other direction with the courts aggressively acting in favor of consumers in all industrial and professional fields.

In order to prove a medical malpractice case today, a suing patient must prove four elements of a case:

1. The existence of a duty toward the patient.
2. The breach of that duty by the physician, generally due to a failure to meet the required standard of medical care.
3. A causal relationship between the breach of duty and the injury to the patient.
4. A personal injury to the patient.

The proof of these elements is now made easier for patients than in the past. The duty of physicians to their patients is now well spelled out in the law. The breach of duty can be more readily proved because of expansion in the standard of care to cover states as a whole rather than local communities and, in the case of specialists, to cover all specialists in a particular field nationally. As to the injury and its proof, the lawyers for patients are becoming much more sophisticated in presenting medico-legal evidence in the courts. Nevertheless, malpractice cases are still not a simple matter. They are still difficult to win on the plaintiff's side. Some physicians believe that the laymen juries in the courts are always overly sympathetic toward injured patients. The statistics do not justify this impression. In 1970, for example, in all malpractice cases which went to juries for decision, the doctor-defendant won 80 percent of the verdicts. In only 20 percent did the plaintiff get any money at all for his claims. Yet this also indicates that many of the most meritorious claims were settled out of court by the insurance companies before any trial was held.

Reform in malpractice litigation

A number of proposals are presently being considered for major reform in the medical malpractice field. One of the proposals would move the litigation of claims to informal arbitration hearings rather than continue to use the law courts. Another more radical reform would install a so-called no-fault system of compensation in the field similar to that adopted recently in many states for automobile injuries. Under such a plan, the patient would be able to recover money damages and additional medical care if needed when an injury occurred in the course of medical treatment, whether or not a doctor, nurse, or other medical personnel were at fault. Such a plan would be attractive to both sides in the controversy. It would eliminate the difficulties of proof for plaintiffs and would also eliminate the attack on the doctor's personal reputation, the aspect of the current system most resented by the practicing professionals.

On the patient's side, there are proposals to provide indigent persons with public legal aid and to require medical care facilities to establish patient complaint mechanisms. It is suggested that hospitals retain *patient advocates* or *patient representatives* to help patients in understand what is happening to them in the increasingly complex medical world, to help them to gain benefits to which they are entitled, and to advise them in a possible malpractice situation.

HEALTH LAW: AN INADEQUATE SYSTEM

The practice of health law is only just beginning to be recognized in the United States, largely because of the inadequate nature of the legal system in the health field in this country.

The United States is a federal legal structure. The basic powers in public safety, public health, and other fields are placed with state, not federal, governments. The words *health* and *medicine* do not appear in our federal Constitution. Nearly all authority in Washington, D.C., on health matters of the people is indirect, being derived from specific powers like those which regulate interstate commerce, foreign commerce, and war. For most of our history, we have had no national policy concerning health matters or health protection.

At the state level, the major activities in the health field have been in licensing health professionals and facilities, such as hospitals and nursing homes, and in providing welfare-type medical care for chronic illnesses such as tuberculosis, schizophrenia, and cancer. At the local level, there have been traditional public health programs designed to control epidemic diseases and to regulate sanitary conditions. However, there is no coordinated national system of health care in the United States, and so there are gaps in health programs and regulatory apparatus. Even the gathering of health statistics is sporadic and unreliable because there is no national legal control over the methods of collecting the data or over the kind of information that is gathered.

The federal government has relied more on the power of the purse than on legal powers in health and welfare matters regarding the people. Using federal income tax resources and the direct tax of the federal Social Security program, the Department of Health, Education, and Welfare distributes large amounts of money to the states, private organizations, and individuals for the support of medical care programs, medical research, and the training of health personnel. The government has not recently proposed any increase in the federal health and welfare programs, but has favored a return of some of the federal income tax moneys on an equitable basis to the states to use as they see fit. Such a

The "thalidomide baby" cases

Thalidomide, a tranquilizer developed in western Europe during the mid-1950s, was used extensively, particularly in West Germany, from 1957 until 1961. Its popularity was due to its lack of the common side effects of most other tranquilizers, particularly induced drowsiness. One of the most frequent uses was to offset so-called morning sickness in pregnant women.

In May of 1960 a German neurologist, Dr. Ralf Voss, called attention in a medical paper to the possible relationship of the drug to severe birth defects in children born to mothers who used the drug very early in their pregnancies. Further investigations proved Dr. Voss's suspicions to be devastatingly correct. It is now believed that the drug was responsible for tragic birth defects (mostly of babies without either arms or legs) in 5,000 to 6,000 babies in western Europe, some 4,000 in West Germany alone.

In May of 1969, the longest court trial in the history of West Germany began. It was a criminal action against the Chemie Grünenthal Company, a pharmaceutical concern which manufactured the drug, and personally against a number of the officials of the company. The trial took 283 days and involved 120 witnesses, including 60 experts from all over the world. The criminal charges were dismissed on the grounds that the company and its officials had no knowledge of the harmful nature of the product. However, a civil settlement was achieved in favor of the parents of the deformed children. The court approved settlements of nearly $30 million in 2,000 cases of children who survived with the deformities. The company was also charged with all court costs, amounting to $1.6 million. There are no comparable personal injury cases in the entire annals of Western justice, either in Europe or in North or South America.

Thalidomide was never commercially released in the United States. Before it was brought to this country, the federal Food and Drug Administration, in the person of one physician, Dr. Frances O. Kelsey, read of its possible dangers in European medical journals. On this basis, she forestalled the applications of American companies to market the drug here. The companies protested, but Dr. Kelsey was able to delay matters until more evidence of the European disaster were in. The applications were withdrawn. Nevertheless, a good deal of testing of the drug was done in this country in the early 1960s and over 2.5 million tablets were distributed to over 19,000 patients. The drug was officially banned in August of 1962, but it was not known how much was still in medicine cabinets all over the country.

The alarm over the thalidomide affair in 1962 greatly helped the passage of new and stricter drug laws in the United States that year. The huge problem in Europe proved that even with supposedly good communication, these dangers were not detected soon enough, either in Europe or in the United States. It also showed that problems with drug safety cannot be confined to one country. They are international problems and require international efforts to combat them.

plan has widespread public support in the country since it would undoubtedly mean a reduction in state and local taxes, particularly property taxes. In an overall way it would also mean a reduction in nationally supported programs in the health and welfare fields. As a matter of legal and political philosophy, it would result in a return of activities and authority to the state government level in these fields.

Consumer protection, more or less

Most Americans believe that they can count on adequate consumer protection in regard to the foods they eat and the therapeutic drugs they receive, both in over-the-counter preparations and in drugs prescribed to them by physicians. This trust is often misplaced. The competitive market system itself is still responsible for most of our safety. It is generally good business to sell clean and safe products, but not always. The government agencies responsible for policing the food and drug industries have lacked sufficient funds to do the job they are expected to do. The federal agencies are handicapped by the limited legal powers they can exercise under the Constitution. Furthermore, divisions of responsibility between agencies make comprehensive law enforcement and consumer protection difficult to achieve. For example, the federal Food and Drug Administration (FDA) can prevent impure foods from crossing state lines, but it cannot destroy the contaminated goods. State agencies must do this. The FDA has only limited authority to inspect food and drug processing plants to prevent the manufacture of impure or unsafe products before they get into interstate commerce. The states are expected to do most of this inspection work, but very few have anything like adequate personnel or laws to do the necessary work.

The Federal Trade Commission (FTC) has jurisdiction to regulate unfair (to competitors) trade practices and to assure the truthfulness and fairness (again to competitors, not the public) in advertising. Nevertheless, the legal tools in the hands of the agency are grossly inadequate. Against false advertising the FTC's main weapon has been the "cease and desist order" under which the advertiser is told not to use exactly the same words in exactly the same advertisement again. The advertisers, after delaying the effective date of the orders for periods of months and years in the courts, merely change a few words and continue the round-robin of law suits and orders, if the FTC even persists in trying again. In recent years, some new commissioners have tried to force the agency to become more aggressive in its consumer protection activities and in the use of more and better enforcement methods, such as requiring the false advertisers to run remedial ads telling the truth and correcting the lies in the same media in which the offending materials appeared.

Until 1962, the Food and Drug Administration had no authority concerning the effectiveness of therapeutic drugs. The agency could require only that the product be safe for human consumption. In other words, it made no difference whether the pain-killing drug had any pain-killing qualities provided it didn't make a person sick. The same was true of a drug designed to kill bacteria, prevent conception of children, or relieve bowel constipation. It took the tragedy of the "thalidomide babies" and the great efforts of one senator, Estes Kefauver of Tennessee, to move the Congress to enact the stricter drug laws.

There is still no federal agency with the power to inspect at the source and to ensure the safety and effectiveness of so-called therapeutic devices such as heart pacemakers, heart-lung machines, artificial kidney machines, and the orthopedic nails and screws put into the bodies of thousands of people every year. Well-drafted legislation to control these devices in the public interest has been defeated in Congress every year for nearly a decade.

Compulsory health measures: public protection or individual freedom? Americans highly value their personal freedoms. In recent years, our courts and legislatures have been doing a better job of protecting those freedoms. At times, however, personal freedoms are upheld at the expense of public safety or public health. Which value should we hold dearest?

In earlier times under legal and social philosophies like that of Jeremy Bentham, the greatest good for the greatest number was the accepted criterion of social welfare. Far from being a conservative doctrine, it was the rallying principle of radical social reformers who attacked the laissez-faire ways of the few who controlled industry and the land. In the United States, this philosophy was used to provide legal justification in the courts for many compulsory health laws including smallpox vaccination, quarantine of contagious diseases, and commitment of the dangerously mentally ill. In 1925, the same principle was applied in the U.S. Supreme Court by Justice Oliver Wendell Holmes, Jr., to uphold the compulsory sterilization of a mentally deficient young girl whose mother was also said to be mentally deficient and who had herself borne an illegitimate child said to be deficient. In allowing the sterilization in order to prevent further burdens on the state in caring for such people (the mother, daughter, and infant were all in an institution for the mentally deficient in Virginia) Justice Holmes observed, "Three generations of imbeciles is enough."

But the times have changed. Substantial doubts have been cast in later cases upon the soundness of the Holmes decision noted above. The laws concerning quarantine and smallpox vaccination have been repealed in many jurisdictions as no longer necessary for public protection since many of the contagious diseases have been substantially eliminated in this country. The compulsory laws on mental hospital commitment have been significantly changed to provide more legal protection for mental patients.

The widespread protest movements of the 1960s brought many changes in the laws, particularly the excellent and far-reaching Civil Rights Act of 1964. It also engendered a great deal of disenchantment and disrespect for law and law enforcement in all aspects. Currently the result in the health field is great difficulty in gaining public acceptance of the need for observance of sanitation laws and such personal hygiene measures as venereal disease reporting and control provisions. The prevalence of the latter diseases has, as a consequence, risen sharply throughout the country in recent years.

The challenge for the future in hopefully quieter years will be to achieve an effective accommodation of both of these conflicting values. We do not want to lose the freedoms and the rights which have been won. Nevertheless, we must protect the helpless and the innocent who may be greatly harmed by unnecessary flaunting of sensible precautions in the interest of the public safety and health.

MEDICAL ADVANCES: PUZZLES FOR HEALTH LAW

A main problem for any effective legal system is keeping up with the changes in the society it is designed to protect. This problem is particularly acute in such fields as health law where the biomedical sciences are making important advances at a fairly regular pace. There tends to be a cultural and, consequently, a legal lag in public reaction to these scientific changes. The legal reactions generally do occur, however, after the medical advances have proved significant and lasting and have been accepted by both the professions and the people. Some recent examples will help to illustrate the methods of legislative and judicial change.

Transplants

The transplantation of human tissues and organs is now quite well accepted as a therapeutic, clinical procedure. It has had its greatest success with blood, with tissues such as skin, and with organs such as the cornea and the kidney. The procedure is still in experimental stages for other organs such as the heart, lung, and liver. The transplant of neurological tissues and the cortex of the brain are in even less advanced stages with study limited at present to some animal experimentation. As little as ten years ago, transplant procedures were handicapped by law. Now, however, every state has passed a consolidated set of legal provisions which facilitate developments in the field. The provisions are known as the Uniform Anatomical Gift Act. They allow any person eighteen years or over to donate human tissues or organs during life when it is possible, as in giving one kidney or allowing a skin graft, or to make provisions for a gift to take effect after death. The postmortem gift is binding on next of kin. The law also allows a next of kin of a dead person to donate tissue or organs of the deceased and permits postmortem gifts of the entire body to anatomical science. In cases which involve an ethical judgment, the act requires that two physicians concur in a pronouncement of the death of a donor and that a physician who participates in the transplanting surgery cannot be one of the doctors pronouncing death. Both of these provisions are intended to avoid any conflict of interest in the medical teams over the welfare of the dying donor and that of any potential donee of organs or tissues.

The heart-lung machine

Another aspect of medical science causing problems for the law has been technology rather than a medical or surgical procedure—the widespread use of the so-called heart-lung machine. The apparatus has made possible the great advance in open-heart operations. The legal problems are created by the fact that the machine can keep people "alive" who may not have the capacity to regain natural heart and lung function after an operative procedure. Also, the machines can keep people "alive" even when all brain function and consciousness have been irreversibly lost, as in an automobile accident.

Under traditional law, a human being could be pronounced "dead" only if all vital signs from all systems of the body were permanently ended. This principle was, of course, quite proper until these machines came into widespread use. After being placed on the machines, patients

Legal document for making an anatomical gift

UNIFORM DONATION CARD

DONOR CARD OF

_____

(print or type name of donor)

In the hope that my gift may help others, I hereby make this anatomical gift
to take effect upon my death. The words and marks below indicate my desires.

I give:

(a) _____ any needed organs or parts

(b) _____ only the following organs or parts

_____

(specify the organ(s) or part(s)

(c) _____ my entire body for anatomical study

For the purposes of transplantation, therapy, medical research or education.

Limitations: _____

(specify limitations, if any)

This is a legal document under the Uniform Anatomical Gift Act or similar laws.

(Other side of card)
Signed by the Donor in the presence of the following two witnesses:

_____   _____
Witness   *Signature of Donor*

_____   _____
Witness   *Date of Birth*

_____   _____
                                              Date Signed

This space available to refer to the group distributing the card and the telephone number and/or address where further information may be obtained.

could not legally be taken off, even though there was no possibility
that they could recover. Families were drained financially and emotionally in greatly prolonged death watches until, in sheer exhaustion, they
consented to ending the agonies by the turning off of the pumps. While
the person was on the machine, it could not be used in open-heart
operations or other procedures to help people who could be saved.
Furthermore, these patients with loss of brain function but without

damage to internal organs could be excellent candidates for donation of healthy organs to save many lives.

In 1968, a committee was formed of Harvard University faculty members involved in various aspects of medicine related to brain function, transplantation of organs and tissue, and other medical specialties, along with a theologian, a historian of science, and a lawyer. This group examined experiences worldwide in patients who had had irreversible loss of consciousness. A new medical definition of "brain death" was developed, and recommendations were made for legal change. Since that time, the new definition has been accepted by medical groups throughout the world and set forth in a declaration by the World Medical Association. Legal change has come more slowly. The definition has been adopted by legislation in two American states, Kansas and Maryland, and has been accepted in legal cases in one Canadian province, British Columbia, and in one American state, Virginia.

CORONERS AND MEDICAL EXAMINERS

The most traditional area of medicolegal relations is the public investigation of violent, accidental, and unexplained death. Very little upsets a community more than a murder, a suicide, or other untimely death. One of the primary functions of any organized society is to investigate these deaths, find their causes, apprehend any wrongdoers, and work to prevent similar tragedies.

The method of investigation in these cases which the American colonies inherited from Great Britain is the coroner system. Coroners were first appointed in England in 1194 by King Richard the Lionhearted. In early America, the coroners were more apt to be elected local officials than appointees of the governments. They also tended to have other duties such as sheriff or public prosecutor. In Mississippi the coroner was also the county ranger and was required to care for stray animals. In Wisconsin he was a deputy fish and game warden. All of the coroners in the colonies and in most of the states in the early years of the Republic were laymen without medical qualifications.

It has taken many years to bring about reform in the coroner system in this country. The best systems now in operation are under the direction of trained medicolegal specialists called forensic pathologists. This group is a recognized medical subspecialty of the American Board of Pathology. Most of the reformed systems under such direction are medical examiner's offices with jurisdiction over an entire state or a large metropolitan area. Some of the best of the medical examiner programs are those operating in the states of Maryland and Virginia and in metropolitan areas such as New York City, Philadelphia, Dallas, Miami, and Washington, D.C. There are also excellent systems operating with forensic pathologists in Cleveland, Pittsburgh, San Francisco, and Los Angeles, who still carry the titles of coroner or coroner-medical examiner.

Reform is by no means complete, however. Only 40 percent of the American people currently live in jurisdictions with fully adequate medicolegal death investigating systems. Only ten states have complete, statewide medical examiner systems.

HUMAN RIGHTS IN
MEDICAL CARE

As a result of the civil rights movement, political and legal attention has turned toward procuring the right of persons to many protections, benefits, and opportunities not universally available in past decades. The first efforts were largely political, such as voting rights. Now efforts are being made on economic and social levels in such areas as employment, education, and medical care (see Chap. 19). Currently organized consumer groups are working for more medical benefits for the poor. In response to these demands hospitals have begun to hire patient representatives or patient advocates, as noted earlier, to aid patients in achieving their rights and to handle their complaints. A few hospitals and neighborhood health centers have begun to adopt and publicize a list of patients' rights as a means of educating both patients and medical care personnel about the existence of the rights and to encourage their observance. Some of the lists were accompanied by statements of the patients' obligations as well. These did not go beyond the requirement of paying the medical and hospital bill and telling the truth to the doctors about one's illness.

In March of 1973, the American Hospital Association endorsed the idea of protecting patients' rights in all hospitals and issued its own "Patient's Bill of Rights." There is nothing startling in the list; it restates commonly accepted principles of law and ethics in the health care field. However, like the Hippocratic Oath, it expresses a philosophy and attitude of concern for the human dignity of patients which is sometimes overlooked in the hustle and bustle and the science and technology of modern medical care facilities.

**American Hospital Association—
Patient's Bill of Rights**

1. The patient has the right to considerate and respectful care.
2. The patient has the right to obtain from his physician complete current information concerning his diagnosis, treatment, and prognosis in terms the patient can be reasonably expected to understand.
3. The patient has the right to receive from his physician information necessary to give informed consent prior to the start of any procedure and/or treatment.
4. The patient has the right to refuse treatment to the extent permitted by law, and to be informed of the medical consequences of his action.
5. The patient has the right to every consideration of his privacy concerning his own medical care program.
6. The patient has the right to expect that all communications and records pertaining to his care should be treated as confidential.
7. The patient has the right to expect that within its capacity a hospital must make reasonable response to the request of a patient for services.
8. The patient has the right to obtain information as to any relationship of his hospital to other health care and educational institutions insofar as his care is concerned.
9. The patient has the right to be advised if the hospital proposes to engage in or perform human experimentation affecting his care or treatment. The patient has the right to refuse to participate in such research projects.
10. The patient has the right to expect reasonable continuity of care.
11. The patient has the right to examine and receive an explanation of his bill regardless of source of payment.
12. The patient has the right to know what hospital rules and regulations apply to his conduct as a patient.

The rights of women and the abortion laws

The women's rights movement has been strong for a number of years. One of the areas of greatest activity is health, for women seek and receive more medical care than men, and they are concerned as mothers in the medical care provided to children.

A primary focus of the women's movement in health is on gaining fuller knowledge and understanding about the functions and malfunc-

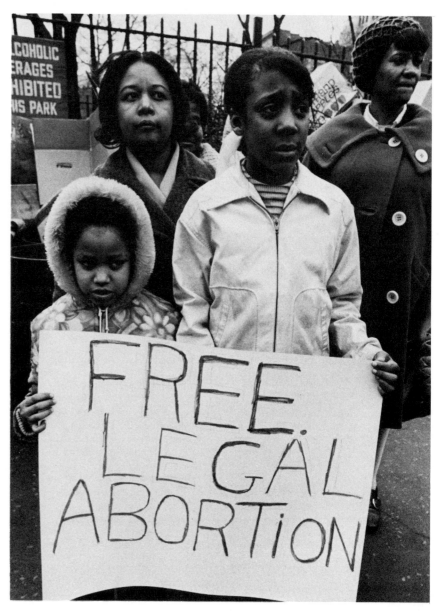

Figure 17.1. The U.S. Supreme Court decisions on abortion in 1973 were a direct response to widespread protest activities and political and legal pressure for change in the country's restrictive abortion laws. (Peter Martens, Nancy Palmer Photo Agency)

tions of their bodies. Many of the women's groups contend that male physicians, particularly obstetricians and gynecologists, have kept women in ignorance of their bodily functions. With increased knowledge, the women believe that they will have more control over their own decisions concerning health care, emotional problems, and childbirth.

The major legal recognition of the changing role of women in health came in 1973 with the U.S. Supreme Court decisions in abortion cases. The decisions were a direct response to widespread protest activities and political and legal pressure for change in the country's restrictive abortion laws. Prior to these decisions, the majority of American states outlawed abortion except where death or serious bodily harm would result to the woman by requiring her to continue the pregnancy. Some states had more liberal laws which allowed "therapeutic abortion" when there was a significant threat to the woman's health, either physically or emotionally. In a few states, abortions could also be performed if there was a likelihood that the child would be severely deformed or mentally deficient. Only in New York and Hawaii were women's groups and a few other pro-abortion organizations such as the Planned Parenthood League able to have "abortion on demand" legislation enacted.

The Supreme Court changed all this. The court ruled that a woman has a constitutional right to the privacy of her decision of whether or not to bear a child, at least during the early period when the fetus is not *viable*, or capable of existence outside the mother. The court described the legally significant periods as the three trimesters of fetal development. During the first three months, no regulation of any kind is allowed. During the second trimester, the states are allowed to regulate the medical practice of abortions in the interest of the safety of the procedure but cannot preclude abortions for any reason. The end of this period roughly coincides with viability, so that in the last trimester the state can take an interest in the fetus and can prevent by law any abortions except where death or serious physical or mental harm is threatened to the mother.

There are still unanswered questions. The court assumed that the fetus aborted during the first six months cannot survive because it is not viable. Yet medical science may soon be able to save fetuses delivered during these early months. Does this change the decision? If it does not, who owns a fetus which a mother aborts and abandons in, let us say, the fourth month but which is saved and grows to maturity in a healthy, normal state? Can this child be let out to adoption? Can it be sacrificed and experimented upon? The court said a fetus is not a "person" entitled to constitutional protection. What then of this abandoned fetus? Can it ever be saved?

The right to health and a healthy environment
Some consumer groups in the medical care field advocate establishing a generalized "right to health" of constitutional status. The significance of

the right as expressed by these groups is essentially economic: it is a right to receive medical care. It would be enforced through the availability of a universal medical care system supported by the government. The care could be rendered by government operated facilities and employees, as in Great Britain and Russia, or in a combination of public facilities and private sources under a government-supported insurance system, as in the Scandinavian countries. At present no such comprehensive system exists in the United States, as indicated in Chapter 19, and therefore no generalized right to health care can be said to exist.

On the other hand, the United States is moving, legally and politically, toward a right to a healthy environment for all persons in our country (see Chap. 21). Unlike the right to medical care, this right to a healthy environment is more in keeping with other constitutionally protected rights. Most other rights, such as the rights of free speech, assembly, and religion, are retained by the individual as an individual, and the government and other people are enjoined from interfering with the exercise of these rights. The right to a healthy environment is similar in that the government and other persons would be prohibited from actions which would unduly pollute the air, water supply, streams and lakes, and so on. No large outlay of money or services would be initially required to assure the individual of his right to a healthy environment as would be necessary to enforce a right to medical and other health care. Many state legislatures are now considering amendments to their state constitutions to establish this environmental right. Enforcement would be by individual suits or class actions (large numbers of people) against polluters to stop harmful conduct and to require corrective action. The defendants could be individuals, large business concerns, public utilities, or even government agencies.

The establishment of the right would be only the beginning, however, of a policy which would require a vast network of other laws, regulations, and enforcement agencies to make it effective. The standards of healthfulness would have to be established for a variety of environments. Many of the standards would have to be varied from one part of the nation to another. Specific enforcement against particular industries would be required in order to apply the standards. Both federal and state laws are now being developed in these areas, and many court actions have been brought to force compliance with these laws.

The most important of the laws on the federal level in recognizing a legal right to a healthy environment is the National Environmental Policy Act of 1969. This law requires the federal government to coordinate all federal agencies in an effort to prevent further degradation of the environment. It also requires all federal agencies to develop plans and programs in the field. All agencies must file with the Congress detailed "environmental impact statements" concerning the effects on the environment of any of their future programs. Section 101(c) of the act states,

The Congress recognizes that each person should enjoy a healthful environment and that each person has a responsibility to contribute to the preservation and enhancement of the environment.

It is clear that the federal government has at least made a start down the road toward establishing the fundamental right of every individual to a healthy world environment.

Questions

1. Describe the basic medical philosophy of the Hippocratic physicians and indicate how it differed from previous methods of medical practitioners.
2. How did the medical etiquette of the nineteenth century physicians differ from the Hippocratic ideal? What were the conditions of the nineteenth century which were said to justify this difference?
3. How has the structure of the American form of government affected the development of health law and a national health policy in this country? Give some examples.
4. Describe the legal requirements for a case of medical malpractice. What are some of the proposed reforms in medical malpractice? Which proposals favor plaintiff-patients? Which proposals favor defendant-doctors?
5. What are the differences between a legal "right to health" and a legal "right to a healthy environment"?

Key Concepts

Hippocratic Oath – an ancient, medical oath upon which the ethical code of modern medical practice is founded. In taking it, the physician was fundamentally promising a continuing devotion to his patients and to the healing process.

Locality rule – an early American regulation which restricted the standard of health care applied when judging a doctor's competence to the quality of health care rendered by other doctors in his locality

Patient's Bill of Rights – a bill drawn up by the American Hospital Association in 1973 to inform the patient in a hospital of his rights as a patient and to protect those rights

Selected Readings

Brennan, J. D. "The Need for Cooperation of Industry, Physicians, and Government in Regulation of Medical Devices," *Business Law*, 26 (1970), pp. 365–71.

Curran, William J., "The Anatomical Gift Act: A Lesson in Uniformity in Health Law," *American Journal of Public Health*, 59 (1969), pp. 1043–44.

———— and E. D. Shapiro. *Law, Medicine, and Forensic Science*, 2d ed. Boston: Little, Brown and Co., 1970.

Morris, R. C. and A. R. Moritz. *Doctor and Patient and the Law*, 5th ed. St. Louis: C. V. Mosby Co., 1971.

Ramsey, Paul. *The Patient as Person*. New Haven: Yale University Press, 1970.

Rish, John, "Federal Control of Bio-Medical Instrumentation," *Food, Drug, and Cosmetic Law Journal*, 27 (1972), pp. 418–30.

Chapter 18

The Delivery of Health Care

There are three reasons why you should know something about how medical care is provided.

1. You and your family will very likely someday be patients.
2. Whether or not you are a patient you pay for medical care through taxes, social security, or insurance premiums. You therefore have a stake in how efficiently medical care is delivered.
3. At some time you may be one of about four million people employed in providing health or medical care.[1]

Today providing health care requires the coordinated efforts of hundreds of different types of personnel working in a wide variety of different settings paid for by very complex financing arrangements. Health personnel require education and equipment, supplies and drugs must be manufactured and distributed, research must be carried out,

---

[1] The words health care and medical care are used interchangeably throughout.

This chapter was contributed by Duncan Neuhauser, Ph.D., Assistant Professor of Health Services Administration, Harvard School of Public Health, and Elinor Neuhauser, M.D. (Pediatrics), Research Assistant, Harvard School of Public Health.

and the whole health care "industry" must be regulated to ensure high quality of care.

In the United States 7.4 cents of every dollar of goods and services produced go to health care. The total bill for health care has been rapidly rising each year, going from 26 billion dollars in 1960 to 83 billion dollars in 1971–1972 (Table 18.1). For each person in this country, an average of $394 was spent on health care in 1971–1972 (Table 18.2). Presently, 39 percent of health care costs are being paid by federal, state, or local government.

Table 18.1 Total and per person national health expenditures, by source of funds, and percent of Gross National Product, selected fiscal years, 1928–1929 through 1971–1972*

| | | Health expenditures | | | | | | | | |
| | Gross National Product[a] (in billions) | Total | | | Private (Nongovernment) | | | Public (Government) | | |
Fiscal year		Amount (in millions)	Per capita	Percent of GNP	Amount (in millions)	Per capita	Percent of total	Amount (in millions)	Per capita	Percent of total
1928–29	$101	$3,589	$29.16	4	$3,112	$25.28	87	$477	$3.88	13.3
1939–40	95	3,863	28.83	4	3,081	22.99	80	782	5.84	20.2
1949–50	263	12,028	78.35	5	8,962	58.38	75	3,065	19.97	25.5
1959–60	496	25,856	141.63	5	19,460	106.60	75	6,395	35.03	24.7
1965–66	719	42,109	211.64	6	31,279	157.21	74	10,830	54.43	25.7
1969–70	955	68,058	328.17	7	42,823	206.49	63	25,235	121.68	37.1
1971–72	1,096	83,417	394.16	8	50,560	238.90	61	32,857	155.25	39.4

* From Barbara S. Cooper and Nancy L. Worthington, "National Health Expenditures, 1929–1972," *Social Security Bulletin*, Vol. 36 (Jan., 1973), p. 5.
[a] Gross National Product is the total value of all goods and services produced in the U.S.A. during that year.

Table 18.2 Where the health care dollar goes, fiscal year 1971–1972*

Health care service	Dollars per person in the U.S.A.
Hospitals	153
Doctors	76
Dentists	24
Other professional services	8
Drugs	37
Eyeglasses and appliances	10
Nursing homes	17
Costs of administering insurance and prepayment programs	14
Government public health	10
Other health services	17
Research	10
Construction	19
Total	394[a]

* From Barbara S. Cooper and Nancy L. Worthington, "National Health Expenditures, 1929–1972," *Social Security Bulletin*, Vol. 36 (Jan. 1973), p. 12.
[a] Errors due to rounding.

Responsibility for the provision of health services is shared by federal, state, and local governments, and various private, nongovernmental agencies. All four levels are involved in direct patient care and in financing health care, and often their functions are interrelated. For example, the federal government finances health care for the elderly with the Medicare program which is supported by Social Security payments made by workers. The federal government also provides Medicaid money to pay for the care of poor people; this money is administered by states which choose to participate in compliance with federal guidelines. Drugs are subject to federal regulation, and state governments regulate pharmacies which, like the drug manufacturers, are private

Table 18.3 Who does what in health services

	Provision of care	Financing care	Drug industry	Education and research	Other
Federal government	Armed services Veterans Administration Indian health services	Medicare Medicaid	FDA regulations Patents Trademarks	Research and educational support National Institutes of Health	Public Health Service
State government	Mental hospitals Centers for the retarded	Administration of welfare and Medicaid programs State insurance regulation	Licensure Regulation of pharmacies	State universities Medical schools	State public health departments Facility licensure Regional planning
Local government	City hospitals County hospitals Homes Ambulances School health programs	Support of local facilities Local welfare			Local public health departments Comprehensive health planning
Nongovernment private sector	Hospitals Nursing homes Clinics Doctor and dentist offices Ambulances HMOs	Insurance companies Blue Cross Blue Shield HMOs Associations United Fund	Manufacturers Distributors Pharmacies	Universities Colleges Schools Research by medical schools Hospitals Drug companies	Hospital supply industry Voluntary associations J.C.A.H.

companies. The federal government supports education and research carried out in state and private universities, medical schools, hospitals, and other facilities.

Health care personnel are employed at all four levels, and public health services are provided by federal, state, and local governments. Licensure of doctors, nurses, and others is administered at the state level. There are numerous private associations of health personnel including the American Medical Association. In the private sector are voluntary associations like the Red Cross, the American Cancer Association, the American Heart Association, and many others.

Table 18.3 summarizes the major functions performed in the delivery of health care services at the four levels. Many of the programs mentioned could fall into more than one box. For example, some programs are supported by matching federal, state, and local funds.

Compared to other countries, the delivery of medical care in America is extremely varied and complex. In the following pages descriptions are given of the training and role of health care personnel, the structure and function of health care facilities, and the financing of health care. While these descriptions are typical of the kind of health care that is found in the United States, it should be noted that there are exceptions to almost everything below.

HEALTH CARE PERSONNEL

Table 18.4 lists the fifteen largest occupational categories in health care. There are about 4 million health care workers who vary widely in skill level and required education. Although the focus here is on the education and functions of nurses and doctors, there are hundreds of other types of health personnel who are also important.

Physicians

Medical doctors (MD degree) and osteopathic doctors (DO degree) alone are called "physicians" while dentists (DMD or DDS degree) and others with doctorate degrees are usually referred to as "doctor." The education and practice of the two types of physicians are so much the same today that they will be considered together here.

PHYSICIAN EDUCATION Admission to medical school usually requires four years of college and a BA degree which includes a number of premedical college courses. These required courses vary somewhat according to the medical school but usually include basic chemistry, organic chemistry, biology, and physics. The Medical College Admissions Test (MCAT) is also used to evaluate the applicant's potential.

There are over 100 medical schools and six osteopathic schools in the United States. Medical schools are either state or privately owned and almost always part of a larger university. The MD degree usually

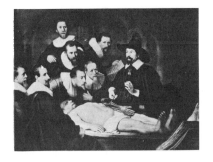

Figure 18.1. The Anatomy Lesson (1632), by Rembrandt. The life-size painting shows Tulp, the Dutch physician and anatomist, lecturing to medical students on the parts of the body. (*Mauritshuis*)

Table 18.4 *The 15 most numerous jobs in the health care industry**

Occupation	Number	Percent of total
Nursing and related services	1,825,000	50
Medicine and osteopathy	313,000	8
Secretarial and office services	250,000–275,000	7
Dentistry and allied services	237,000	6
Environmental control[a]	217,500	6
Pharmacy	130,100	4
Clinical laboratory services	108,000	3
Radiologic technology	75,000–100,000	3
Optometry, opticianry, and ocular services	53,450	1
Administration of health services	39,000–45,000	1
Medical records	38,500	1
Dietetic and nutritional services	36,000	1
Miscellaneous health services[b]	35,000–37,000	1
Veterinary medicine	25,000	1
Social work	24,200	1

* U.S., Congress, Committee on Ways and Means, 92d Congress, June 28, 1971, p. 4. This table excludes occupations indirectly associated with health care such as those in the manufacture of drugs.

[a] Environmental engineers, scientists, technicians, and aides working on air and water pollution, sewage, radiation hazards, etc.

[b] Includes surgical technical aides and inhalation therapy, electrocardiograph, and electroencephalograph technicians.

requires four years. There are half a dozen two-year medical schools that provide basic medical sciences for students who then transfer to four-year medical schools.

The first two years of medical training (the preclinical years) have traditionally emphasized the laboratory sciences and include anatomy, pathology, histology, biochemistry, physiology, pharmacology and so on. The second two years (clinical years) provide education in hospitals and ambulatory facilities where the student learns to diagnose and treat disease. After medical school a year of internship in a hospital is customary although there is a growing trend toward going directly into residency programs.

SPECIALIZATION After completion of an internship, the physician may go on to take further practical training in a residency. The length of a residency depends on the specialty. Both interns and residents are called house staff or house officers.

Internship and residency are called graduate medical education. Further education beyond this point, including fellowships (usually for research or special studies) or other short term nondegree courses, are included under the term postgraduate medical education. Most male physicians have been required to serve for two years or more in the armed services or in Public Health Service.

Physician specialties

Anesthesiology: Administration of local and general anesthetics

Colon and Rectal Surgery (Proctology): Diagnosis and treatment of disorders and diseases of the lower digestive tract

Dermatology: Treatment of skin diseases

Internal Medicine: Treatment of diseases nonsurgically

Neurological Surgery (Neuro-Surgery): Diagnosis and surgical treatment of the brain, spinal cord, and nervous disorders

Neurology: Nonsurgical treatment of the nervous system

Obstetrics-Gynecology: Surgical treatment of the female reproductive organs and the care of women during and immediately following pregnancy

Occupational Medicine: Treatment of conditions relating to industry and other places of employment

Opthalmology: Surgical and non-surgical treatment of the eye

Orthopedic Surgery: Treatment of diseases, fractures, and deformities of bones and joints

Otolaryngology: Surgical treatment of diseases of ear, nose, and throat

Pathology: Study and interpretation of changes in organs, tissues, cells, and body chemistry

Pediatrics: Medical care of children

Physical Medicine and **Rehabilitation:** Treatment by means of physical procedures which include heat, water, electricity, exercise, etc., to restore useful activities to convalescent, disabled, or physically handicapped patients

Plastic Surgery: Surgical correction and repair of skin and soft tissues

Preventive Medicine and **Public Health:** Prevention and protection against disease and promotion of maximum health through all appropriate measures but with emphasis on measures applicable through broad scale action for large groups of people

Psychiatry: Nonsurgical treatment of emotional disturbances and mental disorders

Radiology: Diagnosis and treatment (radiotherapy) of disease by means of X-ray, radium, and other radioactive sources

Urology: Surgical treatment of diseases of urinary and urogenital tracts and the male reproductive organs

Membership in *specialty boards* has various requirements beyond the residency including varying years of practice and written and oral examinations. Completion of the residency requirements makes a physician board-eligible for from three to seven years (renewable) while he completes the rest of the board requirements. Completing all these requirements makes the physician board-certified or a diplomate of that board.

FAMILY PRACTICE AND GENERAL PRACTICE On completion of medical school and internship and after obtaining a state license to practice, a physician may legally perform all types of medical and surgical treatment. A physician who has completed an internship and has not gone on to further specialty training is called a general practitioner. Nearly all new medical school graduates now go on to specialty training, so the number of general practitioners has been steadily declining. Their work is now often being carried out by internists, pediatricians, obstetricians, and other specialists.

This increase in specialization has advantages and disadvantages. On the one hand, the content of medical science is so vast that many feel that a physician must concentrate on one special part of it. On the other hand, there is a need for a family doctor with a long-term relationship with families. The right combination of these two approaches has yet to be completely achieved. A fairly new development is residency training in family practice which provides special training in primary or basic medical care. Thus, family practice is now developing into a specialty itself.

PHYSICIAN PRACTICE SETTING On completion of training a physician may practice medicine as a solo practitioner, that is, by himself or herself in a private office; in group practice, where a number of doctors share office space and income and help each other out; or as a full-time salaried doctor, employed by a hospital, medical school, government agency, or other institution.

Nurses

Professional nurses, or registered nurses (RN degree), may receive their training beyond high school in a hospital-based three-year diploma nursing school, in a two-year program in a community or junior college called an associate degree program, or in a three- to five-year baccalaureate program in a college or university. In addition, masters and doctorate degrees in nursing are given. Traditionally most nurses have received their training in hospital-based nursing schools, but the two-year associate degree programs are rapidly growing.

Practical, or vocational, nurses need two or more years of high school and obtain the LPN usually after one year of training. Both RNs and LPNs are licensed by the states in which they practice. LPNs primarily do bedside nursing in hospitals under the supervision of RNs.

Most nurses work in hospitals and are responsible for the day-to-day care of patients under the supervision of physicians. They see to it that doctors' orders are carried out, and look to the physical and psycho-

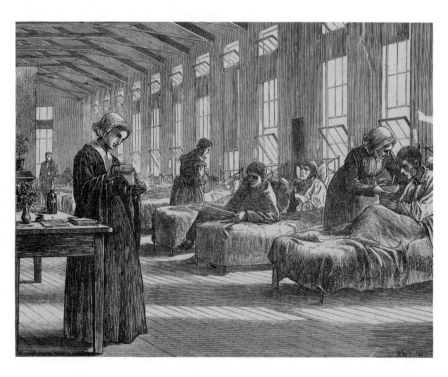

Figure 18.2. A ward in the Hampstead Smallpox Hospital, London, 1871. During this period nurses had a higher risk of dying from disease than women in other occupations because of hospital-based infections. At the time it was thought that infections came from vapors rising out of the ground and walls, and windows were kept open to remedy this. (Courtesy New York Library Picture Collection)

logical well-being of their patients. In addition there are a wide variety of specialized nursing occupations including public health and occupational nursing.

The tasks of health personnel—a case study

The interdependency of different kinds of health personnel is perhaps most clear in a hospital setting, in which literally hundreds of skilled people work to deliver health care services. The example that follows illustrates what some of these tasks are and how they are performed in a typical hospital case.

INITIAL DIAGNOSIS A sixty-year-old man goes to a general practitioner because he has a hernia. (A small part of the intestinal tract protrudes through a defect in the abdominal wall producing a visible bulge below the skin. This makes it painful for him to lift things, and there is a possibility that the intestine might sometime be pinched off with serious or even fatal consequences.) His doctor carries out a physical examination and refers him to a surgeon for an operation. The surgeon also examines him and then calls the hospital to arrange for his admission and to schedule his operation.

Other health personnel requiring college-level training

Years in parentheses indicate length of training beyond high school

Biochemist: (7+ years) Studies biochemical characteristics to detect disease

Blood Bank Technologist: (5–6 years) Processes, types, and analyzes blood and plasma for transfusion

Cytotechnologist: (3 years) Analyzes human tissue specimens for disease, especially cancer

Dental Hygienist: (4 years) Works under the supervision of dentists treating patients

Dentist: (6–8 years) Treats dental diseases; includes several types of specialty training

Dietician: (5+ years) Develops special diets for patients and supervises their preparation

Hospital Administrator: (4 or 6 years) Manages hospital plants, equipment, and personnel

Medical Librarian: (5 years) Maintains a library of scientific publications

Medical Record Librarian: (3–4 years) Supervises processing, storage, and retrieval of patient records

Medical or Psychiatric Social Worker: (6 years) Counsels patients on social and emotional problems

Medical Technologist: (4–5+ years) Analyzes sample specimens to detect disease

Occupational Therapist: (5 years) Teaches patients new work-related skills; works with handicapped patients

Optometrist: (5–7 years) Fits eyeglasses; an independent practitioner

Pharmacist: (5–7+ years) Provides prescription drugs and medications

Physical Therapist: (4–5+ years) Uses exercise, heat, and other treatment forms to help patient regain the ability to carry out activities of daily living

Physician Assistant: (*Medex, Physician Extender, Nurse Practitioner,* and other names are also used) (3–6 years, no clear pattern) Works under the direction of physicians providing screening, counseling, and treatment of patients, leaving the physician time to concentrate on patients with more complex problems; a newly growing category of personnel

Psychologist: (7+ years) Does research, evaluation, and therapy related to mental development and mental illness

Figure 18.3. Doctors, nurses, clerks, and other personnel working in an internal medicine clinic in a hospital outpatient department. A substantial amount of personnel time is required to maintain a patient's medical record, which may include upwards of a hundred pages describing illnesses and treatments. (Courtesy HUD, Printing and Visual Arts Division)

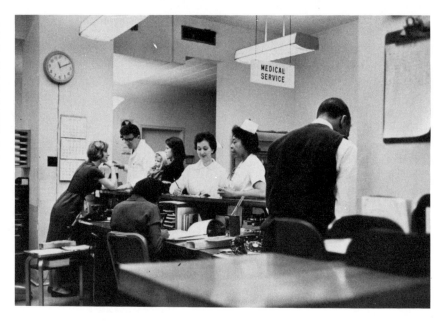

ADMISSION AND PREPARATION On admission his room must be readied by housekeeping personnel, a medical record prepared by the admitting office, and daily checking of his temperature and pulse started, which may be done by a practical nurse under the supervision of the head nurse.

The surgeon orders an ECG (electrocardiogram), a barium enema, and other laboratory tests. The ECG, taken by an ECG technician, graphically measures the heart beat to detect heart disease. It is important to know if heart disease is present because it may greatly increase the risk of operating since the patient's heart might stop during the operation. The ECG tracings are interpreted by a cardiologist, who reports his findings to the surgeon. The barium enema requires inserting a radio-opaque liquid (visible by X-ray) rectally and observing its progress through the intestine by a fluorescope (a type of X-ray which allows the radiologist to observe over time). The barium enema indicates whether there are holes or blockage in the intestine. Other X-rays may also be taken by a radiology technician and interpreted by the radiologist. More tests are carried out by laboratory technicians using in part automated laboratory equipment on samples of blood and urine to check for diabetes, anemia, and so on. If these tests show no illness, the operation can be performed.

SURGERY Preparation for surgery may require medication, minimal diet, and cleaning and shaving the skin around the incision area.

The anesthesia may be given by a nurse anesthetist under the general supervision of an anesthesiologist. Elaborate precautions are taken to maintain sterile conditions in the operating room. The surgeon may be assisted by another doctor, perhaps a surgical resident or intern. Also there will be operating room nurses or surgical technicians to assist with the instruments and equipment.

The operation, a herniorrhaphy, basically consists of cutting through the skin, pushing the intestine back into the abdomen, closing the gap in the abdomen, and stitching the skin back together. The surgeon must use the utmost skill in this process, or there is a chance the hernia will reappear again.

RECOVERY After the operation the patient remains in the hospital to regain his strength. Perhaps this patient will need the help of a physical therapist to learn breathing techniques which will minimize the pain after the operation. He may need a social worker to arrange home care services for him after discharge and perhaps an ambulance to take him home. After discharge he returns to the surgeon's office for removal of the stitches.

Unseen by the patient are numerous other hospital personnel: business office workers who must cope with insurance payments; a medical record librarian who sees to the storage and retrieval of patient records; dieticians who supervise the preparation of special meals; housekeeping, maintenance, and administrative personnel including the hospital administrator. The patient's bill helps pay for all these personnel.

HEALTH CARE FACILITIES Health care facilities include all of the locations where health personnel work: hospitals, nursing homes, institutions for the physically or emotionally handicapped, outpatient clinics, centers for mental health, laboratories, research facilities, schools for the training of health care personnel, drug companies, pharmacies, and many others. Health care facilities include the following listed by type of patient served.

Inpatient and Residential
  Hospital Inpatient Services
  Nursing Homes and Extended Care Facilities
  Personal Care and Domiciliary Homes
  Special Housing for the Aged
  Facilities for the Deaf and Blind
  Facilities for Unwed Mothers
  Facilities for Mentally Retarded
  Facilities for Dependent Children and Orphanages
  Facilities for Drug Addicts
  Homes for Alcoholics
  Juvenile Correctional Facilities
Outpatient
  Ambulance Services
  Organized Home Health Services (visiting nursing, homemaker services, meals-on-wheels)
  Hospital Outpatient Services

Hospital Emergency Department
Special Psychiatric Outpatient Services
Day Facilities for the Mentally Retarded
Sheltered Workshops for the Retarded or Physically Handicapped
Medical Group Practices
Abortion Clinics (also an inpatient service)
Comprehensive Programs
Community Mental Health Centers
Neighborhood Health Centers
Migrant Worker Health Programs
Rehabilitation Centers for the Physically Handicapped
Health Maintenance Organizations
Foundations for Medical Care
Nonpatient Facilities
Research institutions
Universities, colleges, other educational facilities
Clinical laboratories
Dental laboratories
Optician establishments
Drug manufacturers
Pharmacies
Producers of supplies and equipment

These facilities may be government owned or in the private sector. As we have seen, the delivery of health care involves a great number of different personnel; it involves an equally complex variety of facilities. The discussion that follows focuses on one of the most visible of these—the hospital.

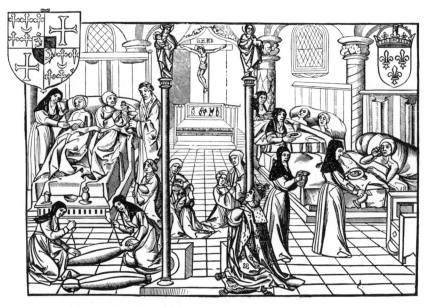

Figure 18.4. A ward in a Paris hospital of the sixteenth century. Early European hospitals were founded by religious orders to care for the poor, and often two patients occupied the same bed. In the lower left corner, nurses are sewing covers on bodies of deceased patients. (Courtesy of New York Public Library Picture Collection)

Hospitals

A hospital can be defined as an institution that maintains inpatient beds; provides diagnostic and treatment services; has a governing authority, an organized medical staff, registered nurses, diagnostic X-ray and clinical laboratory services, a pharmacy, and an operating room; and provides food for patients including special diets.

There are over a million and a half hospital beds in the United States, about eight hospital beds for every 1000 Americans. These beds are located in many different kinds of hospitals. Hospitals are often classified according to whether they are owned by a government agency or a private organization. If government owned, they can be under the jurisdiction of the federal, state, or local government. If privately owned, they can be operated on either a profit ("proprietary") or a nonprofit ("voluntary") basis.

FEDERAL HOSPITALS Each major branch of the military separately operates hospitals which provide care and treatment for its own personnel and their dependents (wives and children). Many former military personnel (called veterans) who require medical attention are eligible for care in Veterans Administration hospitals located throughout the United States. Other persons eligible for care in federal medical facilities include American Merchant Seamen, United States Coast Guard personnel, American Indians, Alaskan Eskimos, and government employees injured on duty; these persons may be cared for in United States Public Health Service (USPHS) hospitals.

STATE HOSPITALS Every state operates one or more hospitals emphasizing long-term institutional care of mentally ill, retarded, and tuberculosis patients. Residents of the state for a certain period of time who are unable to pay for care on a private basis are eligible. These state hospitals are run by departments, boards, or administrative agencies of state governments such as departments of health or welfare. State governments also operate schools for the blind, deaf, and mentally deficient; infirmaries or hospitals connected with state reformatories and prisons; and facilities for short-term care, primarily acute-care general hospitals controlled by state medical schools.

LOCAL HOSPITALS District hospitals are facilities operated within local areas and supported by taxes from the population in the district. They are governed by a board of directors who are elected by district residents, and they are independent of city, state, or county government.

County hospitals are run by county boards of supervisors. They include the large urban hospitals for the poor, such as Cook County Hospital in Chicago, and many smaller rural hospitals which care for both private patients and poor patients.

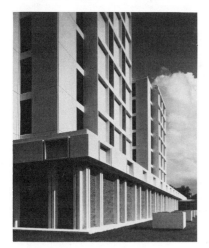

Figure 18.5. Lincoln General Hospital, Lincoln, Nebraska, a modern facility which contains 226 beds. Total cost was $7,250,127, to which the federal government contributed $1,891,054.

City-county hospitals, which are controlled jointly by municipal and county governments, and city hospitals, which are owned by municipal governments and managed by appointed boards of citizens, also often provide care primarily for the poor.

VOLUNTARY HOSPITALS   Voluntary facilities are usually nonprofit. They include a number of hospitals owned and/or operated by religious groups. Roman Catholic hospitals are foremost with respect to numbers and treat patients of all faiths. They are owned and operated by over one hundred different sisterhoods (religious orders). The Mother Provincial of the order is usually president of the hospital governing board. A sister usually administers the hospital (although this is changing), and sisters work in a variety of capacities within the hospital although they are usually only a small fraction of the hospital's total work force. Over a dozen different Protestant denominations also own, operate, or own and operate hospitals. Jewish hospitals are not owned or controlled by religious organizations. Instead, they are independent community hospitals supported by the Jewish community and treat patients of all faiths.

Community hospitals are independent, nonprofit hospital corporations or associations composed of public-spirited citizens who are interested in providing hospital care for their community and who are organized solely for that purpose. These hospitals are governed by nonprofit associations or corporations usually open to any interested citizen who will pay a small yearly contribution. These associations can have up to several thousand members.

HEALTH CARE REGULATION AND QUALITY CONTROL

A great deal of effort is expended to ensure that medical care is of high quality and delivered in an efficient manner to all who can benefit from it. There are few people who think that enough has been done, however. Some of the important means now used to ensure quality are outlined here.

Education

Medical schools, teaching hospitals, and other institutions that are charged with the education of health personnel are committed to high standards in this training. This commitment includes provision for having their students learn appropriate treatment techniques and instilling in them a desire to provide good care.

Because knowledge in the health care fields is continually expanding, the education of health care personnel is an ongoing process. Those who are involved in health care delivery must continue to learn new techniques and new information after they have completed their formal education. There are over 7000 scientific journals related to the health professions that provide current information.

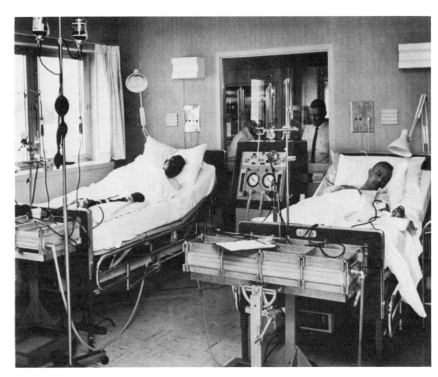

Figure 18.6. An artificial kidney unit, developed by the National Institutes of Health staff, in operation at the Veterans Administration Hospital in Washington, D.C. A lifesaving technique which is very expensive, it is one of many new treatment forms associated with rising health care costs. (E. Hubbard, National Institutes of Health)

Licensure and accreditation

Physicians, nurses, dentists, pharmacists, and other types of health personnel must complete a specified education and pass examinations in order to qualify for state licensure. Licensure grants a legal monopoly to practice. Extreme failure to practice good care can result in revocation of the license. Certification is like licensure in that it signifies a high level of training, experience, and skill. Unlike licensure, failure to be certified does not exclude one from working in the field. One of the weaknesses of present licensing procedures is that licensure, once achieved, is good for life. There is no provision for periodic reexamination of personnel to ensure that they have retained and updated their skills and knowledge.

Hospitals are licensed by the states and must meet minimum federal government standards to qualify for Medicare payments. Educational training programs like medical and nursing schools are inspected by voluntary accrediting agencies which approve the quality of education they provide.

In addition, there are numerous accreditation programs for hospitals. The entire hospital is accredited by the Joint Commission on the Accreditation of Hospitals (JCAH). The JCAH is an independent agency governed by a board mostly appointed by the American Medical Association (representing the doctors) and the American Hospital Association (representing hospitals). This is a voluntary program. About 95 percent of the general hospitals in the U.S. are accredited. In addition there are accrediting agencies for parts of hospitals like blood banks and internship and residency programs. There is also government inspection of boilers, electrical equipment, and fire safety standards.

Consumer control

Most hospitals are governed by laymen rather than medical workers because they are owned either by the government, by religious orders, or by voluntary boards of local citizens. Some of the new neighborhood health centers have consumer advisory boards. Legally the hospital governing board is responsible for the quality of care provided by the doctors in that hospital. To some extent these boards regulate the medical staff in order to promote good care. In some cases, the provider can be sued by a patient who received care that did not meet the standards of practice for the region.

Peer review

Doctors monitor each other's performance to some extent. In hospitals deaths are reviewed and patient medical records are sampled to see if the treatment is appropriate. There is also peer review (called utilization review) of how long the patient stays in the hospital to check to see if it was too long or too short.

Doctors do not want to be associated with other doctors who provide poor care because one bad doctor reflects poorly on the rest. A physician who fails to meet standards of performance acceptable to his colleagues tends to be isolated and ignored but not driven from practice. The respect of their peers is greatly valued by doctors and can be a strong motivating force to conform to the prevailing standards of practice.

Choice and the market place

It is somewhat true that good hospitals and doctors prosper while poor doctors and hospitals do not because patients choose the former and not the latter. Patients are not always knowledgeable enough to make such choices, however. Often the poor and rural people have very little choice. There is much debate as to how effective the market place is in controlling the quality of health care, but more and more people are willing to be critical of health care service delivery and to demand high quality of performance in health care personnel. It has become clear that the regulation of health care services is not always thorough enough to meet the highest standards (see Chap. 19). One area in which many people are able to exercise some consumer control is in their choice of a personal physician and of a hospital.

How to choose a doctor

It is a good idea to select a doctor before you need one. Many people choose a doctor by asking their friends and neighbors to recommend one. People who are moving may ask their present physician to recommend a new doctor to them before they move.

A study of New Jersey doctors and their families showed that when a doctor or a member of his or her family is seriously ill, he sees a board-certified specialist who has a medical school appointment and is on the staff of a medical-school-affiliated teaching hospital.

If you are a stranger in a city, one way of choosing a doctor is to find out if there is a medical school in the area and if so what hospital(s) is affiliated with it. Then call the office of either the chief-of-medicine, chief-of-surgery, or the hospital administrator and say that you wish to find a board-certified specialist. You don't necessarily need to talk directly to the chief-of-medicine or the administrator. An assistant often can answer your questions and will ordinarily be willing to recommend someone.

In addition, a doctor's training can be verified in the *Dictionary of Medical Specialists*, 13th ed. (Chicago, 1965), or by calling the county medical society. Information to consider would be the doctor's age, medical school, hospital(s) of internship and residency training, professional activities, hospital affiliation(s), and whether or not the doctor is on the faculty of a medical school. The quality of a doctor's education is a good guide.

Another good criterion is to look for a group of doctors who have a good reputation, have been practicing for a number of years, and have a record of long-term excellence. The Mayo Clinic is only one of many examples.

After you have made a choice, call the doctor's office and inquire about whether he or she is accepting new patients, the office hours, the charge for a routine office visit, and other pertinent information.

Evaluating medical services

If your doctor should recommend major surgery for you or a member of your family, it is often appropriate for him or her to seek consultation with other doctors before doing the surgery. If your doctor refers you to a surgeon for the operation, you may want to be given more than one surgeon from which to choose. You may also want to check the credentials of the doctors to whom you are referred. If your doctor plans to do the surgery himself and you have any doubt about its necessity, you should feel free to tell your doctor that you would like to consult another doctor who can confirm the need for surgery. Your doctor's willingness to let you do so is a good sign. Your doctor should also be willing to tell you in advance what the bill for the operation will be.

There is a high agreement among doctors and nurses as to which hospitals are good and which are not so good. If you are in a town without a teaching hospital, make sure that the hospital you seek out is accredited by the JCAH. It is also a good sign if the hospital has a high autopsy rate (greater than 35 percent is quite good; less than 25 percent is not so good). If you are going to have major nonemergency surgery, find out how often your doctor and hospital do that operation. The operating team's performance improves with experience.

PAYMENT OF
MEDICAL CARE

American medical care is paid for in one of five ways.

1. Direct "out of pocket" payment by the patient to the provider of care such as doctors and hospitals. These expenses, if large enough, are deductible from the patient's income tax.
2. Provision of service. For example, the government owns and operates hospitals and clinics and they give care to a defined population. The costs are paid for from tax revenues and not from the patients. Veterans Administration hospitals for war veterans or city hospitals for the poor are examples.
3. Insurance plan. The subscriber pays a fixed monthly premium amount to an insurance company. If the subscriber uses medical care the insurer pays him an agreed-upon amount of money toward the medical bill.
4. Prepayment plan. The subscriber pays a fixed monthly premium to Blue Cross-Blue Shield, Social Security (Medicare), or other plan. They in turn pay directly to the provider an agreed-upon amount to cover the costs of care.
5. Prepaid plan. The subscriber pays a fixed monthly amount to the plan which uses this money to pay for the hospitals and clinics it owns and operates. The best-known example is the Kaiser-Permanente Program based in California.

Health insurance

Insurance is protection by written contract between the subscriber and the insurance company against the hazards of specific unpredictable events such as fire, theft, automobile accidents, and illness. Hundreds of different insurance companies write health insurance using thousands of different policies. This health insurance provides protection against the costs of medical care and/or the lost income arising from an illness or injury. The major forms of health insurance include:

1. hospital insurance, which pays for hospital bills
2. surgical insurance, which pays for doctor's operating fees
3. regular medical insurance, which pays for nonsurgical doctor's fees in the hospital and for nonhospital physician care
4. major medical insurance, which pays a percentage of all expenses incurred above a certain cost and is especially designed to cover major illness or injury

5. disability insurance, which compensates for income lost because of time spent in the hospital or time spent out of work or both

The subscriber usually gets his health insurance at his place of employment. Usually his premium, the cost of the insurance, is paid in part by his employer and in part by a deduction from his paycheck. The insurance company determines the cost of the insurance by calculating the risk for each individual or each group of individuals covered. Usually the insurance covers both the subscriber and his family.

The written contract between the subscriber and the insurance company is called a policy. It indicates the conditions of the agreements between the subscriber and the company, including such things as the time that the policy is in effect, the premium to be paid and the time of payment, the types of illness and injury that are covered by the insurance, the amount of money to be paid for each illness or injury, the age limit and other requirements for persons who are insured, and so on.

These arrangements vary with each policy, but it may be helpful to consider a hypothetical example to illustrate the kinds of conditions that are commonly found in such agreements. A typical hospital insurance policy, for example, could be written for subscribers under the age of 65. The policy provides for payment of 100 dollars a day for each day that the insured person is in the hospital up to 50 days. The policy is good for one year. It excludes, or does not pay for, treatment for mental illness, tuberculosis, and medical conditions that exist before the policy goes into effect. Payments are due monthly on the fifth of the month.

Terms commonly used in health insurance policies

coinsurance: a policy provision by which both the insured person and the insurance company share the expenses of illness or injury in a specific proportion. For example, the insurer will pay 80 percent of the hospital bill while the insured pays the remaining 20 percent.

deductible: that portion of covered hospital and medical charges which the insured person must pay before benefits begin. This is in contrast to *first dollar coverage,* in which there is no deductible.

group insurance: a policy protecting a group of persons—usually employees of a firm—rather than a policy providing protection to a policy holder and/or his family. One difference is that the insurer estimates the expected risk for the group as a whole rather than for

each individual. Policies protecting a policy holder and/or his family are called *individual* or *personal insurance.*

indemnity: a benefit paid by a health insurance policy for an insured loss

noncancellable (guaranteed renewable) policy: a policy which the insured has a right to continue in force by the timely payment of premiums set forth in the policy to a specified age during which period the insurer has no right to make unilaterally any change in any provision of the policy while the policy is in force. Usually, the insurance company cannot change the premium rate for an individual insured person.

preexisting conditions: physical conditions of the insured person

which existed prior to the issuance of his policy; they may or may not be covered

premium: the periodic payment required to keep the policy in force

policy term: time period covered by the policy

rider: an amendment to the policy expanding or decreasing benefits

time limits: the period of time in which notice of claim or proof of loss must be filed in order to obtain benefits

upper limits of coverage: limit set in the policy for maximum payment

waiver: an agreement attached to a policy which exempts from coverage certain disabilities normally covered by the policy

The insurance company must receive notice of the hospitalization not more than 30 days after admission to the hospital.

It is common for health insurance policies to provide less than full payment for health care. They also commonly call for the insured person to pay some given amount of the cost of care before benefits begin; this limitation is called the deductible. The policy may also require that the insured person pay a percentage of the cost of the medical care above the deductible amount. Policies usually include an upper limit, a sum beyond which the insurance company is not responsible for payment.

Another hypothetical example may help to make these provisions clear. Note that the figures used in this example have been chosen for ease in calculation and not because they are typical of policies now in use. If a subscriber who has hospital insurance incurs a hospital bill of $1,000, his costs might be apportioned this way: The insurance policy has a $100 deductible, so the subscriber pays the first $100 of the hospital bill directly. An additional $300 of the bill is for costs that are not covered in the policy. The policy also has an upper limit of $600 and provides that the insured will pay 20 percent of covered costs. Table 18.5 indicates the division of payment between the subscriber and the insurance company in this example.

Table 18.5 *Example of insurance coverage for a hospital admission costing $1000*

Dollars		
0	deductible ($100) paid by insured	
100		
200		
300		20% ($100) paid by insured
400	80% ($400) paid by insurance company	
500		
600		
700	Excess of upper limit on policy ($100) paid by insured	
800		
900	uninsured expenses ($300) paid by insured	
1000		

Prepayment plans

Prepayment plans are another kind of contractual agreement in which the subscriber pays for protection against the costs of health care. Both health insurance and the different prepayment plans can be written to cover various kinds of care such as hospital, surgical, major medical, and so on. Premiums for prepayment plans may also be paid in part by the employer of the subscriber and in part by deductions from the subscriber's paycheck. Like health insurance, the plans usually cover both the subscriber and his family.

The difference between health insurance coverage and coverage by a prepayment plan is that health insurance payments are usually paid to the insured person, who then pays the provider of the health care; prepayment plan payments are given directly to the provider of the health care. The most commonly known prepayment plans are Social Security (Medicare), Blue Cross, Blue Shield, and the various groups known as Health Maintenance Organizations. A further feature of HMO's is that they are also the providers of the care in that they own and operate their own hospitals and clinics which serve people who subscribe to the plan.

Blue Cross is a nongovernment, private, nonprofit corporation which provides protection against the costs of hospital care to members of the plan within a limited geographic area. Blue Shield is an independent, nonprofit corporation which provides protection against the costs of surgery and other kinds of medical care to members of the plan within a limited geographical area. Blue Cross and Blue Shield are legally independent of each other, but they often work in close cooperation to offer matched benefit packages to insured groups.

There are approximately seventy Blue Cross organizations in the United States which cover part of a state, an entire state, or several states. They are linked as members of the Blue Cross Association, which provides shared services and arranges for coverage with other Blue Cross plans for travelers who leave their own plan's area. Blue Cross is set up in most states under enabling legislation, generally providing that it should be regulated by the state insurance department. In some states, Blue Cross must submit to public hearings before it can raise its rates.

The distinctive feature of Blue Cross, Blue Shield, and Medicare is that money is paid directly to the provider of care for services rendered to the subscriber of the plan. This is in contrast to indemnity payments, which are made by insurance companies directly to the subscriber. These plans involve a contractual agreement between the provider and the plan (hospitals and Blue Cross, doctors and Blue Shield). Blue Cross contracts usually specify what the hospital is allowed to charge the patient covered by Blue Cross.

Hospitals are not so limited by patients who are covered by commercial health insurance. However, hospitals and other providers of care frequently request that their patients assign their insurance benefits, which means that the patients transfer the insurance benefits from the patient to the hospital. In this case, the hospital is paid directly by the insurance company.

Health Maintenance Organizations combine fixed, periodic payments of subscribers to the plan with ownership and operation of hospitals and clinics. These plans are usually nongovernment and nonprofit, provide group practice by doctors who are salaried by the plan, and include comprehensive benefits in that they pay for and provide a wide range of health services. They serve an enrolled and definable population who subscribe to the plan by making payments to it. The best known and largest of these is the Kaiser-Permanente Plan, which is based in California.

HMO's emphasize outpatient rather than inpatient care. It appears that the patients of these plans are less likely to be admitted to hospitals. A subscriber to these plans may use only the plans' doctors and hospitals, except in an emergency or when the subscriber is traveling outside the plan's territory.

Evaluating insurance and prepayment coverage

One way to judge insurance and prepayment coverage is to ask what part of every dollar you pay in premiums will come back to you and people like you in benefits. The greater the return in benefits and the less taken out in profits and overhead the better the bargain for you. Unfortunately, this information is not easy to obtain.

Group insurance or prepayment coverage usually has much lower overhead than individual insurance and therefore you get more for your money from some form of group coverage. If you work for a large established company, it will probably have negotiated good coverage for the money. A big company or union can take the time to shop for a good plan and to negotiate coverage that suits the needs of its employees. Perhaps there is an employee-employer committee that reviews the benefit structure. The company's personnel office will probably be willing to meet with groups of employees to discuss benefits.

The benefits and exclusions in a policy are also important. If you have diabetes, for example, and your coverage will not pay for preexisting conditions, your future illnesses will probably be related to your diabetes and therefore not be covered.

If you are in a position to choose among various kinds of coverage, you will want to consider whether your premiums are going to subsidize other higher-risk people than you. If so, the high-risk people will get proportionately more benefits. Conversely, are you being subsidized by someone else? If your choice is between insurance and a prepayment plan, you will want to know to what extent your prospective insurer or plan controls utilization and monitors the quality of care. Prepaid plans like Kaiser have lower hospital utilization rates. By keeping their members out of hospitals they can afford to pay for other benefits.

PREVENTION AND
MEDICAL CARE

The prevention of illness includes activities and programs that people do and follow to keep themselves healthy. It also includes activities of health workers such as screening for disease, administering vaccinations, and maintaining sanitation.

The story is told of a bone doctor who worked hard to repair his patients' broken legs. One day he decided that repairing broken bones was not enough so he went out with a shovel and filled up a hole in the street into which his patients were falling. This story illustrates the difference between prevention and medical treatment. Unfortunately it is not always so simple to prevent illness. This is demonstrated by the continued existence of hunger, alcoholism, traffic accidents, battered babies, obesity, smoking, war, drug addiction, absence of fluoridated drinking water, violence, suicide, air pollution, and so on. Medical care is no substitute for reasonable living habits, and often medical care cannot repair the damage done.

Questions

1. How much money should we spend on health care for the United States as a whole? How should we decide?
2. Do you think that doctors should be examined every five years to test their current ability and these scores made available to the public? What about other skilled workers such as teachers, lawyers, T.V. repairmen, and so on?
3. If you were moving to a new city, what would you do to find good medical care?
4. If you were a member of an employee-management insurance committee at your place of employment, what would you do to get good health insurance benefits for the employees?

Key Concepts

Health care services – all of the activities carried out for the prevention and treatment of illness and injury

Physician – a person with an MD or DO degree who practices medicine

Proprietary – run on a profit basis, a term used to describe health care facilities

Voluntary – run on a nonprofit basis, a term used to describe health care facilities

Selected Readings

Anderson, Odin W. *Health Care: Can There Be Equity? The United States, Sweden, and England.* New York: Wiley-Interscience, John Wiley and Sons, 1972.

Burling, Temple, Edith M. Lentz, and Robert N. Wilson. *The Give and Take in Hospitals, A Study of Human Organization in Hospitals.* New York: G. P. Putnam's Sons, 1956.

Freidson, Eliot. *The Hospital in Modern Society.* Glencoe: Free Press, 1963.

———. *Profession of Medicine, A Study of the Sociology of Applied Knowledge.* New York: Dodd, Mead and Company, 1970.

U.S. Department of Labor. *Health Careers Guidebook,* Washington, D.C: Manpower Administration, Bureau of Employment Security, U.S. Employment Service, 1965.

Wilson, Florence and Duncan Neuhauser. *Health Services in the United States.* Cambridge: Ballinger, 1973.

Chapter 19

Human Dilemmas in Health Care

Under the present system of health care delivery in the United States, many important gains have been achieved. A few of these achievements include some decline in the infant mortality rate, a marked decline in the diseases affecting infants, a decrease in maternal mortality, reduction in infectious diseases, improved sanitation, marked improvement in rehabilitative measures, improved care of the mentally ill, and expansion of preventative services. In spite of the advances of medical science and the improvements in the health care delivery system, the health services available to a substantial portion of American society are notably inadequate and medical care is often so expensive that the cost prevents individuals from seeking care or adds a considerable burden to the difficulties caused by illness or injury.

THE COST OF
MEDICAL CARE

The per capita income in America is the highest of any nation, and most Americans are in reasonably good health. Yet when sickness comes,

This chapter was contributed by Elizabeth Prince Rice, M.S., Associate Professor Emerita of Social Work in Public Health, Harvard School of Public Health.

many people who are usually able to support themselves and their families are stripped of their financial resources because of the costs of medical care. Those Americans who do not share the financial security of the majority suffer from a vicious cycle in which their poverty contributes to health problems that they are often neither emotionally or financially equipped to handle. The old saying that "poverty creates illness and illness, poverty" is clearly applicable in America today.

The cost of medical care for an acute illness may use up a family's financial resources, forcing the family to liquidate their assets, such as a car or property, and pushing them into debt from which they cannot easily recover. For a long-term illness or a chronic condition, the indebtedness becomes even worse. One woman suffering from cancer, for example, had had several operations and had used up her savings, borrowed money on her house, and sold the family car to pay for medical costs. When another operation was proposed, she had no assets left but the equity on her house. Since she already owed the hospital over $3,000, she thought she had no choice except to sell her house because the hospital would not admit her with the outstanding debt. Neighbors heard of her predicament and raised enough money to pay the hospital debt and to cover the cost of the new hospital admission.

Another example is that of a twelve-year-old son of an unemployed architect. The boy needed an orthopedic operation on his heel to lengthen the heel cords. Without the operation he would have been lame for life. Delaying the surgery would have lessened his chances for full mobility. The boy's father had always supported his family well, but there had been little house building for some time due to an economic recession and he had been unable to get work. The father was proud and independent. He had already mortgaged his home to raise money for the daily expenses of his family of six. He had no further assets to use for the boy's surgery, and he dared not go further into debt not knowing when the recession would be over. He finally realized that the operation was necessary to save the boy from being handicapped and that his only step was to seek financial assistance from the town where he lived. Financial help was received, but the town put a lien on his house, which caused him anxiety and shattered his feelings of independence. Fortunately, some months after the boy's operation, the recession receded somewhat, and the father was again able to find work and to take the lien off his house.

In addition to the cost of hospitalization, there are often other fees for the physician's services and for x-rays, laboratory tests, medications, and appliances such as braces or eyeglasses. Some of these costs are repeated periodically. Illness may also leave the patient in need of care after hospitalization either at home or elsewhere, thus adding more expense to the family. Many patients cannot secure the care they need at home because there is no one there to care for the patient, because the home is inadequate for the patient's needs, or because no one is able or willing to assume the responsibility for the care. In these situations the patient must be cared for elsewhere, usually in a chronic hospital or a nursing home. Today the cost of care in a licensed nursing home ranges from a low of around $5,000 a year to a high of $20,000 a year in a deluxe setting.

The demands of illness can also contribute to or cause poverty by the changes they make in an individual's way of life. Illness may make it necessary for a person to change or give up his job, or for a child to modify his schooling. Thus earnings or preparation for future work may be jeopardized. For example, a real-estate dealer had an active business that required much time after hours and on weekends. His work included much stair climbing and walking as well as the pressures inherent in making sales in a highly competitive field. When this man left the hospital after a serious illness, he was not encouraged to return to work full time. Several restrictions were placed on his activities by his physician which meant that he could do less work less well. As a result his earnings were less, and in competition with other dealers he ran the risk of losing his business.

Illness can drain a family of its financial resources; it can lessen a family's independence; it can literally push a family into debt and force them to require public assistance. Without a national system of health insurance available to all there will continue to be a substantial number of families who for one reason or another are unprotected financially when illness arises.

Poverty and health care

Poverty also creates illness. Recent studies in the United States have shown that around a third of American families live in poverty, which is defined by the federal government as an income below $3,972 a year for a family of four. When a family is poor, several factors affect the health of its members. The family receives less medical care, postponing care because of the expense and/or distance to medical resources. When they do get medical care, their conditions are usually more severe, sometimes even beyond cure. The poor tend to substitute drugstore treatment for medical care, again because of expense. Thus the people who need most to have immediate and adequate care tend to postpone or delay it. They need it especially in order to lessen incapacity or disability, which they can least afford.

When income is inadequate to buy nourishing food for the family, the general nutritional state of the family tends to be poor. School lunches have been a valuable aid in keeping children healthier than they would be otherwise.

The quality of the housing in which a family lives can also affect health, both physical and mental. An eight-year-old girl with rheumatic fever and rheumatic heart disease had been under treatment in one of the best children's hospitals in the country. She had repeated attacks of

The vicious circle of poverty

Here is one of the most familiar forms of the vicious circle of poverty. The poor get sick more than anyone else in the society. That is because they live in slums, jammed together under unhygienic conditions; they have inadequate diet, and cannot get decent medical care. When they become sick, they are sick longer than any other group in the society. Because they are sick more often and longer than anyone else, they lose wages and work, and find it difficult to hold a steady job. And because of this, they cannot pay for good housing, for a nutritious diet, for doctors. At any given point in the circle, particularly when there is a major illness, their prospect is to move to an even lower level and to begin the cycle, round and round, toward even more suffering. . . .

The individual cannot usually break out of this vicious circle. Neither can the group, for it lacks the social energy and political strength to turn its misery into a cause. Only the larger society, with its help and resources, can really make it possible for these people to help themselves. Yet those who could make the difference too often refuse to act because of their ignorant, smug moralisms. They view the effects of poverty—above all, the warping of the will and spirit that is a consequence of being poor—as choices. Understanding the vicious circle is an important step in breaking down this prejudice.

From Michael Harrington, *The Other America* (Baltimore: Penguin Books, 1963), p. 22.

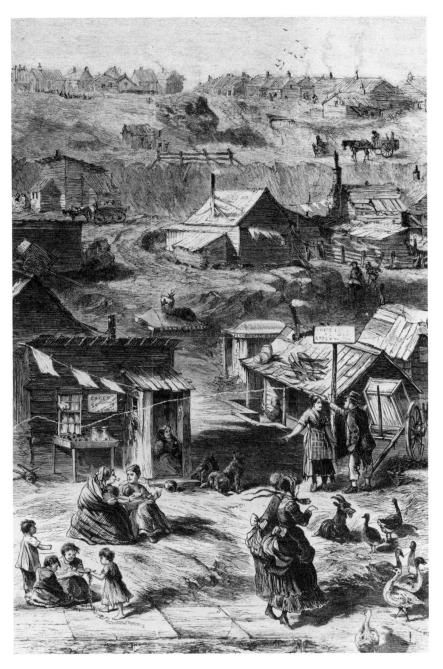

Figure 19.1. Poverty and housing have always been factors affecting health. This wood engraving, which appeared in *Harper's Weekly* in June 1869, depicts a squatters settlement in Central Park, New York City. In such slum conditions, disease rates were high. (Courtesy of National Library of Medicine, Bethesda, Maryland)

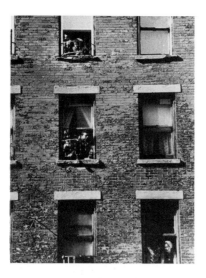

Figure 19.2. Quality of housing affects both physical and mental health. (Courtesy World Health Organization, photo by Jean Mohr)

rheumatic fever and was given medication to prevent the attacks, but in spite of this she was hospitalized several times. A study of the home situation showed that the family of mother, father, and eight children lived in a tenement that had been condemned by the housing authorities and was to be demolished. The apartment the family occupied consisted of a living room, three bedrooms, and a small kitchen. The toilet was in the hall and used by other families on the floor. One of the bedrooms, the one the patient occupied, could not be used in the winter because of dampness that was apparent on the window and walls, which literally dripped water. During the worst of the winter, the family of ten used only two bedrooms, which were also damp. The patient slept in a bed with three siblings and was constantly exposed to their upper respiratory infections. Obviously an important part of the treatment of this girl's illness was to provide the family with a decent place to live. With great difficulty and finally through political and church pressures, the family was relocated in a public housing development where they had an adequate number of bedrooms for the children, privacy for the parents, and the convenience of their own kitchen and bath. The patient's rheumatic fever was then well controlled with medication.

In analyzing the incidence of illness in the population by census

Health care statistics

In 1967 statistics from the Department of Health, Education and Welfare showed the following figures:

1. Of families with incomes less than $2,000, 20 percent have chronic conditions that limit activity as contrasted with 7.5 percent among persons with incomes of $7,000 or more.

a. Within the age group 17–44 years the poor have chronic conditions at twice the rate of the nonpoor.

b. Within the age group 45–64 years the poor have chronic conditions 5½ times greater than the nonpoor.

2. Hospital stays were longer for the poor.

a. With incomes under $2,000, the average hospital stay was 10.2 days.

b. With incomes over $7,000, the average hospital stay was 7.2 days.

3. For those with incomes under $2,000, hospitalizations were more often for nonsurgical conditions than for those with incomes over $2,000.

4. The average length of life for nonwhites was 63.3 years; the aver-

age length of life for whites was 70.19 years. There are more nonwhites among the poor.

5. Maternal mortality rates were 4 times greater for nonwhite mothers than for white mothers. In 1965, 90.2 nonwhite mothers died per 100,000 live births whereas 22.4 white mothers died per 100,000 live births.

6. Infant mortality in 1965 was greater among nonwhites; 40.3 nonwhite infant deaths per 100,000 live births as compared with 21.5 white infant deaths per 100,000 live births.

7. Tuberculosis, influenza and pneumonia, vascular lesions affecting the nervous system, and deaths from homicide were twice as frequent among the nonwhite as the white. There was also a higher nonwhite mortality from cancer of the cervix, a condition in which early diagnosis and treatment are important.

8. Children under 15 years of age saw physicians less often among the poor; with incomes under $2,000 they made an average of 2 visits per

year to the physician, whereas children from families with an income over $7,000 a year made 4 visits a year. Rural children made fewer visits than urban children.

9. Dental care was less frequent according to income. With incomes under $4,000, 22 percent of families had never seen a dentist. With incomes over $10,000, 7.2 percent of families had never seen a dentist. The dental care for the poor in the past has consisted primarily of extractions, with little preventive dentistry.

10. Immunizations also vary by white and nonwhite. In the case of nonwhite children ages 1–4, 22.5 percent had had no DPT immunizations (diphtheria), whereas 8.6 percent of white children had had none.

From George Silver, "Health as a Social Problem—Consequences of Illness," *Encyclopedia of Social Work*, Vol. I (New York: National Association of Social Workers, 1971), pp. 490–99.

tracts, it is interesting to note that the portion of the population with the lowest average income and level of educational attainment have the highest incidence of tuberculosis, venereal diseases, hepatitis, chronic illness, and infant mortality rates. These statistics show the consequences of poor housing, malnutrition, and relatively infrequent medical attention that is often of poorer quality than the attention available to those with better income and education. In addition, studies show that the people in the lower income bracket seek medical care less often, have more hospitalizations, stay in the hospital longer, and are readmitted to hospitals more often within a twelve-month period. An English study made by the National Health Service also showed a greater incidence of deaths and a higher incidence of diseases including whooping cough, measles, mumps, bronchitis, pneumonia, and other respiratory diseases among the poor.

Because one marriage in four in the United States is now broken by death, divorce, separation, or desertion of a parent, more often the father, there are many one-parent families in this country. In broken or single-parent families there are added strains on the one parent who must be both father and mother to the children. Income may be limited, and there may be less attention paid to preventive health care such as periodic physical examinations. Tensions may build up as a result of stresses in the family with only one parent available to cope with all of the demands. Thus, physical or mental health may be affected over a period of time.

Even though illness may not reduce a family to the poverty level, it will inevitably lessen a family's resources and create additional problems. Some will wonder how to continue to live and work with a disability, how to meet the costs of continuing medical care, how to carry on when a family member is handicapped, how to provide for an unwanted child or one who is mentally retarded, or how to care for an elderly relative. Whatever the condition, additional strains are placed on families by illness, and families have difficulty coping with these strains.

DELIVERY OF HEALTH CARE SERVICES

Delivery of health care services refers to the system which provides health care to people; this includes the services which are available, the ways the services are administered, the quality of the services, and the satisfactions of the people who use them. All countries are experiencing a tremendous increase in the demand for health care services. This demand leads to increasing specialization among all types of health care workers, rising costs, and changing morbidity patterns resulting in part from greater longevity and improved medical care.

The right to care

Some people question whether adequate health care is a basic right, and for many years the provision of medical care was not included in the list of the necessities of life—food, shelter, and clothing. However, with the passage of the Social Security Act in 1935 which provided payment for medical care for certain groups and with the later enactment of Medicaid, the right of persons to receive medical care as a part of the basic necessities of life was accepted. It was clearly seen that the cost, not only to the individual but to the public, was markedly increased when an individual was unemployed, unemployable, or required the use of expensive community facilities for long periods of time because of illness or disability.

In spite of the acceptance of health care as a basic right, American health care delivery is far from satisfactory, especially for the poor. Dr. James R. Kimmery, managing editor of the *American Journal of Public Health,* wrote in that journal in October 1972:

> The sensitivity and humanity of a country can be measured by the extent to which health care is accessible and available for the poor. The hard-headed realist will argue that such indicators are too imprecise, too fuzzy, too woolly, too bleeding heart to appraise issues of great complexity. Nevertheless the present state of health care for the poor in the United States indicates a basic insensitivity and inhumanity of our social and political order.

Problems in providing care

What are the problems in this affluent country in providing adequate health care? Why is the delivery of health care referred to as the "health care crisis"? In March and April 1971, several days of hearings were held in Washington before the Subcommittee on Health of the Committee on Labor and Public Welfare of the United States Senate. The major problems in the health care system which evolved from the hearings were:

1. maldistribution and shortage of health manpower
2. inequality in health care
3. rising costs of health care
4. inequality in access to health care including financing
5. too little attention paid to keeping people well
6. lack of coordination in the health care system resulting in waste and duplication.

On behalf of Potomac Associates, a Washington research firm, the Gallup polling organization asked a large sample of the public in 1971 the question: "Do you feel that there is a general 'health crisis' in the United States that will require basic changes in how medical services are made available to the public, or do you think that things are going along pretty well as they are at the present time?" Three out of five persons questioned thought that basic changes were needed in the health care system. This was equally true for men and women of all age groups in all regions of the country. The results of the poll suggest that the feeling that there is a health crisis pervades American society.

*Table 19.1 Results of 1971 Gallup poll on changes needed in medical services**

	Basic changes required	Going along pretty well as is	No opinion
National	61	34	5
Sex			
Men	60	36	4
Women	62	32	6
Race			
White	63	33	4
Nonwhite	49	43	8
Education			
College	68	30	2
High school	63	33	4
Grade school	51	40	9
Occupation			
Professional and business	67	30	3
White collar	67	29	4
Manual	60	35	5
Nonlabor	55	37	8
Age			
18–29 years	64	32	4
30–44 years	62	34	4
45–59 years	66	29	5
60 and over	53	42	5
Region			
East	66	28	6
Midwest	59	36	5
South	57	40	3
West	66	29	5
Income			
$15,000 and over	63	35	2
$10,000–$14,999	63	32	5
$7,000–$9,999	65	30	5
$5,000–$6,999	57	39	4
Under $5,000	60	34	6

* *Health Security News*, December 1972–January 1973, p. 2.

The mobility of our population has tended to expand the central-city ghettos and to create additional problems in providing health care to these areas. Efforts to develop neighborhood health centers have been limited due to lack of funds and personnel. Too many poor families cannot get to health care, cannot afford to pay for it, or do not understand the importance of care, especially early treatment. Emergency care is often at a distant location and carried on under crowded and anxiety-provoking conditions by physicians who are too tired from overwork to give the personal attention the patient wants and needs. Patients are

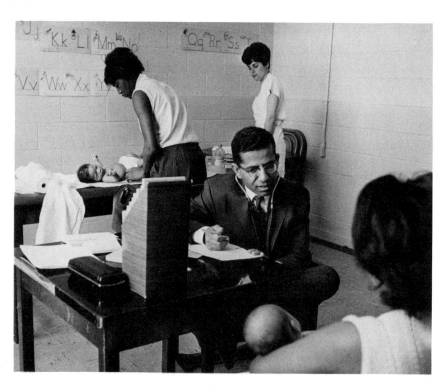

Figure 19.3. A doctor at a Well Baby clinic confers with a mother after examining her baby.

confused by the number of different physicians they are referred to and often become impatient and discouraged.

There are still too many children who die unnecessarily or are left disabled because of insufficient early care. The National Center for Health Statistics estimated that in 1970 there were over 15,000 unnecessary infant deaths. The mortality rate for black children two to eleven months of age was three times that of white children, and the maternal mortality rate was four times greater for black mothers than for white mothers. One-third of all children were getting inadequate care and in addition many children go without dental care, dietary supplements, or corrective appliances.

The problems of delivery of health care, however, are not limited to the poor. Many in the middle and upper income groups are also dismayed, frustrated, and angered by the arrangements for care and rising costs.

FACTORS THAT PREVENT EFFECTIVE HEALTH CARE

Personal attitudes

The attitude of a person toward his health problem is basic to his ability and willingness to use health resources. He may belittle his illness and feel competent to care for himself, perhaps with the help of self-medication. He may be embarrassed because of his illness and hesitate to seek medical care. His illness may come at an inopportune time in his

Cultural and religious biases

Cultural and religious biases affect health. Not only are there groups that refuse to use medical care believing that there is another way to heal, but there are sects that have many strange and varied health practices. These relate often to dietary fads and superstitions. For example, some believe that if a mother eats strawberries during pregnancy, the baby will have a birthmark resembling a strawberry. Or some think that eating raw fruits creates acidity in the stomach causing indigestion. Other superstitions are related to behavior; for example, some believe that a person with eyebrows that grow close together possesses the evil eye and that this can bring bad luck. If the physician or nurse in a clinic possesses these traits, the patient will not be happy to return for further care. There are numerous ideas of this nature, many of which are harmless in themselves but which may, in a crisis of sickness, affect the readiness of the patient to accept or carry out the recommended treatment.

life, and he may be reluctant to take the necessary time off for treatment. He may be fearful of what the doctor will find and unable to face the truth, and unwilling or unable to face the cost of care. A man who refused to have a chest x-ray to rule out the presence of tuberculosis said, "I would rather not know the truth because I can't stop work now anyway, and I would refuse care in a sanatorium."

Attitudes of patients are also dependent on their past experiences with the medical care system and health personnel. If these experiences have been fruitful and pleasant, an individual has a greater chance of seeking medical care again, but if the experiences have been hurried, uncomfortable, or lacking in dignity, he will hesitate to undergo another such experience. The attitude of friends and relatives, based on their experiences with medical care, will also influence the patient to seek or continue care or support his tendency to wait until he feels worse.

The extent of ignorance on health matters and the frequent misinterpretations of health recommendations are barriers to getting care. The confusion in the patient's mind which is created by different, even opposing, recommendations of two or more physicians leaves the patient uncertain and his confidence shaken. The delivery system at present frequently gives little opportunity for the patient to express his concerns and bewilderment, and in the rush of a busy clinic there is often no allotted time for the physician or nurse to listen to the patient's questions, to clarify the recommendations, or to determine whether the patient understands or can carry out the suggested treatment. Thus a patient often comes to believe that no one cares whether he can do what is suggested and feels that no one understands his predicament. Many long for the interest and concern of the family doctor of the past who knew what the patient was able to do and who seemed to care. The *New England Journal of Medicine* in March 1969 reported that "medical care is increasingly fragmented and complex, and the warmth of a long-term association with a single physician has become a luxury for a few rather than a customary setting for the delivery of health care."

Unfortunately, some patients are reluctant to go to a clinic, which now often costs as much as or more than a visit to a physician's office. Often the manner of receiving patients, the crowded waiting rooms, the long periods of sitting, and the rushed examinations leave the patient feeling like a cog in the machinery without any personal identification with anyone in the clinic. Racist, sexist, or other prejudices may be expressed by one of the clinic personnel with whom the patient comes into contact; this will make the patient uncomfortable and resistant to further care.

Health personnel also deplore the delivery system that forces them to give little time to patients, to be unable to do the kind of work they were trained for and want to do. Many doctors and nurses especially regret their inability to give the patient time to discuss his illness and to understand the implications of the treatment. They are pushed by the pressures of great numbers of cases, and often they must deal with medical emergencies in the clinic.

Accessibility and availability of services

To be easily accessible to the patient a health service must be administered so that the patient will be encouraged to seek care. Long waiting lines for services make the patient resistant to seeking care. Some patients find health services difficult because of language barriers. Some people have the unfortunate experience of being denied care until they have paid for it in advance. Rules and regulations established by the clinic are often impossibly difficult for the patient to carry out.

A study made in 1971 by research associates at the Center for Health Administration Studies at the University of Chicago included interviews with 11,800 individuals and showed that relatively high proportions of the group were dissatisfied with the accessibility of their own personal care and with the costs of care. Persons under sixty-five tended to be more dissatisfied than older people, nonwhites more dissatisfied than whites, and the lower income group more dissatisfied than the higher income group. The younger, higher income groups expressed dissatisfaction with accessibility to care at night and on weekends, with getting information about their medical care, and with the coordination of care.

Because of the inaccessibility of care at night and on weekends there has been a conspicuous increase in the use of emergency services in general hospitals. As increasing numbers of people seek help, emergency services become more frequently overcrowded. Service is slow; physi-

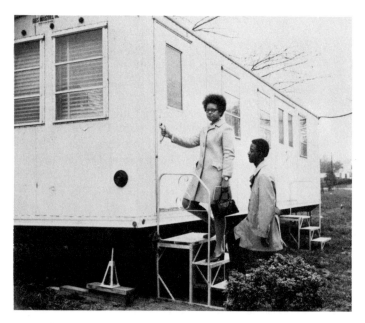

Figure 19.4. A portable x-ray health clinic in Winston-Salem, North Carolina.

cians are under great pressure, often after a full day's work; tensions are high; waiting rooms are chaotic; and patients are exposed to delays, anxieties, and often harrowing experiences.

Families living at some distance from medical care services need time, transportation, and money to get to the services available. Some efforts have been made to reach remote communities by such means as helicopter transportation for physicians, traveling clinics, public health nursing services, or providing transport services to bring patients to medical care.

Comprehensiveness and coordination of care

Specialization in medicine has the tendency to result in treating the patient in parts. Depending on where the patient's care originates, he may or may not receive examination and treatment for his several complaints. In some clinics it is considered advisable to have a patient seen first in a general medical or pediatric clinic where all of his problems can be assessed and a plan for his total care worked out. For special needs, he may then be referred to other clinics. However, with the pressure on clinics many patients are admitted first to a specialized clinic and the patient may never get a comprehensive evaluation. Similarly, in private practice the patient may choose to go to a specialist for a given condition, such as a knee injury, and may never get the complete care desirable.

Many patients, therefore, may be treated for only one condition or may be treated for several conditions in care that may not be coordinated. Very often attention to a preventive program for the patient is omitted since the tendency is to focus on the illness or the disability rather than to include concern for ways of helping the patient to keep healthy.

Coordination of care within the health resources is essential for complete care of the patient. Similarly, coordination between the health staff and the staffs of other community resources is important. The interrelationship of health and disease and the social situation in which the patient and family live is often basic to the patient's health problem. It is essential for the agencies helping the family with problems of housing, financial needs, family relationships, employment, recreation and the like to consider the health needs of the family and to plan together with the health personnel to assure consistency and coordination. In our health delivery system now there is too little coordination between that system and other systems such as the welfare system.

Continuity of care

To be successful a health care delivery system must provide for continuity of care in order to retain the gains resulting from the medical care already provided and to make certain that the patient has received maximum care. To encourage the patient to continue under care as long as

Providing for continuity of care

In a recent study of adolescent health in Harlem, it was found that comprehensive health services were needed to deal with a variety of health problems presented by the adolescents. The young people in the study had the usual problems of adolescence: dental, visual, emotional, weight, and skin difficulties. In addition, they had other problems including high blood pressure, asthma and anemia. The health care made available to them was markedly successful in providing the continuity of care that is essential for complete, successful treatment. This continuity was attributed in part to convenient scheduling and frequent rescheduling of appointments, to personal invitations to appear at the examination, to multiple reminders about the examination appointment, and to the elimination of the requirement for a parent to accompany the adolescent to the examination. The need for flexibility in rescheduling appointments appears to be one of the major findings of the study.

From Ann F. Brunswick and Eric Josephson, "Adolescent Health in Harlem," *American Journal of Public Health*, Oct. 1972 Supplement.

recommended, several factors already referred to are necessary: an acceptable provision of services, an established relationship of trust and confidence, an understanding of the importance of further care, an acceptance of the need for care, and an ability to get and pay for care.

Health personnel encourage continuity when they make clear to the patient his need for further care, help the patient to overcome the barriers to getting care, and provide a method that indicates when a patient has not returned and needs help in continuing care. Without continuity of care some patients will continue to be ill or disabled, and therefore the medical care has been only partially successful.

Probably the greatest dissatisfaction with the delivery of health care is the rising cost of care. Persons in all socioeconomic groups voice their concern, even their anger, about the fees charged by physicians and hospitals. During the 1960s the costs for health and illness in the United States nearly tripled.[1]

In 1929, $3.6 billion was spent for total health care.
In 1960, $26.4 billion was spent for total health care.
In 1969, $60 billion was spent for total health care.

In 1929 the average health expenditure per person was $27 a year while in 1960 the average yearly medical bill was $233, only three-fifths

[1] George Silver, "Costs of National Health," *Encyclopedia of Social Work*, Vol. II, p. 491.

Medicaid and Medicare

Medicaid is a grant-in-aid program in which the federal and state (and sometimes local) governments share the costs of medical care for people with low income. It was authorized in 1965 by Title 19 of the Social Security Act. Its goal ultimately is to make medical care of high quality readily available to those unable to pay for it. The state determines whether an individual or family is eligible according to its definition of need, within certain federal limits. The program is state-administered and is financed in part by the state (or state and local) government and in part (50–83 percent depending on the state's average per capita income) by the federal government. Because each state determines benefits and eligibility within fed-

eral guidelines, there are differences—state by state—in who is eligible and for what benefits.

Medicaid must not be confused with Medicare. Medicare is an insurance program whereas Medicaid is an assistance program. Medicare is a federally administered program offering two kinds of health insurance for people aged 65 or older: hospital insurance and supplementary medical insurance for physicians' services and some other medical services. Benefits are the same throughout the nation. It is financed by deductions from employees' wages and matching taxes by employers and the self-employed. Medical insurance is a voluntary program, financed by monthly premiums paid by the individual and by a matching amount

paid by the federal government. It is administered by the Social Security Administration which also formulates the policies.

Medicaid can pay what Medicare does not pay for those unable to meet the amount uncovered by Medicare. In 1971 Medicaid paid medical bills for more than 18 million people who were aged, blind, disabled, under 21 years, or members of families with dependent children. In addition some states paid medical bills for low-income people not included in the above groups. In July 1972 Medicaid was in every part of the United States except Arizona and Alaska. Medicaid has expanded rapidly since its beginning largely as a result of the rapid rise in hospital costs and physicians' services.

of which was paid for by third-party payments (insurance, government, private funds). In 1950 the percentage of a family's income used for medical care was 4.5 percent; in 1967 it was 6.7 percent. The increase in per capita amounts resulted from the rise in the cost of physicians and hospital services and the increase in demand for health care. The cost of medical care went up faster and greater than any other consumer item during 1965–1968 when medical care prices rose 5.8 percent while consumer prices rose 3.3 percent. Greater use of health facilities was due largely to an increase in the aged population who have more illness, more serious illnesses, more hospitalizations, longer hospitalizations and nursing-home care, and make greater use of physicians' services. The largest increase in medical expenses was in hospital costs, which constituted 43 percent of all costs for medical care.

HEALTH INSURANCE Government funds including Medicare and Medicaid now pay for more than half the costs of hospital care. Insurance benefits pay for a third, and the patient pays for only 12 percent. But the cost to the patient is still more than many families can pay without great sacrifice, unless they carry adequate health insurance.

It has recently been estimated that about 77 percent of the population in the United States has some form of health insurance, but close to 30 million people are without hospital insurance. Moreover, most insurance does not cover all of the costs of health care since policies often have deductibles, expenses that the patient must pay first, or they may cover only certain costs and not others. These costs may be considerable, especially for patients with critical or long-term illnesses. Most insurance policies, furthermore, do not pay for preventive services including immunizations.

Recently insurance rates have increased and benefits have been reduced. This is even true of Medicare, which each year provides less and becomes more costly. Most insurances are geared to help in short-term illnesses but do not cover long-term illnesses, especially in nursing homes or the patient's own home. More than half of all Americans have no coverage for office or home visits by physicians, and after paying the costs of hospital deductibles, many families have no money left to pay physicians' bills. Thus some method more adequate than that which now exists is needed for collective medical financing, regardless of income level. The current system of private insurances supplemented with public funds is costly, inefficient, and incomplete.

One of the reasons for the inadequacies of private insurance plans is that insurance companies use some of their premium income for expenses other than the cost of health care. The AFL-CIO Platform Proposals to the 1972 Democratic and Republican Conventions explained this inadequacy:

> In the year ending June 30, 1971, private insurers took almost 2 billion [dollars] of the 17 billion they received as premiums for advertising, com-

missions, executive salaries, stock options, and profit. Commercial insurers spent 20 cents for every premium dollar on things other than health. In contrast Social Security pays out 98% of tax receipts in cash benefits. Some audits have shown little incentive by insurance companies to hold down health care costs as evidenced by overpayments, payments of unreasonable charges or use of funds for equipment, supplies or services.[2]

PROPOSALS FOR IMPROVING COVERAGE There have been a number of proposals made to meet the cost of health care including those by the American Medical Association, the American Hospital Association, senators and representatives, individuals and consumer groups, and the federal administration. The federal government proposals include four programs:

1. The National Health Insurance Partnership Act (NHIP) for employer–employee groups
2. The Family Health Insurance Plan (FHIP) for the poor and working poor
3. Continuation of Medicaid for the poor, the blind, and disabled
4. Medicare for the aged.

These four together would provide universal availability of limited coverage on a voluntary basis rather than complete coverage for the entire population with broad protection.

There will be many more proposals and modifications of present ones before an adequate plan for health care is formulated and accepted. Probably the greatest interest so far is in a National Health Security Plan, which has bipartisan support and is known as the Kennedy-Griffith bill.

In judging any proposal the following important questions should be considered:

1. Is universal coverage included as a right of all people?
2. Are the benefits comprehensive and complete—that is, without deductibles, coinsurance, cutoff points in amount spent or days of coverage, waiting periods before insurance is effective, requirements for physical examinations to determine eligibility, or exclusion for preexisting conditions? Are preventive services included?
3. Does the plan provide for free choice of physician and hospital?
4. Does the plan include effective cost controls?
5. Does the plan provide for the training of health manpower and for improving the health delivery system?

Pressure from consumer groups for improved health coverage is increasingly more powerful. It is to be expected that some action will be taken in the near future to provide for at least some of the catastrophes of illness that arise when families are least prepared to meet the costs.

[2] *Social Security and Health: The AFL-CIO Platform Proposals.* Presented to the Democratic and Republican Conventions, 1972, p. 34.

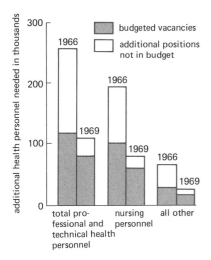

Figure 19.5. Number of additional professional and technical health personnel needed to provide optimum patient care in American Hospital Association registered hospitals in the United States, 1966 and 1969. (From "Health Manpower in Hospitals," U.S. Department of HEW, Public Health Service, National Institutes of Health, U.S. Government Printing Office, 1970)

Health manpower

Another major problem in the delivery of health services is the shortage and poor distribution of health personnel, especially physicians. According to the 1971 Hearings Before the Subcommittee on Health of the Senate Committee on Labor and Public Welfare, 50,000 more physicians, 250,000 more nurses, and 50,000 more dentists are needed. To provide these additional personnel it was suggested that the professional schools should graduate 50 percent more doctors and 20 percent more dentists every year up to 1980. It was also recommended that the number of years required for a medical education be shortened and that nine new medical schools be established in areas that are now without medical schools. Additional proposals included recruiting more students from geographic areas not now sending students to professional schools and more diligent recruitment of minority groups, including women.

The physicians and other health personnel who are available now are not evenly distributed throughout the nation. The average number of nonfederal physicians providing patient care in 1967, for example, was 132 per 100,000 people for the nation as a whole. However, in New York the ratio was 199 per 100,000 people while in Mississippi the ratio was 69 per 100,000. The states with the lowest number of physicians are also the states with the fewest specialists, and in some states there is no specialist available in certain categories. Five states, for example, had no specialist in child psychiatry in 1970. There are generally fewer health personnel of all kinds in rural areas and in areas that lack hospitals and other health care facilities. It is hoped that the new interest in community medicine will encourage new medical school graduates to

Figure 19.6. Active nonfederal physicians in relation to population in each state, 1967. (From *Health Manpower Source Book*, Section 20, U.S. Department of HEW, Public Health Service, National Institutes of Health, U.S. Government Printing Office, 1969)

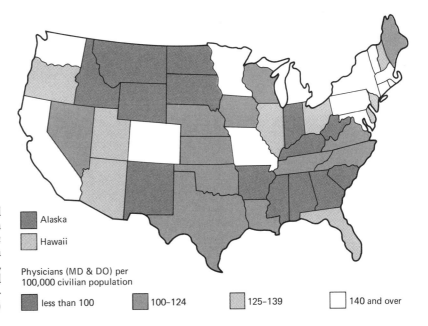

practice away from the larger cities; these young physicians are not likely to seek a practice in an area without a hospital, however.

NURSES In 1971 it was estimated that there were 723,000 registered nurses; 400,000 practical nurses; 848,000 nursing aides, orderlies, or attendants; and 17,000 to 22,000 home-health aides and homemakers employed in America. In 1956 there were 259 registered nurses per 100,000 people. This increased gradually to 353 per 100,000 people in 1971. Nurses are also unevenly distributed throughout the nation.

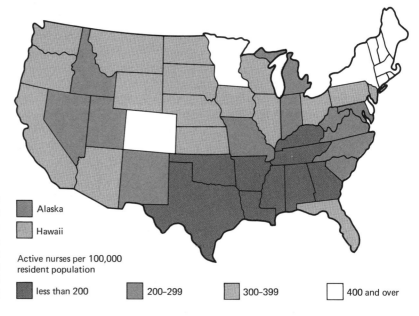

Figure 19.7. Active nurses in relation to population in each state, 1966. (From *Health Manpower Source Book,* Section 20, U.S. Department of HEW, Public Health Service, National Institutes of Health, U.S. Government Printing Office, 1969)

Alaska

Hawaii

Active nurses per 100,000 resident population

less than 200   200–299   300–399   400 and over

OTHER HEALTH PERSONNEL The increase in the numbers of other professionals such as occupational therapists, dieticians, and social workers has not been appreciable. These professions also show similar patterns of shortage and poor distribution.

There has been a movement to develop new types of health personnel. There is an increasing effort to find alternative ways of getting health care work done because of the critical shortages in manpower, because there are tasks that need to be done which now fall into the responsibility of none of the health professionals, and because some tasks now performed by the highly trained professional could be done as well, sometimes better, by less well-trained assistants. The use of registered nurses as physicians' assistants is one step. Further clarification of the task to be performed must precede the definition of the job and the training for it. There will undoubtedly be increasing use for paraprofessionals in the future.

Along with the cost of health services, the shortage of manpower is one of the most serious problems in the delivery of health services as people need and demand more and more health care. Recent curtailment or elimination of funds for medical schools or other schools for health professionals is a serious step when the public is demanding more health professionals to provide the needed care.

Health care facilities

The facilities available for delivery of health care services also are fewer than needed and, again, these facilities tend to be concentrated in certain areas of the country. Areas that lack adequate numbers of health care personnel also generally lack adequate health care facilities, partly because the facilities draw professionals to them as places of employment. A nurse who wishes to work in a community hospital, for example, will go to an area in which there is such a hospital; thus, regions without hospitals have fewer nurses.

Table 19.2 Regional distribution of health care facilities

Facilities	Region	Distribution of care
Hospitals	Northeast	9.0 beds per 1000 people
	North Central	7.5
	South	7.4
	West	6.2
Nursing Homes	Northeast	4,190 homes
	North Central	6,117
	South	4,560
	West	4,043
Day Care Facilities	Northeast	368 facilities
	North Central	799
	South	497
	West	285
Outpatient	Northeast	654 clinics
Psychiatric Services	North Central	508
	South	465
	West	315

NEW PATTERNS OF HEALTH CARE DELIVERY

Many attempts have been made to add to or patch up our present system of delivery of services. Space does not permit an elaboration of all these newer methods, but it will be of interest to make reference to some of them.

Regional planning

Regional planning groups have been formed to identify the problems in health care and the delivery of service for a specific area and plan the ways to make the services available within the region or by agreement with other regions. Efforts are made to lessen manpower shortages and to establish necessary facilities. Decisions are also made as to what services are needed, and plans to coordinate services within an area are developed. Regional planning held promise of being very effective until federal funds were curtailed, hampering further development.

Local planning

At the local level there are usually planning groups that attempt to determine the problems in the health delivery system, to coordinate services, to set standards, and to work with other groups in the community to improve health services. These local groups focus on such problems as the number of beds available in hospitals, the quality of care, the gaps or duplications in services, and so on. In some cities these planning groups are very effective; in others, little is accomplished. The members of the planning committee may be a citizens group, a unit of a health and welfare council, or a group appointed by a mayor or governor. They provide an essential interest in and concern for what is happening in the health field.

The Department of Public Health serves health programs in an advisory and consultative role and has been effective in raising standards for the quality and quantity of care. Also local groups of the American Hospital Association, the American Public Health Association, the National League of Nursing, and the National Association of Social Workers have been both advisory and pressure groups in improving health care services and health legislation.

Increase in group physician practice

There has been an increase in recent years in the number of physicians practicing in medical groups. California has the largest number of groups (785) with New York second (347). With the effort of the American Medical Association to promote the development of Health Maintenance Organizations (HMO) and with increasing interest on the part of many physicians to be in group rather than solo practice, it is expected that more groups will develop.

Local and neighborhood health projects

With encouragement from the federal government largely through health programs for mothers and infants and programs for children and youth, grants were made to some states, to local health departments, and a few to hospitals to provide funds and consultative services in establishing health programs at the neighborhood level. One of the objectives was to bring care closer to where the people live, thus making care more accessible throughout the day and night. Many of these neighborhood centers were an extension of or affiliated with a nearby hospital that provided the direction of the project and the staff and complemented the services. Emphasized in the program were the contributions of a multidisciplinary team approach to health and welfare problems. The re-

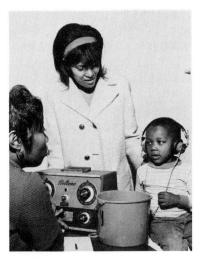

Figure 19.8. A hearing test is one of the services provided for children of low-income families at clinics operated by county health departments.

sults were a more effective and efficient utilization of manpower, more successful programs of reaching out into the community to promote community health, and stronger working relationships between the various health care organizations and social agencies, which in the past had failed to coordinate their services.

Although at first limited to the health needs of children, several of the projects were expanded to include health services for the aged and in some instances, whole families. These neighborhood centers suggest a pattern of providing health care which may be considered in the future organization of health services.

Some hospitals have also extended their services in other ways such as providing manpower for neighborhood "drop-in clinics," free clinics (seen mostly in California), and community rehabilitation programs. Again the objective is to extend health care services into the community and thus to have the care be more accessible to the people. With the renewed interest of medical students in community medicine and with citizen pressure, one may expect further expansion of such programs.

CONSUMER PRESSURE FOR IMPROVEMENT IN HEALTH SERVICES

Consumers on a selected basis have always served on hospital and public health boards and committees and on community planning committees. However, their role has been limited and not clearly defined. Because the consumer often finds it difficult to get health care where and when he needs it at a price he can pay, new consumer pressure groups have been organized and are becoming very vocal about the limitations in our delivery system. It has been suggested that consumer groups can be active in the following ways:

1. Work for legislation to allow consumers to participate in health care policy.
2. Initiate and support legal action to provide consumer representation on health care bodies such as boards of health.
3. Provide technical assistance for consumers to build consumer strength.
4. Support new types of health services.
5. Build coalitions of interested groups to further these goals.

Because of consumer pressures the federal government has encouraged the organization of such groups in each state to be appointed by the governor. The program has been entitled "Partnership for Health."

There was recently organized a "Citizens Board of Inquiry Into the Health Services for Americans." This citizens group, and others like it, believes that the United States has failed to provide adequate health services for the majority of its citizens. Recognizing the problems that exist in the delivery of health services, such groups will undoubtedly bring pressure to create a national health care system with universal financing for comprehensive care. These consumer groups will need the participation of health experts to share with them the situation as it is and to work together towards a solution to the problems in the present system of health care.

The delivery of health care has justifiably been referred to as the health care crisis. The problems in delivery have been identified. The public is aroused and demands that some plan be developed which will provide health care of good quality, accessible to all at costs that can be met through an adequate system of financing. The demand for health care is greater than the present supply of manpower, facilities, and supportive services. Financing for health care costs is incomplete, costly, and not available to all. To continue to add pieces to our present confused picture would only make the system more complex and unmanageable and would still leave gaps. Some single system which will ensure high quality comprehensive care, including preventive care to all at costs that can be met by the people with government help for those unable to pay, seems to be the hope for the future.

Questions

1. Evaluate the health care services that are presently available to you by measuring them against the criteria for adequate care suggested in this chapter.
2. What options for health care are available to you that are not available to others in the same area who are unable to pay for medical care?
3. What are the conditions under which medical care is given in your local public health clinic or hospital emergency room?
4. How would you or your family pay for your medical expenses if you were hospitalized for several months?
5. Why are completeness, coordination, and continuity of health care services important?

Key Concepts

Health care crisis – a term used to indicate the inadequate condition of present health care services in the United States

Poverty – according to the federal government, an annual income below $3,972 for a family of four

Right to care – the concept that adequate health care is a basic human right, analogous to the right to food, clothing, and shelter

Selected Readings

Anderson, O. W. *Health Services in a Land of Plenty.* Chicago: University of Chicago Press, 1968.

Birch, H. G., and J. D. Gussow. *Disadvantaged Children—Health, Nutrition and School Failure.* New York: Harcourt, Brace, Jovanovitch, 1970.

Breslow, Lester. "The Urgency of Social Action for Health," *American Journal of Public Health*, Vol. 60, No. 1 (Jan. 1970), pp. 10–16.

Delivery of Health Services for the Poor, A Program Analysis. Washington, D.C.: Department of Health, Education and Welfare, 1967.

Health Care Crisis in America, 10 vols. Hearings Before Subcommittee on Health of the Committee on Labor and Public Welfare, U.S. Senate. 92nd Congress, 1st session, March and April, 1971.

"Neighborhood Health Centers," *Medical Care*, Vol. 8, No. 2 (Mar.–Apr., 1970), entire issue.

Somers, H. H. and A. R. Somers. *Medicare and Hospitals*. Washington, D.C.: The Brookings Institute, 1967.

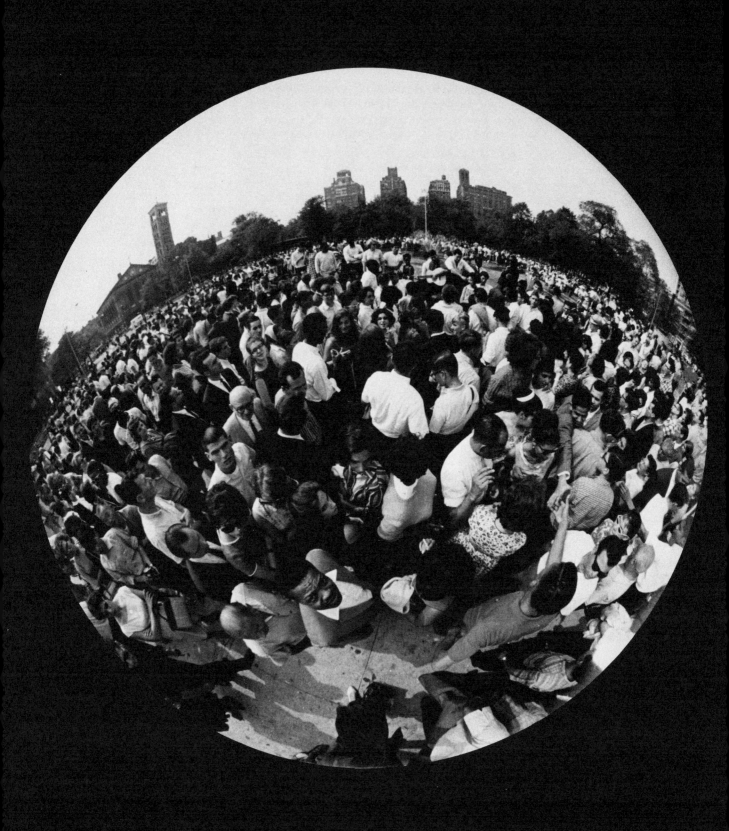

Part IV

HEALTH AND HUMANITY

Chapter 20

Population

The relationship between the health of a human population and its size has been recognized since man first began to wonder about himself. Plato, one of the architects of Western thought, prescribed an ideal size for a society—5040 citizens. Today we would call such a community a small town; America in the 1970s is an urban society most of whose population lives in or near cities of 50,000 or more. Plato's *Laws* and *Republic* are ancient history.

Until recently the relationship between health and population size was thought to be quite simple: a healthy human population grows. This assumption was supported by increasing rates of population growth and life expectancy at birth in most of the nations of the world. In recent years, however, as population problems of crowding, traffic, pollution, and urban unrest afflict rich and poor countries alike, we have begun to question whether humanity may not be reaching its limits of growth.

This chapter was contributed by Henry W. Vaillant, M.D., M.S. Hyg., Lecturer in Population Sciences, Harvard School of Public Health, and physician (internal medicine), Acton Medical Associates, Acton, Massachusetts.

Figure 20.1. In recent years, as population problems have arisen, we have begun to question whether humanity may not be reaching its limits of growth. (Jim Jowers, Nancy Palmer Photo Agency)

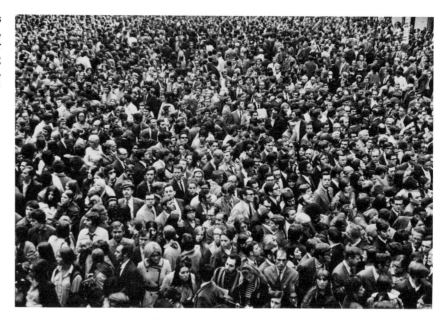

No one has yet established the level at which numbers of people become toxic, and the popularity of the jet plane, football games, mass religious meetings, and discotheques attests to man's desire for togetherness. Many of the most significant developments of our civilization, from the hanging gardens of Babylon to the successful voyage of the Apollo spacecraft, could not have taken place without the facilitating effect of high population density. At the same time, human existence without solitude and privacy is almost unendurable. No committee ever composed a symphony, hatched a hypothesis, or created a poem.

In this chapter we will consider some of the essentials of human population dynamics. Only by understanding what is known of the history, theory, and consequences of human population growth can the student make intelligent decisions about the future of the earth that will shelter his children.

WORLD POPULATION GROWTH AND DISTRIBUTION

At present the population of the world is approximately 3.7 billion, and each year the number increases by approximately 70 million. This large number is distributed over the world's landed surface, 36 billion acres, in a most uneven manner, as is summarized in Table 20.1. The wide disparity between numbers and density has evolved over time for a number of historical and ecologic reasons, which will be developed later in this chapter.

The demographic equation

In order to understand population size and distribution, one must first learn a little of the mathematics of population growth. The current popu-

How is land area used?

The world's land area is composed of approximately 36 billion acres, 56 million square miles, or 150 million square kilometers. A tenth of this area is beneath perpetual snow and ice, leaving 135 million square kilometers as potentially habitable. Half of this area is in turn excluded from cultivation by reason of cold, dryness, or altitude. Of the remaining 16 billion acres, or 67 million square kilometers, only a fifth, or 3.4 billion acres, are presently under cultivation. The remainder is jungle, forest, pasture, or "marginal" land. It is not exactly known how much of the world's land is covered by buildings, asphalt, and concrete, but in the United States as a whole the figure has been reliably estimated at 2 percent, although in the county of Los Angeles the figure is 50 percent.

Table 20.1 Distribution of world's population by continent, numbers, and density*

Name of continent	Number (millions of persons)	Area (million sq. km.)[a]	Density (persons/ sq. km.)
Africa	364	30	12
Asia, including Japan and Australia	2174	36	64
Central and South America	300	21	14
Europe, including the British Isles and Russia	697	27	26
North America	231	22	11

* From United Nations Statistical Yearbook, 1971; and 1972 World Population Data Sheet, Population Reference Bureau, Inc.
[a] 1 sq. km. = 0.386 sq. mile

lation (P_2) of any area at a given time is the result of the births (B), deaths (D), in-migrations (I), and out-migrations (O) that have occurred to the original population (P_1) over a given period of time. This is conveniently expressed by the *demographic equation*, $P_2 = P_1 + B + I - D - O$, which may be applied over any time period. Most nations conduct censuses at regular time intervals. In the United States the Constitution requires a census every ten years, while in Canada, the interval is five years. Births and deaths are recorded as they occur, but many nations of the world do not gather accurate data. In- and out-migration data can be gathered by nations, but town-to-town or city-to-city migration data are exceedingly difficult to obtain and exist only in a few Western European nations.

Each item in the demographic equation, with the exception of P, can be expressed as a rate that is relative to the population as a whole. The *crude birth rate*, for example, is obtained by dividing the number of births that occur during a given year by the total population in the middle of that year. This fraction is then multiplied by 1000 in order to express the rate per 1000 people. The crude death rate is similarly derived, as are in-migration (immigration) and out-migration (emigration) rates. Such rates are termed "crude" for an important reason. Death rates and birth rates vary by the age and sex of a population. Few births occur in an old age home, to cite an extreme example. The crude rates take no account of the age structure of the population, which is one of its most important characteristics. The crude birth rate minus the crude death rate is termed the *rate of natural increase*.

Doubling time

Another way to measure population growth is to determine the *doubling time*, the time it takes a given population to double in size. Although the doubling time for a bacterial population is only a matter of minutes, in the case of human populations it is a matter of decades or even centuries. The doubling time concept enables one to grasp the "compound interest" effects of seemingly tiny annual increments in population. Table 20.2 illustrates this relationship and indicates what a wide variation exists even today among the nations of the world.

*Table 20.2 Relationship between annual population growth rates and time necessary to double population**

Annual growth rate (per thousand)	Doubling time (in years)	Representative countries with such growth rates
1	693	Luxembourg
5	139	Czechoslovakia
10	70	United States
20	35	South Korea (and world rate)
30	23	Peru
40	17	Mexico (some areas)

* From *1972 World Population Data Sheet*, Population Reference Bureau, Inc.

One of the compelling reasons for learning about the dynamics of population growth is evident in Table 20.3, which illustrates the remark-

*Table 20.3 Growth of the world's population over time**

Year	Estimated world population (in millions)	Doubling time (in years)
1,000,000 B.C.	.1	
10,000 B.C.	5	150,000
Birth of Christ	250	1,500
1650 A.D.	500	200
1850 A.D.	1000	80
1930 A.D.	2000	45
1975 A.D.	4000	35

* From United Nations Population Division, *The Determinants and Consequences of Population Trends* (New York: United Nations, 1953). *United Nations Demographic Yearbook*, 1970.

able shortening of doubling time that has occurred during the brief instant of the world's history that man has lived on earth. Almost all human populations that have been studied since recorded history have grown, but rates of growth have varied widely according to the components of the demographic equation given above. When we consider that man in his present form has been inhabiting the earth for a mere one million of its three billion years (two seconds of a 90-minute television special) and that the idea of counting a whole population is only a few centuries old, we can appreciate the changes in growth rate even more. There is good reason to believe that the carrying capacity of what some people have termed "spaceship earth" is being reached, and the idea of the world's present population doubling by the time the children of the readers of this chapter begin to earn a living is disturbing. Many people have reacted to the vision of such a future by forming organizations such as Zero Population Growth.

CULTURAL EVOLUTION One of the most useful ways of understanding the leaps in human population growth that have occurred is to associate each decrease in doubling time with a step in cultural evolution. Although this oversimplifies a very complex process, it serves to highlight several important events. The first such step was the emergence of the

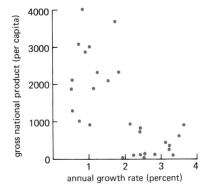

Table 20.4 *Relationship between the wealth of a nation and its rate of population growth: 29 representative nations**

Country	Gross National Product (in U.S. dollars)	Annual growth rate of population (in percent)
Sweden	4052	0.8
Canada	3755	1.7
Denmark	3110	0.7
Germany, West	3027	1.0
France	2906	0.9
Netherlands	2398	1.2
Iceland	2351	1.8
United Kingdom	2172	0.5
New Zealand	2165	1.5
Austria	1936	0.5
Japan	1904	1.1
Ireland	1393	0.5
Greece	1071	0.7
Spain	964	1.0
Singapore	960	2.1
Venezuela	921	3.6
South Africa	805	2.4
Chile	794	2.4
Mexico	662	3.5
Peru	436	3.1
Brazil	364	3.2
Algeria	304	3.2
Korea, South	141	2.4
Pakistan	133	3.3
Zaire	109	2.2
Indonesia	105	2.8
Nigeria	105	2.5
India	96	2.5
Ethiopia	69	1.9

* From *United Nations Demographic Year Book*, 1970.

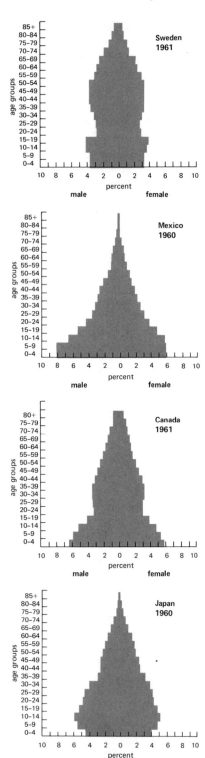

agricultural village as a mode of human settlement rather than a nomadic hunting and foraging existence. This probably occurred simultaneously in about 5000 B.C. in what is now China, India, and Egypt. The next steps included the development of marketing economics and the settlement of Northern Europe. The discovery of the New World in the fifteenth and sixteenth centuries set the stage for another major population advance made possible by the agricultural advances which the blending of European and pre-Columbian cultures allowed and the availability of the rich new lands of the Western Hemisphere for settlement. The final cultural evolutionary development was the Industrial Revolution beginning in the nineteenth century. The increased human and agricultural productivity made possible by harnessing the energy of coal and oil to machines and the astonishing advances in communications and housing which took place at the same time allowed people to live in relative health and wealth in cities as densely populated as Manhattan, Tokyo, and London. Other densely populated areas such as Biafra and Bangladesh, however, have not fared so well.

One of the foremost issues in any current global demographic survey is the fact that there are two populations which coexist on earth—the rich nations and the poor nations. Interestingly enough, the poor populations are growing more rapidly than the rich. This is illustrated in the scatter graph accompanying Table 20.4, on which the rate of population growth is plotted against the per capita income of some of the representative nations.

It is evident that the old axiom "The rich get richer and the poor have children" applies only too appropriately to the nations of the world. The implications for the future of a world in which the citizens of the more economically developed nations occupy a smaller and smaller proportion of the total population are difficult to ponder.

The population pyramid

The economic and social implications of demographic data can be understood in another way by examining the distribution of a country's population by age and sex. Information about the age and sex of a population is often gathered along with other data such as occupation, place of birth, place of residence, and race in the censuses that are conducted periodically by almost all nations. Census data describing the age and sex of a population are customarily expressed graphically as a population pyramid. Representative examples from 1960 and 1961 census data are illustrated in Figure 20.2. Notice the narrow base and relatively wide apex of the Swedish pyramid in contrast to the broad base and sliver-

Figure 20.2. Representative population pyramids. (From Q. H. Stanford, *The World's Population: Problems of Growth*, Oxford University Press, 1972, pp. 9–10. Reprinted by permission.)

shaped apex of Mexico. These are the result of the different demographic forces operating in each country: a low birth rate and low death rate in Sweden, prototype of the developed nation; and a high birth rate and falling death rate in Mexico, prototype of the less developed nation.

The differences between the two are not merely statistical curiosities. A population with many aged such as Sweden will have to provide extensive old-age services, such as pensions and medical care, whereas a nation like Mexico with many young citizens will have to provide a number of educational, maternal, and child-health services. Put another way, the top and bottom of the population pyramid, which are composed of non-workers, will be dependent on the middle layer for their support.

The population pyramids of Canada and Japan offer a different kind of contrast. They show the effect of historical events on population composition. In the case of Canada, the narrow "waist" of persons aged twenty to twenty-nine is the result of the voluntary limitation of birth rates which occurred in all industrialized Western nations during the Great Depression of the 1930s. In Japan the pyramid shows a relative deficiency of men aged thirty-five to forty-nine, a result of the number of soldiers who died in World War II. The Japanese pyramid also shows a rapidly shrinking base, which represents the effect of the promulgation of a liberalized abortion policy in 1948; this policy toppled the crude birth rate from 33 per 1000 population in 1949 to 25 in 1951 and 17 in 1957, the level that has been maintained ever since.

Population pyramids are also useful for predicting the trend of future population growth. In the case of Mexico one may guess that population growth is likely to be sustained when the large numbers of young people at the base reach reproductive age, whereas in Japan industrial planners are already concerned about the shortage of the labor force which is likely to develop in the 1980s.

THE AMERICAN POPULATION

The United States is an excellent illustration of many of the factors that affect population growth. From an initial figure of 4 million in the first census of 1790, the population had grown to 205 million inhabitants in the 1970 census. The most rapid growth took place during the extensive immigration of the nineteenth century and the post-World War II baby boom. The crude death rate has gradually declined over the nineteenth and early twentieth centuries from 30 to about 10 per 1000 inhabitants, as a result of improvements in housing, nutrition, and public health. It is now difficult to believe that outbreaks of malaria, yellow fever, smallpox, diphtheria, and cholera were common events in the United States at the turn of the century, or that pneumonia, influenza, tuberculosis, diarrhea, and enteritis were the major causes of death in 1900, striking children and young adults as their victims. Presently in the United States most deaths occur among the elderly who fall victim to degenerative disorders such as heart disease, cancer, and stroke. The major public health enemy to young adults appears to be the automobile, echoing Pogo's prophecy, "We have met the enemy and he is us."

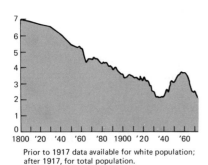

Prior to 1917 data available for white population; after 1917, for total population.

Figure 20.3. Total fertility rate (children per woman) United States—1800 to 1970.

Fertility has also declined over time in the United States, following a pattern similar to that in other industrialized nations. The large rural American family of colonial times has given way to the two-child suburban unit of today. This is illustrated in Figure 20.3, which indicates the gradual decline occurring in the average number of children born to a woman. The steadiness of the decline was interrupted, however, by a twenty-year "mountain" of births between 1945 and 1965, which has been nicknamed the "baby boom." The causes of the boom include the return of military forces from overseas after World War II, an unparalleled period of economic growth and prosperity, and the expansion of the American family's living space in the suburbs.

As the boom generation reaches adulthood, their presence has been felt in a number of ways. The generation first crowded elementary and secondary schools and now universities. They have been blamed for the campus turmoil of the late 1960s, the recent increase in highway accidents, and the increase in crime. Those who point with relief to the remarkable fall in United States births that has occurred in the 1970s must still contend with the enormous impact that the boom generation will have as they move into households of their own and demand employment opportunities.

American population distribution

Population distribution is also of considerable interest in the United States. Americans are a varied people—87.5 percent white, 11.1 percent black, and 1.4 percent other races (American Indian, Japanese, Chinese, Filipino, and many others). Population densities by state vary from

Population density and crime

The crime problems facing urban America will not be solved by increased force or firepower. We are witnessing a breakdown of the social mechanisms that once kept crime in check and gave direction and support to police activity. The small-town environments, rural or urban, which once framed and enforced their own moral codes, have virtually disappeared. We have become strangers sharing the largest collective habitats in human history. Because of the size and density of our newly evolving urban megalopolises, we have become more dependent on each other and more vulnerable to aberrant behavior than we have ever been before.

In our society few neighbors share beliefs or values. Although this heterogeneity may be intellectually desirable, it has crippled our ability to agree on the action required to maintain the social framework necessary to our continued survival. The very winds of liberation that have carried us this far may also have carried with them the seeds for our early demise.

The anonymous cities we have built, for maximum freedom and multiple choice, may have inadvertantly curtailed many of our previous options.... The concentration of population in large metropolitan areas has produced an urban form that makes hapless victims of its defenseless occupants.

From Oscar Newman, *Defensible Space* (New York: Macmillan, 1972).

0.5 per square mile in Alaska to 953 in New Jersey and a whopping 12,321 in the District of Columbia. About 73.5 percent of us live in urban areas which account for only 1.5 percent of the total lands of the United States. In addition, we are a highly mobile population. There is one automobile for every two persons, and it travels approximately 10,000 miles annually. Twenty percent of Americans move each year, and 50 percent have moved within the last five years.

METROPOLITAN DISPERSAL A particular characteristic of United States population distribution is what has been termed "metropolitan dispersal" by the Commission on Population Growth and the American Future appointed by the President in 1969. This term describes the increasing flight of the population within the last two decades from central cities to suburban areas surrounding the metropolis. This population shift, which may geographically be likened to the reaction of a stepped-on ant hill, has left a core city bereft of new investment or industry. Increasingly the core is inhabited only by the poor and unemployed, many of whom are black or relatively recent migrants from areas of rural poverty. Yet new jobs are not opening up in the cities but in suburban shopping malls and industrial parks, areas which are often many miles away from the urban core. This trend is expected to continue over the near term, and the current 22 percent non-white central city population is expected to increase to 40 percent by the year 2000.

Associated with the metropolitan dispersion is the enormous consumption of land in the suburbs by the new arrivals, typically families from the core who have bettered themselves economically or migrants from another metropolitan fringe area. The American ideal of a suburban home, two automobiles, and a half-acre of lawn is beginning to infringe upon land that is needed for farming, forestry, and recreation.

Figure 20.4. A result of "metropolitan dispersal"—a housing development in Queens, New York. (Ron Sherman, Nancy Palmer Photo Agency)

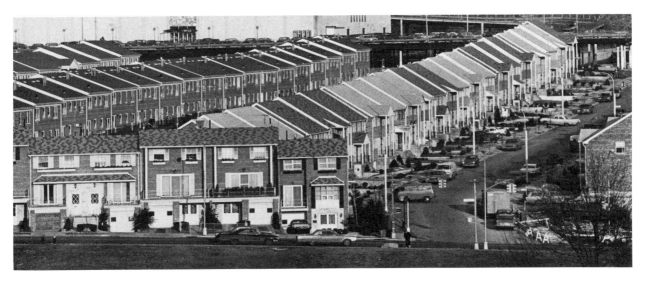

A logical question at this point is what happens next? Predicting future population growth is a hazardous occupation, as many demographers found out in the 1930s when declining birth rates led them to predict actual declines in population. At present the demographers usually make a series of predictions. Table 20.5 is an example of two alternative populations that might be found in the United States in the year 2000 under two different assumptions of population growth—an average two-child versus an average three-child family. It may surprise the reader that the two-child family will result in an increase of 66 million persons over a thirty-year period. Surely two children per couple is what zero population growth is all about! The explanation is, of course, that the large bulge of young persons born during the 1945–1965 baby boom will be producing their children before the death rates that old age brings will be operating upon themselves or their parents. Even if the two-child average (currently a reality) continues, this built-in momentum within the American population pyramid would not smooth out for several generations so that population growth will continue until the middle of the twenty-first century.

Table 20.5 United States population,
*1970 and 2000 (numbers in millions)**

	1970	2000	
		2-child average	3-child average
All ages	205	271	322
Under 5	17	20	34
5 to 17	53	55	80
18 to 21	15	17	24
under 18	70	75	114
18 to 64	115	167	179
65 and over	20	29	29
Dependency ratio[a]	.78	.62	.80

* Data are based on the Census Bureau's *Current Population Reports,* Series P-25, No. 470, "Projections of the United States by Age and Sex: 1970 to 2000." Table modified from *Population and the American Future —The Report of the Commission on Population Growth and the American Future* (New York: New American Library, 1972), p. 20.
[a] Number of persons 65 and over plus persons under 18 per 100 divided by persons aged 18 to 64.

In the case of the three-child family, the growth rate is larger and the geometric aspects of population growth become most evident when we compare the estimates for the year 2000: 271 million for the two-child family versus 322 million for the three-child family, and the estimates for the year 2020: 307 million versus 447 million for the three-child family. By 2070, extrapolation of these figures leads to a two-child expectation of 350 million and a three-child expectation of over 900 million persons.

**CONTROLLING
POPULATION GROWTH**

It is clear from these projections of population growth in the United States that it is appropriate to be concerned with limiting population growth. Controlling human reproduction depends upon an understanding of human fertility as well as upon a number of complex social and psychological issues involved in the personal motivation that leads to voluntary birth control. Once an individual or a couple has decided to limit their reproductive capacity, a number of alternative methods are available to them.

Human fertility

The study of human fertility is complicated by a number of paradoxes. Individual expression of human sexuality is a very private matter, but its natural outcome—reproduction—is the subject of a bevy of laws, sanctions, and other social controls. Sexuality is regulated by taboos against sexual contact in childhood and adolescence, against promiscuity, and against sexual contact among those whom society deems "unfit" such as prisoners and the physically and mentally ill. Such customs have arisen because society relies upon controlled human propagation for its own survival.

There are biological paradoxes, too. Although the *Guinness Book of Records* has authenticated the existence of one remarkable mother of thirty-two children (including four multiple births), the human female can only bear children for about thirty years. The relatively long period of infertility that is imposed by each pregnancy further limits the maximum theoretical number of offspring to fifteen or twenty, at most, assuming that the woman maintains perfect health, experiences regular ovulation, and has an ever present, always willing, biologically capable male partner during her entire reproductive period.

Reproductive capacity of the average woman

Although the earliest known human pregnancy occurred in a five-year-old girl and the latest in a woman over fifty, the average woman does not experience her first menstrual period until age twelve to fourteen and is not capable of bearing children until two years afterwards. Her ability to bear children then remains at a more or less constant level until age thirty-five, when it gradually declines until the menopause (cessation of menstrual periods), which occurs at an average age of forty-five.

The maximum number of pregnancies which can occur during these thirty years is about eighteen, a number which is rarely attained. This maximum is based upon the following assumptions:

The woman and her partner are in good health and are having sexual intercourse regularly without contraception. Under these circumstances, she will usually be pregnant within six months of "exposure."

She will then be infertile during the nine months of pregnancy and, in some women, for approximately six months after childbirth during lactation (breast feeding the newborn baby).

The cycle then begins again with another six months of "exposure," and repeats itself every twenty-one months.

The above assumptions make no allowance for fetal loss (spontaneous abortion, or miscarriage), which occurs in one out of every five pregnancies on the average. They also do not take into account the much longer lactation periods which are customary in many societies or the fact that some women do not remain infertile during lactation.

When one extends these individual limitations to whole societies, however, the "law of averages" begins to operate. This is illustrated by the experience of one of the most fertile populations ever studied, the Hutterites, an agrarian religious sect which inhabits an area located in Montana, North Dakota, and Canada. A careful demographic study found that in this society, where marriage is universally practiced, contraception is entirely eschewed, and maternal welfare is scrupulously supported, the average Hutterite woman produces an average of 10.4 children in her lifetime. This is of course far short of the theoretical maximum but is not likely to be exceeded. Of interest is the strong feeling of community within the sect, the rarity of divorce, the absence of premarital sex, and the extremely low crude death rate of 4.4 per 1000 per year. The latter is the result of the agricultural life style, excellent medical care ($300–$500 is spent per capita on the average Hutterite's health), and most important the broad-based population pyramid that results from such a remarkable reproductive performance. The crude birth rate among the Hutterites is 46 per 1,000 per year.

Other societies that have approached the Hutterites' performance have been the French Canadian immigrants in Quebec and some of the eighteenth-century American colonists. The social conditions of strong religious tradition and an agricultural society with open lands that produced these reproductive rates do not endure for long.

FACTORS LIMITING FERTILITY After citing these biologic maximums, one must consider some of the limiting factors. In most societies women do not engage in sexual intercourse before the age of eighteen and in some cases, such as Ireland, a substantial proportion of women may remain celibate all their lives. Marriage may be interrupted by separation, intercourse may be forbidden at certain times by religious custom, and divorce or widowhood may be extremely common. When one adds to this the frequent practice of contraception (almost universal in the United States at present), the incidence of induced abortion and sterilization, and the high infant mortality that affects so many societies still, it is not difficult to see why the usual number of living children in a family seldom exceeds eight in any society. Infertility is also much more common than generally realized and affects between one out of five and one out of ten couples. Therefore, in most societies today, the average number of births to a couple rarely exceeds six.

BIRTH CONTROL The term *birth control* refers to any action taken by an individual that will limit the number of children produced by that person's sexual activity. There are many methods of birth control, including abstinence from sexual intercourse, sterilization, and the use of various artificial means to prevent conception. *Contraception* refers to the use of drugs or devices to limit fertility.

Birth control has been an important practice since the earliest times

Figure 20.5. Growing population rates have increased the awareness of the need for effective means of birth control. (Courtesy of World Health Organization, photo by Paul Almasy)

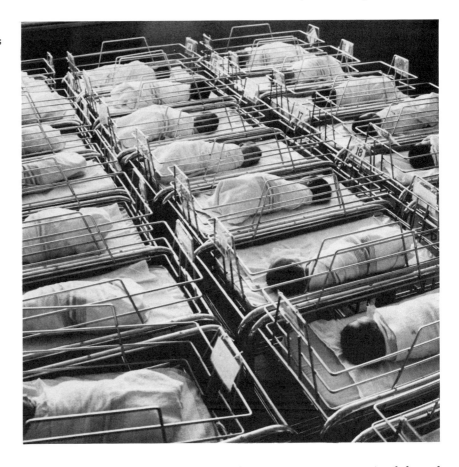

when people relied upon such methods as coitus interruptus (withdrawal of the penis from the vagina before ejaculation), douching (irrigating the vagina with water after intercourse), and occlusive devices made of fibers, gums, and even dung that were inserted into the vagina before intercourse. Similarly, abortion and even infanticide have been regularly practiced although the latter has often been disguised under other names.

Contraception has an interesting and oftentimes colorful history which has featured many women as the leading proponents of reform in the battle to liberalize laws affecting voluntary control of human reproduction. The accomplishments of such figures as Annie Besant, Margaret Sanger, Marie Stopes, and Harriet Pilpel deserve the appreciation of man and woman alike.

Modern contraception had its beginning in the sixteenth century when a condom was developed in the form of impregnated linen sheath. Subsequently, sheep intestine was used, and in 1844 the vulcanization of rubber made mass production possible. Although originally designed to prevent the promiscuous male from contracting venereal disease, the condom was soon popularized as a birth control method by pamphlets

Margaret Sanger

In 1873, Anthony Comstock, head of the New York Society for the Suppression of Vice, persuaded Congress to pass a law against interstate commerce in obscene and pornographic literature. The act of Congress, known as the Comstock Law, specifically classed birth-control information with obscenity and forbade its distribution by mail.

In 1912 a young nurse attended a young woman who had just performed an abortion on herself—the second time the woman had done so in four months. The woman died; and the nurse, Margaret Sanger, resolved to change the destiny of women in America. Specifically, she resolved to provide birth-control information to anyone who wanted it. Sanger was able to get birth-control information only from France (where birth-control had been accepted since the Revolution). She published this information in the U.S.; and, because dissemination of contraceptive information was at that time a federal offense, she was brought to trial. However, her trial was not carried through; and eventually she was released, because Comstock, the leading proponent of the federal statute, had died, and because mounting public pressure in favor of Margaret Sanger made Congress and the courts reluctant to pursue the matter.

After a cross-country lecture tour, Sanger opened this country's first birth-control clinic, in New York. She was soon arrested and her clinic closed, but while in jail she taught birth-control methods to the other prisoners. The Comstock Law was changed, and physicians were allowed to give married women contraceptive advice if it was beneficial to their health. Meanwhile, Sanger campaigned tirelessly. She opened birth-control clinics all over the world. The manufacture and sale of contraceptives and the dissemination of birth-control advice is now permitted in all U.S. states—even in Massachusetts, the last holdout. Margaret Sanger lived to see her life's work succeed.

From Janet J. Lieberman, "A Short History of Contraception," *The American Biology Teacher* (Sept. 1973), pp. 318, 337.

and advertisements. Its acceptance in the English-speaking world at least was attested to by polls in both England and the United States in the late 1950s that indicated that it was the most commonly used method of contraception by married couples.

The development of the diaphragm by Mensinga, a Dutch physician, soon followed in the late 1880s. Its use was pioneered by the feminist birth-control clinic movement which helped to popularize this effective method.

The development of oral contraceptives, surely one of the most remarkable inventions in medicine, was a result of three factors: (1) a greater understanding by endocrinologists of the hormones that control ovulation, (2) inexpensive synthesis of the complicated steroid molecule by chemists and the drug industry, and (3) courageous and imaginative clinical investigations of the newly synthesized components by Drs. John Rock, Gregory Pincus, and Celso Ramon Garcia.

The intrauterine device (IUD) had been known in principle since the nineteenth century when certain surgical devices introduced in the uterus were found to result in sterility. Early in the twentieth century coiled silk thread and silver wire were used for this purpose but occasional serious infections resulted in the abandonment of this practice except in Israel and Japan. The synthesis of polyethylene and biologically inert plastics led to a resurgence of interest in this idea in the 1960s and the development of a number of satisfactory devices of assorted shapes and sizes.

METHODS OF CONTRACEPTION

The condom

What makes the condom a perpetual bestseller in the contraception trade are its availability, low cost, and reliability. Because their manufacture is regulated by the Food and Drug Administration, almost all condoms are of high quality and very unlikely to break or leak. In addition, the condom provides a fairly effective barrier against venereal disease. The condom is a male-responsible method which has almost no side effects other than the interruption of foreplay and a slight dulling of male sensation, a potential advantage in men who are prone to premature ejaculation.

The condom is usually packaged pre-rolled and is best rolled onto the erect penis. Care must be taken to allow the slack and uninflated portion of the device to remain at the tip of the penis. Otherwise the condom may burst, or air may force the ejaculate to leak out at the penile base.

Condom protection is 95 percent effective, which means that a group of married couples using the condom faithfully over a year would experience three to five pregnancies per hundred couples per year. Condom protection can be increased by using it together with a female-responsible method such as a spermicide.

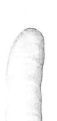

Figure 20.6. Condom.

The diaphragm

The diaphragm is one of the safest and most reliable of all female-responsible contraceptive methods. It is also one of the most difficult to use because of the high degree of motivation and forethought it requires. Diaphragms are made of latex with a coil or flat-spring rim and are invariably used together with a spermicidal cream or jelly. The diaphragm must be fitted by a skilled doctor or midwife, and it must be inserted before intercourse on every occasion.

Before use, the diaphragm is coated on one side with the spermicide; it is then carefully folded and inserted into the vagina in such a way as to completely cover the uterine cervix. After inserting the device, the user must be able to feel the uterine cervix with her finger; the latex dome of the diaphragm should be interposed between the two. If the device has been properly fitted, neither the woman nor her partner should be aware of the diaphragm during intercourse. It is advisable to insert the diaphragm no more than two hours before intercourse because the spermicide loses effectiveness over time. The interruption of foreplay to insert the diaphragm may result in inaccurate placement. The diaphragm should not be removed until eight hours after intercourse. The user should be examined annually so that the diaphragm can be refitted if necessary.

The need for privacy, self exploration, and advance planning makes the diaphragm suitable for only a limited number of couples. Nevertheless, its effectiveness (three to five pregnancies per hundred women per

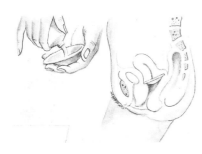

Figure 20.7. Diaphragm and spermicidal jelly.

year) and lack of medical side effects have assured it a permanent place in the contraceptive choices open to today's couples.

Spermicides

Spermicides are so named because they contain chemicals that kill the spermatazoa before they reach the lining of the uterus. They are marketed as foams, jellies, and creams which are sold without a prescription.

They are usually injected into the vagina with a plastic syringe about thirty minutes before intercourse. When used together with a diaphragm or condom, they are thoroughly reliable. When used alone, effectiveness is in the 90 percent category.

Users must be cautioned to reapply a dose if intercourse is repeated and to avoid the more convenient pellet or suppository products, which often do not melt before intercourse takes place.

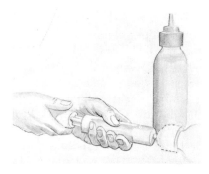

Figure 20.8. Spermicidal vaginal foam and applicator.

The pill

Oral contraceptive steroids, "the pill," are virtually 100 percent effective when taken as directed. Composed of synthetic compounds which have actions similar to the natural female hormones estrogen and progesterone, they are safe for most women to take. However, because they can be dangerous in certain cases they must be prescribed by a physician who has performed a thorough examination of the woman planning to use them.

Oral contraceptives act by preventing ovulation. In almost all women, the ovulatory cycle is restored at once upon stopping the pill or even forgetting one or two.

As with any prescription, the oral contraceptives may cause side effects. Common ones include changes in the menstrual period (usually scantier), weight gain, breast tenderness, and nausea or even vomiting. Less common but more dangerous are circulatory problems such as strokes, blood clots to the lung, and inflamed veins.

Because of its almost total effectiveness and the separation of its use from the sexual act, the pill has become the most popular contraceptive method in many countries, especially among younger women. A high degree of motivation is necessary to use the pill because the woman must remember to take one pill every day without fail for twenty or twenty-one days out of a twenty-eight-day cycle.

There are many different formulas of oral contraceptives on the market. The appropriate one is best chosen by a physician who is thoroughly familiar with the medical history of the user. Anybody using the pill must be examined regularly.

Newer formulations are being actively developed including the "minipill," a low-dose pill which, it is hoped, can achieve the same 100 percent protection with a lower dose hormone. Unfortunately, the data so far indicate that current minipills are associated with menstrual irregularities and a 2 to 3 percent pregnancy rate.

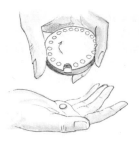

Figure 20.9. Contraceptive pills.

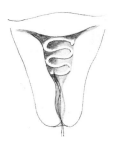

Figure 20.10. Intrauterine contraceptive device.

The intrauterine device

The intrauterine device (IUD) is not a contraceptive method to be adopted lightly. It requires insertion under surgically clean conditions by a pair of expert hands. It is not suitable for all women. It may be expelled or produce unpleasant and even serious side effects.

The IUD is inserted into the uterus via a tube which is passed through the cervix. Insertion causes mild pain, particularly in women who have not borne children. Once in place, it is ordinarily trouble free and provides constant protection against pregnancy by making the uterine lining inhospitable to the implantation of the fertilized egg.

Side effects may include discharge, excess blood loss during menstruation, bleeding between periods, and cramps. Serious side effects are rare but may include infection, perforation of the uterus, or pregnancy and its complications. Occasionally, the IUD is expelled involuntarily by the uterus during the menstrual period, an event which is usually noticed by the user. Most devices have thin threads which protrude through the cervix and allow the user to check that it is still in place. Side effects are more common in women who have not borne children, but many successful users of the IUD have never been pregnant.

The contraceptive effects of the IUD are easily reversed by removal, which is quite simple but must also be done by trained personnel. The effectiveness is in the 97 to 98 percent category. The IUD is cheap, costing less than a dollar wholesale, but the medical supervision that it necessitates makes its cost approximately equal to that of the pill.

Sterilization

When a couple has completed its family and both partners are confident that the marriage is a stable one, sterilization is often the birth control method of choice.

Male sterilization, or vasectomy, refers to cutting and tying of the vas deferens, a surgical procedure which can be done in a clinic in less than half an hour. The effect of the operation is to make the male ejaculate spermatozoa free.

Female sterilization, also called tubal ligation or cautery, requires more time and anaesthesia than the male procedure because the abdomen must be entered with surgical instruments. There are various procedures used which involve burning or tying and cutting of the fallopian tubes.

Sterilization in no way affects the hormone balance of the body, nor does it affect one's sex life. For practical purposes, however, it must be considered irreversible and is not a procedure to be undertaken without careful deliberation.

ABORTION The most common and decisive method of fertility control is abortion. In recent years the legal position on abortion has softened considerably and it is now available to most women who wish it.

There are three types of abortion. *Spontaneous abortion* occurs in about one-fifth of pregnancies and in many cases it must be completed by surgical procedure called dilation and curettage (see below). *Illegal abortions* are those performed by nonphysicians, may be extremely dangerous, and are fortunately less common now than formerly when it was difficult to obtain a legal abortion.

Legal abortions, sometimes called legal termination of pregnancy, are performed by physicians in hospitals or special clinics. They are performed under sterile conditions and are ordinarily quite safe. Typically, they are done during the first three months of pregnancy by one of two methods: dilation and curettage or vacuum aspiration. Dilation and curettage involves dilating the cervix, the neck of the uterus, with special instruments and then scraping the lining of the uterus with a curette, a specially designed scalpel to remove the fetus and membranes. Vacuum aspiration, involves sucking out the tissues with a specially designed suction pump and plastic nozzle. For both techniques local or general anaesthesia is necessary, but the patient can usually go home the same day. Complications are rare, although there is some evidence that premature births may occur more commonly after the procedure. Similarly, there may be an increased risk of Rh sensitization (mother's immunity to the blood cells of subsequent fetuses).

After the third month of pregnancy abortion becomes more complicated and hazardous. The usual method is to inject a salt solution into the pregnant uterus through a needle. This results in the death of the fetus and placenta, and a spontaneous abortion usually ensues within the next 24 to 48 hours. Overnight hospitalization is necessary. Another method involves surgically opening the uterus and removing its contents. Again hospitalization is necessary and the patient will need to deliver any subsequent pregnancies by Caesarian section. Clearly there is no substitute for effective contraception, or if it fails, early diagnosis of pregnancy. Fortunately, current laboratory procedures permit accurate diagnosis of pregnancy within two weeks after the first missed menstrual period.

IN CONCLUSION   Modern man has developed and now has at his disposal a number of safe and effective means of birth control to control population growth. The American population currently exceeds 200 million, and in 1970 it was confidently predicted on the basis of observed birth and death rates that the U.S. population would exceed 300 million by the year 2000. However, no sooner had this prediction become well established than the American birth rate declined quite suddenly to a figure which is only slightly above the rate required to maintain a stable population. However, the growth rate of the world population has not been reduced, and for many reasons it is clear that the populations of the world cannot continue to increase at present rates for an indefinite period and still maintain present standards of living. Thus it is vital and necessary that all people become informed of the population problem and the methods of control. The Rev. Dr. Martin Luther King in a speech delivered on receiving the Margaret Sanger Award in Human Rights in 1966 summed up the essence of the population problem with these words: "Unlike plagues of the dark ages or contemporary diseases we do not yet understand, the modern plague of overpopulation is soluble by means we have discovered and with resources we possess. What is lacking is not sufficient knowledge of the solution but universal consciousness of the gravity of the problem and education of the billions who are its victims."

Questions
1. What is the relationship between population density and the quality of life?
2. Why are crude demographic rates so named? Can you think of a more precise way of expressing death and birth rates?
3. What were some of the cultural developments that led to more rapid rates of population increase?
4. Why do you think that population growth is occurring more rapidly in poor countries? Would national family planning programs be likely to affect birth rates in such countries?
5. What can a population pyramid tell you about demographic events in the past? In the future?
6. What method of contraception would you suggest for: (a) a high school student hitchhiking to a rock festival, (b) a college couple who were going steady, (c) a couple who had been happily married for fifteen years and whose youngest child was six? Justify your answers.

Key Concepts
Census – an official enumeration of the population of a nation
Crude birth rate – the number of births occurring in a population during a calendar year divided by the midyear population; usually expressed as a rate per 1000
Crude death rate – the number of deaths occurring in a population during a calendar year divided by the midyear population; usually expressed as a rate per 1000
Demography – the science which studies vital and social statistics, such as the births, deaths, diseases, marriages, migrations, and other factors, of populations
Life expectancy – a calculation in which the age and specific death rates for a given period are summarized to produce an average length of life of a member of a synthetic population
Population pyramid – a graphic representation of age-sex data of a population

Selected Readings
Commission on Population Growth and the American Future. *Population and the American Future.* New York: New American Library, 1972.
Ehrlich, P. R., and A. H. Ehrlich. *Population, Resources, Environment: Issues in Human Ecology.* San Francisco: W. H. Freeman and Co., 1972.
Heer, D. M. *Society and Population.* Englewood Cliffs, N.J.: Prentice-Hall, 1968.
National Academy of Sciences. *Rapid Population Growth: Consequences and Policy Implications.* Baltimore: Johns Hopkins Press, 1971.
Peel, J., and M. Potts. *Textbook of Contraceptive Practice.* Cambridge: Cambridge University Press, 1969.
Stanford, Q. H. *The World's Population, Problems of Growth.* Toronto: Oxford University Press, 1972.

Chapter 21

Man and his Environment

Ecology is the branch of science concerned with the interrelationship of living organisms and their environment. Within this term it is appropriate to consider both the fitness of an environment to sustain life and the ability of organisms to tolerate their environment. Unfortunately, "the word 'ecology' has come to be used as if it were a slogan, not the name of a branch of science."[1] Although one usually thinks of the changeable external world as the important environment, in reality, we are totally dependent upon the constancy of an inner environment that is unique to man. In a number of very vital ways, the internal environment resists change, called *homeostasis*, to a remarkable degree and this makes it possible for man to live in a variety of external environments,

[1] John Maddox, *The Doomsday Syndrome* (New York: McGraw-Hill, 1972), p. vi.

This chapter was contributed by Melvin W. First, Sc.D., Professor of Environmental Health Engineering, Kresage Center for Environmental Health, Harvard School of Public Health, and Chairman of the Advisory Committee on Environmental Health to the Massachusetts Department of Public Health.

many of them involving extremes of temperature, sunlight, rainfall, and altitude. Man alone has the ability to regulate his external environment in accordance with his own ideas and hence to extend his habitat into physical environments that otherwise would be inhospitable. Nevertheless, it has become possible for modern man to alter adversely his natural environment so greatly that his internal environment becomes unable to maintain its accustomed uniformity and disease results. When this occurs, the environment is called *polluted*. Although man-made ecological catastrophe on a world-wide scale is at least theoretically possible by overpopulation and technological excess, man has proven himself to be a tough and extraordinarily adaptable creature. It is not apparent that his fate is in any way tied to that of the whale, the caribou, or the osprey. For example, the extinction of the passenger pigeon has had no discernible effect on man's survival during the 100-year interval since it occurred. Nonetheless, this experience, among others, has sensitized Americans to the need to preserve as much of the natural environment as possible; for moral and aesthetic reasons, if for no others.

Figure 21.1. (Ron Sherman, Nancy Palmer Photo Agency)

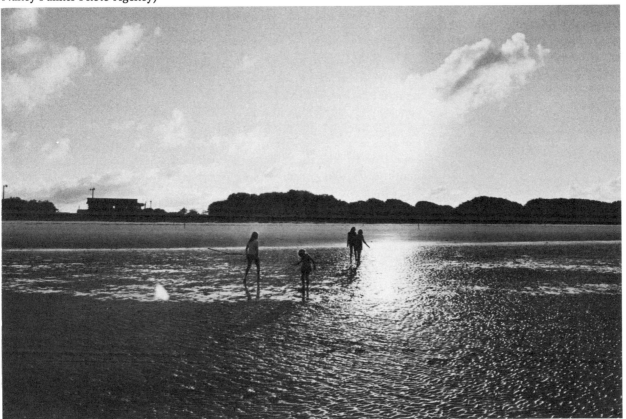

THE NATURAL
ENVIRONMENT

Unity of the environment

When one examines the structure of federal and state environmental protection agencies, public health departments, and universities that have programs concerned with environmental protection, it is apparent that the environment has been subdivided into water, air, radiation and occupational health protection, housing, etc. Although each part of the environment has its special aspects, much of the diversification is historical. In a very real sense, the environment is one.

The concept of the unity of the environment has an important implication for the future—the degradation of one element of the total environment is likely to result in some degree of degradation for all other elements as they interact through time and space.

The resources of the world are fixed and finite. Basically they consist of the substances that compose land and water plus the daily input of energy from the sun. The elements that constitute the earth and the seas may be used in many ways—they may be transmuted into many forms and they may be reused over and over again, as they have been for millions of years—but through it all, the world's supply is neither enhanced nor diminished. It remains the same. This concept is referred to as the *conservation of matter* and it means that the basic physical substance of the world can neither be created nor destroyed, but only converted into new forms with the simultaneous addition or release of energy.

The important conclusion to be drawn from these fundamental considerations of matter and energy is that the resources of the earth are limited to whatever is available today. This concept has been expressed concisely by referring to our world as "spaceship earth." By analogy with the vehicles that transport astronauts to outer space, it emphasizes the idea of a self-contained, self-sufficient closed system. Since this has been true for the earth since its beginnings, why has it now become a matter of serious concern?

The answer is that while the world's resources are fixed, the population is not. This was recognized as long ago as 1798, when Thomas Malthus published his *Essay on the Principle of Population*. This treatise states that population, unrestrained by natural forces, grows much more rapidly than the food supply, with the inevitable result of worldwide starvation. This gloomy conclusion is apparently contradicted by the present record population and record food surpluses, but Malthus's mathematics have not been forgotten. *The Limits to Growth*, by Dennis Meadows and others, not only reiterates Malthus's warning, but also extends his conclusions to now-scarce fuels and mineral resources and considers the detrimental effects of environmental pollution.

However, both Malthus and Meadows base their analyses on the assumption that present trends will continue, and there are many who disagree with that premise. One of the more readable accounts for nonscientists is *The Doomsday Syndrome*, by John Maddox. While it is

The nitrogen and phosphorus cycles

Amino acids, the building blocks of protein, essential structural components of living cells, contain the element nitrogen in combined form. Although the atmosphere contains 80 percent nitrogen, the element in that form is usable only by certain algae, soil bacteria, and a few plants called *legumes* (peas, beans), that are able to extract nitrogen from the air. All plants extract nitrogen from soil and water as dissolved nitrate salts and synthesize plant proteins. Plants are eaten by animals that transform them to animal proteins. Animals excrete nitrogenous wastes during life, such as urea in urine. When animals die, decay bacteria in water and soil convert tissue proteins to ammonia which is converted to nitrites by special bacteria in the soil and these, in turn, are converted to nitrates by other bacteria in the soil. In the form of nitrates, nitrogen can, again, be

utilized by plants and the cycle starts again.

In ways similar to those that apply to nitrogen, other essential elements of life are recycled continuously. The utilization of phosphorus in the oceans illustrates the process on a less than global scale. Phosphorus is believed to be the limiting nutrient in the seas, and the amount of living matter in the oceans expands as the quantity of phosphorus extractable from the water declines. By the time the rapid spring growth period reaches its peak, the phosphorus content of the water has declined to about one-half its maximum value. During summer, fall, and winter, sea organisms die at a faster rate than they are replaced and, in fact, reproduction ceases entirely for most species in northern climates. During this period, the dead bodies settle to the bottom of the sea where they are decomposed by

bacteria to simple salts. In this way, phosphorus, as soluble phosphate, returns to the upper layers of the ocean for reuse the next spring. As a consequence, in northern waters, phosphorus reaches an annual maximum concentration in December or January and a minimum in May or June. The introduction of large new sources of phosphorus from widespread use of phosphate detergents and phosphate fertilizers has upset the natural nutrient balance in some inland lakes and ponds, permitting runaway growth of vegetation that ultimately dies, rots, and turns these waters into foul-smelling cesspools. Other than in the immediate vicinity of sewage discharges from large urban areas, the oceans are too vast to have felt the effects of manmade phosphorus discharges.

reasonable to conclude that the world population cannot continue to increase at present rates while maintaining its present standard of living, it is by no means certain that present population and consumption trends will continue. Recent awareness that careful conservation of materials and energy sources is prudent policy, reinforced by a search for ways to reuse discarded items, cannot fail to become the wave of the future for all responsible citizens.

Dynamic nature of the natural environment

The environment has many ways by which it resists alteration. It is not a fragile system that is easily disturbed. If it were, it would have been destroyed by earthshaking events (such as earthquakes and volcanic eruptions) which, from geological evidence, must have occurred frequently long before man appeared in this world. Nevertheless, modern man has found ways, inadvertently, to produce severe dislocations of the environment that are not easily and rapidly correctable by the forces of nature, with or without the active assistance of humans.

In all but a few outstanding instances, such as DDT and nonbiodegradable detergents, the contaminants discharged to the environment by humans differ only marginally from those produced in nature and, in most cases, naturally produced quantities greatly exceed those gener-

Waste sources

All living organisms affect their external environment by extracting nutrients essential to their growth and reproduction and discharging into it the waste products of their metabolism. Green plants in sunlight extract carbon dioxide from the air for their nutrition and discharge oxygen as a waste product (the same oxygen that is an essential of life for animals). Countless examples of the waste products of one organism becoming the nourishment of another could be cited to emphasize the almost infinite diversity in food requirements that characterizes the biological world. It is highly desirable that this should be so; otherwise the competition among species for a few essential substances would surely have denied to most species a special ecological niche within which each experiences a minimal challenge from competitors for the same or similar nutrients. This not only means that every nutrient must be reused countless times to satisfy the nutritional requirements of the teeming biological world, but, because during some usages the nutrient becomes degraded to simpler compounds with less energy potential, there must be processes whereby the nutrient can be rebuilt for reuse by organisms that are different from those that degraded it. Were this not a fact, essential elements for life would have been exhausted by myriad organisms millions of years before man evolved.

ated by man. More carbon monoxide is emitted from the oceans as a result of underwater decay processes than the total from all the world's automobile tail pipes; more sulfur-containing gases are discharged by volcanic activity, hot springs, and similar geological events than from all the chimneys burning sulfur-bearing coal and oil; more tons of particles are discharged to the air from dust storms, rock erosion, volcanic eruptions, forest fires, sea spray, and similar natural events than from all the steel mills, smelters, rock-crushing plants, and other industries operated by man.

It is reasonable to ask why, if only one-fifth of the emissions to the atmosphere originate with man, we have become so concerned about control of man-made sources. The explanation lies in the severely restricted area within which man discharges his wastes. If man's emissions were distributed evenly throughout the world, as natural emissions tend to be, pollution problems would, once again, recede to the status of localized nuisances. But, of course, populations are not evenly distributed. In the United States, approximately 70 percent of the population lives on less than 1 percent of the total land area. More specifically, the population clusters in a few heavily populated metropolitan areas. The trend toward urbanization has been evident from census figures since the founding of the Republic but this trend has greatly accelerated in recent decades, as may be seen from Table 21.1. It shows that during the 60 year period from 1920 to 1980, the number of people living in cities of 100,000 or greater will have increased from 35 to 150 million. These figures not only reflect a vigorous growth of the total population but, of even greater significance, a tidal wave of migration from farms and small towns into the large cities. In only 200 years, the population of the U.S. has changed from approximately 95 percent farmers to 95 percent town and city dwellers. This trend is shown dramatically in the aerial photographs of Biscayne Bay, Miami, Florida, taken only

*Table 21.1 Land area and population density of U.S.**
(urban areas of 100,000 population or greater)

	1920	1940	1960	1980[a]	2000[a]
No. urbanized areas over 100,000 population	70	98	160	194	223
Total population (in millions)	34.6	52.4	91.0	148	221
Total land area (square miles)	5,261	8,919	21,500	38,592	59,090
Population density per square mile	6,580	5,870	4,230	3,840	3,732

* From Jerome Pickard, *Dimensions of Metropolitanism* (Washington, D.C.: Urban Land Institute, Research Monograph 14, 1967), pp. 48–53.
[a] Estimated.

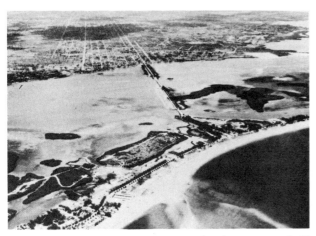 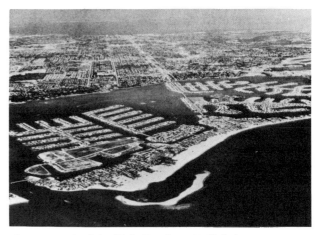

Figure 21.2. Biscayne Bay, Miami, Florida, in 1949 (left) and in 1969 (right). (Bob Graeber, Airflight)

20 years apart (Fig. 21.2). As a consequence, when one travels from coast to coast, the impression is very strong that we live in a vast empty country. Of equal interest in Table 21.1 are the figures that show population density in urban areas declining from 6,600 to 3,800 per square mile during this same 60 year period. This is statistical confirmation that modern cities have grown in area even more rapidly than in population; this growth is usually referred to as *urban sprawl*. One of the consequences of urban sprawl is the total dependence of urban populations on private automobile transportation. Automobiles, in turn, are responsible for many of the plagues of modern life—smog, noise, congestion, accidental deaths—but are also responsible for hitherto unknown freedom of choices for a place to live, to work, and to engage in a wide variety of recreational activities. Another benefit is access to all manner of educational and medical services and facilities. Whatever one's personal evaluation of the relative importance of the many benefits and disadvantages of this strong trend toward worldwide urbanization, it is a fact. It is the most important factor in environmental pollution.

SELF-PURIFYING CAPABILITY The self-purifying capabilities of the natural environment are real, measurable, and effective, but they are finite. When people settle in very large numbers on small land areas, the self-purifying forces are unable to transform wastes into innocuous (harmless) materials at a fast enough rate to avoid pollution. Therefore, the state of the environment at any moment is the result of a balance between the rate at which contaminants are discharged into it and the natural rate at which purifying reactions occur. When the rate of purification exceeds the contamination rate, a clean environment results; when the reverse occurs, pollution results.

The concentration of carbon dioxide in the atmosphere in the days

The biosphere

The totality of life, both seen and unseen, surrounds man, the dominant species. It threatens him on every side while sustaining him in life. Every item of his diet, except water and table salt, is derived from a plant or animal and, until the introduction about 35 years ago of synthetic materials derived entirely from petroleum, the same could be said for all of his clothing. Man's position as the dominant species is of very recent vintage on the evolutionary scale, perhaps only 10,000 to 20,000 years. During prehistory, he experienced severe competition from hordes of larger and stronger beasts but, by developing weapons and sophisticated team hunting techniques, he exterminated the animals that preyed on him and learned to tame those that could be useful to him. He also learned to cultivate grains and a few other food plants that enabled him to secure stocks of stable foodstuffs that could sustain him for long periods. All of this happened when man occupied only a small portion of the world's entire land area and it only required an increase in population for man to take complete and undisputed possession of the entire world.

when the precursor substances that formed coal and oil were alive must have been vastly higher than today to account for the huge amount of carbon that has been locked in the earth for millions of years. Man evolved and adapted to the atmosphere we know today. The burning of coal, oil, and natural gas is returning carbon to the environment in the form of carbon dioxide too rapidly for any possibility of a new adaptive change on the part of man. Carbon dioxide from the burning of carbon-containing fossil fuels accumulates in the atmosphere because the natural removal pathways, principally the oceans by deposition on the ocean bottom as insoluble carbonate rock, are unable to accept more than half the amount produced. Without the oceans, carbon dioxide would accumulate in the atmosphere at double its current rate. If, at some future time, the world's energy needs should be supplied by nuclear, solar, or other forms that do not require the combustion of carbon-containing fuels, the emission of carbon dioxide will decline, but removal in the oceans will continue unchanged. This means that the steady increase in the carbon dioxide content of the atmosphere will be reversed and, after a time (probably many decades) the concentration of this gas in the atmosphere will return to levels that existed before the Industrial Revolution began. For pollutants that produce prompt detrimental effects (carbon dioxide has no known undesirable effect at the levels it is likely to reach within the next hundred or so years), emission limitations are required until the natural purification processes of the atmosphere can change the remaining emissions into innocuous substances with a comfortable margin of safety.

Water, as well as air, can purify itself to an extent, but again there are limits, as the following example will show. By the beginning of the present century, sanitary engineers in Massachusetts had surveyed a sufficient number of streams and evaluated their sanitary quality to establish the self-purification capacity of rivers in terms of dry weather flow and human population density settled on the water shed. They determined that the critical factor in natural purification was the volume of flow in the stream and that a minimum stream flow (that is, during the lowest period of the year) of 56 gallons per second per 1,000 people on the water shed was adequate to preserve the quality of the water for all uses throughout its course. Per person flow rates of this magnitude are no longer attainable in the vicinity of large cities and water purification procedures must be resorted to when remote, protected water supplies of adequate capacity are not available. Nevertheless, the self-purification capacity of natural waters, whether flowing or still, is real and of genuine importance in safeguarding remote water supplies for use by large cities. Further, this self-purification capacity helps establish the degree that wastes must be purified before being emptied into a stream: for example, a flow of 56 gallons per second will be adequate for 10,000 people if the sewage is purified 90 percent before release.

Important purification processes occur on land when solid and liquid wastes are deposited on or under the surface. These include normal soil microorganisms that are capable of converting most waste products to simpler substances that are reusable by plants and the filtration properties of porous soils through which liquids containing suspended matter flow. Large landfills containing municipal wastes often overload the assimilative capabilities of the ground, and contamination, dissolved in rain water, can flow to surface and subsurface water supplies. Intensive animal production at cattle feed lots, poultry farm-factories, and similar activities produce manure in amounts that far exceed the assimilative capacity of nearby farm lands. In Vermont, for example, spring runoff of rain and melted snow from the hills brings a heavy load of contamination to the local streams from the winter's accumulation of wastes from the dairy herds. It is evident, from this, that serious environmental pollution can result from modern methods of intensive animal farming in rural areas as well as from the crowding together of humans in urban centers.

POISONS IN THE ENVIRONMENT   All forms of life discharge wastes into the environment. In all instances, except for man, these wastes are reusable in one form or another, as shown by the nitrogen and phosphorus cycles. These kinds of wastes are known as *biodegradable*, meaning that natural processes are capable of transforming them into useful substances. Farmers put this knowledge to practical use by using animal manures to fertilize the soil. Man, as a consequence of his unique life style, discharges his metabolic (biodegradable) waste products into the water environment, by way of sewage, in enormous quantities but at a relatively few locations. Man also discharges persistent waste products (*nonbiodegradable*) into the water, air, and earth and these generate special dangers that the forces of the natural environment are unable to cope with. A few examples will illustrate the nature of these problems and the solutions that have been found to be appropriate.

DETERGENTS Certain types of synthetic detergents containing alkyl benzene sulfonate (ABS) were used in large quantities during the 1950s and 1960s for clothes and dishwashing. ABS was discovered to be nonbiodegradable when sewage treatment plant effluents, otherwise safe to discharge to streams and estuaries, produced enormous, persistent layers of suds on the surface of the receiving waters. In areas where centralized municipal sanitary services were not available and it was customary for each household to supply its own water from wells and provide for its own sanitary disposal services with septic tanks, tap water acquired a larger and larger head of foam. The solution to this problem was to ban, by law, the sale of nonbiodegradable detergents and, gradually, the problem of foam in streams and tap water abated.

MERCURY   Discharge of mercury into rivers and the ocean from chemical plants that manufacture chlorine (used for water purification) and caustic soda (a starting point for the manufacture of many important industrial chemicals including paper pulp, synthetic fibers, and film) has been responsible for mercury poisonings and deaths from eating fish caught in waters contaminated with this metal. New regulations have required manufacturing plants to eliminate their discharges of mercury to the environment. This has been largely accomplished but mercury is a persistent element and it may be some time before all of the mercury in the environment has been converted to nonavailable compounds.

Consumption of swordfish has been banned in most states for the past few years because of mercury contamination of the edible flesh. The source of mercury in the deep waters inhabited by swordfish is not presently known but mercury emissions to the environment undergo concentration in the *food chain:* a very low level of mercury in sea water is incorporated as a very low level of mercury in the tiny plants that float near the surface of the water and provide the food for small plant-eating animals. These, in turn, provide food for small fish, and the small fish provide food for larger fish in turn. Because mercury tends to concentrate in certain tissues of the body, such as the kidneys and brain, each higher level in a food chain contaminated at the beginning by low levels of mercury receives a larger and larger dose (see Fig. 21.3). Because the fetus is especially susceptible, permissible levels of mercury in fish have been established at very low levels. Deaths from eating fish containing high concentrations of mercury have been reported from Japan, where fish constitutes a large part of the total diet.

There are many unsuspected sources of mercury in the environment. A mysterious mercury contamination of soft shell clams in small areas of Boston Harbor was finally traced to adjacent yacht basins where it was customary to scrape boat hulls coated with mercury-containing antifouling paints in locations where the old paint flakes fall into the ocean. Mud samples from the ocean bottom in the vicinity of these boat yards suggest that there is already sufficient mercury in the bottom slimes to contaminate nearby flats for decades and there is a permanent ban on harvesting clams for human consumption.

LEAD   Most automobile gasolines have contained about 0.065 percent by volume of organic lead (tetraethyl and tetramethyl lead) since the 1920s to improve antiknocking properties when used in high compression engines. This compound is reduced to inorganic lead compounds in the cylinders of the engine and discharged from the tail pipe with the combustion gases. Soil and vegetation on either side of major highways that traverse farming areas are contaminated with lead from automobile exhaust in concentrations that increase as the highway is approached. Root crops and vegetables with inedible husk or pod, such as corn or peas, can accumulate an excessive lead content from the soil in which they are grown. Fruits and leafy vegetables can accumulate lead by direct deposition from the air as well as from the soil. Cows grazing along major highways show an elevated lead concentration in their milk. A farm family that derived a major portion of its food and milk from crops and forage grown close to heavily traveled highways could be dangerously exposed to lead poisoning. Fortunately, town and city dwellers get their food products, including milk, from such a large production area that the danger of lead poisoning from this source is considered negligible and, in fact, the average intake of lead from all sources, principally from drinking water, food products, and air, has been declining for several decades because of the substitution of welded stainless steel for lead-soldered equipment and utensils in food preparation and preservation, replacement of lead pipes in water supply systems, and the abandonment of drinking water supplies found to have excessive amounts of lead extracted from the earth. Occupational exposures to lead have also declined in recent years.

The principal form of lead poisoning seen currently is in small children living in old, dilapidated houses, who eat plaster and chips of lead-based paint. It is thought by some that this occurs because certain lead compounds have a sweet taste, but it is likely that it is related to nutritional deficiency. The name *pica*, from the Latin name of the omnivorous magpie, has been given to this practice. Whatever the causative factors may be, an alarming number of children under 4 years of age from impoverished families dwelling in dilapidated buildings in the core areas of old cities show abnormal intake of lead and some of these are likely to experience permanent mental retardation as a consequence. A permanent solution can be achieved by replacing old housing but this is likely to take many years. In the meantime, education of parents about the dangers of pica and the need for close surveillance of all small children who may be exposed to the risk of eating old lead paint is essential.

DDT The dangers associated with DDT in the environment provide another case history of the peculiar way in which biological concentration occurs in the food chain. DDT is an excellent insecticide partly because it is nonvolatile and only slowly degraded in the environment. Therefore, single applications remain highly effective for many months. Because of this property, plus its low cost, tens of millions of pounds have been applied worldwide since World War II, when it was first used to control mite typhus in American troops stationed in Italy and Southeast Asia. The highly persistent (nonbiodegradable) nature of DDT, a desirable characteristic for an insecticide, produced some entirely unforeseen environmental consequences. After application to orchards and field crops, DDT goes from the soil into nearby streams during rain and snow melting and eventually it reaches the oceans in small amounts. The worldwide distribution of DDT by pathways that are still obscure has been demonstrated by the presence of DDT in the fatty tissues of penguins in Antarctica. It is believed that DDT is brought to this remote area, where DDT has never been applied, by air currents from agricultural zones thousands of miles away and deposited in the waters containing the sea creatures on which penguins feed.

The first step in the food chain involves simple plants that utilize sunlight to synthesize food materials. These plants incorporate chemicals into their cell structure in proportion to their concentration in the environment. Therefore, DDT concentrations found in aquatic plants are normally very small, reflecting the low concentration in the water in which they grow. Herbivores (vegetable-eating animals) eat these plants and retain a high percentage of the ingested DDT in their fatty tissues, in which DDT is soluble. These animals in turn, are eaten by carnivores (meat-eating animals) and the dissolved DDT is largely retained in the fatty tissues of the predators. In this way, DDT becomes concentrated in certain species of animals, including man. A series of measurements of DDT content in plants and animals in a Long Island estuary (arm of the sea at the lower end of a river) showed that bay shrimp that fed on simple aquatic plants contained 0.16 ppm (parts per million). Bullfish that fed on bay shrimp showed 2.1 ppm DDT and green heron that fed on the bullfish showed 3.6 ppm DDT. A more detailed explanation of how DDT becomes distributed in the environment and the biosphere is shown in Figure 21.3.

Similar patterns of biological concentration of DDT have been traced from tree-spraying for Dutch elm disease to earthworms that ate the fallen leaves containing DDT and concentrated this chemical in their bodies. Robins that fed on these worms died and this was one of the events that aroused Rachel Carson to write *Silent Spring*.

By similar methods, man has also accumulated high concentrations of DDT in his fatty tissues over the past two decades but, fortunately, DDT has very low toxicity for man and no known damage has resulted from this increase. However, some species of predatory birds, such as falcons, have accumulated very high DDT levels and this has interfered with their reproduction because it has resulted in laying thin-shelled eggs that do not survive the incubation period. The U.S. imposed a total ban on the use of DDT in 1973 but it is still widely used in many parts of the world for malaria control.

ENERGY AND TRANSPORTATION

Primitive peoples living in a tropical or semitropical climate have little need for energy sources other than their own food supply. The aborigines of America, Australia, and New Guinea, for example, had no beasts of burden before they were introduced by western European explorers. The simple needs of these people were satisfied by foraging and hunting and, in some cases, a simple agriculture which required frequent shifts to new fields to maintain fertility. Clothing and shelter were obtained from plants and animals in the vicinity. Modern man has far more complex needs and unlimited energy is at the heart of most of these. The

Figure 21.3. Distribution of DDT in an estuarian biosphere. Note how the DDT concentration increases in the food chain shown here. The same process occurs for mercury and lead, but in different food chains. (From G. M. Woodwell, "Toxic Substances in Ecological Cycles," *Scientific American* [1967], p. 26)

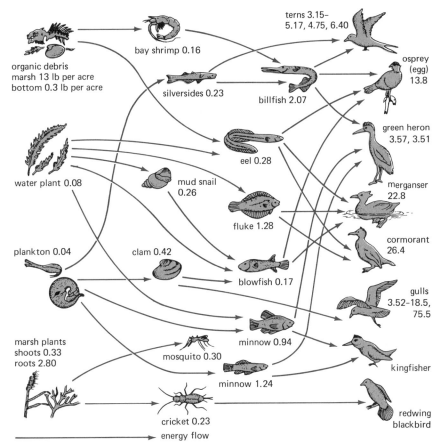

Figure 21.4. Energy use and Gross National Product. (From A. B. Cambel, ed., "Energy R&D and National Programs," prepared for "Interdepartmental Energy Study," U.S. Office of Science and Technology, 1964)

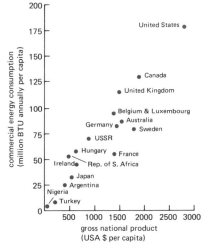

advanced countries of the world have become dependent upon the availability of ample energy supplies. Figure 21.4 shows that the gross national product is directly related to the use of energy. In the 200 years since the founding of the Republic, the major occupations of the nation have changed from growing food, fibers, and hides to the production of the goods and services that make modern city life attractive to the overwhelming majority of citizens.

ENERGY SOURCES Prior to the Industrial Revolution, which began in England at about the time of the American Revolution, man power and beasts of burden, abetted by water wheels, represented the major energy sources other than the burning of wood. Early steam engines burned wood for fuel and, in the newly settled lands of America, close-by forest resources were more than adequate to fuel steamboats, trains, and mills for many decades. In densely settled areas, however, wood was limited and hauling it from remote areas became a serious burden because of its enormous bulk. A cord of maple logs that weighs 2.5 tons and occupies

128 cubic feet gives off no more heat than 0.8 ton of coal that occupies only ¼ that volume. Therefore, coal began to replace wood as the fuel of choice early in the nineteenth century. Oil, a more concentrated fuel than coal, has largely replaced coal for most energy uses except the generation of electricity at central station utility plants. During the second half of the twentieth century, a still more concentrated fuel, uranium, used in nuclear plants, has begun to displace both coal and oil for large scale generation of electricity. A single pound of uranium is capable of producing more electricity than 2.5 million pounds of coal or 250,000 gallons of fuel oil. It is predicted that 60 percent of an enormously greater electricity demand will be supplied by nuclear energy by the year 2000. One of the serious drawbacks to the use of solar energy, which is free and virtually limitless, is that it is not a concentrated energy source—several square miles of heat receptor surface are required to produce the same amount of electricity as a single modern nuclear station. Similar problems are associated with recovering heat from the depths of the earth and energy from the movement of the wind. These are low intensity sources of limitless energy but current requirements place a premium on the concentrated sources with which we are most familiar. Nevertheless, we can expect to see an enlarged research effort directed towards greater use of these sources for the future.

When reviewing the total energy picture for the decades and centuries ahead, it seems clear that clean, compact fuels will be reserved increasingly for domestic (household heating and cooking) and transportation purposes (automobiles and aircraft) while coal and nuclear energy will be reserved for large scale central station generation of electricity. The principle to be applied here is that large fuel consumers have the technical and financial resources to provide all of the protective measures that are required to safeguard public health and safety. Proven coal reserves are believed to be adequate for all demands over the next 200–400 years, including the synthesis of gas and oil when natural reserves of these clean fuels grow scarce. Uranium reserves are thought to be adequate for less than a century of projected requirements but the development of *breeder reactors*, so-called because they generate more fuel than they consume through nuclear transformations of fissionable materials such as thorium, is well advanced. The U.S. is committed to completing the first of a series of large breeder reactors for generating electricity by 1980 and this technology is well advanced in Europe, as well. There is little danger of the world exhausting its energy resources in the foreseeable future, but rapidly increasing demand and competition for readily available supplies of fossil fuels and uranium ore are certain to result in increasing prices. To a considerable extent, increased costs should promote more prudent use of energy and act as a conservative factor.

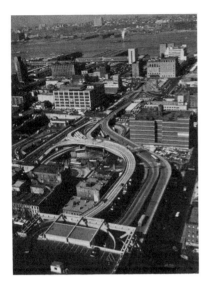

Figure 21.5. Highways and automobiles—interwoven into the fabric of American life.

TRANSPORTATION Approximately 24 percent of the fuel consumed in the U.S. is used for transportation and much of this is for personal travel in private automobiles. The appropriateness of using a 5,000-pound machine to transport one 150-pound person to a daily workplace, to school, or to neighborhood shops has been commented upon endlessly ever since it was recognized that too many automobiles in one place affect the environment adversely in many obvious as well as subtle ways. Nevertheless, personal motor transportation for business, convenience, and pleasure has become so completely interwoven into the fabric of American life that it is difficult to see how significant changes in vehicle usage can be brought about in the foreseeable future other than in the core area of a few large cities. Urban communication patterns are so complex today that after 10 years of construction and the expenditure of many hundreds of millions of dollars to build a brand new Bay Area Rapid Transit System (BART), it has been estimated that it is unlikely to reduce daytime automobile traffic in downtown San Francisco by more than 5 percent. It is no longer uncommon for people to commute daily 25 to 50 miles, or more, and often much of this distance is through areas too lightly populated to support even a rudimentary public transportation system.

On a larger scale, modern life has become totally dependent on transportation networks that carry food from farms and ranches to cities, fuels and metals from mines to refineries, smelters, and factories, and manufactured goods to customers who may be distributed worldwide. In addition to commutation problems in large cities, all types of transportation affect the environment adversely by producing noise, dirt, and undesirable emissions. In addition, transportation is directly responsible for more than 50,000 accidental deaths per year and many times that number of serious injuries. Often, railroads and major highways constructed through wilderness areas have stimulated settlement and growth. The tranquility of the region and the natural habitats of many species have been severely disturbed. Congress and many state legislatures have recognized the seriousness of thoughtless destruction or drastic degradation of environmental quality and have passed laws requiring careful consideration and documentation of every negative effect that might result from each contemplated major project. These reviews, called *environmental impact statements,* are required to demonstrate that no serious environmental damage will result before electric generating stations, major highways, airports, large shopping centers, factories, and many other large enterprises can proceed to the construction stage.

POLITICAL DECISIONS There is no longer any disagreement from any responsible segment of society that serious degradation of the environment must be avoided when planning new or enlarged roads, airports, public transportation systems, or even enterprises that generate substantial traffic flows, such as major sports arenas, but considerable controversy has resulted from attempts to justify some degree of disturbance to the environment on the basis of dire public necessity. Rapidly shrinking open space near to or within large metropolitan centers has made the remaining undeveloped land very precious and has stimulated groups of influential and vocal citizens to oppose further encroachments on these lands for any purpose. It is sometimes forgotten that land can be improved as well as degraded by man's activities and often it is possible to offset some degree of environmental damage by compensating improvements. In many public controversies of this nature it soon becomes clear that there are no absolute criteria on which to base unerring judgments. Instead, after the inevitable compromises have been made, there are offsetting penalties and benefits and it becomes a matter of public policy and, in the end, difficult political decisions (in the best sense of that term) must be made by all of the people or by their elected representatives. A vigorous national debate was conducted for four years over the environmental damage that would occur if a 789-mile trans-Alaska oil pipeline were to be built to bring newly discovered and badly needed oil from Prudhoe Bay, inside the Arctic Circle, to the contiguous states by way of Valdez, a warm water Alaskan port. The opposition of several environmental interest groups persisted in spite of a number of construction modifications that were proposed to permit crossings by migrating animals and minimize the damage from accidental leaks. By the fall of 1973, in the judgment of Congress, the need for additional oil supplies outweighed foreseeable environmental degradation, and pipeline construction was authorized. An earlier public debate involving energy needs concerned proposed construction of the Storm King pumped

Aesthetic degradation of the environment

What traveler has not been shocked and outraged after reaching a remote location and settling to rest beside a charming wilderness stream to observe discarded beer cans and other trash resting on the bottom? The central districts of most of the great cities have become disgustingly filthy, in spite of antilitter campaigns and millions of dollars spent annually to clean streets, alleys, and vacant lots. The edges of major highways accumulate millions of pounds of discarded trash annually, in spite of frequent notices that fines may be imposed for littering. Who are these modern barbarians who are unwilling to respect community needs by carelessly discarding unwanted items or permitting their household animals to foul the public ways? Unfortunately, judging from appearances, they seem to include almost everyone.

A recent study of the rate of littering of vacant lots in a central city district showed that after cleaning by municipal crews, an area remains clean "until someone disposes of a large volume of material at one time. This action tends to 'open the flood gates' and the rate of accumulation of debris increases dramatically."*

It is apparent that after a critical degree of disorderliness is reached, an area becomes the neighborhood dumping ground. The strangest aspect of this behavior is that the areas involved have twice-weekly municipal garbage and trash collections that are without cost to residents. In addition to being an eyesore, litter provides an attractive habitat for rats and other vermin and there is a perpetual demand for rat eradication campaigns in the districts subject to vacant lot littering.

* Lawrence Partridge, Jr., "Quantitative Analysis of Solid Waste Management in Boston, Massachusetts" (Ph.D. diss., Harvard University, 1973), p. v-15.

storage reservoir north of New York City. A utility company proposed to dig a water reservoir on top of Storm King Mountain, located in a large and popular wilderness area, into which it would pump water from the Hudson River at night and on weekends, when electrical demand was normally lowest, and use the stored supply to generate electricity during peak load periods such as hot summer afternoons when demand is at a maximum. Widespread public concern that the proposed construction program would irretrievably damage the area for recreation purposes resulted in a political decision that the benefits to be derived from this project did not outweigh the disadvantages, and permission to proceed was denied. It is interesting to speculate whether the public might reconsider if this same proposal were to be reintroduced after a prolonged and unavoidable series of brownouts and blackouts in New York City resulting from a shortage of power during brief periods of peak demands. This example is not intended to suggest that public decisions in these matters are capricious but, rather, that a new balancing between benefits and environmental damage may sometimes become necessary as a result of unforeseen events. It seems reasonable to believe that the public will be called on with increasing frequency to make decisions of the utmost gravity with respect to environmental affairs and it is essential that mistaken notions that these matters can be resolved conveniently into simple absolutes of "right" and "wrong" be abandoned forever. The environmental problems confronting us have two aspects— the scientific on one hand, and the social, economic, and political on the other. The latter are likely to prove to be the most intractable.

MAN-MADE ENVIRONMENTS

Technology provides the means to control and regulate the environmental stresses to which man is exposed. Modern man can live in comfort in the Arctic, in the tropics, in the desert, and even in orbit around the earth. He can work in safety a thousand feet underground or underwater, near a blast furnace, or in an air-conditioned office or school.

The home

RESIDENTIAL ENVIRONMENT   Man's ability to move permanently from his natural habitat in the trees of tropical Africa to the ends of the earth has depended upon his ability to control his personal environment: first, as simple shelter against the elements and, later, to maintain his thermal environment at an optimum level. The image of the cave dweller crouching before an open fire is a familiar one. Shelter has become more complex. Today, we are concerned with temperature and humidity control, illumination levels, noise insulation, privacy, and suitable areas for family social life. The World Health Organization concluded that housing is more than a physical structure and recommended the term *residential environment*; including in that term "the environs of that structure including all necessary services, facilities, equipment and devices needed

Model housing code

A model housing code recommended by the American Public Health Association and the U.S. Dept. of Health, Education and Welfare provides that "The maximum occupancy of any dwelling unit shall not exceed the following requirements:

For first occupant one hundred fifty (150) square feet of floor space and at least one hundred (100) square feet of floor space for every additional occupant thereof, the floor space to be calculated on the basis of total habitable room area.

A total number of persons equal to two (2) times the number of its habitable rooms.

". . . every room occupied for sleeping purposes shall contain at least seventy (70) square feet of floor space for the first occupant, and at least fifty (50) square feet of floor space for each additional occupant thereof."

and desired for the physical and mental and social well being of the family and the individual."[2]

SPACE Minimum space requirements that provide for normal family living by enabling "occupants to sleep, rest, and relax, read, carry on conversations and listen to radio and watch television without being disturbed by or disturbing other occupants, and to perform efficiently personal and household tasks,"[3] have never been defined adequately, perhaps because there are large personal and cultural differences in human expectations and needs in this area. The amount of space desired increases with duration of occupancy. For travel and vacation needs, minimum facilities are likely to be acceptable but for a permanent home, space requirements are much greater and space separation is much more important. Environmental health considerations can be applied rationally to many aspects of housing such as water supply, waste water removal, temperature regulation, illumination, etc., but space requirements may be approached more logically on the basis of mental health needs. Community space standards have been widely expressed in housing codes which usually specify only the minimum size and maximum occupancy of sleeping rooms.

There does not seem to be any way that recommended space requirements can be applied to old dwellings and, as a consequence, millions of central city and rural slum dwellings are substandard and likely to remain so until they are torn down. Decent replacement housing has been provided in the form of public housing developments, rehabilitation of substandard dwellings, and rent subsidization in private housing but the sum of these programs has not been able to outpace completely the rate of deterioration of existing buildings.

The workplace

CHEMICAL AND PHYSICAL STRESSES Environmental stresses in the workplace can be considered under two broad categories: *chemical* stresses such as mineral dusts, metal fumes, poisonous gases, organic solvents, acids, alkalines, and the thousands of other products that are used in modern industry, and *physical* stresses such as heat, humidity, excessive noise, ionizing and non-ionizing radiations including light from laser beams, xenon flash tubes, and similar bright sources. Less rigid standards of environmental quality are tolerated in the work environment than in the home, school, or out-of-doors because the normal workweek seldom exceeds 40 hours and it is assumed that the working population consists of healthy adults. Generally speaking, this is correct for those employed

[2] World Health Organization, *Expert Committee on the Public Health Aspects of Housing* (Tech. Report Series 225, 1961).
[3] American Public Health Association, *Housing: Basic Health Principles and Recommended Ordinance* (Washington, D.C., APHA, 1971), p. 14.

in the chemical, metallurgical, mineral, and similar industries that are the principal sources of stressful working environments. Whenever the workweek is greatly lengthened over a long period, as may happen during periods of national emergency, standards for safe working environments no longer include all of the safety factors that are associated with briefer exposures. For example, studies of individuals exposed to the vapors of an organic solvent in the workroom environment show that the inhaled vapors accumulate in their blood and body tissues during the work day, often reaching the highest level at the end of the shift. After leaving the job, the concentration in the body declines. When the solvent is entirely gone and the internal environment of the worker has returned to its normal state before the start of work the next morning, this is one of the important indications that the work environment will not produce disease. If, however, the workday is greatly lengthened, say from 8 to 12 hours, two things can occur: 1. the worker will accumulate a higher concentration inside his body while on the job, and 2. there will be less time to get rid of all of the solvent that has accumulated in the body before the next work period begins. Under these conditions, the concentration inside the body becomes slightly greater day by day until a safe level is exceeded and disease results. Restricted periods of exposure to a hazardous work environment, plus adequate recovery periods between exposures, must be observed for safety. For especially hazardous jobs, where the work environment cannot yet be controlled adequately, the maximum daily work period at that particular job may be no more than 2 or 4 hours (with other, nonhazardous, work being provided for the remainder of the normal working day). As Chapter 6 showed, occupational health risks may be reduced by substitution of nontoxic for toxic materials, separation of the worker from the hazard, and personal protective devices (see Chap. 16).

The school

PHYSICAL REQUIREMENTS For children and young adults, school or college is likely to be second only to the home as the most frequently encountered environment. It has two interrelated but distinct functions: the student must be physically comfortable so that he or she can concentrate on the work of education and the school environment must be conducive to learning. Comfort requirements for students and faculty do not differ significantly from those that apply to other assembly places. They are concerned principally with regulation of temperature, humidity, air circulation, illumination, and reduction of noise. Water supply, waste water and solid waste disposal, and lunchroom sanitation follow conventional patterns. The very special aspects of the school environment are associated with its unique role as an institution for mental and physical development and the fact that it is a place of daily assembly for a large transient population.

Some physical environments are more conducive to learning (and teaching) than others. In many schools and colleges, cold weather heating is less of a need than hot weather cooling. Teacher surveys indicate that ability to concentrate, and learning, are improved substantially when air conditioning is installed in overly hot classrooms. Building codes often require mechanical ventilation rates up to 30 cubic feet per minute of outside air per pupil. These high ventilation rates are not for the purpose of replacing oxygen for breathing but to dilute body odors in densely occupied spaces and they reflect normal practices of an earlier time when neither good standards of personal hygiene nor facilities in which to practice them were as widespread or as convenient as they are today. It is generally recognized that obsolete school building codes seriously retard the introduction of air conditioning because they make it too costly. Serious efforts are underway on a national scale by architects, engineers, and building construction contractors to modernize building codes for all types of construction, including schools.

THE LEARNING ENVIRONMENT In addition to caring for the physical needs of students and faculty, a school should strive for a learning environment by its special ambience. This is customarily expressed by the nature and arrangement of the furniture, the use of large windows to admit a lot of natural light, bright colors, clean surroundings, and all other amenities that stimulate mental receptivity. Nevertheless, no amount of favorable environment can substitute for a knowledgeable and enthusiastic teacher inside the classroom.

Eating places

HEALTH RISKS FROM FOOD Food, like water, has been a principal source of illness in man throughout recorded history and it continues to be a problem to this day even though many of the diseases that were widely prevalent years ago have now become rare. For example, transmission of bovine tuberculosis to humans through milk can be completely avoided by pasteurization (heating to 142°F for 20 minutes) and the sale of unpasteurized milk has been outlawed practically everywhere in the U.S. Transmission of tricinosis (infestation by a parasite worm) from pigs to man has been controlled by prohibiting the feeding of uncooked garbage to hogs. This prevents the infection in hogs because they usually contract it from eating raw infected meat scraps.

Proper production, processing, and preservation of foods during transportation and storage are essential steps in the delivery of safe, nutritious, and palatable food to those who prepare it for consumption. By and large, modern food manufacturing and handling methods have proven adequate, although exceptions continue to be brought to public notice with regularity. For nonfarm dwellers, most food comes from the large food producers that are regulated by federal and state public health and agriculture agencies. They are especially active in supervising slaughter houses, meat packing plants, dairies, and frozen food factories.

Unlike the Orient, where human fecal material is used to fertilize food crops, there is no health hazard associated with eating any of the salad vegetables and fruits that are customarily consumed raw. The same statement cannot be made for raw shellfish that have, in recent years, been the source of a number of serious illnesses, including infectious hepatitis, that have their origin in contaminated shellfish beds. The well-publicized fatal cholera epidemic in and around Naples, Italy, during the summer of 1973 from the eating of sewage-contaminated mussels, is a clear warning that consumption of raw shellfish is fraught with serious health hazards in the modern world.

Fortunately, when cooked properly and eaten promptly, all foods are made safe from the transmission of microbiological disease, either through living disease-producing organisms or through their toxic products. The heat of cooking also denatures the botulism toxins that have figured prominently in recent fatalities from eating uncooked canned soups and tuna fish. Many of the toxic chemicals that can enter food during growth (such as mercury contamination of fish) or processing (from the use of unapproved preservatives) survive cooking.

SUMMARY Man is unique among all other creatures in the world because he lives partly in the natural environment, over which he has only very limited control, and partly in a man-made environment, over which he has complete control. In tropical areas, he has the capability of going from his air-cooled home to his air-cooled office in his air-cooled automobile. After work, his air-cooled automobile can take him to his air-cooled club, where he can exercise in an air-cooled gymnasium, and then return him in air-cooled comfort to his air-cooled home. This is illustrative of the ways by which man is capable of insulating himself from external stresses produced by extremes of temperature and noise and from pollution. Nevertheless, man's existence, through his absolute dependence on air, water, food, and shelter, is ultimately tied to the natural environment. His ecological niche as the dominant species on earth is inextricably dependent upon maintaining an environment that is not significantly different from the one that prevailed during the eons of his evolution. Even after he has, at long last, achieved utmost silence and absolute purity of air, water, and land, man is unlikely to be totally satisfied with the natural environment he has recreated and he will want to continue to regulate his own environment according to his own notions of what he believes to be the optimum environment for himself.

Environmental stress crowds in upon man from every side: at home and workplace, while traveling, and during his leisure activities. His long survival celebrates his abilities to resist the impact of these stresses on the constancy of the internal environment that regulates his vital life processes. As the environment in which man lives has become more polluted by his activities, man has flourished and occupied the earth totally. He may be enjoying it less, as has been claimed by many critics of modern life, but it is difficult to confirm this objectively. In former times, when man was one with nature, he strove mightily to free himself from this bondage. Western man has succeeded in this enterprise far beyond his expectations and is fearfully engaged in trying to reverse the process. Hopefully, he will eventually find ways of combining the best features of the natural and the man-made environments for his benefit.

Questions

1. Evaluate your local housing code to see if it contains all of the good practice standards recommended by the World Health Organization and the American Public Health Association.
2. Show how land use planning can play a vital role in preserving environmental quality.
3. Compare the environmental impact of conventional gasoline-powered automobiles with that of electric vehicles (keeping in mind that electrical power must be generated to recharge the batteries).
4. Determine what factors are important for conducting a successful antilitter campaign. How can these principles be put into practice at your school?
5. What are the arguments for and against the worldwide use of DDT for malaria control?

Key Concepts

Biodegradable – capable of being broken down into innocuous compounds by the action of natural processes

Biosphere – living things together with their environment

Ecology – the science concerned with the interrelationships of living things and their environments; it considers both the fitness of an environment to sustain life and the ability of organisms to tolerate their environment

Environment – the complex of climatic and biological factors that act on an organism or a community

Selected Readings

Carson, Rachel. *Silent Spring.* New York: Alfred Knopf, 1962.

Dubos, René. *So Human an Animal.* New York: Scribners, 1968.

Fisher, James, Noel Simon, and Jack Vincent. *Wildlife in Danger.* New York: Viking Press, 1969.

Maddox, John. *The Doomsday Syndrome.* New York: McGraw-Hill, 1972.

Malthus, Thomas. *Essay on the Principle of Population.* New York: Everyman's Library, 1958.

Meadows, Dennis, *et al. The Limits to Growth.* New York: Universe Books, 1971.

Odum, E. P. *Fundamentals of Ecology,* 3d ed. Philadelphia: W. B. Saunders, 1971.

Chapter 22

Managing the Environment

An optimum environment is much more difficult to define than one which is polluted, judging from the large number of definitions of what constitutes intolerable environmental conditions and the few statements about what is considered beneficial. Perhaps this stems from a wide diversity of opinions on the structure of "environmental utopia" and relative unanimity about the exact nature of "environmental hell." Whatever the explanation, there are a number of widely accepted statements about the nature of environmental pollution. Each reflects a special viewpoint and, together, they indicate the wide-ranging effects of environmental pollution.

Pollution has been defined as "a resource out of place," suggesting that economic penalties result from misuse of our natural wealth. *Environmental pollution* has been defined as "the unfavorable accumulation of the metabolic products of civilization." This is a biologist's explanation that emphasizes the fact that natural forces are involved

---

This chapter was contributed by Melvin W. First, Sc.D., Professor of Environmental Health Engineering, Kresage Center for Environmental Health, Harvard School of Public Health, and Chairman of the Advisory Committee on Environmental Health to the Massachusetts Department of Public Health.

and that "every living thing contaminates its environment."[1] A presidential advisory committee defined environmental pollution as:

> the unfavorable alteration of our surroundings, wholly or largely as a by-product of man's actions, through direct or indirect effects of changes in energy patterns, radiation levels, chemical and physical constitution and abundances of organisms. These changes may affect man directly, or through his supplies of water and of agricultural and other biological products, his physical objects or possessions, or his opportunities for recreation and appreciation of nature.[2]

This definition is in conformity with the World Health Organization's statement that health is "not merely the absence of disease or infirmity" but is also "a state of complete physical, mental, and social well-being." It implies that in health, all human functions can be performed effectively and with enthusiasm. It defines pollution as man made, in recognition of the fact that, although major natural sources of environmental pollution exist, such as volcanic eruptions, man is helpless to prevent them. He can do most to avoid pollution when he confines his attention to those sources over which he can exercise control. This definition also indicates that damage must occur before a condition recognized as pollution occurs. Mere emission of substances to the environment is not enough. When emissions cause alterations in the geochemical composition of the environment without producing adverse effects, they are usually designated "contaminants."[3] It is important to recognize that damage to the environment can include degradation of its aesthetic properties, as well as the more obvious ills produced by a polluted environment. Everyone takes great pleasure in sparkling, bright sunny days and clear inviting streams teeming with fish, and all are entitled to enjoy these benefits of a clean environment even though their absence may produce no known disease or economic penalty. It is recognized, therefore, that concern for the preservation of the environment fits into four basic levels in decreasing order of importance, but increasing order of complexity and scope:

1. Insuring the elements of simple survival
2. Preventing disease and poisonings
3. Maintaining an environment suited to man's efficient performance
4. Preserving human comfort and the enjoyment of life.

It has become evident to all that a coherent, thoughtful, and sustained program is required to reverse unfavorable trends in the environment and to safeguard what is yet uncontaminated. There is already

[1] Report of the Air Conservation Commission, *Air Conservation* (Washington, D.C.: American Association for the Advancement of Science, 1965), p. 3.

[2] Report of the Environmental Pollution Panel, President's Science Advisory Committee, *Restoring the Quality of our Environment* (Washington, D.C.: The White House, Nov. 1965), p. 1.

[3] "A Report by the Subcommittee on Environmental Improvement," in *Cleaning our Environment: The Chemical Basis for Action* (Washington, D.C.: American Chemical Society, 1969), p. 6.

Figure 22.1. Preserving the clean environment—Superior National Forest, Minnesota. (Courtesy U. S. Forest Service)

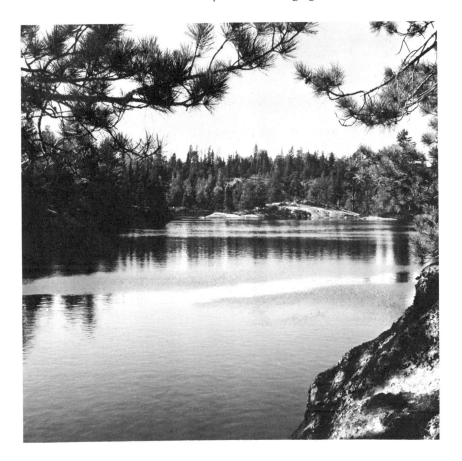

ample evidence that the American public has been sensitized to the vital importance of environmental conservation. The need, now, is to point the way to achievement. Therefore, the emphasis in this chapter will not be to deplore the deficiencies that exist and to point the finger of blame but, rather, to suggest constructive programs for managing the environment in order to preserve all of the natural elements that are considered essential, beneficial, and desirable.

MANAGING THE AIR ENVIRONMENT

Air pollution has been a matter of concern and comment since ancient times and continues as a topic of vital interest to the present day. The Roman philosopher Seneca recorded in A.D. 61 that "As soon as I had gotten out of the heavy air of Rome and from the stink of the smoky chimneys thereof, which, being stirred, poured forth whatever pestilential vapors and soot they had enclosed in them, I felt an alteration of my disposition." In 1306, Edward I, King of England, issued a royal proclamation prohibiting silversmiths from burning sea coal, a smoky fuel containing a high percentage of tar-like volatile matter. It is recorded that at least one silversmith was hanged for disobeying the King's decree.

Atmosphere

The composition of the dry atmosphere is mostly nitrogen (78 percent by volume), a biologically inert gas, and oxygen (21 percent by volume), an essential of life for man. The remaining 1 percent consists of argon (0.93 percent), carbon dioxide (0.03 percent), and a long list of trace gases that include neon, krypton, helium, ozone, hydrogen, and methane. Although the dry gas composition of the atmosphere remains essentially constant, the amount of water vapor in the air varies considerably from place to place and from day to day depending upon temperature and precipitation.

Air is considered to be pure or fresh when it has a normal content of oxygen and carbon dioxide, is invisible, contains no objectionable odors or tastes, and has no substances in sufficient concentration to injure health, even though these may be undetectable by the senses. By technical definition, pure air includes only the normal air gases in the proportions noted above, but this substance exists only in laboratories, if it exists at all. In nature, by common definition, even pure air contains variable quantities of a vast number and variety of substances, some particulate and some gaseous.

Pittsburgh passed its first smoke control ordinance in 1895, and the first intercity smoke control district was formed in Metropolitan Boston in 1911. In each case, the motivation was to reduce soiling from soot deposits, eliminate foul odors from sulfur emissions, and reduce atmospheric smoke that significantly reduced the incidence of sunlight in cities, especially during the winter months. This reduction was associated with a high incidence of a childhood bone disease called rickets, from a lack of vitamin D normally induced by exposure to sunlight. Rickets disappeared with the introduction of vitamin D fortified milk during the 1920s and interest in coal smoke in the atmosphere declined to a low level. During the great depression of the 1930s, concern was directed to the absence of smoking factory chimneys, rather than the reverse, but during this period a tragic episode occurred that had important, although unrecognized, portends for the future. During December 1930, a persistent fog associated with stagnant air conditions settled over the Meuse Valley in Belgium. The deep valley contained many metallurgical industries whose furnace stacks were below the surrounding hilltops. During the four to five days of deep fog and cold, 63 deaths were attributed to the buildup of sulfur-containing gases and fluorides emitted from the factory stacks. This was thought to be a curious but isolated incident until 1948 when an almost identical episode occurred in Donora, Pa., also a deep valley town with a large metallurgical industry. For five days in October of that year, there was air stagnation and a chill, persistent fog in the valley. During this period, 23 excess deaths occurred and about half the population of the town reported respiratory illnesses.

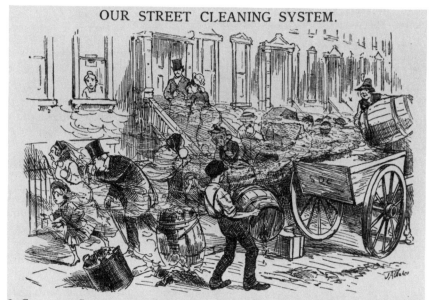

OUR STREET CLEANING SYSTEM.

IT CLEANS THE STREETS—SO IT DOES—BUT WHO IS TO CLEAN THE UNFORTUNATE WAYFARERS?

Figure 22.2. A cartoon on air pollution in the 1870s. (Courtesy of National Library of Medicine, Bethesda, Maryland)

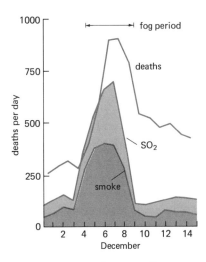

Figure 22.3. Deaths, air pollution, and temperature during December 1952 in Greater London. (From Committee on Air Pollution, *Interim Report*, London: Her Majesty's Stationery Office, December 1953.)

Once again, emissions from metallurgical plants were implicated, but it soon became clear that they were not a necessary factor for air pollution disaster. In December, 1952, one of its notorious "pea soup fogs" settled over London for 5 days and 4000 excess deaths were recorded from air-pollution-induced effects. The relationship between the occurrence of elevated air pollution and excess deaths is shown in Figure 22.3. Sulfur-containing gases and particulate matter emitted from burning coal were implicated. A similar, though less lethal, episode occurred in London during December, 1962 and was a powerful stimulant in motivating the British government to take strong remedial measures, including a ban on the burning of coal.

Acute air pollution episodes are now known to cause premature deaths among the ill, the elderly, and the very young. The effect on health and longevity of low levels of air pollutants over very long periods of time is also a major concern. Whereas deaths that occur during acute episodes are generally blamed on the stress of air pollution added to severe and debilitating pre-existing diseases, long exposure to lower levels of air pollutants may be capable of producing chronic disease of the respiratory system. Evaluations of lung disease among populations residing for many years in communities having different levels of sulfur oxides and particulate matter in the atmosphere show that chronic respiratory disease is more prevalent in communities with higher pollution levels.

Sources and amounts of emissions

Table 22.1 is a summary of nationwide emissions for 1970. It shows that total man-made emissions in the U.S. were 267 million tons in 1970. Carbon monoxide (CO) represented more than 50 percent of this total and most of the CO came from motor vehicles. Hydrocarbons (HC),

Table 22.1 *Summary of nationwide emission estimates, 1970**

Source category	SO_x	Part.	CO	HC	NO_x
Transportation	1.0	0.7	111.0	19.5	11.7
Fuel combustion in stationary sources	26.5	6.8	0.8	0.6	10.0
Industrial process losses	6.0	13.3	11.4	5.5	0.2
Solid waste disposal	0.1	1.4	7.2	2.0	0.4
Agricultural burning	Neg[a]	2.4	13.8	2.8	0.3
Miscellaneous	0.3	1.5	4.5	4.5	0.2
Total	33.9	26.1	149.0	34.9	22.8

* From J. H. Cavender, *et al.*, *Nationwide Air Pollution Emission Trends, 1940–1970.* (Research Triangle Park, N.C.: U.S. Environmental Protection Agency, January, 1973), p. 21.
[a] Negligible (less than 0.05×10^6 tons/year).

derived largely from motor vehicles, is the next largest emission category. Transportation also accounts for more than half of the nitrogen oxides (NO_x) emitted to the atmosphere. Altogether, transportation (largely motor vehicle travel) accounts for 54 percent of all emissions to the atmosphere and for this reason is regarded as the most important air pollutant source in America. If other criteria, such as human toxicity and property damage effects, were used, another source might be considered the most important air pollutant.

Solid waste disposal in urban areas and agricultural burning in rural areas, although intense local sources of air pollution, are responsible for only a small fraction of total U.S. emissions. These operations have a bad reputation because they offend local groups of people very severely. Area wide pollution sources, such as automobile emissions, which affect entire populations, generally provoke less intense reactions because they are not as offensive to the senses. Intense negative reactions are evoked by poorly maintained and badly operated diesel trucks and buses that needlessly emit dense black smoke and acrid, nauseating exhaust fumes. Even though trucks and buses represent only a very small fraction of total vehicles and miles traveled, as shown in Table 22.2, they are often intense local sources of disagreeable air pollution. Passenger cars and light trucks, representing 95 percent of all cars and mileage traveled, are, individually, inoffensive but in the aggregate represent the largest source of air polluting emissions in the U.S.

Table 22.2 *Vehicle miles of travel in the U.S., 1969**

Type of vehicle	Urban	Rural	Total
Passenger cars	455.55	410.51	866.06
Light-duty trucks[a]	33.46	50.20	83.66
Heavy-duty trucks			
Class II[b]	9.34	14.02	23.36
Class III[c]	6.23	9.34	15.57
Class IV[d,e]			
Gasoline	11.72	28.71	40.43
Diesel	9.20	23.10	32.30
Total	525.50	535.88	1,061.38

* From J. H. Cavender, *et al., Nationwide Air Pollution Emission Trends, 1940–1970* (Research Triangle Park, N.C.: U.S. Environmental Protection Agency, January, 1973), p. 28.
[a] Under 6,000 pounds.
[b] 6,000 to 10,000 pounds.
[c] 10,000 to 19,000 pounds.
[d] Over 19,000 pounds.
[e] Includes buses.

Concentrations of pollutants in the atmosphere

MEASUREMENTS Measurements of soot (settlable particulate matter) and sulfur oxides have been made routinely for more than 50 years in many cities. Comparing current air measurements with those taken 40 to 50 years ago, it is clear that modern cities are very much cleaner and far less polluted with sulfur-containing gases. This came about because of the almost universal substitution of clean fuels (distillate oil and natural gas) for dirty, sulfur-containing coal for almost all uses except central station generation of electricity. Although total coal consumption by this single source has risen steadily, central stations using coal have installed highly efficient flyash collectors to prevent release of soiling particles. The technology for removing sulfur oxides from flue gases is under rapid development. In the interim, low-sulfur-containing fuels are favored and the emissions are being discharged from tall stacks to promote effective dilution and dispersion in the atmosphere. A few figures will serve to illustrate the reduction of pollution from coal burning in central city air that has occurred over several decades. In St. Louis, Missouri, sulfur dioxide in the atmosphere averaged 0.25 parts per million by volume (ppm) during the cold months of 1931–1932 and 0.13 ppm during the warm months, whereas in 1964, the annual average for sulfur oxides was only 0.06 ppm, less than half. During this same period, particulate matter in St. Louis air averaged 630 micrograms of dust per cubic meter of air (μg/m^3) whereas in 1964 it averaged only 138 μg/m^3 —one-quarter the amount of dust found three decades earlier.

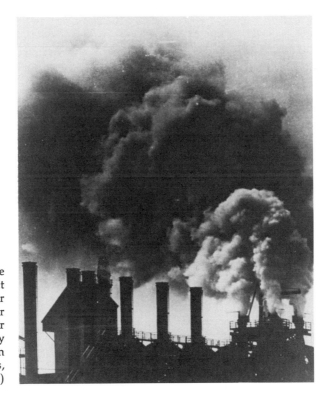

Figure 22.4. A steel plant in the 1960s. The Federal Clean Air Act of 1970 set up guidelines for air management and National Air Quality Standards for all air pollutants of importance. (Courtesy of the Environmental Protection Agency, Office of Public Affairs, Washington, D. C.)

In spite of commendable reductions in dust, soot, and sulfur-containing gases in the core areas of several cities that were formerly badly polluted, the levels were still not sufficiently low and, at the same time, different pollutants—carbon monoxide and nitrogen oxides—principally from automobiles, were increasing rapidly. To provide reliable guidelines for air management, the Federal Clean Air Act of 1970 mandated the establishment of National Air Quality Standards for all air pollutants of importance. These took the form of *primary standards* based on protection of the public health with an adequate margin of safety and *secondary standards* based on protecting the public welfare, that is, avoiding property damage and protecting the aesthetic qualities of the atmosphere.

The primary and secondary air quality standards for the U.S. were published in the Federal Register of April 30, 1971. They are summarized in Table 22.3. The national goal in 1970 was to achieve the primary standards everywhere by 1975 and the secondary some time later. The entire task has proven too difficult to achieve within a five-year period and time extensions have already been granted for meeting the nitrogen oxides, carbon monoxide, and hydrocarbon standards. The current national goal for primary standards is 1977 and achievement of secondary standards is farther in the future. These delays reflect no lack of determination to achieve a satisfactory level of air purity everywhere in the

*Table 22.3 National air quality standards in the U.S.**

Substance	Air-quality standard, $\mu g/m^3$	
	Primary (human health)	Secondary (all other effects)
Sulfur dioxide		
Annual arithmetic mean	80	60
24-hour max[a]	365	260
3-hour max[a]	—	1,300
Particulate matter		
Annual geometric mean	75	60
24-hour max[a]	260	150
Carbon monoxide		
8-hour max[a]	10,000	10,000
1-hour max[a]	40,000	40,000
Oxidant		
1-hour max[a]	160	160
Nitrogen oxides (e.g., NO_2)		
Annual arithmetic mean	100	100
Hydrocarbons		
3-hour max (6–9 A.M.)	160	160

* From A. C. Stern *et al., Fundamentals of Air Pollution* (New York: Academic Press, 1973), p. 159.
[a] Not to be exceeded more than once per year.

Auto emissions

Tailpipe emissions per ton-mile from all uncontrolled cars are approximately the same. This means that a small car, weighing 2500 pounds, emits only half as many pounds of carbon monoxide, unburned hydrocarbons, and nitrogen oxides as a 5000-pound luxury car even though the concentration of pollutants in the tail gases is the same. This seemingly places the small car at a tremendous advantage in achieving limitations based on pounds of emissions per mile of travel, but just the opposite is the case. Luxury cars consistently do better than smaller cars because luxury cars have closer-tolerance engines, better carburetors, and other parts, and are therefore more easily modified and controlled for low emissions. In spite of the ability of heavy cars to meet all forseeable emission limitations, small cars that give double or more miles per gallon are likely to become increasingly popular as the price of gasoline rises.

nation as rapidly as possible, but they are a recognition of the enormity of the tasks involved in reversing the trends and practices of a hundred or more years standing.

In addition to national air quality standards, the U.S. Environmental Protection Agency has been issuing standards for mobile (automobile and airplane) and stationary (industrial plant and power station) emission sources. Although the need for automobile emission controls is confined to large metropolitan areas, national standards have been adopted to simplify manufacturing procedures and to ease administrative control. Nationwide emission controls for stationary sources have already been promulgated for power plants, incinerators, cement manufacturing plants, sulfuric and nitric acid plants, asphalt plants, petroleum refineries, petroleum storage vessels, scrap metal refineries of lead, brass, bronze, iron and steel, and sewage treatment plants.

Progressive national emission standards that have been established for automobiles are summarized in Table 22.4. Crankcase emissions have been totally controlled since 1963 by passing these gases, containing high concentrations of hydrocarbons, through a flow control valve into the fuel intake manifold and then to the cylinders where the hydrocarbons are burnt to carbon dioxide and water vapor with the gasoline. Gasoline evaporative losses from the fuel tank and carborator have also been totally controlled since 1971 by a vapor recovery system. Tail pipe emissions are the only automotive source not yet under complete control. Table 22.4 gives the current control schedule. When all automotive controls are in effect, more than 95 percent of the emissions of an uncontrolled vehicle will have been eliminated.

Air pollution control strategies

Many plans have been proposed for controlling air pollution. Most proposals are based on some method of limiting or eliminating emissions.

Table 22.4 *Federal emission control requirements for light-duty vehicles**

Emissions (grams/mile)	Baseline (Pre-1968[a])	1968	1970	1971	1972	1973	1974	1976
Hydrocarbons	10	3.4	2.2	2.2	3.4	3.4	3.4	0.41[b]
Carbon Monoxide	77	35	23	23	39	39	39	3.4[b]
Nitrogen Oxides	4–6	NR	NR	NR	NR	3.0	3.0	3.0
Evaporative Losses (grams/test)	40	NR	NR	6.0	2.0	2.0	2.0	2.0

* From J. H. Ludwig, et al., "Seminar on Air Pollution from Motor Vehicles" (Unpublished report, Office of Air Programs, U.S. Environmental Protection Agency, 1972), p. 75.
NR—No requirement
[a] Uncontrolled vehicle except for crankcase blowby which was already controlled.
[b] 90 percent reduction compared to 1970 vehicles.

They differ principally in the motivation. The use of legislative controls to obtain compliance was outlined in the previous section. The motivating forces are the penalties that can be assessed for noncompliance with the regulations. Other methods of control have been proposed that are based on reason rather than compulsion, which is generally abhorred by most Americans. The several alternative plans that are outlined below are intended to illustrate the entire range of options available for control.

ECONOMIC CONTROLS President Nixon, appealing to the profit motive, proposed emission charges of 10 cents per pound of sulfur emitted to the atmosphere in order to make it economically expedient to reduce the emission of sulfur-containing gases to the atmosphere. The difficulty with this type of proposal is in arriving at a proper emission charge that will stimulate innovative changes for the better rather than institutionalizing payments for the privilege of polluting the air. Advocates of this strategy proposed it as a means of rapidly attaining secondary air quality standards. They are satisfied to achieve primary standards by legislative fiat. To date, emission fees have been used for control of water pollution but have not been applied to atmospheric emissions.

SOCIAL CONTROLS If we believe that pollution results from too many people living in excessive affluence, a reasonable way of controlling pollution is to reduce the population and return to a simpler life style. This is the policy advocated by those who espouse zero population growth. Basically, it is the "Walden concept," Thoreau's retreat to a wilderness unspoiled by man's presence. This is a romantic and compelling idea but man has eaten the apple of knowledge and no longer has the option of retreating to the innocence of Eden. In short, he must live in the world he has created and he has a moral obligation to make every possible effort through industrialization to raise the underprivileged millions to a decent standard of living.

MEDICAL CONTROLS Although air pollution bears heavily on those with pre-existing respiratory and circulatory diseases, unequivocal evidence that polluted air is, by itself, a primary cause of disease in otherwise healthy individuals is largely lacking. The susceptible population, namely those who respond rapidly and unfavorably to elevations in pollution levels, is relatively small. Since air quality criteria are based on the excellent public health practice of protecting even the most sensitive fraction of the population, established standards are currently far below the threshhold levels that affect the overwhelming majority. This suggests that a very economical control strategy could be instituted by providing state-supported sheltered retreats for the few susceptibles in the population. This could take the form of one or more rooms in the home of each susceptible individual equipped with adequate gas cleaning devices to deliver purified air to the interior. On notification that elevated pollution levels were imminent, the susceptible individual would retire to his protective living space until outdoor levels returned to normal. As air pollution episodes normally occur infrequently, this routine is unlikely to be a serious restriction for those who suffer serious medical disabilities.

Numerous studies have shown conclusively that heavy smokers are much more likely to have diseases that are affected adversely by elevated levels of air pollution. This combination of respiratory stresses (air pollution and smoking) produces what is known as a *potentiating effect*—the damage produced is far greater than a simple adding together of the two effects. Therefore, a potent medical control would be to reduce other stresses, such as smoking, which react with air pollution to produce greatly enhanced physiological damage. Reduction in work exposures to toxic agents would have similar beneficial effects.

This exploration of the potential for medical controls as an air pollution control strategy is not intended as an argument for unrestrained air contamination. It does recognize, however, that attempts to reduce pollution levels to the point where no single individual is ever affected adversely are likely to be financially ruinous, and hence, impractical. Therefore, some lesser standard must be adopted and medical controls provide a responsible solution for the few extraordinarily susceptible individuals who would otherwise be affected adversely.

LAND USE MANAGEMENT   It was pointed out in Chapter 21 that pollution results from an overcrowding of land areas in relation to the natural, self-purifying potential of the local air resource. This refers to the total range of activities conducted by modern urban man, for example, automobile operation, power generation, and manufacture of capital and consumer goods. Therefore, if man's activities can be spread out more evenly, local overburdening of the air resource can be avoided. This has led to the concept of an allowable emission quantity per unit of land area that can be divided among all potential activities. On this basis, a power plant or a steel mill might acquire the air rights of many thousands of acres to avoid excessive air contamination. These air rights could be acquired by extensive land purchases or by lease from neighbors who use their properties in ways that do not emit substances to the atmosphere.

More conventional land use management practices include zoning that reserves certain areas for residences, others for commercial uses, and still others for industrial uses. By this method, land usages that may produce unpleasant emissions are prevented from encroaching upon residential areas. In turn, those in industrial areas are protected from the need to meet the strict community standards that are appropriate for residential districts, but which may be unreasonable for certain types of industrial activity. The danger inherent in this approach to land use management for control of air pollution is that a larger concentration of heavy industry in a restricted area may represent such a large source of emissions that they are carried downwind to remote residential and commercial areas in undiluted form. Nevertheless, modern zoning practices have proven useful for an equitable allocation of the air resource among the several segments of the community.

AIR USE MANAGEMENT If we consider air to be a resource in exactly the same sense as coal, minerals, and land, it is necessary to devise intelligent ways to use it effectively and efficiently. Use of the atmosphere must, of course, be completely consistent with the goals of air pollution control. With this constraint in mind, full use of the air is dependent upon an understanding of the considerable self-purifying properties of the atmosphere. The way in which excess carbon dioxide is removed from the atmosphere was discussed in Chapter 21. Other substances have different modes of removal and different retention times in the atmosphere. Several are summarized in Table 22.5.

Table 22.5   Sources, residence times, and removal mechanisms for common air pollutants

Air pollutant	Sources	Residence times	Principal removal mechanisms
SO_2	Combustion of fossil fuels	4 days	Conversion in the atmosphere to particulate sulfates, incorporation into precipitation.
CO	Auto exhaust	several years	Conversion in the atmosphere to CO_2 by reaction with ozone.
NO, NO_2	Auto exhaust and fossil fuel combustion	5 days	Conversion in the atmosphere to solid or liquid nitrates and incorporation into precipitation.
Hydrocarbons	Auto exhaust and industrial processing	7 days	Conversion in the atmosphere to solid and liquid particles and incorporation into precipitation.
Solid particles	Industrial processing and fossil fuel combustion	Minutes to 2 days, depending on size	Gravitational settling, impaction on trees and buildings, incorporation into precipitation.

Sulfur dioxide gas from combustion of coal and heavy oil, oil refining, and metal smelting reacts in the atmosphere with particles of metal oxides such as rust and with ammonia to form solid sulfite and sulfate particles that settle to the earth under the action of gravity, become incorporated into rain and snow when water condenses around them, or are washed out of the air by falling rain or snow. Retention time of sulfur dioxide in the atmosphere is approximately four days.

Particles emitted from sources at or near ground level seldom reach high altitudes. The largest particles settle to earth rapidly; others are impacted on trees, buildings, and natural ground features that extend above the ground as they are carried downwind. The very finest particles reach higher altitudes and are eventually brought to earth in precipitation. Atmospheric residence times for particles range from seconds, for the largest, to hours, for the smallest. Particles formed in the atmosphere from gases include eye irritating photochemical haze (smog) particles characteristic of Los Angeles-type air pollution. These haze particles are formed from hydrocarbons (emitted from automobiles and stationary sources such as dry cleaning establishments and large gasoline storage tanks) and nitrogen oxides (emitted by automobiles and power plants). These particles are liquid. They reflect and absorb the different colors in sunlight. When seen from certain angles relative to the sun's position, the haze appears white, blue, or reddish brown. These particles are about 0.00001 inches in diameter. They are too small to respond to the settling force of gravity but can be swept from the atmosphere by precipitation.

Carbon monoxide emitted from automobile tailpipes has a relatively long life in the atmosphere of about three years because it is not chemically reactive at ordinary temperatures. The exact way in which it is removed is not known for certain, but it is believed that it diffuses upward into the stratosphere where it reacts with high concentrations of ozone to form carbon dioxide. Carbon dioxide has an equally long residence time in the atmosphere because the rate of solution in the oceans is slow. Carbon dioxide is not considered an air pollutant because it is a normal constituent of the atmosphere. Concern over increases in carbon dioxide in the atmosphere has not been associated with its toxic properties, but rather with its effects on worldwide climate. A significant increase in carbon dioxide in the atmosphere could warm the earth's

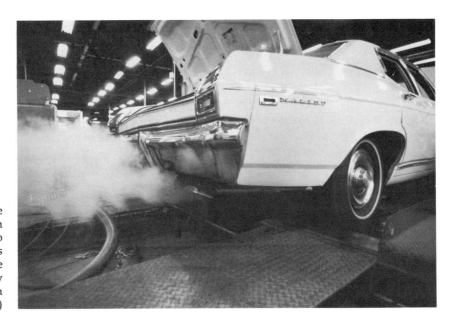

Figure 22.5. A new way to use an old device. This is a car run on steam. The system has a way to go before being adopted for mass production but holds some promise of reducing pollution. (Courtesy of J. Mohr and the World Health Organization)

temperature and result in a melting of the polar ice caps, a rise in the level of the oceans, and inundation of all coastal plains. Fortunately, any such event is at least 100–200 years off and there is ample time to take such protective action as resorting to nuclear or solar power in place of burning fossil fuels.

A way in which the air resource can be used intelligently is by enlisting the dilution and dispersive powers of the wind. All emissions to the atmosphere can be made odorless, invisible, and harmless by dilution. This principle has been employed by emitting air contaminants to the atmosphere through tall stacks to take advantage of the superior dispersive powers associated with height. Power plant stacks as tall as 1,000-feet (equivalent to a 100-story building) have been constructed for this purpose.

Other ways in which use of the air resource may be maximized are through a recognition that atmospheric capacity to absorb, dilute, and disperse emissions is highly variable. It depends upon wind velocity and air turbulence. On a bright, breezy day, atmospheric dilution and dispersion may be 1,000 or more times as effective as during periods of atmospheric stagnation that have been responsible for fatal air pollution episodes. Therefore, more stack discharges are permissable during periods of good atmospheric mixing. In many sections of the country, good mixing conditions are normal and periods of atmospheric stagnation, abnormal. In these areas, it may be feasible to increase and decrease emissions depending upon atmospheric conditions. This is the basis for plans to conserve scarce low sulfur-containing fuels by using readily available high sulfur fuels during periods of excellent atmospheric ventilation and switching to low-sulfur fuels when stagnation periods are predicted by the weather services.

Full use of the assimilative capacities of the atmosphere is often criticized because it does not reduce greatly the total quantity of substances emitted to the air. This is correct, but there are two counter arguments to consider: 1. by definition, a condition of air pollution exists only when some damage occurs; and 2. the self-purifying properties of the atmosphere expel these substances from the air before damaging concentrations can accumulate.

ENGINEERING CONTROL AT THE SOURCE　Without question, the most satisfactory way of controlling air pollution is to eliminate all emissions to the atmosphere by changing products or altering the process. This can be done in a number of ways. Sulfur gas emissions can be eliminated by switching from sulfur containing fuels such as coal and heavy oil to sulfur-free fuels such as natural gas and nuclear power. Lead emissions to the environment from gasoline driven motor vehicles can be eliminated by switching to electric battery-operated machines. An example of a profitable process change is the installation of condensing vapor traps on large gasoline and other volatile liquid storage tanks that collect and return to the product pool sufficient liquid to more than pay for the installation that prevents emission to the atmosphere.

Unfortunately, only a few examples can be cited of pollution controls that return a cash profit to the one who pays for their installation. Usually, one collects a waste product at high cost and then pays to dispose of it. This is not considered objectionable when the one who pays is a utility or a large industry, but the general public has been less enthusiastic about the substitution of sanitary methods of waste disposal for backyard burning and mandatory motor vehicle emission controls, each of which has been personally costly to a great many people. Nevertheless, the American public's determination to achieve and maintain a clean atmosphere has remained steadfast; all automobile emission controls are scheduled to become fully effective in the 1970s.

MANAGING THE
WATER ENVIRONMENT

Public water supplies are derived from rivers and lakes, from underground waters, and from remote upland sources. Upland water is collected from rural tributary regions where there is little or no pollution because of an absence of population. Boston and New York City, for example, have sources which originate in northern mountainous areas one hundred or more miles distant. Water from remote areas is generally of excellent quality and, until relatively recently, was supplied with no treatment beyond the self-purifying effects of long storage in protected reservoirs. The Boston water supply, for example, is stored in protected reservoirs for an average of three years before consumption.

Rivers are the largest source of water supplies but though river water is available to many communities in sufficient quantity, quality is often poor. The Ohio River, the water supply for innumerable communities along its banks, is estimated to be 15 percent sewage effluent at low flow, and the Rhine River, in even worse condition, has a low-flow sewage content of about 40 percent. It is frequently said that every glass of water withdrawn from the Rhine River at Amsterdam has already passed through nine Germans. This grim joke dramatizes the deplorable condition of most of the world's rivers that pass through densely populated regions.

Degradation of the water supply

THERMAL DEGRADATION Thermal degradation of natural waters occurs when power generating stations and manufacturing plants use them for cooling purposes and raise the temperature sufficiently to change the balance of naturally-occurring plant and animal species for the worse. Moderate warming of a cold stream may favor the growth of bass at the expense of trout and salmon, and whether or not this constitutes thermal degradation depends on one's preference for catching trout or bass. Biologists recognize that most plant and animal species grow faster and reproduce earlier in moderately warm water as opposed to icy cold water, and it has been observed that enormous numbers of fish congregate and

Water usage

Nationwide, water usage is currently about 400 billion gallons per day from municipal supplies and for industrial usage and irrigation. Approximately three times this amount flows to the oceans unused by man. Future needs, estimated to become 1,000 billion gallons per day by the year 2000, must somehow be withdrawn from this presently unused supply or effective ways must be found to reuse current supplies several fold. About 40 percent of total rainfall over the U.S. directly sustains crop farms and pastures, forests, and grazing lands. Although not included in the figures for daily water consumption, this usage represents a vital water resource for the nation inasmuch as all but a very small fraction of our food, natural fiber, and wood supplies are totally dependent upon this water source.

Public water supply use in the U.S. averages 150 gallons per person per day. About one-third is used in the home (domestic supplies) and most of the remainder is used by industry. Surprisingly, 25 of the 150 gallons is lost through leakage in the supply system. Of the 50 gallons of water used per person per day in the average home, 80 percent is accounted for by toilet flushing and personal washing. The most vital use, drinking, requires only 1/20 of the total. Nevertheless, all of the water supplied must be maintained at or above drinking water standards to avoid accidental entry of impure water into the drinking water supply. This is a costly safety measure as most industrial and domestic requirements (e.g., steam condensation and toilet flushing) could be met adequately by water of greatly inferior quality but experience has demonstrated repeatedly that this is an essential precaution to protect the public health.

thrive around the warm water outlets of power plants. Large fish kills have occurred following a sudden shut down of the power plant because of the inability of the fish to withstand the temperature shock of the abrupt cooling of their habitat.

Any water body can become overloaded with waste heat. When too many power plants and industries use a single stream to discharge their waste heat, its temperature can rise to the point where inadequate amounts of oxygen can be dissolved to sustain marine life: all fish disappear, the stream becomes black and foul smelling, and is no longer useful for recreational purposes. This condition can be avoided by discharging waste heat to the atmosphere instead of into natural waters with the use of land-based heat exchangers. For power plants, steel mills, and similar large industries, these are usually huge hyperbolic towers that induce continuous flow of outside air from the bottom upward, while hot water falls downward and is cooled by countercurrent contact with the air. The construction cost of such a tower for a moderately-sized modern power station is 3 million dollars, and its operation reduces the energy developed by the power station by 5 percent.

As there is no danger of overheating the oceans, except locally in shallow estuaries, ocean front sites are favored by industries requiring very large waste heat removal capacity.

WATER POLLUTION Water pollution, meaning the introduction by man of substances that interfere with the full use and enjoyment of a stream or lake, arises from three sources: the discharge of domestic sewage containing mostly human excrement; industrial wastes containing a variety of chemicals, some of which are toxic; and agricultural wastes that include animal excrement, fertilizers and insecticides from cultivated land, and the liquid wastes from slaughter houses, canning and packing plants. The main naturally-occurring discharge to water bodies is silt which is carried into streams with runoff of precipitation from the land and is deposited in the stream bed. Wherever the stream empties into a body of still water, silt, in suspension, prevents the penetration of sunlight, and when deposited on the bottom, smothers the bottom-dwelling organisms. Man can accelerate this process by denuding the watershed of trees, grass, and other vegetation that absorbs precipitation and prevents rapid runoff, but wise agricultural practices, including contour plowing of crop lands and maintenance of forested areas along river banks, reduces silting.

The annual human discharge to sewage in the U.S. is 1.4 pounds of phosphorus and 11 pounds of nitrogen per person. Added to this is the phosphorus contained in sewage water that accounts for about half of the total. Phosphorus and nitrogen are essential elements for biological growth and are the principal active components of most agricultural chemicals. The settled sewage sludge retains only a small fraction of these elements that are essential to growth. Most is discharged to the rivers and lakes that receive the clear effluent from the treatment plant and act as powerful stimulators of marine plant growth. For many lakes and streams, some growth stimulation can be beneficial in increasing the productivity of the waters, but when fertilization is overdone, undesirable consequences result. One of these is an enormous increase in the numbers of microscopic plants (algae) that form a scum on the surface and make the water cloudy. This interferes with its use for drinking and swimming, and after the growth becomes extreme, the algae die, and drift onto adjacent shores where they decay and produce foul odors.

In agricultural areas, additional phosphorus and nitrogen enter these waters from leaching of excess fertilizers applied to the soil and from animal excrement. Domestic animals excrete from 17 to 45 pounds of phosphorus per 1000 pounds of animal per year and equivalent quantities of nitrogen. These also find their way into waters and provide additional fertilization of the aquatic plants. It has been estimated that the production of animal wastes is almost six times that of the human population in the Potomac River basin.

Excessive enrichment of natural waters with nutrients is called *eutrophication*. When this results in massive overgrowths of green plants and the troubles described above, the water body is called *eutrophic*. The shallow, inshore areas of Lake Erie have been eutrophic for several decades from massive inflows of sewage from the large cities lining its shores, such as Cleveland, and from agricultural wastes that drain from the rich farm lands surrounding it. So bad has this condition become, that Lake Erie has been called a "dead lake." Nevertheless, the offshore, deeper portions of the lake are still clear and produce 50 million pounds of fish a year, indicating that Lake Erie may be ill but it is far from "dead." For it to be really "killed" would require that it receive so much toxic waste that nothing would grow. This obviously has not yet occurred and, in fact, remedial measures have been taken in recent years that seem to be slowing the rate of deterioration and, perhaps, to have reversed it.

Industrial wastes can differ greatly from municipal domestic wastes. Often they contain toxic metals and chemicals that interfere with or totally destroy the microorganisms that transform human and animal wastes to simple, innocuous compounds. This destruction of the biological purification process can take place in natural waters and in the sewage treatment plant. Cyanide-containing chemical wastes from electroplating operations are an example of the kinds of poisonous industrial wastes that must be kept out of natural water bodies and municipal waste treatment facilities by requiring the industries that produce these materials to remove them at the source of the waste discharge.

Oil is another important water pollutant. Approximately half of the more than 2 billion tons of oil produced annually is shipped by sea, and approximately 0.1 percent, or more than a million tons per year, is lost at sea by leakage, accident, and other causes. Natural oil seepage into the oceans through fissures in the ocean bottom is probably larger in volume, and the two sources together represent a serious contamination of the oceans. Figures for worldwide leakage and seepage fail to dramatize the tragedies associated with man-made oil leakage as well as did the breakup of the *Torrey Canyon,* a loaded oil tanker, on the western coast of Great Britain a few years ago. Considerable damage to marine and bird life resulted from the extensive coverage of water and beach with tar-like crude oil, and even greater damage to plants and animals resulted from the use of toxic detergents to clean up the oil deposits on land and sea. After the Santa Barbara oil release from producing wells offshore, straw was used instead of detergents for cleanup and much less damage to marine life resulted. The effect on most sea birds of immersion in major oil spills is almost always lethal, but the common seagull seems to be able to survive even this threat. Current U.S. laws provide for strict financial accountability for oil spills from ships and ocean oil drilling rigs.

Pure water

Chemically pure water, like pure air, exists only as a laboratory curiosity that is difficult to produce and maintain in its uncontaminated state. In fact, chemically pure water is insipid to the taste, as it lacks the dissolved minerals and gases that give water its characteristic refreshing flavor. In the ordinary use of the term, pure water is "potable," that is, safe and pleasant to drink. During the centuries that it took to open up a vast empty continent, folklore had it that "running water is pure water." Doubtless, this was true during those times because it was unlikely that there was anyone higher up to contaminate it. This is no longer true in our crowded world and it is a sad fact that even running water can become contaminated. Virtually all of our municipal supplies are currently safe to drink but many are not especially pleasant because of the presence of traces of industrial chemicals or large amounts of chlorine that have been added at the treatment station to insure the destruction of disease organisms that might have entered from sewage contamination.

Water and sewage treatment

From the standpoint of preventing human disease, protection from water-borne infection can be achieved by two processes: purification of the supply and treatment of waste waters prior to discharge to the receiving water bodies. Until recently, only treatment of supplies has been extensively practiced, but this is no longer satisfactory. Under the stimulus of an urgent need to reverse the rapid degradation of our lakes and streams, plus the promise of substantial monetary assistance for this purpose from the federal government, enormous improvements in waste treatment facilities are scheduled to occur nationwide during the next ten years.

WATER TREATMENT Drinking water standards have been established by the U.S. Public Health Service and they have been widely adopted. These standards include color, taste, odor, and turbidity as well as chemical, radiological, and bacteriological criteria for acceptable drinking water quality.

A complete system of water supply treatment includes: 1. chemical coagulation by the addition of a flocculating agent such as alum; 2. sedimentation to remove the flocs that enclose and retain bacteria, sediment, and some dissolved substances; 3. filtration through several feet of graded sand and crushed stone to remove residual floc; 4. disinfection by addition of chlorine, ozone, or some other bacteria-killing chemical. Chlorine is the usual disinfecting agent. A small excess, called residual chlorine, is customarily added at the treatment plant to preserve the bacteriological safety of the water as it flows to the consumer through the distribution system. Drinking water supplies from deep wells and

Figure 22.6. A modern waste treatment plant. (Courtesy of Permutit Co., Division of Sybron Corp., Paramus, N. J.)

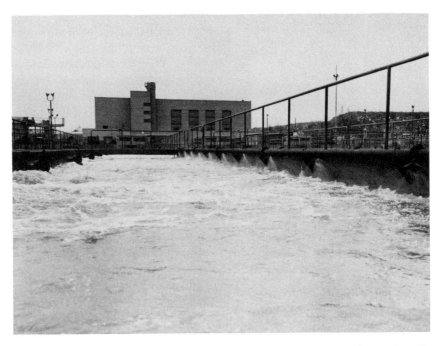

from protected remote upland ground water sources are often of sufficiently high quality to require only disinfection as a precaution against the possibility of unknown contamination in the distribution system. On the other hand, a badly contaminated source may require taste and odor removal by aeration, ozonation, or passage through activated charcoal in addition to the entire four-step purification process.

Water for industrial use may undergo additional treatment to remove special minerals and other components that may be detrimental. Calcium and magnesium salts and dissolved oxygen and carbon dioxide must be removed from boiler waters, iron must be removed from laundry waters, all organisms, including those that are harmless to man, must be removed from water used for brewing and canning.

SEWAGE TREATMENT Municipal waste water treatment plants carry out in a confined area, under controlled conditions, the normal chemical, physical, and biological purification processes that would occur naturally, but more slowly, in nature.

Sewage treatment starts with the removal of large solids by screening and the skimming of floating oils and grease. Next, settleable solids are removed by sedimentation, or gravity settling, in holding tanks for an hour or more. Next, the partially clarified sewage is subjected to biological treatment. This is done by putting the sewage in direct contact with an enormous mass of biologically active organisms that use the dissolved and suspended sewage materials as their food. Biological conversion of the sewage is hastened by providing adequate oxygen and other conditions for maximum biological growth. After biological treatment, a clarified water is obtained that can be discharged to rivers and lakes after chlorination for disinfection.

When the receiving water body is subject to eutrophication, phosphate removal may be undertaken as well. Eutrophication was observed before the introduction of phosphate detergents, but their use has made a troublesome condition very much worse. Therefore, in addition to phosphate removal at the sewage plant, restrictions on the use of phosphate-rich detergents in those areas where phosphate-caused eutrophication is already a serious problem would be beneficial. Phosphorus is not the only element that can cause eutrophication when it is present in excess—large amounts of nitrogen can have a similar effect. Nonetheless, phosphorus is a limiting element for growth and reproduction and has the important advantage of being the one essential element in municipal waste waters that can be removed efficiently. Therefore, phosphorus removal has become the method of choice for control of eutrophication even in those instances when it is primarily caused by the addition of an excess of a different element.

Sewage treatment plant sludge, a wet, slimy mass composed of microbiological organisms, accumulates in large volumes as a result of the forced feeding of sewage to the slime organisms and presents problems in disposal. In some cities it is incinerated in large, high temperature furnaces; in others, it is spread on drying beds, dewatered, and buried or used for fill. The city of Milwaukee for decades has been drying their sewage sludge and selling it bagged as garden fertilizer under the name "Millorganite." So popular has this product become that Milwaukee purchases the sewage sludge from other communities for processing into Millorganite. Normally, sewage sludge is not rich enough in essential minerals to be used as a fertilizer without the addition of agricultural chemicals. In Switzerland, attempts are being made to add sewage sludge to ground solid waste collections and prepare an agricultural compost that will be valuable to local farmers, thereby simultaneously solving difficult solid waste and sewage disposal problems. Under the stimulus of fuel shortages, old technologies for decomposing sewage sludge microbiologically in closed tanks in the absence of air to produce methane, the principal component of natural gas, are being revived.

MANAGING THE LAND ENVIRONMENT

Public-health aspects

The public-health aspects of solid wastes (refuse) are not as well defined as those for liquid wastes or sewage, and public-health authorities in the United States have been content in recent years to delegate handling of solid wastes to departments of public works. Although it is commonly understood that accumulations of garbage and rubbish that have been poorly handled are likely to attract and provide breeding places for vermin and to produce malodors and unsightly dumps, evidence that disease is spread from such sources is largely lacking. Rats, insects, and birds are known to be carriers of disease under certain circumstances but in none of these cases is the poorly handled waste the reservoir of the disease, with the exception of the transmission of trichinosis to man through the feeding of uncooked garbage to hogs. Other reasons why public-health directors have been reluctant to accept collection and disposal of garbage and trash as a health-department function are, first of all, that the costs of municipal solid-waste handling usually far exceed those of all public-health functions combined.

Inadequacy of current waste-handling methods

The traditional method of handling domestic food wastes has been to use them as feed for animals, usually hogs. Solid, nonfood wastes have been dumped into conveniently located, but useless, land sites such as marshes, old quarry pits, or ravines.

It has already been pointed out that the United States is now an urban society, and that with the exception of dogs and cats, animals have disappeared from daily life. Although aesthetic considerations have played a large part in making the population acutely aware of environmental problems, other changes of a fundamental nature that have occurred in recent years have had a direct and generally detrimental effect on solid-waste management. These are as follows:

1. The concentration of population into high-density, geographically extensive metropolitan areas has engulfed once remote trash-disposal sites in a sea of residential and commercial developments. Traditional disposal practices are resented by the new neighbors at their gates. In addition, because dump sites often represent a major fraction of all remaining open urban land available for recreational, residential, commercial and industrial use, there are strong pressures to convert them to these higher economic uses as rapidly as possible.
2. The population explosion has increased the number of people generating wastes.
3. Prosperity has increased per capita waste production enormously. Modern packaging practices, a spate of periodical literature, almost instant obsolescence of an endless variety of material acquisitions and the enormous growth of industry have combined to nearly double solid-waste production.
4. Effective research and development programs for solid-waste handling were virtually nonexistent up to five or ten years ago.

Research on solid-waste technology has never been a "respectable" activity at universities, technical schools and research foundations although, fortunately, this attitude is undergoing rapid alteration. The penalty for this lack of vision is the current dependence on solid-waste handling methods that are largely obsolescent (when not totally obsolete), inadequate for coping with the quantities of material that will be generated soon, and unsuitable for the rapid and safe disposal of many new materials rapidly coming into common use. Examples of substances in this category are fire- and decay-resistant plastic and aluminum, which, unlike iron and steel, resist rusting and disintegration for very long periods, even when buried in the ground or under water.

It has been recognized, belatedly, that although solid wastes may rate low on a scale of sources of transmissible disease, improper disposal practices can cause serious air, water, and land pollution.

Solid Waste Disposal Act of 1965

Recognition of a worsening situation regarding the level of technology associated with solid-waste collection and disposal practices and an awareness that it is no longer possible in a crowded urban society to treat the three broad classifications of pollution (air, water, and land) separately have directed advanced thinking along channels that can be most accurately labeled *solid-waste management*.

The situation in research on problems of solid-waste management and technologic development improved enormously with the passage and signing of the Solid Waste Disposal Act in October, 1965. Substantial funds were then designated for the following activities: research and development in new and improved methods of disposal, including studies directed toward the conservation of natural resources by reducing the amount of waste and unsalvageable materials and by recovery and use of potential resources in solid wastes; and technical and financial assistance to state and local governments for planning, development, and conduct of solid-waste disposal programs. Appropriations up to $60,000,000 were authorized for the period October 20, 1965, to June 30, 1969, to carry out the provisions of this act although lesser sums were appropriated and expended.

Waste-disposal methods

All procedures for solving solid-waste problems involve the use of one or more of three basic methods: reduction of waste production; reclamation, utilization and recycling of waste products; and returning the wastes to the environment via land, air, or water. There seems to be little quarrel with the first two proposals, and, indeed, conservationists have been advocating them for many years, but major problems arise in attempting to put them into practice. For example, complex product distribution and sales mechanisms favor the extravagant use of packaging materials for preservation and selling appeal. In many cases the cost of packaging is a small proportion of the total price, and this is more than compensated for by a reduction in spoilage, breakage, soiling, and other losses. It is difficult to foresee any factor in the immediate future that is likely to reverse this trend.

It seems clear that for the foreseeable future all but a small fraction of the total quantity of solid wastes will be returned to the environment as a means of final disposal. The current tendency to regard each element of the environment as a resource makes it very clear that each becomes most valuable when exploited to the maximum degree compatible with prudent safeguards for human health, well-being, and preservation of property. It is naive to maintain that nothing whatsoever can be added to the environment, for even if it became technically possible to achieve such an ideal, the human and material resources that would have to be committed to this single purpose would be so great that the quality of daily life would be substantially impoverished. Instead, the objective should be to utilize to the fullest the self-purifying properties of the environment, which are enormous when properly understood and managed.

At present, there are two satisfactory methods in general use for disposing of the fraction of municipal wastes not flushed into the sewer via the garbage grinder. Both methods return wastes to the environment. One is the sanitary landfill, and the other high-temperature incineration and ground disposal of the residue.

SANITARY LANDFILL Sanitary landfill, often referred to as cut-and-cover burial, overcomes almost all the objectionable features associated with open dumping. When the process is properly operated, each day's refuse collections are compacted and completely covered with at least 6 inches of compacted clean fill. This prevents fires, suppresses odors of decomposition and putrefaction, eliminates much of the unsightliness associated with open dumps, and destroys feeding and breeding places that would otherwise be open to rodents, birds, and insects. This method of waste disposal produces no air pollution problems, except for the generation of some local dustiness during periods of prolonged dryness. Problems of water pollution can be avoided by provision of drainage for the site, the waters being conducted to an adjacent waste-water disposal facility. This is an important feature of a sanitary landfill since it guards against water pollution and prevents erosion of the landfill by surface runoff of rainwater and melting snow.

Sanitary landfilling, when suitable land is available, is the cheapest method of solid waste disposal that is entirely satisfactory from sanitary and esthetic considerations. When properly graded, finished with loam, seeded and planted, a site may be converted to public use or sold for commercial development. The increased value of the filled land, whether retained for public use or sold, may properly be treated as a credit when the net cost of refuse disposal is calculated.

INCINERATION Incineration reduces refuse to between one-fifth and one-tenth its original volume and thereby decreases many times the land area required for final disposal. This means that during the combustion process, 80 to 90 percent of the volume (50 to 75 percent by weight) is converted to gaseous products that are discharged to the air environ-

Oregon's "Bottle Bill"

The State of Oregon, in October, 1972, put into effect a novel law—the so-called bottle bill—designed to reduce litter. The bill requires 2-cent to 5-cent deposits on all "certified" containers, and prohibits the sale of pull-tab beverage containers. The law's constitutionality has been upheld, despite the court actions of the beverage industry.

Preliminary comparisons between the winter before (1971–1972) and the winter after (1972–1973) enactment show that the law has had a significant and positive impact on litter in Oregon. Litter data for 1971–1972 showed an average of 269 beverage containers per mile of highway per month; data for 1972–1973 showed 51 per mile per month. This represents an 81% reduction. The number of beverage containers as a percentage of the total number of items of roadside litter decreased from 37% before enactment to 19% after enactment—a reduction of about 50%.

The bill has been attended by some disruption in the beverage and beverage container industries. The effect has been greatest on manufacturers forced to change production from throw-away to refillable containers, and on out-of-state brewers and soft-drink producers who have not been able to ship refillable containers profitably. It is estimated that a total of 142 jobs have been lost as a result, but a sizeable number of new jobs may be created in the bottling industry. Retailers face problems due to the space requirements of large numbers of empty containers, and find that their handling costs have increased. However, there has been no effect on price or demand for beverages.

Oregon's experience shows how economic and legislative controls can be applied to the problems of solid-waste management. The bill deals effectively with a specific problem, and minimizes the disruptions inherent in any change from equilibrium.

ment. When incineration is complete, well over 99 percent of the gases formed by combustion are carbon dioxide and water vapor. These two compounds are not usually considered to be pollutants although, there is considerable current interest in the long-term (one hundred to three hundred years) climatologic effects that may result from an increase in the carbon dioxide content of the atmosphere.

Many new incineration processes are under development. One, a converted iron-melting blast furnace, reduces the residue from all wastes to a glass-like slag that may be broken up and used for clean fill in road building or as an aggregate for cement. The ability to handle wastes that are ordinarily classed as incombustible and the compactness of the residue are noteworthy, but the need to purchase supplementary fuel (coke) to melt these refractory materials may lead to excessive costs. In addition, severe flue-gas cleaning problems are created by the blast of hot air that rises when the falling refuse is fed into the top of the furnace. Methods for cleaning the stack discharges to a satisfactory sanitary standard are available commercially, but the cost will be high.

Pyrolysis of solid wastes in a high temperature, inert atmosphere chamber produces combustible gases that can be used for fuel, a char that has all of the characteristics of coke, and clean scrap metals that are principally iron and aluminum cans. Because of the nonoxidizing atmosphere inside the pyrolyzer, aluminum and iron cans are discharged as elemental metal and are easily salvageable. The small gas volumes emitted to the atmosphere by this process can be cleaned to a very high standard of purity at moderate cost.

Fossil fuel shortages have generated a keen interest in utilizing the heat value of solid wastes, about one-half that of coal on an equal weight basis, for generating steam and electricity. Connecticut has adopted a statewide solid waste management plan that contemplates the construction of regional waste incinerators to feed recovered heat to adjacent power stations.

Solid-waste collection

Although disposal creates most of the solid-waste problems, collection and transportation of refuse to a disposal site represents up to 80 percent of the total system cost. It has been noted that "it costs more to dispose of the New York Sunday *Times* than it does a subscriber to buy it."

Plans for the future include development of mobile incinerators that can travel the streets and combine the collection and disposal function into one operation.

The millions of junked automobiles present special problems. Each automobile contains about 1.5 tons of metals, principally iron and steel. The copper radiator, lead battery, cast-iron motor block and some other special parts are easily removed and find a ready market, but the steel body shell has little value to steel makers until it is separated from glass, upholstery, rubber and other nonferrous materials that make up the usual automobile body. For many years, it was customary in junk yards to drain the gasoline from the junk car, pour it inside the body and ignite it. The resulting fire consumed the upholstery, shattered the windows and otherwise removed sufficient nonferrous materials to make the product clean enough to be acceptable to steel manufacturers. These fires produced enormous clouds of black, sooty smoke and were severe local air-pollution nuisances. Consequently, open burning of automobiles is prohibited in most urban areas, and, specially designed incinerators, continuous and batch type, with gas-fired afterburners and tall stacks were developed for this purpose. These proved to be satisfactory from the air-pollution-control standpoint but are costly to operate because of fuel requirements and low production rate. The increase in processing cost caused by more stringent air-pollution control regulations, combined with a reduction in demand (and price) for steel scrap because of technologic changes in steel-making methods, resulted in the buildup of large inventories in junk car yards.

A newer way of handling stripped automobile body shells (called the Proler process) is to place them in giant hammer mills and reduce them to small pieces of steel, cloth, rubber and so forth that can be separated magnetically. The product is clean steel scrap in the form of fist-sized fragments that are easily handled for loading and unloading, pack well for economical shipment and melt easily in the steel furnace. The nonsteel residue is buried. A single full-scale plant of this kind can handle 1000 body shells per day.

Figure 22.7. Over half of municipal wastes consist of salvageable commodities.

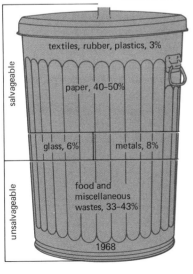

Nonurban solid-waste problems

Worrisome solid-waste problems also exist outside metropolitan areas. These include mining refuse of all kinds and the severe disturbances to ground and water caused by large-scale strip mining. Agricultural waste-disposal problems are countrywide, ranging from long standing and severe pollution of Long Island's inland bays by duck-raising farms and duck-packing plants to enormous accumulations of manure in California's cattle-raising western valleys. However, these special problems are outside the scope of urban solid-waste management.

SUMMARY   Managing the environment to maintain healthful, safe, and aesthetically pleasing conditions involves substantial costs to the nation, most of which are paid for by all citizens in taxes and higher prices for goods and services. A substantial part of this cost is recovered in the form of better health, less soiling, and reduced destruction of vegetation and materials. The remainder of the cost is likely to be considered money well spent if it preserves and sustains the pleasure and pride of all Americans in their magnificent and bountiful land.

All the technology needed to achieve clean air, pure water, and an undefiled land is available now. Doubtless, better methods will be developed in the future. Faith in the ability of engineers and scientists to respond to the obvious worldwide need makes us hesitate sometimes to commit now the huge resources necessary to achieve environmental goals lest better and cheaper methods become available tomorrow. Nevertheless, experience demonstrated that progress was slow until national goals were announced and timetables for achievement were established. The several recent congressional acts pertaining to air, water, and solid wastes are a clear indication that the nation has resolved to make prompt and substantial improvements in the management of its environmental affairs and has committed major funding for this purpose.

The energy crisis is likely to result in some temporary environmental regression and to extend the time for achieving national goals. Although this is regrettable from many aspects—a loss of momentum being one of the more obvious—an enforced temporary slowdown can be put to good purpose if the time is used to reassess objectives and refine techniques for more rapid achievements after present difficulties have been resolved. The obvious fact that most college students consider the environment a subject of concern and serious study is a substantial guarantee that environmental matters will receive intelligent handling on the part of the citizenry for the foreseeable future.

Questions   1. Discuss the effects of a heavy tax on atmospheric pollutants. Consider in your answer the economic effects of higher prices or unemployment should the affected companies find they are losing money.

2. What is a "dead lake"? What are some measures that can prevent or lessen eutrophication?

3. How do industrial wastes in sewage differ from municipal wastes? Why is it essential that industrial wastes be treated at the source?

4. Describe your priorities for dealing with environmental pollution. For example, is productivity more important than air quality? Is cleaner water worth a higher water bill?

Key Concepts

Air quality standards – the levels of atmospheric pollutants considered safe, as determined by the Federal Clean Air Act of 1970 for each pollutant; *primary standards* are levels below which little or no damage occurs to public health, and *secondary standards* are levels below which little or no damage occurs to property or to the aesthetic qualities of the atmosphere

Eutrophication – the excessive enrichment of natural waters with nutrients; this leads to an undesirable level of plant growth and results in degradation of the quality of natural bodies of water

Heat recovery – the use of municipal refuse as a fuel source, mainly to generate electricity; it is expected that this process will be used more as the price of other fuels (oil, gas, and coal) rises

Pollution – the unfavorable alteration of the environment through man's actions

Thermal degradation – the warming, by man, of natural waters to such an extent that an unfavorable change in the balance of naturally-occurring plant and animal species results

Selected Readings

ACS Committee on Chemistry and Public Affairs. *Cleaning Our Environment: The Chemical Basis for Action*. Washington, D.C.: American Chemical Society, 1969.

National Academy of Sciences–National Research Council, Committee on Pollution. *Waste Management and Control: A Report to the Federal Council for Science and Technology*. Washington, D.C.: National Research Council, 1966. (Pub. No. 1400.)

President's Council on Recreation and Natural Beauty. *From Sea to Shining Sea*. Washington, D.C.: U.S. Government Printing Office, 1968.

President's Science Advisory Committee, Environmental Pollution Panel. *Restoring the Quality of Our Environment*. Washington, D.C.: The White House, November, 1965.

Report of the Air Conservation Commission. *Air Conservation*. Washington, D.C.: American Association for the Advancement of Science, 1965.

Index

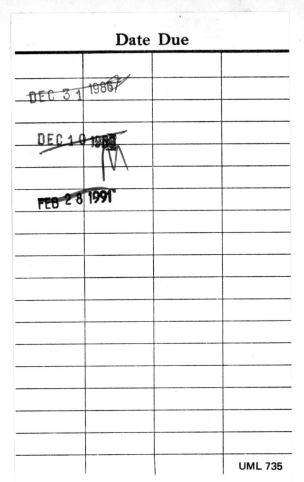
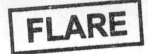

FLARE